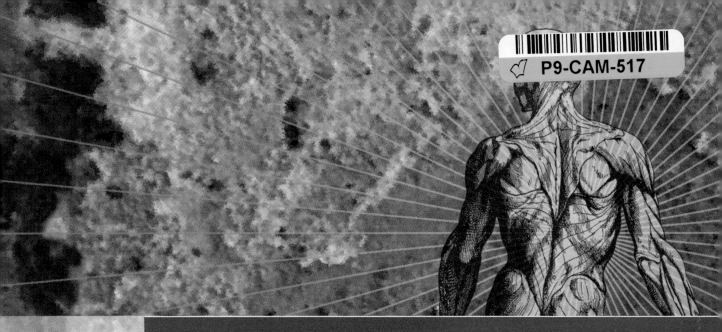

Diseases of the Human Body

THIRD EDITION

Carol D. Tamparo, PhD, CMA-A

Dean, Business & Allied Health
Lake Washington Technical College
Kirkland, Washington

Marcia A. Lewis, EdD, RN, CMA-AC

Associate Dean, Mathematics, Engineering Sciences, and Health
Adjunct Instructor, Medical Assisting
Olympic College
Bremerton, Washington

F.A. Davis Company   •   Philadelphia

F.A. Davis Company
1915 Arch Street
Philadelphia, PA 19103

Copyright © 2000 by F.A. Davis Company

Printed in the United States of America

Last digit indicates print number: 10 9 8 7 6 5 4 4 3 2 1

Publisher: Jean François Vilain
Senior Editor: Lynn Borders Caldwell
Developmental Editor: Christa Fratantoro
Production Editor: Elena Coler
Designer: Bill Donnelly

As new scientific information becomes available through basic and clinical research, recommended treatments and drug therapies undergo changes. The author(s) and publisher have done everything possible to make this book accurate, up to date, and in accord with accepted standards at the time of publication. The authors, editors, and publisher are not responsible for errors or omissions or for consequences from application of the book, and make no warranty, expressed or implied, in regard to the contents of the book. Any practice described in this book should be applied by the reader in accordance with professional standards of care used in regard to the unique circumstances that may apply in each situation. The reader is advised always to check product information (package inserts) for changes and new information regarding dose and contraindications before administering any drug. Caution is especially urged when using new or infrequently ordered drugs.

Library of Congress Cataloging in Publication Data

Tamparo, Carol D., 1940–
    Diseases of the human body / Carol D. Tamparo, Marcia A. Lewis.—3rd ed.
      p. cm.
    Includes bibliographical references and index.
    ISBN 0-8036-0564-1
      1. Diseases. 2. Pathology. I. Lewis, Marcia A. II. Title.
    [DNLM: I. Disease—Handbooks. 2. Pathology—Handbooks. 3. Internal
Medicine—Handbooks. WB 39 T159d2000]
    RC46.T27 2000
    616—dc21
                                                        99-054159

Note to Instructors

Every reasonable effort has been made to ensure the information in *Diseases of the Human Body,* third edition, is accurate, up to date, and in accord with accepted standards. Not all authorities agree, however, on the etiologies, the signs and symptoms, or the diagnostic and treatment procedures or the prognosis/prevention for many of the medical conditions presented here. In cases in which conflicting information was noted, the authors attempted to present the consensus from among the authorities consulted.

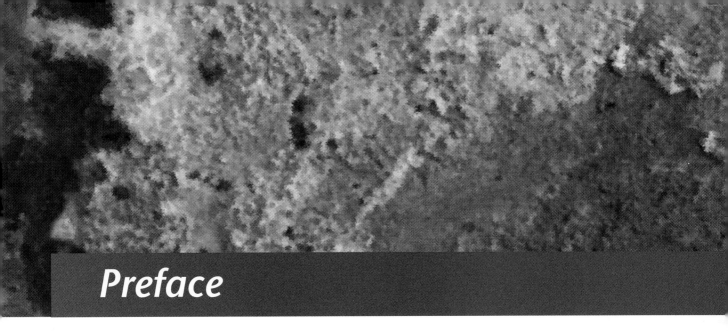

Preface

This text provides clear, succinct, and basic information about common medical conditions. *Diseases of the Human Body,* third edition, is carefully designed to meet the unique educational and professional needs of health care personnel. The book focuses on human diseases that are frequently first diagnosed or treated in ambulatory health care. Each entry considers what the disease is, how the physician might diagnose and treat the disease, and the likely consequences of the disease for the person experiencing it.

Following an overview of the disease process, infectious diseases, neoplasms, and congenital diseases, the coverage of major conditions is organized by body system. This pattern of organization is easily integrated with medical terminology or anatomy and physiology courses that health care professional students often take concurrently with their study of human disease. Within the body system chapters, each disease condition is highlighted following a logical, seven-part format consisting of:

- Description
- Etiology
- Signs and Symptoms
- Diagnostic Procedures
- Treatment
- Prognosis
- Prevention

The balance of information in each of these subsections varies according to the relative frequency and severity of the condition. In every case, however, the information selected is chosen to reflect the health care professional's need for thorough yet concise information about the condition in question. Each prevention entry, as well as the concluding chapters on pain management and holistic health, can be usefully combined with units on client teaching within the students' curriculum.

The organization of the text is thoroughly contemporary and designed to help students retain and understand basic concepts within the context of their professions. The addition of color to the interior further enhances its appeal. These features include clear chapter outlines, chapter learning objectives, pronunciation of key terms, study questions, references, and bibliography for further study. In most chapters, **Special Focus** sections present detailed coverage of important concerns related to the body system under discussion, including the most prevalent and/or serious childhood diseases. Throughout the text are references to **Alternative Medicine** treatment modalities that are increasingly becoming more integrated with traditional medicine.

We have added **Case Studies** to the system chapters to allow for discussion and critical thinking. (Answers to Case Study questions can be found in the *Instructor's Guide* to this textbook.) The comprehensive glossary appears at the end of the text. The authors use *Taber's Cyclopedic Medical Dictionary,* 18th edition, as their reference. Throughout the text, carefully chosen illustrations help students visualize body structures and conditions. For this edition, we have included over 100 full color illustrations. The expanded appendixes, which include succinct descriptions of most of the diagnostic procedures mentioned in the text, the organ function tests, and an exhaustive listing of normal laboratory values, help make *Diseases of the Human Body,* third edition, a valuable and useful reference after the student has begun his or her professional career. Finally, in addition to a general Subject Index, a specialized **Index of Diseases Covered** (beginning on page 403) directs the reader to the seven-part presentation of each disease covered.

The study of human disease is never easy. We have, however, attempted in every instance to make it clear and accessible by presenting information that will benefit both students and health care professionals. To assist instructors, we have developed an Instructor's Guide and an Electronic Test Bank, and a Power Point presentation, which are available to adoptors.

Carol D. Tamparo

Marcia A. Lewis

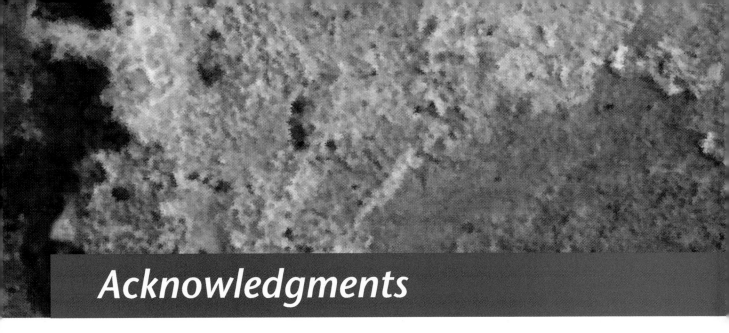

Acknowledgments

We are colleagues in the medical assistant profession. We are educators and administrators in community and technical colleges. We write as a team. We share our homes and meals, good times of laughter, and play. We write to the accompaniment of great music. We share sad times and tedious times. We agree and we disagree. Always we are friends and mentors of one another. We are co-authors.

We could not exist as such without the support of many individuals. Our publishers at the F.A. Davis Company, especially Jean-François Vilain and our editors Lynn Borders Caldwell, Christa Fratantoro, and Elena Coler, have always been encouraging, supportive, and dedicated to excellence for this project. Ginny Torres and Patricia VonBehren worked tirelessly to produce a readable manuscript out of our collection of changes, corrections, deletions, and additions. Since the book's inception, a great many dedicated, expert reviewers have added their wisdom and knowledge; our heartfelt appreciation to Marty Hitchcock, CMA, Gwinnett Technical Institute; Laura B. Burcham, RN, CMA, Shelby Baptist Medical Center; Michael Lewis Decker, BS, MA, Omaha College of Health Careers; Desmyrna R. Taylor, PT, Loma Linda University; Harriet L. Carlin, CMA-AC, Pacific Medical Services; Juanita Bryant, CMA-AC, Cabrillo College; Ann Frazier, RN, BS, MA, Detroit College of Business; Barbara Herlihy, RN, PhD, Incarnate Word College; Thomas R. Klobchar, PA-C, MS, Gannon University; and Phyllis E. Barks, BS, MA, CMA-AC, Northwestern Michigan College.

No writing project could be undertaken without the support of our families, who allowed us time to work on the weekends and gave us the moral support and encouragement that is so vital. Thank you, Tom, Les, Jayne, Duuana, and Martiann.

We also owe a debt of gratitude to our students and peers who continually challenge us. They remind us that their desire for knowledge is the most important reason for this textbook.

Finally, we acknowledge all the authors of the many reference resources we used in this edition. The content of this text cannot be entirely new, because it is based on the work of a community of researchers, clinicians, and authors; it is our hope that we have presented it in a unique manner and style.

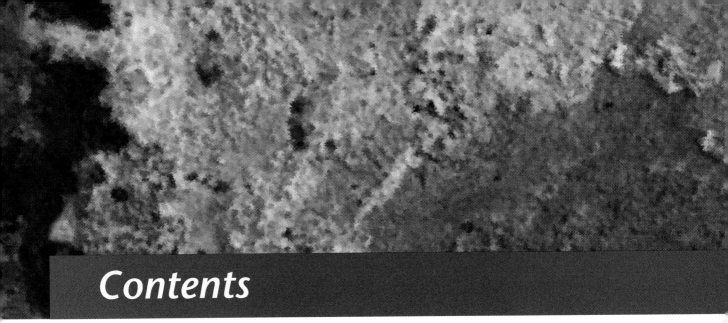

Contents

Preface . . . .*v*

Acknowledgments . . . .*vii*

chapter 1
The Disease Process *1*

Predisposing Factors   3
Hereditary Diseases   3
Classification of Hereditary Diseases   4
Inflammation and Infections   6
Trauma   9
   Head Trauma   10
   Trauma to the Chest   11
   Abdominopelvic Trauma   11
   Trauma to the Neck and Spine   11
   Trauma to the Extremities   11
Effects of Physical and Chemical Agents   11
   Extreme Heat and Cold   11
   Ionizing Radiation   12
   Extreme Atmospheric Pressure   12
   Electric Shock   12
   Poisoning   12
   Near-Drowning   12
   Bites of Insects, Spiders, and Snakes   13
   Asphyxiation   13
   Burns   13
Neoplasia and Cancer   13
Immune-Related Factors in Disease   15
   The Immune Response   15
   Allergy   15
   Autoimmune Disease   16

Immunodeficiency   17
Mental and Emotional Factors in Disease   17
Nutritional Imbalance   18
   Starvation   18
   Malnourishment   18
   Obesity   18
   Vitamin Deficiencies and Excesses   18
   Mineral Deficiencies and Excesses   18
Idiopathic and Iatrogenic Diseases   19
Summary   19
References   19
Bibliography   19
Review Questions   19

chapter 2

Infectious Diseases *23*

Infectious and Communicable Diseases   24
   Common Cold   26
   Influenza   29
   Alternative Medicine   29
   Chronic Fatigue Syndrome   29
   Acquired Immunodeficiency Syndrome (AIDS)   30
   Lyme Disease   32
   Escherichia Coli 0157:H7   32
Communicable Diseases of Childhood and Adolescence   33
   Measles (Rubeola)   34
   Rubella (German Measles)   34
   Mumps   37
   Varicella (Chickenpox)   37
   Diphtheria   38
   Pertussis (Whooping Cough)   39
   Tetanus (Lockjaw)   39
Summary   40
References   40
Bibliography   40
Review Questions   41

chapter 3

Neoplasms *43*

Cancer Risk Factors and Preventive Measures   46
Classification of Neoplasms   47
Grading and Staging of Neoplasms   48
Etiology of Neoplasms   48
Diagnosis of Neoplasms   49
Treatment of Neoplasms   49
   Surgery   49
   Radiation Therapy   50
   Chemotherapy   50
   Immunotherapy (Biotherapy)   51

Hormonal Therapy 51
Alternative Medicine 51
Summary 52
References 52
Bibliography 52
Review Questions 52

chapter 4

Congenital Diseases *55*

Nervous System Diseases 57
Cerebral Palsy 57
Neural Tube Defects: Spina Bifida, Meningocele, Myelomeningocele 57
Hydrocephalus 58
Digestive System Diseases 59
Pyloric Stenosis 59
Hirschsprung's Disease (Congenital Aganglionic Megacolon) 59
Cardiovascular Diseases 60
Erythroblastosis Fetalis (Hemolytic Disease of the Newborn) 60
Congenital Heart Defects 61
Genitourinary Diseases 64
Undescended Testes (Cryptorchidism) 64
Congenital Defects of the Ureter, Bladder, and Urethra 64
Musculoskeletal Diseases 65
Clubfoot (Talipes) 65
Congenital Hip Dysplasia 65
Metabolic Factors 66
Cystic Fibrosis 66
Phenylketonuria (PKU) 67
Bibliography 67
Review Questions 67

chapter 5

Urinary System Diseases *71*

Kidney Diseases 73
Polycystic Kidney Disease 73
Pyelonephritis (Acute) 78
Glomerulonephritis (Acute) 79
Nephrotic Syndrome 79
Chronic Renal Failure (Uremia) 80
Acute Tubular Necrosis (ATN) 81
Renal Calculi (Uroliths or Kidney Stones) 81
Hydronephrosis 83
Lower Urinary Tract Diseases 83
Cystitis and Urethritis 83
Neurogenic Bladder 84
Tumors of the Urinary System 85
Adenocarcinoma of the Kidney (Hypernephroma) 85
Tumors of the Bladder 85
Special Focus: Treatment of Renal Failure 86

    Dialysis 86
        Kidney Transplantation 88
    Common Symptoms of Urinary System Diseases 88
    References 88
    Bibliography 88
    Case Studies 89
    Review Questions 89

chapter 6

Reproductive System Diseases *93*
    Sexual Dysfunction 96
        Dyspareunia (Painful Intercourse) 96
        Erectile Dysfunction (Impotence) 96
        Arousal and Orgasmic Dysfunction in Women 97
        Premature Ejaculation 97
        Male and Female Infertility 98
    Sexually Transmitted Diseases (STDs) 99
        Gonorrhea 99
        Genital Herpes 99
        Genital Warts 101
        Syphilis 101
        Trichomoniasis 103
        Chlamydial Infections 104
        Common Symptoms of STDs 104
    Male Reproductive Diseases 104
        Prostatitis 104
        Epididymitis 105
        Orchitis 106
        Benign Prostatic Hyperplasia (BPH) 107
        Prostatic Cancer 107
        Testicular Cancer 108
        Common Symptoms of Male Reproductive Diseases 108
    Female Reproductive Diseases 109
        Premenstrual Syndrome (PMS) 109
        Amenorrhea 111
        Dysmenorrhea 111
        Ovarian Cysts and Tumors 111
        Endometriosis 112
        Uterine Leiomyomas 113
        Pelvic Inflammatory Disease (PID) 113
        Menopause 114
        Abnormal Premenopausal and Postmenopausal Bleeding 114
        Common Symptoms of Female Reproductive System Diseases 114
    Diseases of the Breasts 115
        Mammary Dysplasia or Fibrocystic Disease 115
        Benign Fibroadenoma 116
        Carcinoma of the Breast 116
    Special Focus: Breast Reconstruction 117
    Disorders of Pregnancy and Delivery 118

Spontaneous Abortion 118
Ectopic Pregnancy 118
Toxemias of Pregnancy (Preeclampsia and Eclampsia) 118
Placenta Previa 120
Abruptio Placentae 121
Premature Labor/Premature Rupture of Membranes (PROM) 121
Common Symptoms and Disorders of Pregnancy and Delivery 122
Special Focus: Cesarean Birth 122
References 122
Bibliography 122
Case Studies 123
Review Questions 123

chapter 7

Digestive System Diseases 127

Upper Gastrointestinal Tract 129
  Stomatitis 129
  Gastritis 129
  Gastroenteritis 130
  Gastric Ulcer (Peptic Ulcer of the Stomach) 131
  Hiatal Hernia 132
Lower Gastrointestinal Tract 134
  Malabsorption Syndrome 134
  Celiac Sprue (Gluten-Induced Enteropathy) 134
  Duodenal Ulcer (Peptic Ulcer of the Duodenum) 135
  Acute Appendicitis 135
  Irritable Bowel Syndrome (IBS) 136
  Crohn's Disease (Regional Enteritis, Granulomatous Colitis) 137
  Ulcerative Colitis 137
  Diverticulitis 138
  Hemorrhoids 139
  Abdominal Hernias 140
  Colorectal Cancer 141
  Diarrhea 142
Accessory Organs of Digestion: Pancreas, Gallbladder, and Liver 142
  Acute Pancreatitis 142
  Chronic Pancreatitis 143
  Pancreatic Cancer 144
  Cholelithiasis 144
  Acute Cholecystitis 146
  Cirrhosis 147
  Acute Viral Hepatitis 147
Special Focus: Eating Disorders 149
  Anorexia Nervosa 149
  Bulimia 149
Special Focus: Digestive Diseases Common in Children 150
  Infantile Colic 150
  Diarrhea 151
  Vomiting 151

    Food Allergies 151
    Helminths (Worms) 151
  Common Symptoms of Digestive System Diseases 152
    Alternative Medicine 152
  References 152
  Bibliography 152
  Case Studies 153
  Review Questions 153

chapter 8
Respiratory System Diseases *157*
  Epistaxis (Nosebleed) 160
  Sinusitis 160
  Acute and Chronic Pharyngitis 160
  Acute and Chronic Laryngitis 161
  Infectious Mononucleosis 161
  Pneumonia 162
  Legionella Infections (Legionnaires' Disease) 164
  Lung Abscess 164
  Pneumothorax 165
  Pleurisy (Pleuritis) 166
  Pleural Effusion 166
  Chronic Obstructive Pulmonary Disease (COPD) 167
  Chronic Bronchitis 167
  Chronic Pulmonary Emphysema 168
  Asthma 168
  Pulmonary Tuberculosis (TB) 169
  Pneumoconiosis 171
    Silicosis 171
    Asbestosis 171
    Berylliosis 171
    Anthracosis 172
  Respiratory Mycoses 172
  Pulmonary Edema 173
  Cor Pulmonale 173
  Pulmonary Embolism 174
  Respiratory Acidosis (Hypercapnia) 175
  Respiratory Alkalosis (Hypocapnia) 175
  Atelectasis 175
  Bronchiectasis 176
  Lung Cancer 176
  Special Focus: Respiratory Diseases of Childhood 177
    Sudden Infant Death Syndrome (SIDS) 177
    Acute Tonsillitis 177
    Adenoid Hyperplasia 178
    Croup 178
    Acute Epiglottitis 178
  Common Symptoms of Lung Diseases 179
  References 179

Bibliography   179
Case Studies   180
Review Questions   180

chapter 9
Circulatory System Diseases *183*
Rheumatic Fever and Rheumatic Heart Disease   185
Carditis   187
Pericarditis   187
Myocarditis   188
Endocarditis   189
Valvular Heart Disease   190
Mitral Insufficiency/Stenosis   190
Tricuspid Insufficiency/Stenosis   191
Pulmonic Insufficiency/Stenosis   192
Aortic Insufficiency/Stenosis   192
Hypertensive Heart Disease   193
Essential Hypertension   193
Coronary Diseases   194
Coronary Artery Disease   194
Angina Pectoris   195
Myocardial Infarction (Heart Attack)   195
Congestive Heart Failure (CHF)   197
Cardiac Arrest   198
Special Focus: Cardiac Advances   198
Blood Vessel Diseases   199
Aneurysms: Abdominal, Thoracic, and Peripheral Arteries   199
Arteriosclerosis and Atherosclerosis   200
Thrombophlebitis   201
Varicose Veins   202
Anemias and Other Red Blood Cell Disorders   202
Iron Deficiency Anemia   203
Folic Acid Deficiency Anemia   204
Pernicious Anemia   205
Aplastic Anemia   205
Sickle Cell Anemia   206
Polycythemia Vera   206
Leukemias   207
Acute Myeloblastic (Myelogenous) Leukemia (AML)   207
Acute Lymphoblastic (Lymphocytic) Leukemia (ALL)   208
Acute Monoblastic (Monocytic) Leukemia   208
Chronic Myelocytic Leukemia (CML)   208
Chronic Lymphocytic Leukemia (CLL)   209
Lymphatic Diseases   209
Lymphedema   209
Hodgkin's Disease   211
Lymphosarcoma   211
Special Focus: Bone Marrow Transplantation   212
Special Focus: Circulatory Disease of Childhood   212

Reye's Syndrome   212
Common Symptoms of Circulatory System Diseases   213
   Alternative Medicine   213
Bibliography   213
Case Studies   214
Review Questions   214

chapter 10

Nervous System Diseases 219
   Headaches   221
      Acute and Chronic Headache   221
      Migraine Headache   224
      Alternative Medicine   225
   Head Trauma   225
      Epidural and Subdural Hematoma (Acute)   225
      Cerebral Concussion   227
      Cerebral Contusion   227
   Paralysis   228
      Hemiplegia   228
      Spinal Cord Injuries: Paraplegia and Quadriplegia   228
   Infections of the Central Nervous System   230
      Acute Bacterial Meningitis   230
      Encephalitis   231
      Brain Abscess   232
   Peripheral Nerve Diseases   233
      Peripheral Neuritis   233
      Bell's Palsy   234
   Cerebral Diseases/Disorders   234
      Cerebrovascular Accident (Stroke)   234
      Transient Ischemic Attacks (TIAs)   235
      Epilepsy   235
   Degenerative Diseases   236
      Alzheimer's Disease   236
      Parkinson's Disease   237
      Multiple Sclerosis   237
      Amyotrophic Lateral Sclerosis (ALS)   238
   Cancer   239
      Tumors of the Brain   239
   Common Symptoms of Nervous System Diseases   239
   Bibliography   239
   Case Studies   240
   Review Questions   240

chapter 11

Endocrine System Diseases 243
   Pituitary Gland Diseases   247
      Hyperpituitarism (Gigantism, Acromegaly)   247
      Hypopituitarism   248

Diabetes Insipidus   249
Thyroid Gland Diseases   250
  Simple Goiter   250
  Hashimoto's Thyroiditis   251
  Hyperthyroidism (Graves' Disease)   251
  Hypothyroidism (Cretinism, Myxedema)   253
Parathyroid Gland Diseases   254
  Hyperparathyroidism (Hypercalcemia)   254
  Hypoparathyroidism (Hypocalcemia)   254
Adrenal Gland Disease   255
  Cushing's Syndrome   255
Endocrine Dysfunction of the Pancreas   256
  Diabetes Mellitus   256
Common Symptoms of Endocrine System Diseases   258
Bibliography   258
Case Studies   258
Review Questions   259

chapter 12

Musculoskeletal Diseases *261*
Bones   262
  Deformities of the Spine: Lordosis, Kyphosis, Scoliosis   262
  Herniated Intervertebral Disk   266
  Osteoporosis   267
  Osteomalacia   268
  Osteomyelitis   269
  Paget's Disease (Osteitis Deformans)   270
  Fractures   270
Joints   272
  Osteoarthritis   272
  Rheumatoid Arthritis (RA)   272
  Gout   274
  Alternative Medicine   274
Muscles and Connective Tissue   275
  Sprains and Strains   275
  Bursitis   275
  Carpal Tunnel Syndrome   275
  Alternative Medicine   276
  Tendonitis   276
  Myasthenia Gravis   276
  Polymyositis   277
  Systemic Lupus Erythematosus (SLE)   278
Neoplasms   279
Special Focus: Childhood Disease of the Musculoskeletal System   279
  Duchenne's Muscular Dystrophy   279
Common Symptoms of Musculoskeletal Diseases   280
Bibliography   280
Case Studies   280
Review Questions   280

chapter 13

Skin Diseases *283*

Psoriasis   287
Urticaria (Hives)   287
Acne Vulgaris   288
Alopecia   289
Impetigo   291
Furuncles and Carbuncles   291
Pediculosis   292
Decubitus Ulcers   293
Dermatophytoses   293
Corns and Calluses   296
Warts   296
Discoid Lupus Erythematosus   297
Scleroderma   298
Dermatitis   298
  Seborrheic Dermatitis   298
  Contact Dermatitis   299
  Atopic Dermatitis (Eczema)   299
Herpes-Related Skin Lesions   301
  Cold Sores and Fever Blisters   301
  Herpes Zoster (Shingles)   302
Cancer   303
  Skin Carcinomas   303
  Malignant Melanoma   303
Special Focus: Childhood Diseases of the Skin   304
  Atopic Dermatitis   304
  Diaper Rash   304
  Pediculosis   305
  Dermatophytosis   305
Common Symptoms of Skin Diseases   306
Bibliography   306
Case Studies   307
Review Questions   307

chapter 14

Eye and Ear Diseases *309*

Eye Diseases   311
  Refractive Errors   311
  Nystagmus   313
  Stye (Hordeolum)   313
  Corneal Abrasion   314
  Cataract   314
  Glaucoma   315
  Retinal Detachment   315
  Macular Degeneration   316
Eye Inflammations   317
  Conjunctivitis   317
  Uveitis   317

Blepharitis 317
Keratitis 318
Special Focus: Childhood Disease of the Eye 318
Strabismus 318
Common Symptoms of Eye Diseases 319
Ear Diseases 319
Impacted Cerumen 319
External Otitis (Swimmer's Ear) 319
Otitis Media 321
Otosclerosis 322
Motion Sickness 322
Ménière's Disease 322
Special Focus: Childhood Diseases of the Ear 323
Deafness 323
Otitis Media 323
Common Symptoms of Ear Diseases 323
Bibliography 323
Case Studies 324
Review Questions 324

chapter 15
Pain and Its Management *327*
What Is Pain? 328
Definition of Pain 328
Purpose of Pain 329
Pathophysiology of Pain 329
Assessment of Pain 330
Acute, Chronic, and Terminal Pain 330
Treatment of Pain 331
Medications 331
Surgery 331
Biofeedback 332
Relaxation 332
Imagery 332
Autohypnosis 332
Transcutaneous Electrical Nerve Stimulation (TENS) 332
Massage 332
Humor, Laughter, and Play 332
Music 333
Alternative Medicine 333
Conclusion 334
References 334
Bibliography 334
Review Questions 334

chapter 16
The Holistic Approach to Disease *337*
The Mind's Connection with Health and Disease 338
Holistic Health and Holistic Medicine Defined 338

Personal Responsibility   339
The Influence of Lifestyle   339
   Environmental Influences-External and Internal   339
   The Value of Good Nutrition   340
   Stress and Distress   340
Managing Negative Emotions   341
Laughter and Play   341
Love, Friendship, and Faith   342
References   343
Bibliography   343
Review Questions   343

Glossary *347*

appendix 1
Diagnostic Procedures *361*

appendix 2
Organ Function Tests *369*

appendix 3
Profile or Panel Sample Groupings and Laboratory Tests *375*

appendix 4
Associations Concerned with Diseases of the Human Body *381*

appendix 5
Normal Reference Laboratory Values *389*

Subject Index *403*

Index of Diseases Covered *423*

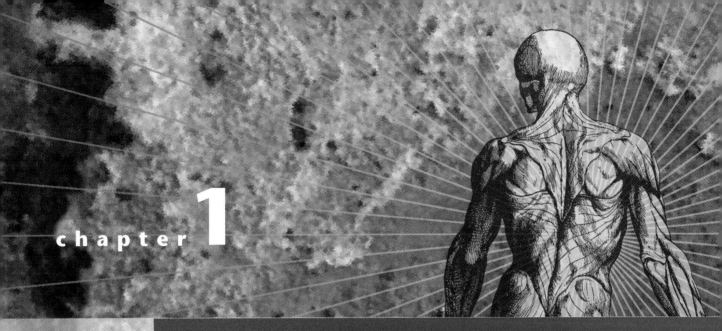

The Disease Process

CHAPTER OUTLINE

Predisposing Factors

Hereditary Diseases
Classification of Hereditary Diseases

Inflammation and Infections

Trauma
Head Trauma
Trauma to the Chest
Abdominopelvic Trauma
Trauma to the Neck and Spine
Trauma to Extremities

Effects of Physical and Chemical Agents
Extreme Heat and Cold
Ionizing Radiation
Extremes of Atmospheric Pressure
Electric Shock
Poisoning
Near-drowning
Bites of Insects, Spiders, and Snakes
Asphyxiation
Burns

Neoplasia and Cancer

Immune-Related Factors in Disease
The Immune Response
Allergy
Autoimmune Disease
Immunodeficiency

Mental and Emotional Factors in Disease

Nutritional Imbalance
Starvation
Malnourishment
Obesity
Vitamin Deficiencies and Excesses
Mineral Deficiencies and Excesses

Idiopathic and Iatrogenic Diseases

Summary

References

Bibliography

Review Questions

LEARNING OBJECTIVES

Upon successful completion of this chapter, you will:

- Define disease.
- Contrast illness and disease.
- Restate at least three predisposing factors of disease.
- Identify the three classifications of hereditary diseases.
- Describe DNA's genetic activity.
- Distinguish between genotype and phenotype.
- Identify the process of inflammation.
- Describe how infections are transmitted.
- Name at least four groups of microorganisms.
- Identify the most likely anatomic sites for traumatic injuries.
- Recall at least six physical and chemical agents that may cause disease.
- Contrast neoplasm and cancer.
- Define benign and malignant tumors.
- Identify three means of protection afforded by the immune system.
- Differentiate between:
    Natural and acquired immunity
    Humoral and cell-mediated immunity
    B-cell and T-cell immunity
- Name three classifications of immune-related diseases.
- Identify allergic reactions.
- Describe how anaphylactic shock can occur in any of the allergic reactions.
- Name four categories of immunodeficiency diseases.
- Explain mental and emotional factors as a cause of illness.
- Give three examples of nutritional imbalance.
- Define idiopathic and iatrogenic causes of disease.

KEY WORDS

Acute (ă•kūt')
Allergen (ăl'ĕr•jĕn)
Amino acid (ă•mē'nō ă'sĭd)
Analgesic (ăn•ăl•jē'sĭk)
Anaphylaxis (ăn•ă•fĭ•lăk'sĭs)
Antibody (ăn'tĭ•bŏd•ē)
Antiemetic (ăn•tĭ•ē•mĕt'ĭk)
Antigen (ăn'tĭ•jĕn)
Biopsy (bī'ŏp•sē)
Carpal tunnel syndrome (kăr'păl tŭn'ĕl sĭn'drōm)
Chromosome (krō'mō•sōm)
Chronic (krŏn'ĭk)
Diuretic (dī•ū•rĕt'ĭk)
Dyspnea (dĭsp•nē'ă)
Edema (ĕ•dē'mă)
Erythema (ĕr•ĭ•thē'mă)
Exocrine (ĕks'ō•krĭn)
Gene (jēn)
Genotype (jĕn'ō•tīp)
Heterozygous (hĕt•ĕr•ō•zī'gŭs)
Homeostasis (hō•mē•ō•stā'sĭs)
Homozygous (hŏm•ō•zī'gŭs)
Hypoventilation (hī•pō•vĕnt•ĭ•lā'shŭn)

Hypovolemic shock (hī•pō•vō•lē'mĭk shŏk)
Hypoxemia (hī•pŏks•ē'mē•ă)
Immunoglobulin (ĭm•ū•nō•glŏb'ū•lĭn)
Incontinence (ĭn•kŏn'tĭ•nĕns)
Lipid (lĭp'ĭd)
Lymphadenopathy (lĭm•făd•ĕ•nŏp'ă•thē)
Macrophage (măk'rō•fāj)
Metastasis (mĕ•tăs'tă•sĭs)
Mutation (mū•tā'shŭn)
Myocardium (mī•ō•kăr'dē•ŭm)
Pathogenic (păth•ō•jĕn'ĭk)
pH (pē•aitch')
Phagocytosis (făg•ō•sī•tō'sĭs)
Phenotype (fē'nō•tīp)
Pleura (ploo'ră)
Polymorphonuclear leukocyte (pŏl•ē•mŏr•fō•nū'klē•ăr loo'kō•sīt)
Pruritus (proo•rī'tŭs)
Stridor (strī'dŏr)
Syncope (sĭn'kō•pē)
Systemic (sĭs•tĕm'ĭk)
Tachycardia (tăk•ē•kăr'dē•ă)
Urticaria (ŭr•tĭ•kā'rē•ă)
Wheal (hwēl)

E ven though a rapid growth in medical research and a phenomenal development in technology have been accompanied by society's increased awareness of wellness and health, we have not been able to eradicate disease from our lives. *Disease* is a pathological condition of the body in response to an alteration in the normal body harmony. It may be the direct result of trauma, physical agents, and poisons or the indirect result of genetic anomalies and metabolic and nutritional disturbances.

Keep in mind that there is a difference between illness and disease. *Illness* describes the condition of a person who is experiencing a disease. It encompasses the way in which individuals perceive themselves as suffering from a disease. A disease, on the other hand, is known by its medical classification and distinguishing features. For most health-care providers, a disease is easier to treat than an illness. Proper and effective medical management should deal with both the disease and the illness.

Fear, anxiety, embarrassment, or concern about the cost of treatment or about possible disfigurement may be some of the troubling emotions persons feel when faced with an illness. Some will desire to know everything about their particular disease; others will choose complete ignorance. Most expect the medical community to have a "cure"; few fully understand the importance of their participation in the "getting well" process.

This chapter provides a brief synopsis of the causes of disease. When considering the disharmony that occurs in the body in the form of disease, remember the harmony that exists most of the time.

PREDISPOSING FACTORS

A *predisposing factor* is a condition or situation that may make a person more susceptible to disease. Some predisposing factors include age, sex, heredity, and environment. For example, an infant's immune system is not fully developed and functioning at birth. Consequently, any undue exposure to disease-producing agents could cause drastic effects. For a short time, a newborn does have residual immunity provided by its mother, but the infant needs to be protected by immunization shortly after birth.

Elderly people have unique problems that arise from the aging process itself. Physiological changes occur in the body systems, and some of these changes can cause functional impairment. Elderly persons experience problems with temperature extremes, have lowered resistance to disease as the result of decreased immunity, and have less physical activity tolerance. Certain conditions and diseases are more common in the elderly population. They include degenerative arthritis, presbyopia, atrophy of the ovaries and testes, hyperplasia of the prostate, osteoporosis, senile dementia, and Alzheimer's disease.

Men have gout more frequently than women, whereas osteoporosis is more common in women. However, sex is a predisposing factor only when the disease is physiologically based. For example, lung cancer is as prevalent in women as in men. Women suffer from heart disease as often as men.

Hereditary influences will be discussed later in this chapter. If hereditary risks are known, individuals can be better prepared to prevent, treat, or cope with possible problems.

Environmental hazards may have an effect on health. Exposure to air, noise, and other environmental pollutants may predispose individuals to disease. Living close to a heavily traveled thoroughfare in a city may be a predisposition to respiratory disease. Some geographical locations have a higher incidence of insect bites and exposure to venoms. Living in rural areas where fertilizers and pesticides are commonly used can predispose one to disease. Conditions and diseases once endemic to only one area of the world are crossing borders to invade an unsuspecting and unprepared society. This invasion is due largely to the increased mobility of the world's inhabitants. Even the office employee may be affected by environmental or occupational health problems: for instance, **carpal tunnel syndrome** and eye problems are the result of heavy use of computer technology.

HEREDITARY DISEASES

Hereditary diseases are the result of a person's genetic makeup. It is uncertain to what extent environmental factors influence the course of a hereditary disease, but the two do interact. Hereditary diseases do not always appear at birth. Mild hemophilia and muscular dystrophy may go undetected until adolescence or adulthood.

Genetic diseases are the result of monogenic (Mendelian) alterations, chromosome aberrations, and multifactorial errors. There are over 5,000 genetic diseases identified in humans—some are fatal.[1] All genetic information is contained in deoxyribonucleic acid (DNA), a complex molecular structure found in the nucleus of cells. The DNA itself is incorporated into structures called **chromosomes.** The normal number of chromosomes in humans is 46 (23 pairs). In the formation of the ovum and sperm cells (sex cells, or gametes), this number is reduced by half, with each gamete having 23 chromosomes. When the two sex cells unite at the time of fertilization, the 23 chromosomes from the ovum combine randomly with the 23 chromosomes from the sperm, producing a cell with a full complement of 46 chromosomes. Two of these chromosomes are responsible for our sex (X, Y).

A **gene** is the basic unit of heredity. Each gene consists of a fixed segment of the DNA on a specific chromosome. Our physical traits result from the expression of pairs of genes. Gene pairs are **homozygous** when they are both dominant or both recessive in their expression of a trait. Gene pairs are **heterozygous** if one gene is dominant and one recessive. Recessive genes are expressed only when the gene pair is homozygous, whereas dominant genes are expressed whether the gene pair is homozygous or heterozygous. When trying to determine genetic makeup, a family history is taken to determine a person's **genotype.** Genotype includes all the genes you have inherited from your parents. Your **phenotype** is revealed in your appearance: the color and texture of your hair, the shape of your nose, how tall you are, and so on.

A sex-linked hereditary disease can occur when one of the parents contributes a defective gene from the sex chromosome. In color blindness, the inability to distinguish reds from greens is the result of a recessive gene located on the X chromosome. The trait shows up when there is no dominant gene for normal color vision to override the recessive gene.

Changes in the structure of genes, called **mutations,** may cause functional disturbances in the body. Mutations occur when the normal sequence of DNA units is disrupted. How such a disruption is manifested depends on whether the affected gene is dominant or recessive and whether it is homozygous or heterozygous. What causes mutations is largely unknown, but they could be the result of environmental factors, such as exposure to certain chemicals or radiation.

Classification of Hereditary Diseases

The conventional method of classifying hereditary diseases is to group them into monogenic or mendelian alterations, chromosomal alterations, and multifactorial errors.

Monogenic (Mendelian) Disorders

Monogenic disorders are those caused by mutation in a single gene. The way in which the disorder is passed on to succeeding generations (the pattern of inheritance) is determined by whether the gene is dominant, recessive, or sex-linked. (A sex-linked gene is carried on the X chromosome. Because males have only one X chromosome, a sex-linked gene will be expressed in males whether it is dominant or recessive). Figure 1–1 illustrates the three most common patterns of inheritance of monogenic disorders.

AUTOSOMAL RECESSIVE

- *Cystic fibrosis.* A **chronic,** generalized disease of the **exocrine glands,** primarily affecting the pancreas, respiratory system, and sweat glands (see Chapter 4).
- *Tay-Sachs disease.* A rare **lipid** abnormality distinguished by progressive neurologic deterioration and a cherry-red spot with a gray border on both retinae. It chiefly affects Jewish infants, resulting in deafness, blindness, and paralysis. Recurrent bronchopneumonia usually causes death before the age of 5.
- *Cretinism* (or hypothyroidism). An undersecretion of hormones from the thyroid gland (see Chapter 11).
- *Phenylketonuria* (PKU). An inability to metabolize an essential **amino acid,** phenylalanine. Mental retardation results unless a special diet is followed (see Chapter 4).
- *Sickle cell anemia.* A disease affecting mostly African and black populations. It occurs because the body produces a defective form of hemoglobin that causes red blood cells to

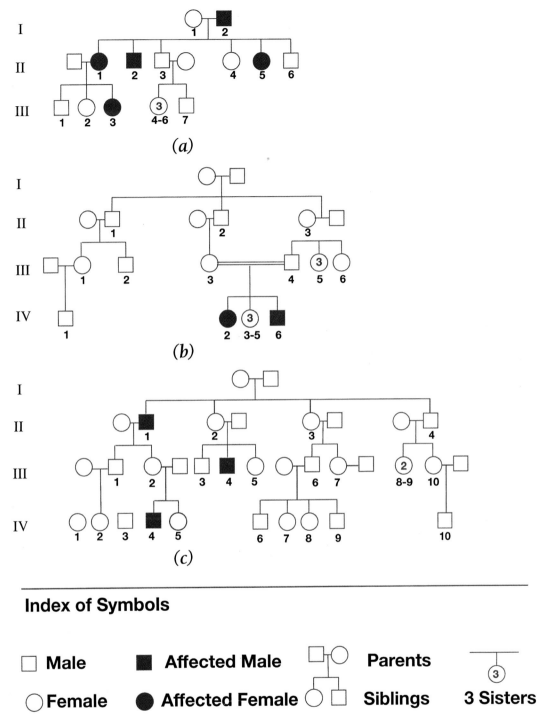

Index of Symbols

☐ **Male**	■ **Affected Male**	☐○ **Parents**
○ **Female**	● **Affected Female**	○☐ **Siblings**

3 Sisters

Figure 1–1 Patterns of inheritance. (*a*) Pedigree illustrating inheritance of autosomal dominant character. Individual is a male heterozygous for the mutant trait; if he were homozygous, all of the progeny in generation II would show the trait. None of the individuals in generation II or III can be homozygotes, because each has received a normal recessive allele from one parent. Note the large number of affected individuals (50% in generation II). (*b*) Pedigree illustrating inheritance of an autosomal recessive character. If the trait were dominant rather than recessive, then either III-3 of III-4 would have to show the trait for IV-2 and IV-6 to have inherited it. There is no indication of sex linkage. (*c*) Pedigree illustrating inheritance of sex-linked recessive character. The affected individuals (II-1, III-4, and IV-4) are all males. Individuals II-2 (and her mother), III-2, and the wife of II-1 must all be carriers. (Adapted from Purves, WK: Life: The Science of Biology, ed 2. Sinauer Associates, Sutherland, Mass., 1987, p 284, with permission.)

roughen and become sickle-shaped (see Chapter 9).

AUTOSOMAL DOMINANT

- *Diabetes insipidus.* A condition that results from insufficient secretion of vasopressin by the posterior portion of the pituitary gland (see Chapter 11).
- *Retinoblastoma.* A rare cancer usually present at birth (see Chapter 3).

X- OR SEX-LINKED

- *Hemophilia.* A bleeding disorder caused by a deficiency of specific types of serum proteins called *clotting factors.*
- *Duchenne-type muscular dystrophy.* A progressive bilateral wasting of skeletal muscles (see Chapter 12).

Chromosomal Disorders

Chromosomal disorders are caused by abnormalities in the number of chromosomes or by changes in chromosomal structure, such as deletions (missing genes) or translocations (genes shifted from one chromosome to another or to a different location on the same chromosome).

Diseases caused by chromosomal alterations include:

- *Klinefelter's syndrome.* A condition that occurs when there is an additional X chromosome in males. The body shape is elongated, the testes are small, the mammary glands are abnormally large, and mental retardation is common.
- *Turner's syndrome.* A condition caused by the loss of the X chromosome in either the ovum or the sperm. This syndrome is often characterized by shortened stature, swollen hands and feet, and coarse, enlarged, prominent ears.
- *Trisomy 21 or Down syndrome.* A condition in which an individual has three number 21 chromosomes instead of the normal two. The condition is more likely to occur in babies born to women older than 40 years. Infants with this condition typically have sloping foreheads, folds of skin over the inner corners of their eyes, and other physical abnormalities. They generally become moderately to severely retarded.

Multifactorial Disorders

Multifactorial disorders result from the interaction of many factors, both hereditary and environmental. Among the multifactorial diseases are:

- *Rheumatoid arthritis.* A chronic, **systemic,** inflammatory disease affecting the joints (see Chapter 12).
- *Gout.* A metabolic disturbance causing the excessive accumulation of uric acid in the body (see Chapter 12).
- *Diabetes mellitus.* A disorder of carbohydrate, fat, and protein metabolism. The disease is due primarily to insufficient insulin production by the pancreas (see Chapter 11).
- *Congenital heart anomalies.* This category includes six major anatomic defects that cause circulatory problems (see Chapter 4).

INFLAMMATION AND INFECTIONS

Inflammation is the body's response to trauma, physical agents (temperature extremes, radiation) or chemical agents (poisons, venoms), allergens, and pathogenic organisms (bacteria, viruses, fungi). It is a process that begins with the physical irritant and ends with healing. How well the body responds to inflammation depends on (1) an individual's general health, nutritional state, and age, (2) tissue factors, and (3) type of physical irritant.

Inflammation may be **acute** or chronic. In its acute phase, there is redness, swelling, pain, heat, and loss of function. At the site of injury, there will be a large number of **polymorphonuclear leukocytes.** Examples of acute inflammation include insect bites, mild burns, and minor abrasions and cuts. The inflammation may persist, spread to adjacent or distant tissue, and become chronic. In chronic inflammation, there is an increase in the number of lymphocytes, monocytes, and plasma cells.

A typical injury results from microorganisms gaining entry through a cut in the skin. The microorganisms release a toxin that causes the capillaries of the host to become permeable and allow access to white blood cells; hence, the redness, swelling, heat, and pain. Factors that help in abating the inflammatory response include adequate nutrition, rest, and good blood supply.

Inflammation is a beneficial biological response in most instances; however, if it becomes chronic, inflammation can be debilitating, as is the case, for example, in rheumatoid arthritis. Whatever the cause of inflammation, it is the body's protective response.

Infection is the invasion and multiplication of **pathogenic** microorganisms in the body. Most microorganisms in our bodies are nonpathogenic and, in fact, are often necessary to maintain **homeostasis.** When one or more of the requisite factors in the infectious process are present, a microorganism can become a potential pathogen.

People serve as hosts for organisms, as do animals. A host does not necessarily have to be "diseased" or "sick," but simply serves as a reservoir for the microorganisms. Transmission can be from coughing, sneezing, or touching something contaminated from the infected host, as well as from direct contact with the microorganism. If the receiving host is not susceptible, then the microorganism

has little chance of becoming a pathogen. The susceptible host, however, may have low resistance or provide the microorganism with an unusual means of entry such as an open wound.

Whenever a pathogenic microorganism finds a suitable environment for growth in an appropriate host, disease may result. Growth factors for microorganisms vary and include the presence or absence of oxygen, a ready source of food, an optimal temperature, moisture, darkness, and a specific **pH.**

Microorganisms, including those that cause disease, can be classified into six general groups:

FUNGI This group includes yeasts and molds that may be present in the soil, air, and water; however, only a few species cause disease (Fig. 1–2). Fungal diseases, called *mycoses,* usually develop slowly, are resistant to treatment, and are rarely fatal. The more common mycoses include histoplasmosis,

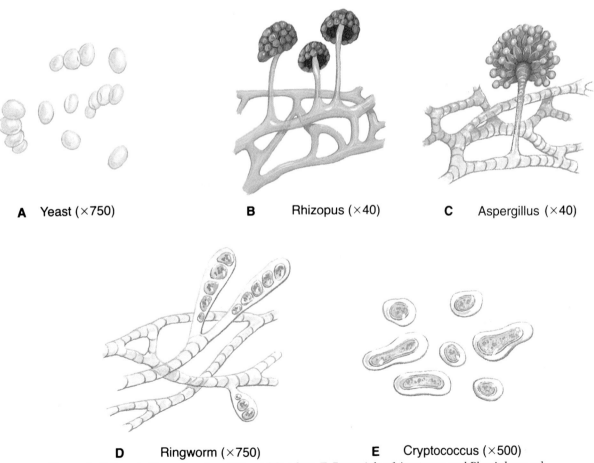

A   Yeast (×750)   **B**   Rhizopus (×40)   **C**   Aspergillus (×40)

D   Ringworm (×750)   **E**   Cryptococcus (×500)

Figure 1–2 Fungi. (From Scanlon, VC, and Sanders, T: Essentials of Anatomy and Physiology, ed 3. FA Davis, Philadelphia, 1999, p 498, with permission.)

coccidioidomycosis (see Chapter 8), ringworm, athlete's foot, and thrush.

RICKETTSIAE This group of bacterialike organisms live parasitically inside living cells. They are transmitted by bites from infected lice, fleas, ticks, and mites. Rickettsial diseases include Rocky Mountain spotted fever, typhus, and trench fever. These diseases are more likely to occur where unsanitary conditions prevail.

PROTOZOA These are single-celled organisms with animal-like characteristics (Fig. 1–3). Malaria, amebic dysentery, and African sleeping sickness are examples of protozoal diseases. *Trichomonas vaginalis* is a protozoon that causes trichomoniasis or vaginitis, a disease fairly common among women.

VIRUSES These are the smallest microorganisms, visible only through electron microscopy (Fig. 1–4).

They are independent of host cells, they are difficult to isolate, and few are susceptible to drug therapy. Viruses may remain dormant in a host for long periods before becoming active. Viral infections include the common cold, yellow fever, measles, mumps, rabies, chickenpox, herpes, poliomyelitis, hepatitis, influenza, and certain types of pneumonia and encephalitis.

BACTERIA These are single-celled organisms of many varieties. Most are nonpathogenic and useful. Bacteria, including those that cause disease, are classified according to their shape (Fig. 1–5):

- *Bacilli* are rod-shaped bacteria. Diseases caused by bacilli include tuberculosis, whooping cough, tetanus, typhoid fever, and diphtheria.
- *Spirilla* are spiral-shaped bacteria. Diseases caused by spirilla include syphilis and cholera.

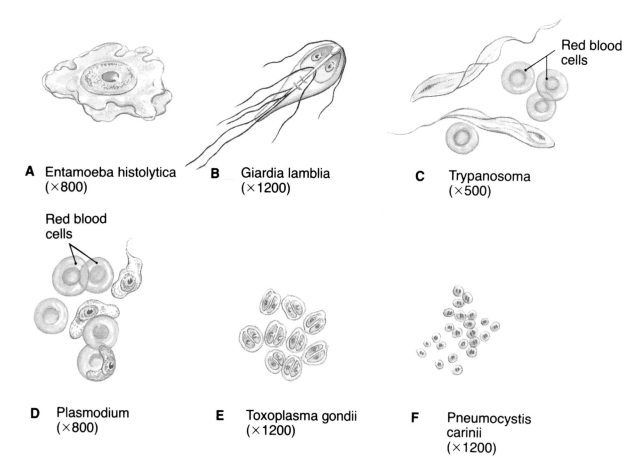

A Entamoeba histolytica (×800)

B Giardia lamblia (×1200)

C Trypanosoma (×500) Red blood cells

D Plasmodium (×800) Red blood cells

E Toxoplasma gondii (×1200)

F Pneumocystis carinii (×1200)

Figure 1–3 Protozoa. (From Scanlon, VC and Sanders, T: Essentials of Anatomy and Physiology, ed 3. FA Davis, Philadelphia, 1999, p 499, with permission.)

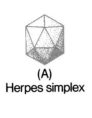

(A)
Herpes simplex

(B)
Influenza virus

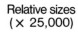

Relative sizes
(× 25,000)

E. coli

Rabies

Influenza

Polio

Figure 1–4 Viruses. (From Scanlon, VC, and Sanders, T: Essentials of Anatomy and Physiology, ed 3. FA Davis, Philadelphia, 1999, p 496, with permission.)

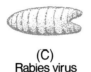

(C)
Rabies virus

- *Cocci* are dot-shaped bacteria. Diseases caused by cocci include gonorrhea, meningitis, tonsillitis, bacterial pneumonia, boils, scarlet fever, sore throats, and certain skin and urinary infections.

PARASITES A group of host-requiring organisms that include external and internal parasites. External parasites include lice and mites (insects) and are discussed in Chapter 13. Helminths are wormlike internal parasites that are typically transmitted from person to person via fecal contamination of food, water, or soil. Three classes of helminths may infect humans (Fig. 1–6):

- *Roundworms* resemble earthworms in appearance. Those most frequently affecting humans are pinworms.

- *Tapeworms* are long and narrow, as their name indicates, and they depend on two hosts, one human and one animal, from the development of the egg to the larva to the adult. The easiest way to remember their names is by the name of the animal that acts as the second host: that is, beef tapeworm, pork tapeworm, fish tapeworm, and dog tapeworm.

- *Flukes* are small, leaf-shaped, flat, unsegmented worms. They are not common in the United States, but they may become a problem for individuals traveling in Asian countries.

TRAUMA

The leading cause of death in the United States for persons younger than 35 is *physical trauma,* an in-

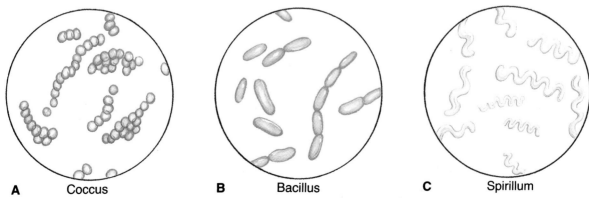

| A | Coccus | B | Bacillus | C | Spirillum |

Figure 1–5 Bacteria. (From Scanlon, VC, and Sanders, T: Essentials of Anatomy and Physiology, ed 3. FA Davis, Philadelphia, 1999, p 494, with permission.)

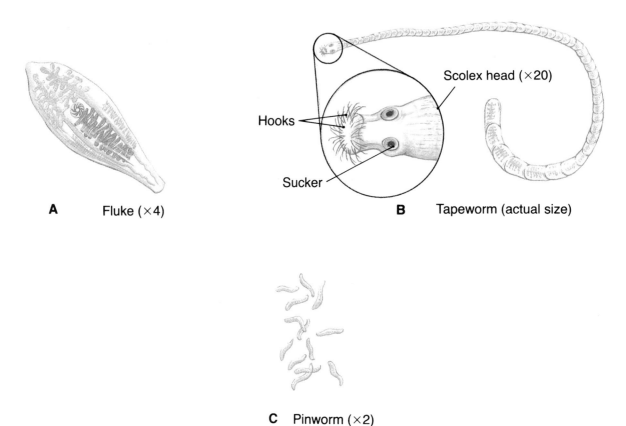

Figure 1–6 Worms. (From Scanlon, VC, and Sanders, T: Essentials of Anatomy and Physiology, ed 3. FA Davis, Philadelphia, 1999, p 500, with permission.)

jury or wound caused by external force or violence. Overall, it is the third leading cause of death in the United States, following cardiovascular disease and cancer.[2]

Head Trauma

Injuries to the head include concussion; cerebral contusion; skull, nose, and jaw fractures; and perforated eardrum.

Cerebral contusions and *concussions* cause the brain to be jostled inside the skull. Cerebral contusions are more serious than concussions because contusions bruise the brain tissue and disrupt normal nerve function. Contusions may cause loss of consciousness, hemorrhage, and even death. Concussions cause temporary neural dysfunction but are not severe enough to cause a contusion. This kind of trauma is normally the result of falls, severe blows to the head area, and automobile accidents. If unconsciousness, convulsions, forceful and persistent vomiting, blurred vision, staggering walk, or hemorrhage occur, the person should be taken to a hospital immediately. A physician should determine the seriousness of the event and the proper treatment needed.

Skull fractures often are accompanied by scalp wounds and profuse bleeding. The concern in skull fractures is possible damage to the brain. Fractures generally are accompanied by pain, tenderness, and swelling of the affected areas. Surgery may be required to remove foreign bodies or bone fragments. The patient will be closely monitored in a hospital.

Perforated eardrums normally result from the insertion of sharp objects into the ear canal or from a severe blow to the side of the head. Sudden and excessive changes in air pressure can cause perforation. Children suffering from acute otitis media (earache) may suffer a perforated eardrum as a complication of this disease.

Trauma to the Chest

Penetrating chest injuries are often caused by knife and gunshot wounds. Penetrating chest wounds typically cause a sucking sound as air enters the chest cavity through the chest wall opening. The patient may be in severe pain. **Tachycardia** is apt to occur. There may be a weak pulse, blood loss, and possible **hypovolemic shock.** It is important to control blood loss in penetration wounds.

Nonpenetrating chest injuries such as rib fractures usually result from an automobile accident in which the driver is thrown against the steering wheel. There is a sensation of tenderness and pain that worsens with deep breathing or exertion. A potential complication of rib fractures is the penetration of a rib into the **pleura,** lung tissue, or **myocardium.**

X-ray examination is necessary to determine the extent and location of the damage. An electrocardiogram (ECG) and blood studies help assess cardiac damage. Immediate assessment and attendance by a physician are paramount. Surgical repair is often necessary.

Abdominopelvic Trauma

Injuries to the abdominopelvic region may cause hemorrhages within the liver, spleen, pancreas, and kidneys, and/or rupture of the stomach, intestine, gallbladder, and urinary bladder. Rupture of the organs results in the spilling of the organs' contents (including bacteria) into the abdominopelvic cavity. This is a major cause of infection. Blood loss and hypovolemic shock are also a concern. Emergency attention is necessary to determine the extent of the damage and the necessary treatment. Most abdominal injuries require surgical repair. The prognosis depends on the extent of the injury, but prompt attention generally improves the outcome.

Trauma to the Neck and Spine

Neck and spine injuries include fractures, contusions, and compressions of the vertebral column. The greatest concern with this type of trauma is damage to the spinal cord and paralysis. Spinal cord injuries are discussed in connection with the nervous system, in Chapter 10.

Trauma to Extremities

Sprains, strains, and fractures to the arms and legs are common. They are discussed with musculoskeletal diseases in Chapter 12.

EFFECTS OF PHYSICAL AND CHEMICAL AGENTS

Physical and chemical agents can adversely affect the body. The degree to which this occurs depends on many factors. If the exposure to the irritant is short in duration and frequency and is fairly localized, and if the person is healthy, the damage may be unnoticed or reversible; however, the irritant may cause irreversible systemic damage if the person is debilitated, diseased, very young or elderly, has lowered resistance, or is on some medication.

Some of the more common physical and chemical agents include extreme heat and cold, ionizing radiation, extremes in atmospheric pressure, electric shock, poisonings, near-drowning, bites from insects and snakes, asphyxiation, and burns.

Extreme Heat and Cold

Extreme heat may occasion **syncope,** heat exhaustion, heat cramps, and heatstroke. Causes of these heat disorders include overexertion in heat, prolonged heat exposure, salt depletion, dehydration, failure of the body's heat-regulating mechanisms, or a combination of these. Heat exhaustion, sometimes resulting in syncope, is caused by overexposure to heat, insufficient water intake, insufficient salt intake, and deficiency of sweat production. Heat cramps in the legs and abdomen result from heavy salt loss. The person is usually pale and clammy, with a rapid, weak pulse and shallow breathing. Individuals treated at this stage generally respond promptly to rest, cooling, and weak salt liquids administered orally. If the person does not respond or is not treated, heat exhaustion may lead to heatstroke when the body's temperature control mechanism malfunctions. Sweating ceases and the body temperature rises. The skin becomes hot, dry, and flushed. This is a life-threatening condition that may require hospitalization with intravenous (IV) therapy, cooling therapy, increased fluid intake, temperature monitoring, and muscle massaging. Hypersensitivity to heat may remain for some time. Any of these heat disorders can be fatal.

Extreme cold may occasion disorders such as chilblain, frostbite, and hypothermia. Causes include overexposure to cold air, wind, or water. *Chilblain,* a mild frostbite, produces red, itching skin lesions, usually on the extremities, whereas *frostbite,* the freezing of exposed areas, causes tingling and redness followed by paleness and numbness of the affected areas. Untreated, either condition can lead to gangrene and may necessitate amputation. *Hypothermia* is a systemic reaction; it can be fatal. Treatment of any of the cold disorders includes gradually warming the person, monitoring body temperature, protecting the affected part, preventing infection, and administering **analgesics** as necessary.

Ionizing Radiation

Depending on the duration and intensity of exposure and the form of the irradiating agent, the effects of ionizing radiation range from mild skin burns to fatal tissue destruction. The exposure to radiation may be due to ingestion, inhalation, or direct contact. Causes may include occupational or accidental exposure, or the misuse of radiation for diagnostic or treatment purposes. Persons at risk include those with cancer receiving radiation therapy and employees in nuclear power plants. The harmful effects of radiation may be immediate or delayed, acute or chronic. Treatment is symptomatic and supportive and may include **antiemetics,** simple and palatable foods, blood transfusions, and emotional support.

Extremes of Atmospheric Pressure

Extremes of atmospheric pressure result from changing too rapidly from a high-pressure to low-pressure environment or from a low-pressure to high-pressure environment. Decompression sickness is an occupational hazard for deep-sea divers and airplane pilots, who descend ascend too quickly, or for hospital personnel who work in hy-

perbaric chambers. Systemic damage occurs following rapid decompression when gases dissolved in the blood and other tissues escape faster than they can be diffused through respiration. Nitrogen gas bubbles form in the blood and tissue causing respiratory problems and pain. Treatment consists of emergency oxygen until the person can be transported to a hyperbaric chamber, where recompression is followed by slow decompression. Supportive measures are also employed.

Electric Shock

Electric shock can occur anywhere there is electricity—home, work, or school. The causes of electric shock can be natural (as from lightning) or contrived (due to carelessness or ignorance, or from faulty equipment). The victim must be freed from the source of electric current without the rescuer contacting the current, and treatment must begin immediately. Cardiopulmonary resuscitation (CPR) may be necessary. If the damage is severe, hospitalization may be required to observe the patient, treat any burns, and prevent infection.

Poisoning

Poisoning is a common occurrence, especially among curious children. Recently, our society has become increasingly aware of poisonous chemicals that have been dumped or buried. Such chemicals cause soil and water contamination that results in ecological and personal damage.

Poisons may be accidentally ingested, inhaled, injected, or absorbed through the skin, but poisoning can also be the result of occupational exposure when working with toxic chemicals, improper cooking and canning of food, and drug overdoses or drug abuse. Treatment consists of first aid measures, identifying and providing the correct antidote if one exists, and supportive measures. The local poison control center offers valuable help. Prompt, correct treatment can save a life.

Near-drowning

Near-drowning is a common occurrence during the warm summer months and could be prevented in many cases by following water safety precautions. In near-drowning, the person generally aspirates fluid, or the person may have an obstructed airway caused by a spasm of the larynx when gasping under water, resulting in **hypoxemia.** Later, within minutes or possibly days of near-drowning, the person may experience respiratory distress. Emergency treatment is critical. Hospitalization may be required for oxygenation, airway maintenance, observation of the cardiovascular status of the patient, and prevention of further complications.

Bites of Insects, Spiders, and Snakes

Insect, spider, and snake bites occur more often during the warm summer months. Bee, yellow jacket, wasp, and hornet stings may cause localized pain, but they usually require little more than symptomatic treatment. Allergic reactions and multiple stings or bites, however, are a more serious matter and should be treated as a medical emergency. Poisonous bites require quick emergency measures to prevent venom absorption and life-threatening symptoms from occurring. The victim should be immobilized and transported immediately to a hospital, where the specific antidote can be administered. Whether the bite is considered serious or mild, close observation of the victim is essential.

Asphyxiation

Asphyxiation, or lack of oxygen coupled with accumulating carbon dioxide in the blood, may result from near-drowning, **hypoventilation,** airway obstruction, or inhalation of toxic substances. Emergency treatment is generally required, and it may involve removal of any obstruction, CPR, oxygenation, and intubation. Hospitalization may be necessary to stabilize the victim's vital signs. Obviously, any breathing difficulty is frightening to the victim, so reassurance and encouragement are needed.

Burns

Tragically, burns are a leading cause of death among children. They usually are preventable by following fire safety guidelines. Burns are classified by extent, depth, person's age, and associated ill-

ness and injury. The rule of nines is useful for assessing the extent of burns. Figure 1–7 illustrates the rule of nines and burn classification criteria. Emergency measures may be necessary to maintain the burn victim's airway, cool the wound, and prevent serious loss of body fluids. Once the victim has been transported to a hospital, frequently a special burn center, the focus is on maintaining fluid balance, prevention of infection, and patient support. Severe burns can be extremely painful and require a lengthy rehabilitation period, including possible skin grafting and plastic surgery. Emotional support is essential.

Neoplasia and Cancer

Neoplasia means new formation or new growth. The terms *tumor* and *neoplasm* are commonly used synonymously and are thus used herein. Specific neoplastic diseases will be dealt with in Chapter 3. Here we discuss etiologic factors and their results.

The actual cause of neoplasms is not known; however, alteration in genes does occur, allowing independent and uncontrollable growth. As was discussed earlier under Hereditary Diseases, an alteration in a gene on a chromosome is a *mutation.* The mutant cell differs from the normal cell in that the abnormal cell is no longer subject to normal control mechanisms. Apparently, mutations such as this occur relatively frequently, but the body usually is able to destroy the resulting mutant cells as soon as they appear. Therefore, a tumor may represent a failure on the part of the body's immune system. The harmful effects of the neoplastic growth may be from the growth itself or from destruction of surrounding tissue.

The neoplasm may be benign or malignant, depending on its growth pattern. A *benign* tumor is one that remains circumscribed, although it may vary in size from small to large. A *malignant* tumor, or cancer, is one that spreads to other cells, tissues, and parts of the body through the bloodstream or lymphatic system. The spreading process is called **metastasis.**

Cancer is a general term for more than 100 diseases, all of which are characterized by the uncontrollable growth of cells. The diagnosis, treatment, prognosis, and prevention of cancer are discussed in Chapter 3.

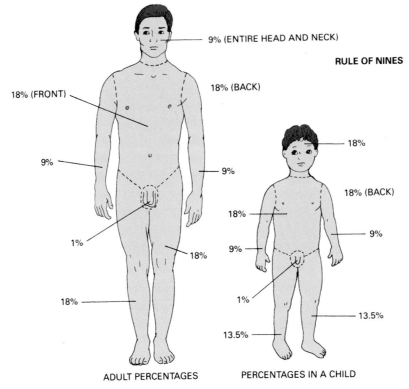

RULE OF NINES

9% (ENTIRE HEAD AND NECK)

18% (FRONT)

18% (BACK)

9%

9%

1%

18%

18%

ADULT PERCENTAGES

18%

18% (BACK)

18%

9%

9%

1%

13.5%

13.5%

PERCENTAGES IN A CHILD

CLASSIFICATION OF BURNS

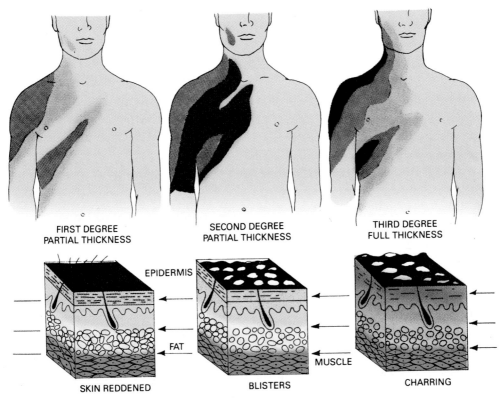

FIRST DEGREE
PARTIAL THICKNESS

SECOND DEGREE
PARTIAL THICKNESS

THIRD DEGREE
FULL THICKNESS

EPIDERMIS

FAT

MUSCLE

SKIN REDDENED

BLISTERS

CHARRING

Figure 1–7 Rule of nines and burn classification. (From Thomas, CL [ed]: Taber's Cyclopedic Medical Dictionary, ed. 15. FA Davis, Philadelphia, 1985, p 243, with permission.)

IMMUNE-RELATED FACTORS IN DISEASE

The Immune Response

An ideally designed body would be free of disease. A careful study of body chemistry and cellular function reveals a blueprint for maintaining a disease-free state. The body is protected in three ways:

- Normal body structures function to block the entry of germs, by means of tears, mucous membranes, intact skin, cilia, and body pH.
- The inflammatory response rushes leukocytes to a site of infection, where invading organisms are engulfed in a process called **phagocytosis.**
- A specific immune response causes a protective reaction to a foreign antigen.

The body's immune system is both natural and acquired. Natural immunity is a genetic feature specific to race, sex, and the individual's ability to respond. The body's normal structure and function are natural defenses. For example, the skin is a barrier to invading organisms, the gastric juices destroy swallowed organisms, and the white blood cells, through phagocytosis, destroy bacteria. The term *acquired immunity* indicates that the body has developed the ability to defend itself against a specific agent. This can occur after actually having a disease or after receiving immunization against a disease. Although the human body does not begin developing **antibodies** until 3 to 6 weeks of age, an infant receives temporary immunity because it receives antibodies produced by its mother's immune system in utero.

There are two different types of acquired immunity[3]:

- *Humoral immunity* is the body's major defense against bacteria. Here the body produces antibodies or **immunoglobulins** that combine with and eliminate the foreign substance or **antigen.** These antibodies are formed by white blood cells called B-cell lymphocytes. The humoral response is rapid, beginning immediately, or within 48 hours of antigen contact. Humoral immunity, in the presence of an antigen, causes an antibody to be released, which, in turn, reacts exclusively with that antigen. This binding of antibody to antigen encourages phagocytosis of the antigen and activates the complement system. The complement system is responsible for enzyme development, which helps remove the antigen from the body.
- *Cell-mediated immunity* is action by another group of white cells, called *T-cell lymphocytes.* These are the main protection against viruses, fungi, parasites, some bacteria, and tumors. The T cells mature in the thymus and are stored in the lymphatic system and spleen. Cell-mediated immunity is initiated when a T lymphocyte becomes sensitized by contact with a specific antigen. In response to additional contacts with the antigen, the T lymphocyte releases sensitized lymphocytes, which migrate to the inflammation site. These lymphocytes help to transform local **macrophages** into "killer" T lymphocytes that are highly phagocytic. The migration of antigens also is prohibited. Some normal tissue can be destroyed during this process, which is very intense.

The ability to generate an immune response is controlled by genetics. Immune response genes regulate B-cell and T-cell proliferation; therefore, they influence resistance to infection and tumors. The immune response normally recognizes its own body cells, thereby preventing damage to tissue.

While this complex system to protect the body is an example of the disease-free design of the body, the immune response can malfunction. Immunologic malfunctions are classified as (1) allergy, when the immune response is inappropriate; (2) autoimmunity, when the immune response is misdirected; and (3) immunodeficiency, when the immune response is inadequate.

Allergy

Allergic reactions that reflect malfunctioning immunity include **urticaria,** or hives (Fig. 1–8). The symptoms include **wheals** surrounded by a reddened area that may cover a small area or the entire body. Causative factors may include foods (especially milk, fish, and strawberries), the presence of pets, insect bites, certain fabrics, inhalants, and cosmetics. Familial history, stress, and general physical condition may predispose to allergies.

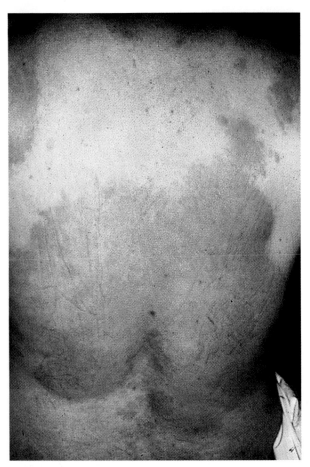

Figure 1–8 Urticaria (hives). Huge wheals in a patient allergic to penicillin. (From Reeves, JRT, and Maibach, H: Clinical Dermatology Illustrated: A Regional Approach. FA Davis, Philadelphia, 1991, p 212, with permission.)

Another allergic reaction results from the transfusion of the wrong type of blood or blood components, which become toxic to the body's cells. Transfusion reactions may be mild or severe, depending on the amount of transfused fluid and the person's condition. Symptoms of transfusion reaction range from chills and fever, pain, nausea, and vomiting, to **anaphylaxis** and congestive heart failure. Blood and laboratory tests have to be performed to confirm the type and severity of reaction. The attention of a physician is necessary to prevent complications.

Allergy is also seen in hypersensitivity reactions to drugs. Certain drugs in some people may act as antigens, stimulating the formation of sensitizing antibodies. Although any drug can be the offender, common ones include penicillin, sulfa drugs, and aspirin. The degree of hypersensitivity depends on the extent and duration of exposure to the drug, the person's genetic background, age, sex, and the presence of underlying disease. Symptoms range from a local rash, **pruritus,** flulike symptoms, and **erythema** to more severe conditions such as asthma, anemia, or anaphylaxis.

Anaphylactic shock is considered by some authorities as an allergic reaction. This reaction is acute and potentially life-threatening. It may be caused by drug hypersensitivity, foods (the most likely offenders are nuts, legumes, berries, and seafoods), and insect stings (honeybees, wasps, yellow jackets, mosquitoes, ants, and certain spiders). Anaphylaxis may occur after a single exposure to an antigen or following repeated exposures. For this reason, it is important to be alert for an allergic reaction in any person at any time. In some cases, the reaction may occur within seconds, but it is usually no later than 40 to 50 minutes following contact with the **allergen.** Cardiovascular symptoms may include hypotension, shock, and cardiac irregularities. Respiratory symptoms may include nasal congestion, profuse watery rhinorrhea, itching, and sudden sneezing. **Edema** of the nose or throat can cause **stridor, dyspnea,** or acute respiratory failure. Gastrointestinal and genitourinary symptoms include stomach cramping, nausea, diarrhea, and urinary urgency and **incontinence.**

Anaphylactic shock is an emergency. It requires immediate countermeasures, which may include injection of epinephrine. It is important to maintain the individual's airway and to administer CPR in the event of cardiac arrest.

Autoimmune Disease

In autoimmune disease, self-antigens, or abnormal immune cells, develop that incite the immune response into abnormal or excessive activity of T cells or B cells.

In this book, most of the autoimmune diseases are discussed in conjunction with the specific organ systems affected; however, a brief summary of five types follows:

- *Gastrointestinal:* Primary biliary cirrhosis, chronic active hepatitis, ulcerative colitis, and atrophic gastritis (see Chapter 7).
- *Cardiovascular:* Rheumatic fever, pernicious anemia, hemolytic anemia, idiopathic thrombocytopenia, and leukopenia (see Chapter 9).
- *Endocrine:* Juvenile autoimmune diabetes, thyrotoxicosis, and Hashimoto's thyroiditis (see Chapter 11).
- *Musculoskeletal:* Mixed connective-tissue diseases, systemic lupus erythematosus (SLE), and myasthenia gravis (see Chapter 12).
- *Dermatologic:* Dermatomyositis and scleroderma (see Chapter 13).

Immunodeficiency

The immunodeficiency diseases are a result of B-cell and/or T-cell deficiency or some unknown immunodeficient factor. The majority of immunodeficient diseases are diagnosed by immunologic analyses, as many persons are asymptomatic except for recurrent infections. Most immunodeficient patients have impaired resistance to infections, and it is these infectious conditions that may cause death.

Acquired immunodeficiency syndrome (AIDS) is an important, highly publicized, and severe form of acquired immune deficiency. Another immunodeficiency disease is *Hodgkin's disease,* a neoplastic malignancy of the lymph system. The immunodeficiency is thought to be due to impaired T-cell function, which leaves the person more susceptible to infections. Once a fatal disease, it is now potentially curable, even in advanced stages. Hodgkin's disease will be discussed in detail in Chapter 8, under the lymphatic system.

Non-Hodgkin's lymphomas, and sometimes lymphosarcomas, are malignant neoplasms of the lymphoreticular system. Persons with genetic, or acquired, immunodeficiency disorders clearly are predisposed to these malignant neoplasms. A symptom is swelling of lymph glands. Diagnosis is chiefly by lymph node **biopsy** to differentiate lymphoma from Hodgkin's disease and other causes of **lymphadenopathy.** Identification of the disease is necessary for proper treatment, and chemotherapy and radiation are used with some success. Non-Hodgkin's lymphomas cause more deaths than Hodgkin's disease; death usually results from complications such as anemia and infections.

MENTAL AND EMOTIONAL FACTORS IN DISEASE

To this point, disease etiologies have been traditional and readily identifiable. Almost everyone is affected by some form of mental disorder sometime in his or her life. Such emotional and mental disorders are related to organic disease in three ways:

1. An emotional response to a physical illness or injury that may result in depression, anxiety, or some transient situational disturbance.
2. Mental illness may occur secondarily to an organic disease such as Alzheimer's.
3. Physical ailments that are considered psychophysiological disorders because they frequently are associated with emotional disturbances.

Whatever the cause of the mental and emotional factors, a person's adaptation ability will strongly influence the course of the illness.

From the moment of birth, each person begins a process of developing a sense of self and self-esteem. Adaptations and adjustments are necessary. When the stimuli are stressful, adaptation occurs to keep the body in a state of well-being. How adaptation occurs is the key to mental health.

Laurence J. Peter and Bill Dana, in their book, *The Laughter Prescription,* say:

> Emotional stress can cause physical deterioration by setting off a complex process that starts in the cerebrum, the thinking part of the brain. Thoughts in the cerebrum can affect the hypothalamus, the part of the brain that regulates body temperature, certain metabolic processes, the autonomic nervous system and chemical balance. Your feelings literally can make you sick or well. Emotional stress is just as real as any kind of physical stress. When you experience sustained anxiety, anger or fear, your physical processes are out of balance and your body cells actually are deteriorating. If degenerative trends are not corrected, you will become susceptible to colds, coronaries, and a host of diseases. It is, therefore, important that downward spirals be reversed immediately.[4]

It becomes important, therefore, in considering the etiology of disease, to consider the emotional and mental state of the individual as the direct or indirect cause of a particular ailment. Refer to Chapter 16 for further information on the mind's connection to health and disease.

NUTRITIONAL IMBALANCE

Nutritional imbalance can cause growth problems, specific diseases, and even death. Nutritional imbalances, deficiencies, and excesses are becoming more apparent as causes of health problems. Nutritional deficiencies can cause grave intellectual and physical impairments as well as affect an individual's overall well-being. Causes of nutritional imbalances include starvation, malnourishment, obesity, and vitamin and mineral deficiencies and excesses.

Starvation

Causes of starvation include lack of food, or an unbalanced diet over a long period of time, causing metabolic and physiological body changes. A starved person generally is one who does not have adequate food, whereas someone who is malnourished generally has adequate food available, but of inadequate nutritive value. Starvation is seen at any age; however, infants and children from 1 to 3 years of age suffer more severely than adults.

Malnourishment

Malnourishment may be due to:

- Improper intake of foodstuffs in both quality and quantity, as seen in people suffering from alcoholism, anorexia nervosa, and bulimia, or in those who engage in diet faddism.
- Improper intake of foodstuffs because of gastrointestinal problems, as exhibited in the person who has no taste or smell, the postoperative anorexic, or the person who has a lesion in the throat.
- Malabsorption or poor utilization of foodstuffs, as seen when an individual is unable to absorb nutrients properly.
- Increased need for food, as seen in a marathon runner, a person in a febrile state, and a person

with cancer increased needs for certain nutrients.
- Impaired metabolism of foodstuffs, as in both hereditary and acquired biochemical disorders.
- Food and drug interactions, as seen in those taking corticosteroid medications, which are known to deplete muscle protein, lower glucose tolerance, and induce osteoporosis.[5]

Obesity

Obesity has been defined as a condition where body weight is 10 to 20 percent above the ideal. Of course, "ideal" is difficult to determine, and factors such as family history and body build need to be considered. The cause of obesity may be too many calories, too little activity, or, less frequently, an endocrine and metabolic problem. Fluid retention may cause an increase in weight, too. Treatment may include lowering caloric intake, increasing physical activity, or in the case of metabolic disorders, correcting the error. If fluid retention is a problem, **diuretics** may be prescribed, and any underlying cause of the retention should be detected and treated. The prognosis for obesity is not good. Although a small percentage of obese individuals are able to lose weight, an even smaller percentage are able to maintain permanent weight reduction. Obesity poses a serious risk for development of diabetes mellitus, hypertension, gallbladder disease, and heart disease.

Vitamin Deficiencies and Excesses

Early signs of *vitamin deficiency* are generally vague and nonspecific. Vitamin-deficiency diseases include *scurvy,* which is caused by a lack of vitamin C and is characterized by abnormal bone formation and hemorrhages of mucous membranes; *rickets,* which is due to a lack of vitamin D (see Chapter 12); and *beriberi,* in which a lack of vitamin B$_1$ causes neurological damage. Treatment typically consists of a diet high in protein and the required vitamin. Vitamin excess may occur when people take vitamins in an attempt to cover missed or inadequate meals, when they hope to prevent some disease (e.g., the common cold), or when they self-treat a condition. Large doses of some vitamins are toxic and may cause illness, especially when taken over a long period of time.

Mineral Deficiencies and Excesses

Minerals are a vital component of a balanced diet. *Mineral deficiencies* of chloride, potassium, sodium, calcium, and magnesium are the more common ones. Causes include dietary deficiencies and metabolic disorders. Treatment may involve increasing the intake of a deficient mineral through foodstuffs or medication, or addressing any underlying metabolic disorder. *Mineral excess* also may be caused by diet, medication, or a metabolic error. Treatment consists of locating the cause and correcting the problem.

IDIOPATHIC AND IATROGENIC DISEASES

Some diseases, having no known cause, are described as *idiopathic.* Of course, when the cause is unknown, the disease can only be treated symptomatically.

Some diseases are *iatrogenic:* that is, caused by medical treatment and its effects. This can be seen in the treatment of some cancers, where the chemotherapy drugs used may cause severe anemia, or when hepatitis develops as a result of blood transfusion.

SUMMARY

The disease process is varied, complex, and sometimes unknown. When the body is out of harmony, there is a need for care and treatment. Only when the disease process is understood is the best care and treatment possible.

REFERENCES

1. Professional Guide to Diseases, ed 6. Springhouse Corporation, Springhouse, Pa., 1998, p 2.
2. Diseases. Springhouse Corporation, Springhouse, Pa., 1993, p 213.
3. Mulvihill, ML: Human Diseases, A Systemic Approach, ed 4. Appleton & Lange, Stamford, Conn., 1995, pp 17–18.
4. Peter, LJ, and Dana, B: The Laughter Prescription. Ballantine Books, New York, 1982, p 22.
5. Chatton, MJ, and Ullman, PM: Nutrition: Nutritional and metabolic disorders. In Current Medical Diagnosis and Treatment, Lange Medical Publications, Los Altos, Calif., 1985, p 794.

BIBLIOGRAPHY

Fauci, AS, et al: Harrison's Principles of Internal Medicine, ed 14. McGraw-Hill, New York, 1998.
Frazier, MS, et al: Essentials of Human Diseases & Conditions. WB Saunders, Philadelphia, 1996.
Kent, TH, and Hart, MN: Introduction to Human Disease, ed 3. Appleton & Lange, Stamford, Conn., 1993.
Mulvihill, ML: Human Diseases, A Systemic Approach, ed 4. Appleton & Lange, Stamford, Conn., 1995.

REVIEW QUESTIONS

MATCHING

_____ 1. Genetic constitution of organism

_____ 2. Describes condition of a sick person

_____ 3. DNA sequence is disrupted

_____ 4. The smallest microorganism

_____ 5. Not in harmony

_____ 6. Contains all hereditary information

_____ 7. Worms

_____ 8. Leukocytes rush to site and phagocytize invading organism

_____ 9. Caused by treatment

a. Disease

b. Illness

c. Genotype

d. DNA

e. Mutation

f. Virus

g. Helminths

h. "Rule of nines"

i. Phagocytosis

_____ 10. Helps assess extent of burns

j. Iatrogenic

k. Homeostasis

l. Phenotype

SHORT ANSWER

1. List nine causes of diseases and/or disorders:

   a.

   b.

   c.

   d.

   e.

   f.

   g.

   h.

   i.

2. The leading cause of death in the United States for those under 35 is _____.

3. Predisposing factors in disease are:

   a.

   b.

   c.

   d.

TRUE/FALSE

T   F   1. Some of the disorders caused by exposure to extreme cold are chilblain, frostbite, and hypothermia.

T   F   2. Burns are a leading cause of death in children.

T   F   3. Neoplasia is defined as cancer.

T   F   4. Humoral immunity is the body's major defense against bacteria.

T   F   5. Allergy is an example of an inappropriate immune response.

MULTIPLE CHOICE

Place a checkmark next to all the correct answers.

1. Phagocytosis
   a. Is a process of devouring foreign substances.
   b. Is accomplished by neutrophils and macrophages.
   c. Depends on the lymphatic system.
   d. Activates the complement system.

2. B-cell lymphocytes
   a. Provide cell-mediated immunity.
   b. Are responsible for acquired humoral immunity.
   c. Are the first and most rapid response of antigen contact.
   d. Are processed in the thymus.

3. Cell-mediated immunity
   a. Is responsible for rejection of transplanted organs.
   b. May be referred to as T-cell immunity.
   c. Is initiated when a T lymphocyte is sensitized by contact with a specific antigen.
   d. Is highly effective against fungal and viral invasion and cancer.

4. Three main classifications of immunity gone wrong are:
   a. Allergy
   b. Pneumoconiosis
   c. Autoimmunity
   d. Immunodeficiency

ANSWERS

MATCHING

1. c	4. f	7. g	10. h
2. b	5. a	8. i	
3. e	6. d	9. j	

SHORT ANSWER

1. a. Genetic factors
   b. Infections
   c. Trauma
   d. Chemical agents and irritants
   e. Neoplasia and cancer
   f. Immune-related factors
   g. Mental and emotional factors
   h. Nutritional imbalance
   i. Idiopathic and iatrogenic
2. Trauma
3. a. Age
   b. Gender
   c. Heredity
   d. Environment

TRUE/FALSE

1. T	4. T
2. T	5. T
3. F	

MULTIPLE CHOICE

1. a, b, and d	3. a, b, c, and d
2. b and c	4. a, c, and d

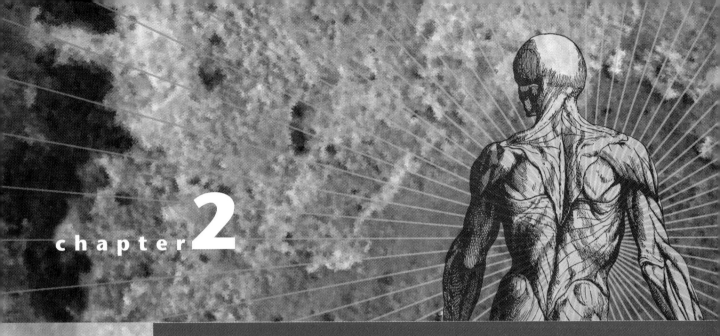

chapter 2

Infectious Diseases

CHAPTER OUTLINE

Infectious and Communicable Diseases
Common Cold
Influenza
☐ ALTERNATIVE MEDICINE
Chronic Fatigue Syndrome
Acquired Immunodeficiency Syndrome (AIDS)
Lyme Disease
Escherichia coli 0157:H7

Communicable Diseases of Childhood and Adolescence
Measles (Rubeola)
Rubella (German Measles)
Mumps
Varicella (Chickenpox)
Diphtheria
Pertussis (Whooping Cough)
Tetanus (Lockjaw)

Summary

References

Bibliography

Review Questions

LEARNING OBJECTIVES

Upon successful completion of this chapter, you will:
- Recall the symptoms of colds.
- Describe the treatment of influenza.
- Define chronic fatigue syndrome.
- Restate at least six signs or symptoms of chronic fatigue syndrome.
- Discuss the etiology of AIDS.
- Recall the prevention of AIDS.
- Identify the etiology and three stages of Lyme disease.
- Discuss the foodborne infection *Escherichia coli* 0157:H7.
- List the most common communicable diseases of childhood and adolescence.
- Recall the signs and symptoms of measles.
- Distinguish measles and rubella.
- Define the classic symptoms of mumps.
- Describe the treatment of varicella.
- Explain measures to prevent diphtheria.
- Discuss the two stages of pertussis.
- Describe the signs and symptoms of tetanus.

KEY WORDS

Acute (ă•kūt′)
Analgesic (ăn•ăl•jē′sĭk)
Anorexia (ăn•ō•rĕk′sē•ă)
Antibody (ăn′tĭ•bŏd•ē)
Antipruritic (ăn•tĭ•proo•rĭt′ĭk)
Antipyretic (ăn•tĭ•pī•rĕt′ĭk)
Arthralgia (ăr•thrăl′jē•ă)
Endemic (ĕn•dĕm′ĭk)
Epididymo-orchitis
   (ĕp•ĕ•dĭd•ĭm•ō•ŏr•kī′tĭs)
Fibrin (fī′brĭn)
Gamma globulin (găm′ă glŏb′ū•lĭn)
Koplik's spots
Leukopenia (loo•kō•pē′nē•ă)
Macule (măk′ūl)

Maculopapular (măk•ū•lō•păp′ū•lăr)
Malaise (mă•lāz′)
Myalgia (mī•ăl′jē•ă)
Nonvirulent (nōn•vĭr′ū•lĕnt)
Opportunistic infection (ŏp•ŏr•tū•nĭs′tĭk
   ĭn•fĕk′shŭn)
Papule (păp′ūl)
Photophobia (fō•tō•fō′bē•ă)
Retrovirus (rĕt′rō•vī•rŭs)
Rhinitis (rī•nī′tĭs)
Seroconversion (sē•rō•kŏn•vĕr′zhŭn)
Spirochete (spī′rō-kēt)
Transient visual scotomata (tran′zhŭnt
   vĭ′zhū•ăl skō•tō′mă•tă)
Universal precautions
Vesicle (vĕs′ĭ•kl)

Infectious and Communicable Diseases

As we saw in Chapter 1, infection is a major cause of disease. An infectious disease occurs whenever a pathogenic microorganism finds a suitable environment for growth in an appropriate host. A *communicable* (or *contagious*) *disease* is an infectious disease that is readily transmitted from one individual to another, either directly or indirectly. Table 2–1 lists several communicable diseases and their methods of transmission.

Modern sanitation methods, immunizations, and potent antibiotics have not eradicated infectious diseases. Persons can refuse immunizations, and some infections are resistant to antibiotics; hence, infections flourish. No matter what precautions we take, microbes continue to be virulent, appear in unsuspected places, and cause infection to be a serious illness.

Table 2–1 Methods of Transmission of Some Common Communicable Diseases

Disease	How Agent Leaves the Bodies of the Sick	How Organisms May Be Transmitted	Method of Entry into the Body
Acquired immunodeficiency syndrome (AIDS)	Blood, semen, or other body fluids, including breast milk	Sexual contact Contact with blood or mucous membranes or by way of contaminated syringes Placental transmission	Reproductive tract Contact with blood Placental transmission Breastfeeding
Cholera	Feces	Water or food contaminated with feces	Mouth to intestine
Diphtheria	Sputum and discharges from nose and throat Skin lesions (rare)	Droplet infection from patient coughing	Through mouth or nose to throat
Gonococcal disease	Lesions Discharges from infected mucous membranes	Sexual activity Hands of infected persons soiled with their own discharges	Reproductive tract or any mucous membrane
Hepatitis A, viral	Feces	Food or water contaminated with feces	Mouth to intestine
Hepatitis B, viral and delta hepatitis	Blood and serum-derived fluids, including semen and vaginal fluids	Contact with blood and body fluids	Exposure to body fluids including during sexual activity Contact with blood
Hepatitis C	Blood and other body fluids	Parenteral drug use Laboratory exposures to blood Health care workers exposed to blood (i.e., dentists and their assistants, and clinical and laboratory staff)	Infected blood Contaminated needles
Hookworm	Feces	Cutaneous contact with soil polluted with feces Eggs in feces hatch in sandy soil	Larvae enter through skin (esp. of feet), migrate through the body, and settle in small intestine
Influenza	As in pneumonia	Respiratory droplets or objects contaminated with discharges	As in pneumonia
Leprosy	Cutaneous or mucosal lesions that contain bacilli Respiratory droplets	Cutaneous contact or nasal discharges of untreated patients	Nose or broken skin
Measles (rubeola)	As in streptococcal pharyngitis	As in streptococcal pharyngitis	As in streptococcal pharyngitis
Meningitis, meningococcal	Discharges from nose and throat	Respiratory droplets	
Mumps	Discharges from infected glands and mouth	Respiratory droplets and saliva	Mouth and nose
Ophthalmia neo-natorum (gono-coccal infection of eyes of newborn)	Vaginal secretions of infected mother	Contact with infected areas of vagina of infected mother during birth	Mouth and nose
Pertussis	Discharges from respiratory tract	Respiratory droplets	Mouth and nose

Table continued on following page

Table 2–1 Methods of Transmission of Some Common Communicable Diseases (*Continued*)

Disease	How Agent Leaves the Bodies of the Sick	How Organisms May Be Transmitted	Method of Entry into the Body
Pneumonia	Sputum and discharges from nose and throat	Respiratory droplets	Through mouth and nose to lungs
Poliomyelitis	Discharges from nose and throat, and via feces	Respiratory droplets Contaminated water	Through mouth and nose
Rubella	As in streptococcal pharyngitis	As in streptococcal pharyngitis	As in streptococcal pharyngitis
Streptococcal pharyngitis	Discharges from nose and throat	Respiratory droplets	Through mouth and nose
Syphilis	Lesions Blood Transfer through placenta to fetus	Kissing or sexual intercourse Contaminated needles and syringes	Directly into blood and tissues through breaks in skin or membrane Contaminated needles and syringes
Trachoma	Discharges from infected eyes	Cutaneous contact Hands, towels, handkerchiefs	Directly on conjunctiva
Tuberculosis, bovine		Milk from infected cow	Mouth to intestine
Tuberculosis, human	Sputum Lesions Feces	Droplet infection from person coughing with mouth uncovered Sputum from mouth to fingers, thence to food and other things	Through nose to lungs or intestines From intestines via lymph channels to lymph vessels and to tissues
Typhoid fever	Feces and urine	Food or water contaminated with feces, or urine from patients	Through mouth via infected food or water and thence to intestinal tract

Source: Thomas, CL (ed): Taber's Cyclopedic Medical Dictionary, ed 18. FA Davis, Philadelphia, 1997, pp 422–423, with permission.

Communicable diseases demand an extra measure of caution. It is helpful to know what the infectious period is for the disease, so that anyone who has been exposed can be alerted. Isolation may be necessary to prevent further exposure. Table 2–2 shows the incubation period, the onset and duration, and the suggested isolation period for several contagious infections.

Medical personnel and hospital staff members are required to notify county and state health departments of confirmed cases of certain communicable diseases. Such reporting helps monitor epidemics and alerts the medical community to special problems.

Immunizations are important for protection against certain communicable diseases. Medical personnel keep accurate records of immunizations, but in the mobile society of the present-day United States, parents should keep a separate and complete record of their children's and their own immunizations. Additional health immunizations are required for travel to some other countries. County health departments have specific information on recommended or required immunizations for world travel.

■ COMMON COLD

DESCRIPTION The *common cold* is an **acute** infection causing inflammation of the upper respiratory tract. Colds occur more frequently in children and account for more time lost from work or school than any other cause. The highest incidence of colds is during the winter months.

Table 2–2 Incubation and Isolation Periods for Common Infections*

Infection	Incubation Period	Isolation of Patient†
AIDS	Unclear; antibodies appear within 1–3 mo of infection; T-cell counts probably drop in 1–3 yr. Symptoms appear in 5–12 yr. Median incubation in infants is shorter than in adults.	Protective isolation if T-cell count is very low; enteric precautions with severe diarrhea; private room only necessary with severe diarrhea, bleeding, copious blood tinged sputum if patient has poor personal hygiene habits
Bloodstream (bacteremia fungemia)	Variable; usually 2–5 days	Contact: private room; gloves and masks; gowns, as needed for dealing with drainage or body fluids
Brucellosis	Highly variable; usually 5–21 days; may be months	None
Chickenpox	2–3 wk	1 wk after vesicles appear or until vesicles become dry
Cholera	A few hours to 5 days	Enteric precautions
Common cold	12 hr–5 days	None
Diphtheria	Usually 2–5 days	Until two cultures from nose and throat, taken at least 24 hr apart, are negative; cultures to be taken after cessation of antibiotic therapy
Dysentery, amebic	From a few days to several months, commonly 2–4 wk	None
Dysentery, bacillary (shigellosis)	12–96 hr	As long as stools remain positive
Encephalitis, mosquito-borne	5–15 days	None
Giardiasis	3–25 days or longer; median 7–10 days	Enteric precautions
Gonorrhea	2–7 days; may be longer	No sexual contact until cured
Hepatitis A	15–50 days	Enteric (gloves with infected material; gowns as needed to protect clothing)
Hepatitis B	45–180 days	Blood and body fluid precautions (gloves and plastic gowns for contact with infective materials; mask if risk of coughing or sneezing exists)
Hepatitis C	14–180 days	As for hepatitis B
Hepatitis D	2–8 wk	As for hepatitis B
Hepatitis E	15–64 days	Enteric precautions
Influenza	1–3 days	As practical
Legionella	2–10 days	None
Lyme disease	3–32 days after tick bite	None
Malaria	12 days for *Plasmodium falciparum;* 8–14 days for *P. vivax, P. ovale;* 7–30 days for *P. malariae*	Protection from mosquitoes
Measles (rubeola)	8–13 days from exposure to onset of fever; 14 days until rash appears	From diagnosis to 7 days after appearance of rash; strict isolation from children under 3 yr
Meningitis, meningococcal	2–10 days	Until 24 hr after start of chemotherapy
Mononucleosis, infectious	4–6 wk	None; disinfection of articles soiled with nose and throat discharges
Mumps	12–25 days	Until the glands recede

Table continued on following page

Table 2–2 **Incubation and Isolation Periods in Common Infections*** (*Continued*)

Infection	Incubation Period	Isolation of Patient†
Paratyphoid fevers	3 days–3 mo; usually 1–3 wk; 1–10 days for gastroenteritis	Until 3 stools are negative
Plague	2–8 days	Strict; danger of airborne spread (pneumoniae plague)
Pneumonia, pneumococcal	Believed to be 1–3 days	Enteric precautions in hospital. Respiratory isolation may be required
Poliomyelitis	3–35 days	1 week from onset
Puerperal fever, streptococcal	1–3 days	Transfer from maternity ward
Rabies	Usually 2–8 wk; rarely as short as 9 days or as long as 7 yr	Strict for duration of illness; danger to attendants
Rubella (German measles)	16–18 days with range of 14–23 days	None; no contact with nonimmune pregnant women
Salmonellosis	6–72 hr, usually 12–36 hr	Until stool cultures are salmonella free on two consecutive specimens collected in 24-hr period
Scabies	2–6 wk before onset of itching in patients without previous infections; 1–4 days after re-exposed	Patient is excused from school or work until day after treatment
Scarlet fever	1–3 days	7 days; may be ended in 24 hr
Syphilis	10 days–10 wk; usually 3 wk	None; but for hospitalized patients, universal precautions for body secretions
Tetanus	4 days–3 wk	None
Toxic shock syndrome	Unknown but may be as brief as several hours	None
Trachoma	5–12 days	Until lesions disappear, but usually not practical
Tuberculosis	4–12 wk to demonstrable primary lesion or significant tuberculin reactions	Variable, depending on conversion of sputum to negative after specific therapy and on ability of patient to understand and carry out personal hygiene methods
Tularemia	2–14 days	None
Typhoid fever	Usually 1–3 wk	Until 3 cultures of feces and urine are negative. These should be taken not earlier than 1 month after onset.
Typhus fever	7–14 days	None
Whooping cough	Usually 6–20 days	Respiratory isolation for known cases; for suspected cases, removal from contact with infants and young children

*Universal precautions and handwashing are assumed.

Source: Thomas, CL (ed): Taber's Cyclopedic Medical Dictionary, ed 18. FA Davis, Philadelphia, 1997, pp 980–983, with permission.

ETIOLOGY Colds are usually caused by viruses. Some colds, however, result from infection by a group of microorganisms called *Mycoplasma*. These microorganisms are transmitted by airborne respiratory droplets.

SIGNS AND SYMPTOMS Common symptoms include nasal congestion, pharyngitis, headache, **malaise,** burning and watery eyes, and low-grade fever. A productive or nonproductive cough may be present. The symptoms commonly last from 2 to 4 days, but nasal congestion may persist for an indefinite period. Reinfection is common, but complications are rare. The cold is contagious for 2 to 3 days after onset.

DIAGNOSTIC PROCEDURES There is no specific diagnostic test for the common cold. A throat culture may be done to rule out other diseases.

TREATMENT Treatment of the cold is symptomatic and includes mild analgesics, ample fluid intake, and rest. Decongestants, nasal sprays, throat lozenges, and steam may be helpful. If secondary bacterial infections are suspected, antibiotics may be prescribed, but they are not a cure for the common cold.

PROGNOSIS The disease is self-limiting, but it can lead to secondary bacterial infection.

PREVENTION There is no known prevention. Handwashing and avoiding crowds may lessen the likelihood of contracting a cold.

◼ INFLUENZA

DESCRIPTION *Influenza (flu)* is an acute, contagious respiratory disease characterized by fever, chills, headache, and **myalgia.** The disease may affect anyone, but school-age children and elderly persons are especially susceptible. Flu often occurs in epidemic outbreaks, particularly in the winter and spring.

ETIOLOGY Flu is caused by viruses that are members of the *Orthomyxoviridae* family. For diagnostic and treatment purposes, the viruses are classified as either type A, B, or C based on their antigenic properties. Influenza viruses frequently mutate, creating new strains that easily infect populations that had acquired immunity to previous strains of the virus. Transmission generally occurs via cough, sneeze, hand-to-hand contact, and other personal contact.

SIGNS AND SYMPTOMS The onset generally is abrupt, with fever, chills, croup in children, malaise, muscular aching, headache, nasal congestion, laryngitis, and a cough.

DIAGNOSTIC PROCEDURES Because the signs and symptoms of flu resemble so many other illnesses, it is frequently difficult to diagnose solely on the basis of symptomatology, unless there is an on-

going epidemic. A throat culture may be performed to isolate the virus, or various immunofluorescence techniques may be performed to detect viral antigens.

TREATMENT Treatment consists of bed rest, adequate fluid intake, and administering analgesics and antipyretics. *Note:* Aspirin should *not* be used to treat fever and muscle pain in children and adolescents with flu, because of its association with an increased incidence of Reye's syndrome (see Reye's Syndrome, Chapter 9). The use of antibiotics is not indicated, and therefore they are to be avoided. Any overuse of antibiotics makes them less effective when they really are necessary.

PROGNOSIS The prognosis is good with proper care. Complications include sinusitis, otitis media, bronchitis, and pneumonia.

PREVENTION Influenza vaccines prepared from the most recent strains of A and B type viruses are useful in preventing flu. The vaccines may produce reactions in some, especially people who are allergic to egg products. The U.S. Public Health Service recommends inoculation against influenza for those with chronic cardiac and respiratory conditions, for those with serious systemic diseases, and for elderly persons.

ALTERNATIVE MEDICINE

Stress can increase susceptibility to colds and flu. The more stress there is, the greater the chance of viral infection. It is logical, then, to seek ways to reduce stress. It is also helpful to get extra sleep and drink large amounts of herbal tea, water, vegetable juices, and broths. Saline nasal sprays will keep nasal passages moist. Baths with eucalyptus, lavender, lemon, or peppermint can be soothing to someone with a cold or the flu.

◼ CHRONIC FATIGUE SYNDROME

DESCRIPTION *Chronic fatigue syndrome* (CFS), while not fully understood, is aptly named. Individuals suffer from debilitating chronic fatigue, and the illness presents a host of syndromes. Another name for the illness is myalgic encephalomyelitis. The symptoms are many and varied, and individuals may suffer for weeks or even years from CFS. It is twice as prevalent in women as it is in men, and generally it affects persons 25 to 45 years of age.

ETIOLOGY There is no current agreement on the cause of CSF. It is most likely multifactorial. It was once thought to be attributed to the Epstein-Barr virus, but that hypothesis has been set aside. Viruses suspected include human herpesvirus 6, enteroviruses, or **retroviruses.** Other predisposing factors that may be partly responsible include the state of a person's immune system, the individual's genetic makeup, age, hormonal balance, sex, environment, and previous illness.

SIGNS AND SYMPTOMS Symptoms arise suddenly and include a prolonged, unbearable exhaustion in association with the following symptoms:

- Fever or chills
- Sore throat; nonexudative pharyngitis
- Painful cervical or axillary lymph nodes
- Unexplained generalized muscle weakness
- Muscle discomfort and myalgia
- Migratory **arthralgia** without joint swelling or redness
- **Photophobia,** forgetfulness, **transient visual scotomata,** irritability, confusion, depression, inability to concentrate
- Sleep disturbance

DIAGNOSTIC PROCEDURES A complete history and physical examination are essential for diagnosis. Laboratory testing is used to rule out other possible causes. The challenge in diagnosing is that CFS remains a syndrome of symptoms and a diagnosis of exclusion.

TREATMENT Treatment is supportive. The person with CFS needs to know about the illness; therefore, information sharing is paramount. The physician will want to reassess the disease process frequently so that new symptoms can be treated. Nonsteroidal anti-inflammatory drugs may be beneficial in the treatment of headache, pain, and fever. Medications to improve energy and emotional state may be used. At times, a psychiatric evaluation may be necessary if the person becomes depressed. Lifestyle changes may be needed in the areas of sleeping and exercise. Lastly, unproven treatments should be avoided.

PROGNOSIS The disease is debilitating and may last for months. Some individuals respond to a variety of treatment protocols. With research under way, the future for persons with CSF is brighter.

PREVENTION None known.

ACQUIRED IMMUNODEFICIENCY SYNDROME (AIDS)

DESCRIPTION *Acquired immunodeficiency syndrome (AIDS)* is a severe illness associated with a human immunodeficiency virus (HIV) infection. Sexual contact is the major mode of transmission of HIV, but it can also be transmitted by blood and blood products. In addition, transplacental, parturition, or postpartum transmission can occur, and the virus can be transmitted via breast milk from an infected mother. In the United States, the majority of individuals suffering from AIDS are male homosexuals and bisexuals; the next largest group consists of intravenous drug users. Other individuals at risk are children born to mothers infected with HIV, sexual partners of those infected with HIV, and persons who have received blood products and transfusions infected with HIV (before screening of blood and blood products was possible). Recent studies, however, indicate that teens and young adults (regardless of sexual orientation) are the fastest growing group of persons testing positive for HIV.

ETIOLOGY AIDS, which was first diagnosed in the United States in 1981, is caused by the human immunodeficiency virus (HIV). HIV is a member of the class of retroviruses. These very simple viruses carry their genetic material in the form of ribonucleic acid (RNA) rather than DNA. HIV predominantly infects cells called helper T-4 cell lymphocytes, which are critical to the operation of the body's immune system. An HIV virus replicates itself by taking over the genetic machinery of the T cell it invades. The replication process continues until the host cell is destroyed. The newly produced HIV viruses can then infect other T-4 lymphocytes. This progressive and inevitable destruction of T-4 cells leaves the body open to opportunistic infections.

SIGNS AND SYMPTOMS AIDS usually produces a spectrum of clinical manifestations. The mean time from exposure to the clinical manifestations of the disease is 10 years.[1]

After high-risk exposure to HIV, the majority of individuals experience no recognizable symptoms. Some persons, however, may develop a mononucleosislike syndrome characterized by fever and flulike symptoms. The syndrome resolves spontaneously, with **seroconversion** usually occurring 8 to 10 weeks later. When symptoms of HIV occur later, the most common are generalized persistent lymphadenopathy, weight loss, fever, fatigue, neurological symptoms, **opportunistic infections,** and malignancy.

The pulmonary, gastrointestinal, and neurological systems may be involved, and several forms of malignancy and chronic illnesses may result:

- *Pulmonary symptoms* include shortness of breath, dyspnea, coughing, chest pain, and fever; these are caused by a variety of opportunistic infections. The most common pulmonary infection is *Pneumocystis carinii* pneumonia, which has a mortality rate of 60 percent. There is an increased incidence of tuberculosis.
- *Gastrointestinal symptoms* of AIDS may include loss of appetite, nausea, vomiting, oral candidiasis, and chronic diarrhea. Diarrhea occurs in over half of all AIDS clients.
- *Neurological symptoms* may include memory loss, headache, depression, fever, confusion, and visual disturbances. Dementia and depression may also be seen.
- *Malignancies* commonly associated with AIDS include Kaposi's sarcoma, a neoplasm evidenced by multiple vascular nodules in the skin and other organs. This malignant neoplasm is especially prevalent in the lymph nodes, the gastrointestinal tract, and the lungs. The purple lesions characterizing Kaposi's sarcoma may appear on the skin and grow rapidly until wounds are produced that increase the client's susceptibility to infections.
- *Chronic illness* results because AIDS sufferers are often severely immunocompromised. Nearly all eventually develop one or more chronic opportunistic infections during the course of the disease. Such illnesses may complicate treatment and produce debilitating symptoms.

DIAGNOSTIC PROCEDURES It is necessary to obtain a complete client history (including risk factors) and to perform a physical examination. Laboratory studies are essential to determine the extent of immune system impairment, the presence of any opportunistic infections, and the presence of HIV antibodies.

The most widely used screening test is the enzyme-linked immunosorbent assay (ELISA), followed by the Western blot test for confirmation. Additional tests to help evaluate the severity of immunosuppression may be performed.

According to the Centers for Disease Control (CDC), the disease progression of HIV can be measured even before symptoms occur. When HIV establishes itself in the body, the number of CD4 lymphocytes begins to decline. If the number falls below 300, individuals are at heightened risk for one or more opportunistic infections. If the CD4 cell number drops below 200, an individual is said to have AIDS.

TREATMENT Currently there is no effective treatment to stop the HIV infection and the immunodeficiency it causes. Research has developed zidovudine (AZT), didanosine (DDI), and other antiretroviral drugs, which impair HIV's ability to insert itself into a host cell. Protease inhibitors, another class of antiretroviral agents, has greatly increased life expectancy for persons with AIDS. It is important to manage the opportunistic infections and malignancies as aggressively as possible, using antimicrobial agents for infections and radiation therapy or chemotherapy for the malignancies. Chronic illnesses may require symptomatic treatment for malnutrition, weakness, immobility, diarrhea, skin lesions, and altered mental state.

PROGNOSIS Recurrent bouts of opportunistic infections, with or without malignancies, usually cause the death of individuals with AIDS.

PREVENTION Education is the first defense against this epidemic. To avoid exposure to HIV, a person should practice safe sex. The use of latex condoms for any form of sexual intercourse is essential. Body fluids and items such as used hypodermic needles should be considered potentially infective. Healthcare workers must practice **universal precautions** when handling blood and body fluids. Eliminating risk factors for HIV-infected people can be as beneficial as treating the HIV infection. Eliminating drug abuse and malnutrition is extremely important, and purifying blood-clotting factors for hemophiliacs has been very beneficial.

◼ LYME DISEASE

DESCRIPTION Lyme disease is caused by a tick-transmitted **spirochete.** The disease occurs in stages. Each stage has different clinical manifestations, and between stages there may be remissions and exacerbations. Lyme disease was named for Lyme, Connecticut, a town in which it was first recognized in 1975. The incidence has increased, but although the disease has spread west, most cases have occurred in the northeastern United States.

ETIOLOGY Lyme disease is caused by a bacterium known as *Borrelia burgdorferi,* which is carried by pinhead-sized ticks found on the white-tailed deer, the white-footed mouse, and even raccoons, rabbits, dogs, horses, cattle, migrating birds, mosquitoes, and flies. The tick injects its saliva into the host's bloodstream, or it deposits fecal material on the skin (Fig. 2–1).

SIGNS AND SYMPTOMS Stage I signs include a rash called *erythema chronicum migrans* (*ECM*), which appears at the site of the bite. ECM is very distinct, with a dark-red rim and faded center. Often, however, ECM does not occur. Other signs of stage I include flulike symptoms such as fatigue, headache, fever, chills, stiff neck, and joint and muscle pain, which can last from several weeks to several months. Stage II symptoms affect the central nervous system, causing such diverse problems as meningitis, nerve damage, and facial palsy. Stage III symptoms include chronic arthritis and continuing neurological problems. Stage I usually lasts for several weeks; stage II occurs during the following several months; and stage III occurs months to years after the onset of the initial infection. Except for fatigue and lethargy, which are often constant, the early signs of the disease are typically intermittent and changing.

DIAGNOSTIC PROCEDURES Blood tests will be used to assist in diagnosis; however, it can take more than 6 weeks for the **antibodies** to appear in the blood, making diagnosis by this method alone inconclusive. The most common laboratory abnormalities are a high erythrocyte sedimentation rate (ESR), an elevated total serum immunoglobulin M (IgM) level, or an increased aspartate aminotransferase level.

TREATMENT The treatment of choice in all three stages is the use of antibiotics and/or parenteral penicillin.

PROGNOSIS Although minor recurrences of headaches, musculoskeletal pain, or lethargy are consistent with the disease, eventually, complete recovery occurs with proper treatment.

PREVENTION The best prevention is to cover as much of the body as possible when in the woods. Look for tiny pinpoint specks on your body and clothing. Use an insect repellent on clothes and exposed areas of arms and hands as directed. Make certain pets who go outside have protection against fleas and ticks and inspect them after outings.

◼ *ESCHERICHIA COLI* 0157:H7

DESCRIPTION *E. coli* 0157:H7 is only one of hundreds of strains of the bacterium *E. coli.* Most strains are harmless and live in the intestinal tract of healthy humans and animals, but the 0157:H7 strain produces a powerful toxin and can cause serious illness. *E. coli* 0157:H7 is an emerging cause of foodborne illness, with an estimated 10,000 to 20,000 cases of infection in the United States each

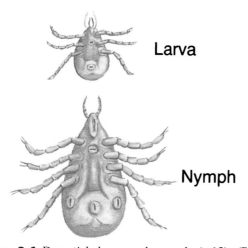

Larva

Nymph

Figure 2–1 Deer tick larva and nymph (×12). (From Scanlon, VC, and Sanders, T: Essentials of Anatomy and Physiology, ed 3. FA Davis, Philadelphia, 1999, p 501, with permission.)

year. The infection, associated with eating under-cooked, contaminated ground beef or drinking un-pasteurized milk and fruit juices, often leads to bloody diarrhea.

ETIOLOGY The organism, which can be found on some cattle ranches, lives in the intestines of healthy cattle. Meat may become contaminated during slaughter. Organisms can be thoroughly mixed into beef when it is ground. Bacteria present on the cow's udders or on equipment may get into raw milk. Swimming in sewage-contaminated water can also cause infection. Bacteria in the diarrheal stools of infected persons can be passed from one person to another if handwashing and personal hygiene is inadequate.

SIGNS AND SYMPTOMS The infection causes bloody diarrhea and abdominal cramps; sometimes the infection causes nonbloody diarrhea or no symptoms. Usually no fever is present and the illness will resolve in 5 to 10 days. In elderly persons and children, the infection can cause a complication called *hemolytic uremic syndrome*. This syndrome is the leading cause of acute kidney failure in children in the United States. The syndrome is associated with death and long-term complications in a small percentage of individuals. Complications in-clude endstage renal disease, hypertension, or seizures, blindness, and paralysis.

DIAGNOSTIC PROCEDURES The infection from *E. coli* 0157:H7 is diagnosed by detecting the bacteria in the stool. Some laboratories in the United States do not test for this bacteria, and it is not considered a reportable disease in some states. Therefore, it may be necessary to request that the stool specimen be tested for the organism for all individuals who suddenly have bloody diarrhea.

TREATMENT Persons with only diarrhea usually recover without specific treatment in 5 to 10 days. However, hemolytic uremic syndrome is life-threatening and treated in an intensive care unit. Blood transfusions and kidney dialysis are usually required.

PROGNOSIS The prognosis is good with bloody diarrhea symptoms only; it is guarded if hemolytic uremic syndrome develops.

PREVENTION Consumers can prevent the illness by cooking all ground beef thoroughly, by consuming only pasteurized milk and fruit juices, and by making certain that all persons, especially children, wash their hands carefully with soap and water to reduce the spread of infection.

Communicable Diseases of Childhood and Adolescence

The incidence of certain communicable diseases in the United States has steadily decreased over recent decades. Children and adolescents are no longer the routine victims of many diseases, thanks to advances in medical knowledge, general improvements in living conditions, and government-mandated immunization programs. Poliomyelitis, for example, once **endemic** in the United States, occurs only rarely since the advent of the Salk vaccine.

Caution cannot be thrown to the wind, however. A serious outbreak of rubeola occurred recently on a college campus, where a substantial number of students had not been vaccinated against the disease owing to their religious beliefs. In the inner cities of the United States, limited access to medical care, lack of knowledge, and distrust of government-sponsored health outreach programs have conspired to leave significant numbers of children unprotected by vaccines. In the absence of the effective immunization provided by vaccines, communicable disease can still cause major epidemics.

A *vaccine* is a suspension of infectious agents or some part of them. It is given for the purpose of establishing resistance to an infectious disease. There are four general classes of vaccines:

- Those containing living infectious organisms. The organisms are either disabled or otherwise **nonvirulent** strains.
- Infectious agents killed by physical or chemical means.
- Those containing solutions of toxins from microorganisms. The toxins may be used directly,

but usually they are treated to neutralize their toxic potential.

- Those containing substances extracted from a portion of an infectious agent. Effective antiviral vaccines often are made by extracting only a small portion of the virus's protein coat.

Whatever its makeup, a vaccine stimulates the development of specific defensive mechanisms that result in more or less permanent protection from the disease. Table 2–3 lists the vaccines commonly administered during childhood and adolescence.

■ MEASLES (Rubeola)

DESCRIPTION *Measles* is a highly communicable disease whose diagnostic signs are fever and the appearance of a characteristic rash. The disease is most common in school-age children, with outbreaks occurring in the winter and spring. Recently, though, the disease has occurred with increasing frequency among high school and college students who were not vaccinated as children or who were vaccinated between 1957 and 1980 with an ineffective vaccine.

ETIOLOGY Measles is caused by the rubeola virus. The virus has an incubation period of 10 to 20 days.

SIGNS AND SYMPTOMS The onset of symptoms is usually gradual. Initial symptoms may include **rhinitis,** drowsiness, **anorexia,** and a slow but progressive rise in temperature to 101°F or 103°F by the second day. **Koplik's spots** appear on the oral mucosa by the second or third day. Photophobia and cough soon follow. By about the fourth day, the fever usually reaches its maximum (as high as 104°F to 106°F) and the characteristic rash appears. The rash first appears on the face as tiny **maculopapular** lesions. These rapidly enlarge and spread to other areas of the body. The lesions may be so densely clustered in certain areas that the skin surface appears generally swollen and red.

DIAGNOSTIC PROCEDURES The clinical picture of symptoms is usually a sufficient basis for a diagnosis of measles. Blood testing may reveal **leukopenia,** and various tests are available to detect the presence of measles antibody.

TREATMENT Treatment for measles is essentially symptomatic. Bed rest is indicated, usually in a darkened room to alleviate the discomfort of photophobia. **Antipyretics** and liquids may be recommended. The affected individual should be kept isolated until the rash disappears.

PROGNOSIS Measles is usually a benign disease, running its course in about 5 days after the rash appears. An attack of measles usually confers permanent immunity. Complications may arise, however; these include croup, conjunctivitis, myocarditis, hepatitis, and opportunistic respiratory tract infections from staphylococci, streptococci, or *H. influenzae.* Measles infection during pregnancy may result in the death of the fetus, but it does not seem to produce birth defects, as does rubella (see Rubella).

PREVENTION Measles can be prevented within 5 days of exposure by administration of **gamma globulin.** Active immunization can be produced by administration of measles vaccine, preferably containing the live attenuated virus.

■ RUBELLA (German Measles)

DESCRIPTION *Rubella* is an acute infectious disease characterized by fever and rash. It closely resembles measles, but it differs in its short course, mild fever, and relative freedom from complications. Rubella is not as contagious as measles, and it now occurs most frequently among teenagers and young adults.

ETIOLOGY The disease is caused by the rubella virus. This virus has an incubation period of 14 to 21 days.

SIGNS AND SYMPTOMS The onset of the disease is sometimes characterized by malaise, headache, slight fever, and sore throat. These symptoms may be entirely absent, however, especially among children. The rash typically appears the first or second day after onset. It may be composed of pale red, slightly elevated, discrete **papules,** or the rash may be highly diffuse and bright red. The rash begins on the face, spreads rapidly to other portions of the body, and usually fades so rapidly that the face may clear before the extremities are affected. Rash-covered portions of skin may itch or peel.

DIAGNOSTIC PROCEDURES Because rubella can be easily confused with other diseases, a definitive diag-

Table 2–3 Vaccines

Name	Age Administered	Booster Schedule	Comments
BCG (bacillus of Calmette and Guérin)	In epidemic conditions, administered to infants as soon as possible after birth.	None	The only contraindications are symptomatic human immunodeficiency virus (HIV) infection or other illnesses known to suppress immunity.
Cholera	See Comments	Every 3–6 mo for those who remain in epidemic areas	Only those traveling to countries where cholera is present need to be vaccinated. Whole cell vaccines provide partial protection for 3–6 mo.
DPT (diphtheria, pertussis, tetanus)	At 2 mo, 4 mo, 6 mo, and 15–18 mo. A fifth dose may be given at 4–6 yr.	Tetanus and diphtheria immunization every 10 yr, esp. for people over 50. Persons who have received 5 doses of tetanus toxoid in childhood may not need a booster until age 50.	Tetanus booster may be required following a wound even though all routine and booster immunizations have been received. Booster of diphtheria toxoid should be given if a child under 6 is exposed to diphtheria. Vaccine is contraindicated in cases of acute infection, previous central nervous system damage, or convulsions.
Haemophilus influenzae b (polysaccharide or conjugate)	At 2 mo, 4 mo, discretionally at 6 mo, and at 12–15 mo.	None	SEE: *Haemophilus influenzae type b infection.*
Hepatitis B	At birth, 2 mo, and 6–18 mo, or at 1–2 mo, 4 mo, and 6–18 mo. All ages if risk is present.	None	Recommended as a routine childhood vaccine. All health care workers should receive it. Immune globulin or hepatitis B globulin may be given to produce passive immunity in exposed contacts. They are contraindicated for those allergic to yeast products.
Influenza (flu)	All ages	Annually, given prior to time influenza is expected.	Recommended for elderly persons, health-care professionals, residents of long-term care facilities, and those of any age who have chronic disease of the heart or lungs, metabolic diseases such as diabetes, or immuno-suppression.
MMR (measles [live attenuated rubeola], mumps, rubella)	12–15 mo	4–6 yr or 11–12 yr	Vaccine will usually prevent measles if given within 2 days after a child has been exposed to the disease. Not given to adults. Contraindicated for those with allergy to egg or neomycin, active infection, or severe immunosuppression.

Table continued on following page

Table 2–3 **Vaccines** (*Continued*)

Name	Age Administered	Booster Schedule	Comments
Plague	See Comments	See Comments	Recommended for those traveling to Southeast Asia, persons who work closely with wild rodents in plague areas, and laboratory personnel working with *Yersinia pestis* organisms.
Pneumococcal vaccine, polyvalent	Should not be given to children under age 2 or to pregnant women.	None	Vaccine is effective against the 23 most prevalent types of pneumococci. Administered to those who have an increased risk of developing pneumococcal pneumonia. Included are those who have chronic diseases, have had a splenectomy, are in chronic care facilities, or are 65 years of age or older.
Polio (live oral trivalent vaccine)	At 2 mo, 4 mo, and 6–18 mo	At 4–6 mo or 11–12 yr	Administration is postponed in those with persistent vomiting, diarrhea, acute illness, or immunosuppression and in those who live in the same household as an immunosuppressed person. An alternative polio vaccine is available for immunosuppressed children.
Rabies	See Comments	See Comments	Each exposure to rabies needs to be evaluated on an individual basis by the physician. Postexposure prophylaxis includes the human diploid cell vaccine and rabies immune globulin.
Typhoid	See Comments	See Comments	Immunization is indicated when a person has come into contact with a known typhoid carrier, if there is an outbreak of typhoid fever, or prior to traveling to an area where typhoid is endemic.
Varicella zoster (chickenpox)	12–18 mo	None	Immunizes against chickenpox in adulthood as well as childhood. The illness is much more serious in adults than in children.
Yellow fever	See Comments	Every 10 yr	Vaccine should be given to all persons traveling or living in areas where yellow fever is present.

Source: Thomas, CD (ed): Taber's Cyclopedic Medical Dictionary, ed 18. FA Davis, Philadelphia, 1997, pp 2051–2053, with permission.

nosis can only be reached by isolating the virus or detecting its antibody.

TREATMENT Treatment is nonspecific and symptomatic. Bed rest is indicated. Topical **antipruritics** or warm water baths may be recommended to relieve itching. Antipyretics may be prescribed.

PROGNOSIS The prognosis for an individual with rubella is usually good. The disease is benign, seldom produces complications, and runs its course in 3 days. Rubella is dangerous, however, when it occurs in pregnant women, especially during the first trimester of pregnancy. The virus is capable of producing severe fetal malformation.

PREVENTION Lasting immunization can be conferred through use of a live rubella vaccine. This vaccine must not be administered to pregnant women or to those who may become pregnant within 3 months after immunization. Administration of gamma globulin shortly after exposure may prevent development of the disease, but it still may not prevent transfer of the virus to the fetus if exposure occurs during pregnancy.

◼ MUMPS

DESCRIPTION *Mumps* is an acute contagious disease characterized by fever and inflammation of the parotid salivary glands. The disease is most common among children and young adults.

ETIOLOGY The disease is caused by the mumps virus, which has an incubation period of 18 days. The disease is transmitted by little droplets of saliva.

SIGNS AND SYMPTOMS The classic symptoms of mumps are unilateral or bilateral swollen parotid glands. Headache, malaise, fever, and earache may occur, and other salivary glands may become swollen.

DIAGNOSTIC PROCEDURES The clinical picture of mumps and a history of recent exposure usually is sufficient for diagnosis.

TREATMENT Analgesics, antipyretics, and adequate fluid intake may be recommended. Isolation of the affected individual is important during the contagious period.

PROGNOSIS The prognosis for an individual with mumps is good. Complications can occur, how-

ever, and include **epididymo-orchitis,** pancreatitis, and various central nervous system (CNS) manifestations. Epididymo-orchitis, which causes swelling of the testes in adult males, is extremely uncomfortable but rarely causes sterility, as is often feared.

PREVENTION The best prevention is to receive the mumps vaccine and avoid exposure to the disease during its period of communicability.

◼ VARICELLA (Chickenpox)

DESCRIPTION *Varicella* (*chickenpox*) is a highly contagious disease characterized by the appearance of a distinctive rash that passes through stages of **macules,** papules, **vesicles,** and crusts. The disease occurs most commonly among children and may occur in epidemic outbreaks in winter and spring.

ETIOLOGY The disease is caused by the varicella-zoster virus (VZV). Its incubation period is 2 to 3 weeks, usually between 13 and 17 days via the respiratory route.

SIGNS AND SYMPTOMS The signs of chickenpox are a pruritic rash, which begins as erythematous macules that produce papules and then clear vesicles. The rash usually contains a combination of papules, vesicles, and scabs in all stages. Anorexia, malaise, and fever may accompany the rash (Fig. 2–2).

DIAGNOSTIC PROCEDURES The clinical signs are usually sufficient for the diagnosis. A history that indicates recent exposure helps confirm the diagnosis.

TREATMENT Isolation is important during the infectious period—usually until all the scabs disappear. The only treatment necessary is to reduce the itching. Calamine lotion or cool bicarbonate of soda baths can be very helpful. It is best not to scratch the lesions. *Note:* Aspirin should *not* be used to treat fever in cases of chickenpox among children and adolescents because of its association with an increased incidence of Reye's syndrome (see Reye's Syndrome, Chapter 9).

PROGNOSIS The prognosis for an individual with varicella is good. The disease runs its course in about 2 to 3 weeks. Complications may include secondary bacterial infections of the skin as a result of scratching open lesions.

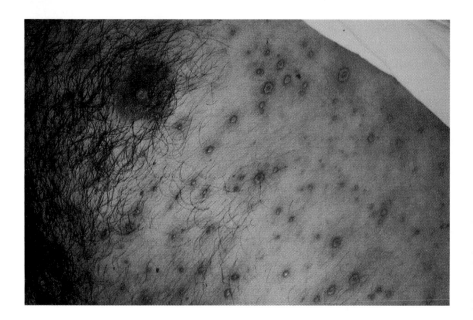

Figure 2–2 Chickenpox (varicella). (From Goldsmith, LA, Lazarus, GS, and Tharp, MD: Adult and Pediatric Dermatology: A Color Guide to Diagnosis and Treatment. FA Davis, Philadelphia, 1997, p 312, with permission.)

PREVENTION In certain situations, varicella-zoster immune globulin (VZIG) may be administered within 72 hours of exposure to stop the development of the disease.

DIPHTHERIA

DESCRIPTION *Diphtheria* is an acute, life-threatening infectious disease. It is characterized by a membranelike coating that forms over mucous membrane surfaces, particularly along the respiratory tract, and by a toxic reaction primarily affecting the heart and peripheral nerves. The disease may occasionally involve the skin. Most cases occur in children younger than age 10, but older children and adults also may be affected. Diphtheria used to be a frequent affliction of children in the United States, but because of diligent immunization efforts, the disease now appears only sporadically.

ETIOLOGY Diphtheria is caused by *Cornebacterium diphtheriae.* The bacterium has an incubation period of 2 to 5 days. *C. diphtheriae* has two principal pathogenic effects. As it multiplies along mucous membrane surfaces, the bacterium forms a distinctive, leathery, blue-white membrane composed of bacteria, necrotized tissue, inflammatory cells, and **fibrin.** This false membrane may enlarge to the extent that it impairs respiratory function. Most strains of *C. diphtheriae* also release a highly potent

toxin capable of damaging the heart, kidneys, and peripheral nerves.

SIGNS AND SYMPTOMS The specific symptoms vary with the site of infection. In typical cases, diphtheria may first present as a slight headache and malaise. A mild fever (100°F to 101°F) may ensue, followed by the appearance of the characteristic membrane adhering to the tonsils or the walls of the pharynx. If the bacterium localizes in the nasal passages, fever may be more pronounced, and a steady, blood-tinged discharge may appear from the nostrils. There may be a strong, foul odor to the breath. Manifestations of myocarditis and neuritis commonly develop as late symptoms. Some individuals infected with *C. diphtheriae* remain asymptomatic but become carriers of the disease.

DIAGNOSTIC PROCEDURES The appearance of the characteristic membrane may be enough to establish a diagnosis of diphtheria. A definitive diagnosis can be made only by identifying the bacterium in smears or cultures.

TREATMENT The only specific treatment is administration of sufficient quantities of diphtheria antitoxin as early in the course of the disease as possible. The affected individual must be isolated, and bed rest is required. A soft or liquid diet is recommended. Emergency measures may be required to maintain an airway or control cardiac complications. Carriers of diphtheria are usually treated with antibiotics.

PROGNOSIS The prognosis for an individual with diphtheria varies according to the severity of the disease. Mild cases of diphtheria resolve in 3 to 4 days, or a week in moderate cases. Even with effective antitoxin therapy, however, death may result from extension of the diphtherial membrane into the lower respiratory tract or from organ system damage produced by the diphtheria toxin.

PREVENTION Diphtheria is highly preventable. Innoculation with diphtheria toxoid at the age of 3 months is normally routine. Booster doses should be administered at appropriate intervals during early childhood (see Table 2–3). Diphtheria toxoid is usually administered along with the vaccine for pertussis and the toxoid for tetanus (the DPT shot), because higher levels of antibodies are produced when all three vaccines are administered simultaneously rather than individually.

PERTUSSIS (Whooping Cough)

DESCRIPTION *Pertussis* is an acute, highly infectious respiratory tract disease characterized by a repetitious, paroxysmal cough and a prolonged, harsh or shrill sound during inspiration (the "whoop"). Prior to effective immunization, pertussis caused more deaths among infants and young children than any other communicable childhood disease. Pertussis still affects infants and children more frequently and more severely than it does adults, although the incidence of the disease among adults has recently increased.

ETIOLOGY Most cases of pertussis are caused by *Bordetella pertussis*. This bacterium has an incubation period of 7 to 10 days. *B. pertussis* multiplies along the surfaces of airways, most often affecting the bronchi and bronchioles, less frequently affecting the trachea, larynx, and nasopharynx. The bacterium induces a mucopurulent secretion and hampers the natural ability of the respiratory tract to clear such secretions. Consequently, mucus accumulates in the airways and obstructs airflow. The bacterium also may produce a mild toxic reaction.

SIGNS AND SYMPTOMS The signs and symptoms of pertussis can be divided into three stages. The *catarrhal stage* is marked by the gradual onset of coldlike symptoms: mild fever, running nose, dry cough, irritability, and anorexia. This stage lasts from 1 to 2 weeks, during which the disease is highly communicable. The *paroxysmal stage* is marked by the onset of the classic cough, consisting of a series of several short, severe coughs in rapid succession followed by a slow, strained inspiration, during which a "whoop" (stridor) may be heard. The coughing occurs in periodic attacks. This stage, lasting 3 to 4 weeks, may be accompanied by weight loss, dehydration, vomiting, epistaxis, and hypoxia. After several weeks, a period of *decline* begins, marked by the gradual diminishment of coughing.

DIAGNOSTIC PROCEDURES A history of exposure to another infected individual and the presence of the classic cough may be enough to establish the diagnosis. A very high white blood cell count is a further distinguishing feature of pertussis. A definitive diagnosis may depend on identifying the bacteria in respiratory secretions.

TREATMENT Antibiotics administered during the catarrhal stage may check the development of the disease; if administration is delayed past this stage, antibiotics have little effect. The individual with pertussis requires meticulous care to ensure adequate nutrition, hydration, and clearance of mucous secretions.

PROGNOSIS The prognosis for an individual with pertussis varies from case to case. Uncomplicated pertussis may run its course in 12 weeks. Recovery may be considerably extended, however, particularly among infants. Death can occur as a result of pneumonia, produced by *B. pertussis* itself or by a secondary infection.

PREVENTION A child can be rendered less susceptible to pertussis by receiving a series of immunizations with pertussis vaccine, starting around the age of 3 months. Receiving the vaccine or having the disease, however, does not guarantee lasting immunity from pertussis.

TETANUS (Lockjaw)

DESCRIPTION *Tetanus* is an acute, life-threatening infectious disease characterized by persistent, painful contractions of skeletal muscles. The disease may affect any person at any time, but children are at greater risk because of their tendency to develop skin wounds as a result of play activities.

ETIOLOGY The disease is caused by *Clostridium tetani,* a bacterium commonly found in soil. The bacillus becomes pathogenic when its spores enter the body through a puncture wound. Burns, surgical incisions, and chronic skin ulcers may also provide opportunities for *C. tetani* spores to enter the body, as may generalized conditions such as otitis media and dental infections. The spores produce a powerful toxin that attacks the central nervous system and that also acts directly on voluntary muscles to produce contraction.

SIGNS AND SYMPTOMS The onset of symptoms may be either gradual or abrupt. Stiffness of the jaw, esophageal muscles, and some neck muscles is often the first sign of the disease. Later, in the most common manifestation of tetanus, the jaws become rigidly fixed (lockjaw), the voice is altered, and the facial muscles contract, contorting the individual's face into a grimace. Finally, the muscles of the back and the extremities may become rigid or the individual may experience extremely severe convulsive spasms of muscles. This final phase of the disease often is accompanied by high fever, profuse sweating, tachycardia, dysphagia, and intense pain.

DIAGNOSTIC PROCEDURES Tetanus is diagnosed on the basis of its classic symptomatology.

TREATMENT The site of the wound or the point of infection must be thoroughly cleaned and debrided. Human tetanus immune globulin (TIG) often will be administered. Muscle relaxants may be prescribed. A tetanus patient requires meticulous care and support to maintain adequate nutrition and hydration and to avoid developing decubitus ulcers. Tracheostomy is routinely performed in moderate to severe cases of tetanus to prevent choking.

PROGNOSIS Despite effective treatment measures, tetanus is frequently fatal, especially among unimmunized people. It is the most common cause of neonatal deaths in developing countries where the umbilical cord is cut with an unclean machete or knife. Death may result from asphyxiation, a host of possible complications, and sometimes from sheer exhaustion. In cases of tetanus in which the individual survives, the disease usually runs its course in about 6 to 7 weeks, seldom producing any lasting disability.

PREVENTION Surprisingly enough, having tetanus does not confer future immunity to the disease. Immunization with tetanus toxoid should be routinely started at 3 months of age. Boosters are required periodically throughout life. The risk of contracting tetanus also can be minimized by wearing protective clothing and by prompt cleansing and care of wounds and other skin lesions.

SUMMARY

Communicable diseases demand an extra measure of caution. It is helpful to know the infectious period for the disease so that anyone who has been exposed can be alerted. Isolation is necessary to prevent further exposure. Table 2–2 outlines the incubation period, the onset and duration, and the suggested isolation period for several contagious infections.

Medical personnel and hospital staff members are required to notify county and state health departments of confirmed cases of certain communicable diseases. This helps monitor epidemics and alerts the medical community to special problems.

The incidence of certain communicable diseases in the United States has steadily decreased over recent decades. Children and adolescents are no longer the routine victims of many diseases because of advances in medical knowledge, general improvements in living conditions, and government-mandated immunization programs. Poliomyelitis, for example, once endemic in the United States, is now considered rare since the advent of the Salk vaccine.

In the absence of the effective immunization provided by vaccines, communicable disease can still cause major epidemics. It is advised that continuous caution be exercised.

REFERENCES

1. Fauci, AS, et al: Harrison's Principles of Internal Medicine. McGraw-Hill, 1998, pp 1818–1819.

BIBLIOGRAPHY

Altekruse, SF, Cohen, ML, and Swendlow, DL: Emerging Foodborne Diseases. Centers for Disease Control and Prevention, Atlanta, 1996.

Kent, TH, and Hart, MN: Introduction to Human Disease, ed 4. Appleton & Lange, Stamford, Conn., 1998.

Lewis, MA, and Tamparo, CD: Medical Law, Ethics, and Bioethics for Ambulatory Health Care, ed 4. FA Davis, Philadelphia, 1998.

Mulvihill, ML: Human Diseases, A Systemic Approach, ed 4. Appleton & Lange, Stamford, Conn., 1995.

REVIEW QUESTIONS

FILL IN THE BLANKS

1. Koplik's spots are characteristic of what childhood disease? _____

2. Another name for German measles is _____ .

3. Another name for tetanus is _____ .

4. The _____ virus causes mumps.

5. Another name for chickenpox is _____ . It is caused by _____ .

6. DPT stands for _____ , _____ , and _____ . All are caused by _____ .

DISCUSSION/FURTHER STUDY

1. Contact your county health department to determine the number of diagnosed AIDS cases in your geographic location. How does this number compare with the previous 2 years? What percent of increase or decrease is indicated? What might be the cause of this increase or decrease?

2. Contact your county health department to ascertain which communicable diseases must be reported in your geographic location. What vaccinations are required before being permitted to start school? Do pediatricians in your area recommend or require hepatitis B vaccination for newborns?

ANSWERS

FILL IN THE BLANKS

1. Rubeola
2. Rubella
3. Lockjaw
4. Paramyxovirus
5. Varicella; varicella-zostervirus (VZV)
6. Diphtheria, pertussis, tetanus; bacteria

DISCUSSION/FURTHER STUDY

Answers will vary.

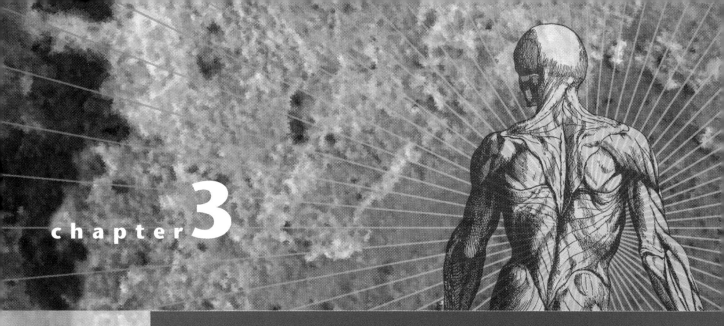

chapter 3

Neoplasms

CHAPTER OUTLINE

Cancer Risk Factors and Preventive Measures

Classification of Neoplasms

Grading and Staging of Neoplasms

Etiology of Neoplasms

Diagnosis of Neoplasms

Treatment of Neoplasms
Surgery
Radiation Therapy

Chemotherapy
Immunotherapy (Biotherapy)
Hormonal Therapy
□ ALTERNATIVE MEDICINE

Summary

References

Bibliography

Review Questions

LEARNING OBJECTIVES
Upon successful completion of this chapter, you will:
* Define neoplasm.
* Compare benign and malignant tumors.
* Recall death statistics on cancer.
* Identify at least eight suggestions for cancer prevention.
* List the seven warning signals of cancer.
* Describe the three main classifications for cancer.
* Identify the grading and staging of neoplasms and their use.
* List at least four possible causes of cancer.
* Discuss four major forms of cancer treatment and their advantages and disadvantages
* Describe circumstances in which a physician and patient may choose a combination of the four major cancer treatments.

KEY WORDS
Anaplasia (ăn•ă•plā′zē•ă)
Anorexia (ăn•ō•rĕk′sē•ă)
Biopsy (bī′ŏp•sē)
Carcinogen (kăr•sĭn′ō•jĭn)
Choriocarcinoma (kō•rē•ō•kăr•sĭ•nō′mă)
Differentiation (dĭf•ĕr•ĕn•shē•ā′shŭn)
Dysplasia (dĭs•plā′zē•ă)
En bloc (ĕn blŏk′)
Encapsulation (ĕn•kăp•sŭ•lā′shŭn)
Epithelial (ĕp•ĭ•thē′lē•ăl)
Erythema (ĕr•ĭ•thē′mă)
Excretion (ĕks•krē′shŭn)

Exfoliative cytology (ĕks•fō′lē•ă•tĭv sī•tŏl′ō•jē)
Hyperplasia (hī•pĕr•plā′zē•ă)
Leukocyte (loo′kō•sīt)
Leukopenia (loo•kō•pē′nē•ă)
Mammogram (măm′ō•grăm)
Metastasis (mĕ•tăs′tă•sĭs)
Neoplasm (nē′ō•plăzm)
Osteolytic (ŏs•tē•ō•lĭ′tĭc)
Palliative (păl′ē•ă•tĭv)
Papanicolaou test
Radioisotope (rā•dē•ō•ī′sō•tōp)
Reed-Sternberg cells

Some new growth in our bodies is necessary and advantageous. Bone and skin repair is an example. Other new growth (**neoplasm**) can be frightening, perplexing, and life-threatening. *Neoplasm* is a new formation or new growth that serves no useful purpose. In fact, the growth is uncontrollable and progressive, and it may be detrimental to other parts of the body. The term *tumor,* a swelling or enlargement, may be used interchangeably with neoplasm.

A tumor may be benign or malignant depending on its growth pattern, cell characteristics, potential for **metastasis,** tendency to recur, and capacity to cause death. A *benign* tumor is one that grows slowly, and whose cells closely resemble normal cells of the tissue from which the tumor originated. The tumor usually is **encapsulated** and does not infiltrate surrounding tissue; it does not tend to recur when removed. A favorable recovery is likely.

A *malignant* tumor, by comparison, is one that is invasive, grows rather rapidly, is sometimes **anaplastic,** and has the capability of metastasizing through the blood or lymph. These tumor cells are not normal. If untreated, a malignancy generally will progress, and death frequently results. We commonly refer to malignant tumors as cancer. Henceforth in this chapter, the two terms will be used interchangeably (see Table 3–1).

Cancer is a focus of attention in American society because of its toll in lives, the suffering it causes, and the economic losses it produces. Cancer strikes people of all ages, both men and women, and is the second leading cause of death in the United States, preceded only by heart disease. According to the American Cancer Society, the disease strikes approximately one in three Americans. Figure 3–1 illustrates the estimated incidence of cancer by site and sex.

Table 3–1 Benign and Malignant Tumors

	Growth Pattern	Appearance
Benign	Grows slowly Remains localized (no metastasis) Expands	Cells closely resemble mature, normal cells Cells are well differentiated In many cases, the tumor is encapsulated

Malignant
  Carcinoma
  Sarcoma
  Leukemias
	Grows rapidly
	Infiltrates surrounding tissues
	Spreads via blood and lymph
	Establishes secondary tumors
		Cells are not well differentiated
		Tumor is seldom encapsulated

In the United States, more than 1 million new cases of cancer are diagnosed each year. Cancer is the cause of death for more than 550,000 people in this country every year. Almost half of all deaths from cancer are from the four most frequently diagnosed kinds: prostate, lung, breast, and colorectal cancer. For males, prostate cancer is the most frequently diagnosed kind of cancer; for women, breast cancer is the most frequently diagnosed. Lung cancer remains the leading cause of cancer death for both men and women. Colorectal cancer occurs at about the same frequency in men and women.

One way to measure the overall success of cancer treatment is to see how many patients remain alive at specific time intervals (for example, 5, 10, and

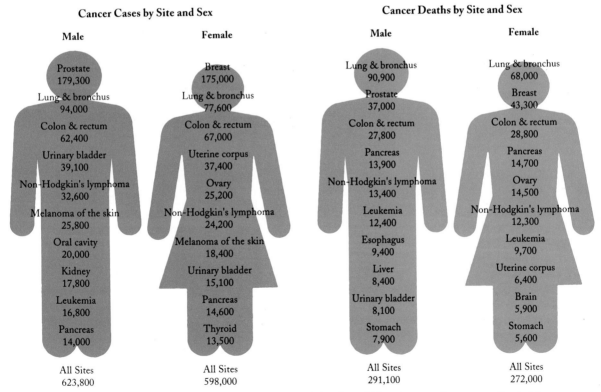

Figure 3–1 Leading sites of new cancer cases and deaths: 1999 estimates. Rates are adjusted for normal life expectancy and are based on cases diagnosed from 1989 to 1994, followed through 1995. (From Cancer Facts and Figures: 1999. American Cancer Society, Atlanta, 1999, p 9, with permission.)

15 years) after they are diagnosed. The 5-year survival rate is a widely used marker. In treating cancer, much depends on the *stage* of the cancer at the time it is diagnosed. A *localized* cancer is one in which the cancer cells have not yet spread from the site of the original tumor. In the *regional* stage, the cancer has spread to sites within the same region of the body. The cancer is said to be in the *distant* stage when cancerous cells have entered the bloodstream and been carried to other sites in the body (metastasis). Successful treatment is more likely with localized tumors, least likely in the distant stage.

Medical researchers continue to develop improved treatment procedures for various forms of cancer. "About 468,000 Americans, or 4 out of 10 patients who get cancer this year, will be alive 5 years after diagnosis."[1] Table 3–2 shows the survival rate for various kinds of cancer.

CANCER RISK FACTORS AND PREVENTIVE MEASURES

There is no single cause of cancer. Research indicates a genetic factor. It is widely accepted, however, that some substances or agents to which humans are exposed increase the risk of developing cancer. Such an element is termed a **carcinogen.** Carcinogens include many kinds of chemicals and certain kinds of radioaction (such as x-rays).

The use of tobacco is a significant factor in the cause of respiratory cancers. "All cancers caused by cigarette smoking and heavy use of alcohol could be prevented completely."[2] A high incidence of colon

Table 3–2 Five-Year Relative Survival Rates* by Stage at Diagnosis, 1989–1994

Site	All Stages %	Local %	Regional %	Distant %
Breast (female)	85	97	77	22
Uterine cervix	70	91	48	11
Colon and rectum	62	91	66	9
Uterine corpus	84	96	66	27
Esophagus	12	24	12	2
Kidney	61	89	62	10
Larynx	66	83	54	44
Liver	5	15	5	2
Lung and bronchus	14	50	20	2
Melanoma	88	96	59	12
Oral cavity	53	82	42	20
Ovary	50	95	79	28
Pancreas	4	17	6	1
Prostate	93	100	99	33
Stomach	21	60	21	2
Testis	95	99	98	73
Thyroid	95	100	94	44
Urinary bladder	82	95	50	6

*Rates are adjusted for normal life expectancy and are based on cases diagnosed from 1989 to 1994, followed through 1995.

Local: An invasive malignant cancer confined entirely to the organ of origin. **Regional:** A malignant cancer that 1) has extended beyond the limits of the organ of origin directly into surrounding organs or tissues; 2) involves regional lymph nodes by way of lymphatic system; or 3) has both regional extension and involvement of regional lymph nodes. **Distant:** A malignant cancer that has spread to parts of the body remote from the primary tumor either by direct extension or by discontinuous metastasis to distant organs, tissues, or via the lymphatic system to distant lymph nodes.

Data source: NCI, Surveillance, Epidemiology, and End Results Program, 1998.

Source: Cancer Facts and Figures—1999. American Cancer Society, Atlanta, 1999, p 14, with permission.

cancer may be linked to a high-fat, low-fiber diet, which is very popular in American households.

About 1 million skin cancers diagnosed in 1993 could have been prevented by protection from the sun's rays.[3]

The American Cancer Society recommends the following preventive measures:

- Do not smoke. The risk of developing lung cancer increases 15 to 25 times for the smoker.
- Limit alcoholic intake. Heavy drinking increases the risk of cancer of the esophagus, mouth, throat, larynx, and liver.
- Protect the skin from excessive sun exposure.
- Refuse needless x-rays. Special precautions must be taken to protect the unborn child if x-rays are necessary.
- Limit exposure to chemicals such as asbestos, aniline dyes, arsenic, chromium, nickel compounds, vinyl chloride, benzene, and certain products of coal, lignite, oil shale, and petroleum.
- Take hormone therapy to relieve menopausal symptoms only as long as necessary. However, the use of progesterone with estrogen helps decrease the cancer risk.
- Avoid heavily polluted air and long exposure to household solvent cleaners, paint thinners, and so on.
- Follow label instructions carefully when using pesticides, fungicides, and other home, garden, and lawn chemicals.
- Monitor caloric intake, and exercise properly. Eat less fatty foods and more high-fiber foods such as bran, whole grains, and fibrous vegetables and fruits.
- Regular screening and self-exams can detect cancers of the breast, tongue, mouth, colon, rectum, cervix, prostate, testes, and skin.
- Limit consumption of salt-cured, smoked, and nitrite-cured foods.
- Have regular checkups by physicians. For women over 50, the doctor may recommend a **mammogram** as part of the routine examination. Also, the **Papanicolaou test** (also known as the *Pap smear* or *Pap test*) should be performed at regular intervals. Men should be regularly checked for prostate cancer. A rectal examination should be part of every medical checkup for men and women, and stool sam-

ples should be examined for blood, which may be an indication of colon cancer.

CLASSIFICATION OF NEOPLASMS

Neoplasms are classified for diagnostic, treatment, and research purposes, as well as to aid in reporting cancer statistics. One commonly accepted system classifies neoplasms according to the type of body tissue in which they appear. Using this method, neoplasms are divided into three categories: carcinomas, sarcomas, and blood and lymph neoplasms.

Carcinomas, the largest group, are solid tumors of **epithelial** tissue of external and internal body surfaces. Benign tumors of epithelial origin usually are named using the suffix *-oma* added to the type of tissue involved. For example, an *adenoma* is a benign tumor of a gland. Malignant tumors of epithelial origin, however, are named using the term *-carcinoma* added to the type of tissue involved. An *adenocarcinoma* is a malignant tumor of a gland. Such terminology often is confusing for the layperson, who may believe that *all* tumors are cancerous.

Sarcomas, less common than carcinomas, arise from supportive and connective tissue such as bone, fat, muscle, and cartilage. Again, benign tumors of connective tissue are named by appending the suffix *-oma* to the type of tissue involved, and malignant tumors of connective tissue are named by adding the term *-sarcoma* to the type of tissue involved. Thus, *osteoma* is a benign tumor of bone; *osteosarcoma* is a malignant tumor of bone.

Neoplasms of blood and lymph include leukemias, Hodgkin's disease, and non-Hodgkin's lymphoma.

Leukemias are sometimes considered to be sarcomas. But the fact that leukemias do not form solid tumors suggests the need for a separate category. Leukemias rise from the body's blood-forming tissues within the bone marrow. The abnormal tissue proliferates, crowding out normal blood-forming cells, and releases large quantities of abnormal **leukocytes** into the circulating blood.

Leukemias are further subdivided into chronic and acute forms. (See Chapter 9.) The chronic leukemias include chronic myelocytic leukemia and chronic lymphocytic leukemia. The acute leukemias include acute myeloblastic leukemia.

The pathological course of leukemia is characterized by the infiltration of leukemic cells into numerous organs, which subsequently become enlarged, soft, and pale. The lymph nodes, spleen, and bone marrow are particularly susceptible. No organ is exempt from this infiltration, however.

Hodgkin's disease is a lymphoma characterized by an unusual giant cell, the **Reed-Sternberg cell.** The disease is characterized by painless enlargement of lymph nodes beginning in the cervical region and moving to all lymphoid structures.

Non-Hodgkin's lymphomas, more common than Hodgkin's disease and increasing in incidence, especially in patients with autoimmune disorders, is characterized by painless lymph node swelling. The difference between Hodgkin's disease and non-Hodgkin's lymphoma, other than the Reed-Sternberg cell, is that non-Hodgkin's lymphoma may involve lymphoid tissue other than lymph nodes, such as the gut and skin.

GRADING AND STAGING OF NEOPLASMS

Pathologists grade neoplasms by studying the microscopic appearance of suspected tumor cells to determine their degree of **anaplasia.** The grading helps in the diagnosis and in treatment planning. Usually four grades are used, as follows:

- Grade 1: Tumor cells are well **differentiated,** closely resembling normal parent tissue.
- Grades 2 and 3: Tumor cells are intermediate in appearance, moderately or poorly differentiated.
- Grade 4: Tumor cells are so anaplastic that recognition of the tumor's tissue origin is difficult.

Persons with grade 1 tumors typically have a high survival rate, whereas persons with grade 4 tumors have a much poorer likelihood of survival. Grading also is used when evaluating cells from body fluids in preventive screening tests, such as Pap smears of the uterine cervix.

Staging neoplasms involves estimating the extent to which a tumor has spread. As with grading, staging is important in determining a proper course of treatment. For this purpose, the *TNM system* was developed by the International Union Against Cancer and the American Joint Committee on Cancer Staging and End-Stage Reporting. This system stages tumors according to three basic criteria: *T* refers to the size and extent of the primary tumor, *N* indicates the number of area lymph nodes involved, and *M* refers to any metastasis of the primary tumor. The grading and staging system will be specific and more greatly detailed according to the site of the disease.

ETIOLOGY OF NEOPLASMS

As discussed in Chapter 1, the actual cause of neoplasms is not known, but some alteration in the cell chromosomes does occur, allowing independent and uncontrollable cell growth. Such a mutated cell is abnormal in that it is not subject to normal control mechanisms. It is suspected that mutations occur fairly frequently, but that the body's immune response is able to destroy the abnormal cells as soon as they occur. Therefore, a malignancy may represent a failure of the body's immune system.

There is some evidence that viruses may cause some kinds of cancers, and this is an area of active research. It has been shown that viruses can cause tumors in animals, but the situation is not so clear in humans. A herpeslike virus, the Epstein-Barr virus, often associated with infectious mononucleosis, is thought to be a causative factor in Burkitt's lymphoma.* The herpes simplex virus appears to be more common in individuals with cervical cancer.

It is a debatable issue whether heredity has any importance in the cause of cancer. There are, however, a few examples deserving of discussion. Cancer of the breast generally is more common in female relatives of affected women than in the general population. The uncommon condition polyposis coli† is inherited through an autosomal dominant gene and eventually leads to carcinoma of the colon. Another rare cancer, retinoblastoma,‡

---

*A malignant neoplasm composed of undifferentiated lymphoreticular cells that form a large **osteolytic** lesion in the jaw or an abdominal mass. It is seen chiefly in Africa.

†A highly malignant condition marked by multiple adenomatous polyps lining the intestinal mucosa, beginning about puberty.

‡A tumor arising from retinal germ cells, a common malignancy of the eye in childhood.

is inherited as a Mendelian dominant trait and usually is present at birth.

Carcinogens were mentioned briefly earlier in this chapter. Hundreds of carcinogenic compounds have been identified. *Carcinogenesis* is the process by which compounds act directly on cells to cause cancer. The process may take many years to occur in humans; it may stop at any point and occasionally may be reversible. Generally, there will be a progressive evolution of cancer cells through different states—**hyperplasia, dysplasia,** carcinoma in situ, to carcinomas that metastasize.

Chronic irritation is not usually considered to be a cause of cancer, but it is thought to be a precursor in some instances. A chronic irritation that is not eliminated can cause abnormal cell changes that may become cancerous. For example, chronic skin ulcers sometimes are complicated by the development of squamous cell carcinomas.

DIAGNOSIS OF NEOPLASMS

Early recognition of the cancer warning signals is essential to diagnosis. The American Cancer Society lists several signs of cancer, the initial letters of which form the acronym **CAUTION:**

- **C**hange in bowel or bladder habits
- **A** sore that does not heal
- **U**nusual bleeding or discharge
- **T**hickening or lump in breast or elsewhere
- **I**ndigestion or difficulty in swallowing
- **O**bvious change in a wart or mole
- **N**agging cough or hoarseness

Responsibility for early detection lies with the individual. Because any delay in the diagnosis and treatment of cancer can significantly alter the disease course, the American Cancer Society recommends:

- A cancer-related checkup by a physician every 3 years for persons aged 20 to 39, and annually for those aged 40 and over.
- Persons at greater risk for certain cancers may require more frequent testing.
- Checkups should include health counseling on topics such as cessation of smoking, use of sun blocks and so on.
- Checkups should include exams for cancer of the breast, uterus, cervix, ovaries, prostate, testes, colon, rectum, mouth, skin, thyroid, and lymph nodes.

To help in the diagnosis of the disease, a Pap test and a biopsy may be performed. The Pap test was developed by Dr. George N. Papanicolaou (1883–1962) to detect cancer, commonly of the uterus and cervix. It is a simple test using an **exfoliative cytology** staining procedure, and it can be performed on any body **excretion,** such as urine and feces; secretion, such as sputum, prostatic fluid, and vaginal fluid; or tissue scrapings such as from the uterus or the stomach. The specimen sample is placed on a slide, stained, and studied under the microscope for abnormal cells. For a person at average risk who has had two negative Pap tests 1 year apart, the American Cancer Society recommends subsequent Pap tests every 3 years. The Pap test is highly effective in detecting early cancer of the cervix or the uterus.

In a **biopsy,** a live tissue sample is taken for microscopic examination. The tissue may be obtained by needle aspiration, endoscopy, or surgical excision. In needle aspiration, the tissue is obtained by application of suction through a needle attached to a syringe. In endoscopy, the tissue is removed by the appropriate instrument, such as a bronchoscope or cytoscope. In surgical excision, the tissue is removed from the body by surgery; sometimes the entire tumor is removed.

TREATMENT OF NEOPLASMS

Treatment of cancer is continually changing as new technology develops. The treatment may offer symptomatic relief to the patient, be used in conjunction with some primary course of treatment, and, perhaps, cure the cancer. The five major types of treatment against cancer include surgery, radiation therapy, chemotherapy, immunotherapy or biotherapy, and hormonal therapy. The physician may recommend one or any combination of these treatment procedures in order to combat a particular form of cancer.

Surgery

Surgery now is more precise because of improved diagnostic equipment and operating procedures and advances in preoperative and postoperative care. Surgery for cancer may be specific, **palliative,** or preventive.

Specific surgery is done to remove all the cancerous tissue and hopefully cure the patient. The types of cancers that respond well to this type of surgery are those of the lung, skin, stomach, large intestine, breast, and endometrium.

Palliative surgery is done to sustain the cancer patient or to alleviate the pain that directly or indirectly results from the cancer. Examples include treating complications of cancer such as abscesses, intestinal perforation and bleeding, or intestinal obstructions. In advanced cancers, palliative surgery may be done to sever nerves to alleviate pain.

Preventive surgery may be done to prevent the development of cancer. For example, polyps of the colon may be removed because they are thought to be precancerous.

Types of surgery include excisional, or **en bloc,** which is done during a radical mastectomy, colectomy, or gastrectomy. *Electrocautery* is the burning of cancer tissue with electric current. This is the preferred method of treating cancers of the rectum.

Radiation Therapy

Radiation may be used alone or in combination with other forms of cancer treatment. About half of all cancer victims receive some type of radiation therapy. The radiation may be externally or internally applied. In the external mode, an x-ray machine or **radioisotopes** may be used. In the internal mode, a radioisotope is placed into catheters, beads, seeds, ribbons, or needles and implanted inside the body.

The goal of radiation therapy is to destroy as much of the tumor as possible without affecting surrounding healthy tissue. Unfortunately, some cancers are situated where radiation would cause serious harm to surrounding tissues. Moreover, some cancers are *radioresistant,* meaning they are not affected by radiation within the safe dosage range.

The effects of radiation on the body include cell death, because ionizing radiation disrupts DNA and interferes with cell replication and growth. Recovery from radiation damage to normal tissue does occur between doses, but the degree varies, depending on the radiosensitivity of the normal

tissue. The radiation dose is determined by the size, type, and location of the tumor.

The adverse effects of radiation generally occur in the skin, mucous membranes, and bone marrow. Hair may begin to fall out, **erythema** may develop, and eating may be difficult because of the nausea, vomiting, and mucosal damage to the mouth and stomach. These distressing side effects generally subside, either between radiation treatments or after the therapy is complete.

New developments in cancer radiology are continually appearing for both curative and palliative purposes. For example, *particle beam therapy,* which produces an intense beam of fast neutrons, emits a precise localization of energy. The neutrons deposit 50 to 100 times more energy in cells than do the x-rays used in conventional radiotherapy treatments, and the depth of particle penetration can be accurately controlled, thus sparing normal tissue.

Chemotherapy

Chemotherapy may be used alone or in combination with other cancer treatments. It is especially effective against cancers that spread, such as leukemias and some solid cancers, including **choriocarcinoma** and Hodgkin's disease. As with radiation, chemotherapeutic drugs affect normal cellular growth and replication, especially of rapidly proliferating cells. There are nearly 50 chemotherapeutic agents, used alone or in combination, for the treatment of malignancy. Many of the chemotherapeutic drugs are experimental and can be used only by oncologists. Chemotherapeutic drugs of similar action generally are grouped together. For example, taxol, an agent from the bark of Pacific yew trees, has been found to be effective in the treatment of ovarian cancer. Currently the drug is approved by the FDA in a semisynthetic form.

Most of these drugs are toxic and have adverse effects on the gastrointestinal tract, skin, and bone marrow. The most common side effects of chemotherapeutic drugs include nausea, vomiting, **anorexia,** anemia, **leukopenia,** and loss of hair. The person receiving chemotherapy will be monitored closely with laboratory testing and physical examination in order to evaluate the efficacy of the treatment and to detect potentially serious side effects.

Immunotherapy (Biotherapy)

A treatment that is used in combination with radiation and chemotherapy is *immunotherapy* or *biotherapy*—treatment of tumors by stimulating the body's own immune defenses. Some tumors overwhelm the body's immune system; radiation and chemotherapy may also suppress the immune system. Thus, treatment to enhance the immune system's response may be indicated. Biotherapy is most effective in the early stages of cancer. Much of the work in this area is experimental, but the use of interferon, a naturally occurring body protein that is capable of killing cancer cells or stopping their growth in some types of leukemias, has been useful. Bone marrow transplantation has proved effective in restoring hematologic and immunologic properties in patients suffering from some cancers.

Hormonal Therapy

Hormonal therapy is based upon research that shows that certain hormones affect the growth of certain cancers. For example, hormonal therapy may be used to treat prostate cancer and breast cancer either by administering or removing certain hormones.

 ## ALTERNATIVE MEDICINE

Very few individuals diagnosed with cancer have not considered or participated in some form of alternative medicine therapy. In some circles, the debate rages on with traditional therapies on one side and alternative therapies on another. Although traditional therapies are the treatment of choice, persons who have cancer continue to seek alternative treatment methods.

Alternative medicine identifies the same cause factors as traditional medicine, but it stresses the effects of diet and nutrition, smoking and tobacco use, environmental toxicity and radiation, oxygen deficiency, stress and related psychological factors, and viruses.

Prevention and treatment modalities common to alternative therapies for cancer are likely to include a diet consisting largely of organically grown foods with little or no fat or meat. Another important cancer-fighting nutrient or element is beta-carotene, which is found in carrots, sweet potatoes, spinach, and leafy green vegetables. All of the major vitamins are encouraged. Minerals such as selenium, folic acid, calcium, iodine, magnesium, and zinc also are identified as having cancer-fighting properties. Garlic is touted as fighting against cancer in general.

In looking at the treatment of cancer, it is helpful to recognize that traditional physicians view cancers as tumors that, if not aggressively treated, will spread through the body and eventually cause death. Alternative medicine views cancer as the manifestation of an unhealthy body whose defenses are so imbalanced that they can no longer destroy cancerous cells. The line of separation between these two treatment modalities becomes less obvious with the passage of time.

A few alternative medicine therapies are identified here:

- *Antineoplaston therapy:* This treatment is based on the theory that the body has a parallel biochemical defense system independent of the immune system. Stanislaw Burznski, MD, PhD, uses this therapy to change the program inside defective cells so they will function normally.
- *714X:* Biologist Gaston Nessens explains that 714X treatment and injections of nitrogen-rich camphor and organic salts into the lymphatic system attract the cancer cells and this enables the immune system to recover and fight off the cancer. Nessens was criminally charged with practicing illegal therapies, but he was acquitted. Harvey Bigelson, MD, in Scottsdale, Arizona, treats cancer patients with a combination of 714X and other alternative therapies with 60 to 80 percent success, he states.
- *Hydrazine sulfate:* This therapy has been documented to shrink some tumors and reverse cachexia. *Cachexia* is the wasting away of the body that so often accompanies life-threatening cancers. Hydrazine sulfate, which can be toxic if not used in its purest form, has shown promise in giving the body extra strength to fight disease.

Several other therapies can be researched by contacting the Cancer Control Society, 2043 North Berendo Street, Los Angeles, CA 90027.

The best approach for the person with cancer to take is to learn as much as possible about all kinds of cancer therapies. Read, explore, and research. Talk to physicians and persons they have treated, especially those persons with similar cancers. Treatment is clearly a choice; inform your primary caregiver of all the therapies being used.

SUMMARY

Cancer is a life-threatening disease that can strike any person at any age. It can strike with or without warning. Early detection and prompt treatment are the best course of action. If the spread is not controlled or checked, cancer can result in death; however, many cancers can be cured if detected and treated promptly. Research marches on and includes therapies to "starve" tumors, confine cancer cells to one area, inhibit the growth of cancer cells, engineer viruses to infect cancer cells, and develop vaccines that goad white blood cells into attacking cancer cells.

REFERENCES

1. American Cancer Society: Cancer Facts and Figures— 1998, p 2.
2. Ibid.
3. Ibid.

BIBLIOGRAPHY

Alternative Medicine: The Definitive Guide. Burton Goldberg Group, Future Medicine Publishing, Fife, Wa., 1995.
Burns, Mary V: Pathophysiology. Appleton & Lange, Stamford, Conn., 1998.
Curing cancer—The hype and the hope. Time 151(19), 1998.
Mulvihill, ML: Human Diseases, A Systemic Approach, ed 4. Appleton & Lange, Stamford, Conn., 1995.
Professional Guide to Diseases, ed 6. Springhouse Corporation, Springhouse, Pa., 1998.

REVIEW QUESTIONS

SHORT ANSWER

1. _____ is a new formation that serves no useful purpose; it is uncontrollable and progressive.

2. _____ is a new formation that grows slowly; cells resemble cells of tissue from which the tumor originates.

3. _____ is a new formation that is invasive, grows rather rapidly, is anaplastic, and is capable of metastasis.

4. Cancer of the _____ is the leading cause of cancer death in both men and women.

5. _____ , _____ , and _____ are the three most common cancer sites for females.

6. List the seven warning signs of cancer that make the acronym CAUTION:

    C

    A

    U

    T

I

O

N

7. Name at least three recommendations for prevention of cancer:

   a.

   b.

   c.

MATCHING

Match the following definitions with their correct cancer classification.

a. Carcinomas
b. Sarcomas
c. Leukemias
d. Blood and lymph neoplasms

_____ 1. Largest group of cancers, solid tumors of epithelial tissue

_____ 2. Neoplasms of blood-forming tissues

_____ 3. Cancers made up of supportive and connective tissue

4. Define TNM:

   T:

   N:

   M:

MULTIPLE CHOICE

Place a checkmark next to all the correct answers.

1. Which of the following are diagnostic tools of neoplasms?
   a. Early recognition of cancer warning signals
   b. Breast self-examination
   c. Testicular self-examination
   d. Pap test
   e. Biopsy by needle aspiration, endoscopy, or surgical incision

2. Which of the following are treatments for cancer?
   a. Surgery
   b. Radiation
   c. Chemotherapy
   d. Biopsy
   e. Immunotherapy/biotherapy
   f. Hormonal therapy

ANSWERS

SHORT ANSWER

1. Neoplasm
2. Benign neoplasm
3. Malignant neoplasm
4. Lung
5. Lung, breast, and colorectal
6. Change in bowel or bladder habits
   A sore that does not heal
   Unusual bleeding or discharge
   Thickening or lump in breast or elsewhere
   Indigestion or difficulty in swallowing
   Obvious change in a wart or mole
   Nagging cough or hoarseness
7. a. Don't smoke.
   b. Limit alcohol intake.
   c. Protect your skin from excessive sun exposure.
   d. Refuse needless x-rays.
   e. Limit exposure to chemicals.
   f. Avoid heavily polluted air.
   g. Follow label instructions carefully on all containers.
   h. Monitor caloric intake and exercise properly.

MATCHING

1. a
2. c and d
3. b
4. The TNM system relates to staging of neoplasms for more accurate diagnosis and treatment of the cancer. T refers to the size and extent of the primary tumor. N refers to the number of area lymph nodes involved. M refers to any metastasis of the primary tumor.

MULTIPLE CHOICE

1. All are correct.
2. a, b, c, e, and f

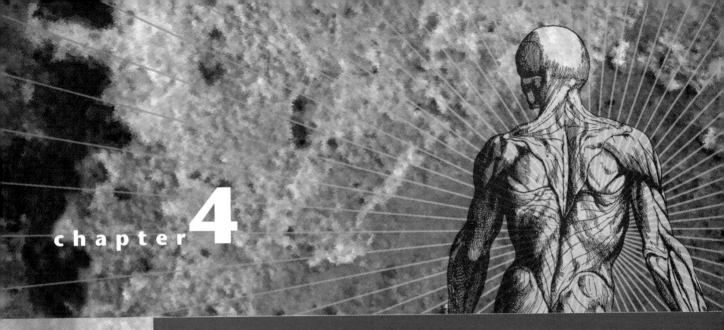

chapter 4

Congenital Diseases

CHAPTER OUTLINE

Nervous System Diseases
Cerebral Palsy
Neural Tube Defects: Spina Bifida,
    Meningocele, Myelomeningocele
Hydrocephalus

Digestive System Diseases
Pyloric Stenosis
Hirschsprung's Disease (Congenital
    Aganglionic Megacolon)

Cardiovascular Diseases
Erythroblastosis Fetalis (Hemolytic Disease of
    the Newborn)
Congenital Heart Defects

Genitourinary Diseases
Undescended Testes (Cryptorchidism)
Congenital Defects of the Ureter, Bladder,
    and Urethra

Musculoskeletal Diseases
Clubfoot (Talipes)
Congenital Hip Dysplasia

Metabolic Errors
Cystic Fibrosis
Phenylketonuria (PKU)

Bibliography

Review Questions

LEARNING OBJECTIVES

Upon successful completion of this chapter, you will:

- Describe the three types of cerebral palsy.
- Identify the signs and symptoms of spina bifida, meningocele, and myelomeningocele.
- Recall the diagnostic procedures used for hydrocephalus.
- Identify the etiology of pyloric stenosis.
- Discuss Hirschsprung's disease.
- Review the prevention of erythroblastosis fetalis.
- Compare and contrast the various congenital defects of the heart.
- Define cryptorchidism.
- Compare and contrast the congenital defects of the ureter, bladder, and urethra.
- List the four common forms of clubfoot.
- Recall the etiology of congenital hip dysplasia.
- Describe the signs and symptoms of cystic fibrosis.
- Restate the diagnostic procedures for PKU.

KEY WORDS

Acetabulum (ăs•ĕ•tăb′ū•lŭm)
Alveoli (sing. *alveolus*) (ăl•vē′ō•lī)
Amniotic Fluid (ăm•nē•ŏt′ĭk floo′ĭd)
Anastomosis (ă•năs•tō•mō′sĭs)
Angiography (ăn•jē•ŏg′ră•fē)
Anoxia (ăn•ŏk′sē•ă)
Arrhythmia (ă•rĭth′mē•ă)
Atelectasis (ăt•ĕ•lĕk′tă•sĭs)
Auscultation (aws•kŭl•tā′shŭn)
Autosomal recessive trait (aw•tō•sō′măl rē•sĕ′sĭv trāt)
Bilirubin (bĭl•ĭ•rōo′bĭn)
Bronchiole (brong′kē•ŏl)
Cardiomegaly (kăr•dē•ō•mĕg′ă•lē)
Chyme (kīm)
Claudication (klaw•dĭ′•kā′shŭn)
Colostomy (kō•lŏs′tō•mē)
Computerized tomography (tŏ•mŏg′ră•fē) scan
Cyanosis (sī•ăn•ō′sĭs)
Ductus arteriosus (dŭk′tus ăr•tē•rē•ō′sĭs)
Dysplasia (dĭs•plā′zē•ă)
Dyspnea (dĭsp′nē•ă)
Dystonia (dĭs•tō′nē•ă)
Epigastrium (ĕp•ĭ•găs′trē•ŭm)
Epistaxis (ĕp•ĭ•stăk′sĭs)
Exchange transfusion
Excoriation (ĕks•kō•rē•ā′shŭn)
Excretory urography (ĕks′krē•tŏ-rē ū′rŏg′ră-fē)
Exocrine (ĕks′ō•krĭn)
Femoral head (fĕm′ŏr•ăl hĕd)
Fontanelle (fŏn•tă•nĕl′)
Ganglion (găng′lē•ŏn)
Hematuria (hē•mă•tū′rē•ă)

Hemolysis (hē•mŏl′ĭ•sĭs)
Hydronephrosis (hī•drō•nĕf•rō′sĭs)
Hydroureter (hī•drō•ū•rē′tĕr)
Hypertrophy (hī•pĕr′trŏ•fē)
Ileostomy (ĭl•ē•ŏs′tō•mē)
Isoimmunization (ī•sō•ĭm•ū•nĭ•zā′shŭn)
Lumen (lū′mĕn)
Macrocephaly (măk•rō•sĕf′ă•lē)
Magnetic resonance imaging
Meninges (mĕn•ĕn′jēz)
Nephrectomy (nĕf•rĕk′tō•mē)
Neuroblastoma (nū•rō•blăs•tō′mă)
Nevus (nē′vŭs)
Nystagmus (nĭs•tăg′mŭs)
Ortolani's sign
Pallor (păl′ŏr)
Parasympathetic (păr•ă•sĭm•pă•thĕt′ĭk)
Peristalsis (pĕr•ĭ•stăl′sĭs)
Petechiae (sing. *petechia*) (pē•tē′kē•ē)
Phototherapy (fō•tō•thĕr′ă•pē)
Postnatal (pŏst•nā′tl)
Prenatal (prē-nā′tl)
Projectile vomiting (prō•jĕk′tīl vom′ĭ•tĭng)
Pylorus (pyloric sphincter) (pī•lŏr′ŭs)
Reflux (rē′flŭks)
Renal calculi (rē′năl kăl′kū•lī)
Resection (rē•sĕk′shŭn)
Rubella (roo•bĕl′lă)
Septum (sĕp′tŭm)
Shunt (shŭnt)
Stenosis (stĕ•nō′sĭs)
Tachypnea (tăk•ĭp•nē′ă)
Teratogen (tĕr-ăt′ōjĭn)
Thrill (thrĭl)
Toxemia (tŏks•ē′mē•ă)
Ventricle (vĕn′trĭk•l)

I n Chapter 1, a basic description of genetic factors relating to the body's disease processes was given. Here the term *congenital diseases* refers to those problems that are present at birth and have genetic causes, nongenetic causes, or a combination of the two. The clinical manifestations of congenital disease may be minor and inconsequential, or they may be life-threatening. Some may be detected at birth; others are not apparent until later in infancy or childhood. All congenital diseases, however, require the attention of physicians and the involvement of the entire family.

Nervous System Diseases

■ CEREBRAL PALSY

DESCRIPTION *Cerebral palsy* is bilateral, symmetrical, nonprogressive paralysis resulting from developmental defects of the brain or trauma at birth.

ETIOLOGY Cerebral palsy is caused by central nervous system damage prior to, during, or following birth. **Prenatal** causes may include maternal rubella (especially in the first trimester), maternal diabetes, **toxemia,** or **anoxia.** Causes related to the birth process include trauma during delivery, prematurity, or asphyxia from the umbilical cord becoming wrapped around the infant's neck. **Postnatal** causes may include head trauma, meningitis, or poisoning. The occurrence of cerebral palsy is highest in premature infants, and it is the most common cause of crippling in children. There are three types: spastic, athetoid, and ataxis.

SIGNS AND SYMPTOMS *Spastic cerebral palsy* affects the majority of children and is characterized by hyperactive reflexes, rapid muscle contraction, muscle weakness, and underdevelopment of limbs. Children with this form of cerebral palsy typically walk on their toes, crossing one foot in front of the other.

Athetoid cerebral palsy affects far fewer children and is characterized by involuntary muscle movements and **dystonia.** The arms are more often affected than the legs, and speech may be difficult. The body movements in athetoid cerebral palsy are increased during times of stress and are not apparent during sleep.

Even fewer persons show signs of *ataxic cerebral palsy.* They have difficulty with balance and coordination and show signs of **nystagmus,** muscle weakness, and tremor. Sudden movements are almost always impossible.

A few children will exhibit signs of all three types of cerebral palsy. Mental retardation, seizure disorders, and impaired speech or vision often are present.

DIAGNOSTIC PROCEDURES Careful neurological assessment, including examination and history, is necessary. The spontaneous movement and behavior of the child are observed for characteristic signs, such as (1) inability to suck or keep food in the mouth, (2) difficulty in voluntary movements, (3) difficulty in separating the legs during diaper changes, and (4) use of only one hand or both hands, but not the legs. An electroencephalogram (EEG) may be done to determine the source of any seizure activity.

TREATMENT Cerebral palsy has no cure, and treatment is directed toward helping children overcome any functional or intellectual disability. The treatment process typically involves the entire family. Treatment may include the use of braces and special appliances, range-of-motion exercises, orthopedic surgery, and medications to decrease seizures and spasticity. The family may benefit from a referral to the local chapter of the United Cerebral Palsy Association.

PROGNOSIS The prognosis varies. If impairment is mild, a near-normal life may be possible.

PREVENTION Early prenatal care and good maternal health are preventive measures.

■ NEURAL TUBE DEFECTS: SPINA BIFIDA, MENINGOCELE, MYELOMENINGOCELE

DESCRIPTION *Spina bifida, meningocele,* and *myelomeningocele* (Fig. 4–1) are developmental defects of the first trimester of pregnancy that are characterized by incomplete closure of the bones encasing the spinal cord. *Spina bifida occulta* is the most

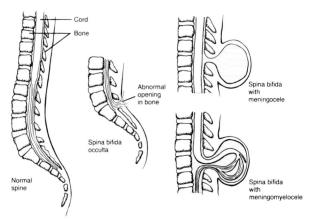

Figure 4–1 Neural tube defects. (Adapted from Rothstein, JM, Roy, SH, and Wolf, SL: The Rehabilitation Specialist's Handbook ed 2. FA Davis, Philadelphia, 1998, p 704, with permission.)

common but least severe of these defects. It is marked by an incomplete closure of one or more vertebrae, with no protrusion of the spinal cord or **meninges.** In *meningocele,* the incomplete closure of the vertebra is accompanied by a protrusion of the spinal fluid and meninges into an external sac. *Myelomeningocele* results when the external sac contains meninges, cerebrospinal fluid, and a portion of the spinal cord or its nerve roots.

ETIOLOGY Between 20 and 23 days of gestation, the neural tube should be complete except for the opening at each end. What causes the failure to close or a later reopening is essentially unknown. Neural tube defects may be isolated birth defects or they may result from exposure to a **teratogen.** Risk factors associated with these conditions include exposure to radiation and viruses. There may also be genetic factors. Recent research has identified a lack of folic acid in the pregnant woman's diet. Spina bifida affects about 5 percent of the population.

SIGNS AND SYMPTOMS Spina bifida occulta may show no visible signs or may be manifested by a dimple in the skin, hair tuft, or a port-wine **nevus** along the posterior surface of the body, in the midline above the buttocks. In meningocele and myelomeningocele, a saclike structure protrudes from the spinal area. Spina bifida and meningocele may cause little or no neurological deficit, but

myelomeningocele frequently results in permanent neurological difficulties.

DIAGNOSTIC PROCEDURES Prenatal detection of some open neural tube defects is possible through ultrasound examination between the 14th and 16th weeks of gestation or through amniocentesis, which shows high levels of acetylcholinesterase. Following birth, meningocele and myelomeningocele are obvious upon examination. Spina bifida occulta may show as a dimple, depression, tuft of hair, soft fatty deposits, or a combination of these, or it may not be evident upon visual inspection. Accordingly, x-rays, pinprick examination of the legs and trunk, and myelography are other procedures used to diagnose the condition and show the level of sensory and motor involvement.

TREATMENT Spina bifida occulta usually requires no treatment. Meningocele and myelomeningocele require surgical repair of the sac and supportive measures to promote independence and to decrease the possibility of complications.

PROGNOSIS The prognosis is dependent on the extent of neurological deficit that accompanies the condition. The prognosis is worse for individuals with large open spinal lesions, neurogenic bladder, or leg paralysis, and much better for those with only spina bifida occulta. In the latter, many affected individuals may be able to live a normal life. In the most severe cases of spina bifida, waist supports, leg braces, and management of fecal incontinence and neurogenic bladder are necessary.

PREVENTION Because spinal cord defects occur more often in offspring of women who have previously had a child with a similar defect, genetic counseling may be helpful.

■ HYDROCEPHALUS

DESCRIPTION *Hydrocephalus* is a condition marked by too much cerebrospinal fluid in the **ventricles** of the brain. The condition is called *noncommmunicating hydrocephalus* when there is an obstruction in cerebrospinal fluid flow. If the problem is faulty absorption of cerebrospinal fluid, the condition is called *communicating hydrocephalus.* This condition is more common in newborns but may occur in adults as the result of injury or disease.

ETIOLOGY Noncommunicating hydrocephalus may result from problems in fetal development, an infection, a tumor, or a blood clot. In communicating hydrocephalus, faulty absorption of the cerebrospinal fluid may be a consequence of surgery to repair myelomeningocele or a meningeal hemorrhage.

SIGNS AND SYMPTOMS The classic symptom of noncommunicating hydrocephalus is the enlarged head; communicating hydrocephalus produces bulging **fontanelles** as the only visible sign. The scalp skin may be thin and fragile-looking, with the veins clearly visible. Hydrocephalic infants often have high-pitched cries and abnormal muscle tone in their legs. **Projectile vomiting** often occurs.

DIAGNOSTIC PROCEDURES The abnormally large head suggests the diagnosis. A measurement of head circumference is done. Skull x-rays, **angiography,** computed tomography (CT) scan, and magnetic resonance imaging (MRI) also may be used.

TREATMENT Surgical correction is the treatment of choice for hydrocephalus. A **shunt** is usually placed from the affected ventricles of the brain into the peritoneal cavity or into the right atrium of the heart, where the excess fluid makes its way into the venous circulation.

PROGNOSIS The prognosis is guarded even with early detection and surgical correction. Mental retardation, vision loss, and impaired motor function often occur. Without surgery, the mortality rate is high.

PREVENTION There is no known prevention.

Digestive System Diseases

■ PYLORIC STENOSIS

DESCRIPTION *Pyloric stenosis* is narrowing of the **pylorus (pyloric sphincter)**. This condition causes obstruction of the flow of **chyme** into the small intestine. Pyloric stenosis is much more common in male than in female infants and adolescents.

ETIOLOGY The cause is unknown, but the disease may be hereditary.

SIGNS AND SYMPTOMS The classic symptom is projectile vomiting, beginning about the second to fourth week after birth. The infant may eject vomitus a distance of 3 to 4 feet. Signs of dehydration and starvation may be evident if the pyloric sphincter closes completely. There may be decreased elasticity of the skin, abdominal distension, and a palpable tumor in the **epigastrium.**

DIAGNOSTIC PROCEDURES The history and physical examination may suggest the condition. Other studies may include upper gastrointestinal x-rays and laboratory tests, with the latter being used to detect dehydration and electrolyte imbalances. Pyloric stenosis must be distinguished from feeding difficulties associated with colic or disturbed mother-child relationships.

TREATMENT The standard treatment is incision and suture of the pyloric sphincter. The procedure, called *pyloromyotomy,* is relatively simple, safe, and effective.

PROGNOSIS The prognosis is excellent with proper care and surgical correction.

PREVENTION There is no known prevention.

■ HIRSCHSPRUNG'S DISEASE (Congenital Aganglionic Megacolon)

DESCRIPTION Hirschsprung's disease is the obstruction and dilation of the colon with feces as a result of inadequate intestinal motility. The condition is due to an absence of autonomic **parasympathetic ganglion** cells in the colorectal walls, resulting in the absence of **peristalsis** in the affected portion. Consequently, feces are not moved past the aganglionic segment of the colon. Pressure from accumulating feces then distends the preceding portion of the colon. The amount of intestinal wall affected varies; involvement may be limited to the internal sphincter or may extend to the entire colon. The disease more frequently affects white female infants and adolescents. Often, the disease occurs with other congenital anomalies.

ETIOLOGY The cause of the disease is unknown, but it appears to be a hereditary, usually familial disease. Hirschsprung's disease may occur with other congenital anomalies, such as trisomy-21 (see Chapter 1).

SIGNS AND SYMPTOMS Clinical manifestations typically appear during infancy, but they may not appear until adolescence. In infancy, signs and symptoms include severe abdominal distension, feeding difficulties, fever, failure to thrive, and explosive watery diarrhea. In adolescence, symptoms may include chronic constipation, abdominal distention, and palpable fecal masses. The child also may be anemic and appear poorly nourished.

DIAGNOSTIC PROCEDURES Diagnosis is confirmed by a rectal biopsy revealing the absence of ganglion cells in the colorectal wall. A barium enema, upright x-rays of the abdomen, or rectal manometry may be ordered.

TREATMENT Medical or surgical treatment may be tried. Medical treatment includes enemas, stool softeners, and a low-residue diet. Surgery may be performed to remove the aganglionic portion of the bowel and to improve functioning of the internal sphincter. A temporary **colostomy** or **ileostomy** may be necessary.

PROGNOSIS With prompt treatment, the prognosis is good. If untreated, death is likely from enterocolitis, severe diarrhea, and shock.

PREVENTION There is no known prevention.

Cardiovascular Diseases

■ ERYTHROBLASTOSIS FETALIS
(Hemolytic Disease of the Newborn)

DESCRIPTION *Erythroblastosis fetalis* is a disease of the newborn characterized by excessive rates of red blood cell destruction (**hemolysis**) (Fig. 4–2). The condition is caused by an incompatibility between maternal and fetal blood, especially an Rh factor or ABO incompatibility. Generally, the maternal antibodies offer the fetus immune protection, which the fetus is unable to provide for itself. During a first pregnancy, an Rh-negative woman becomes sensitized to Rh-positive blood antigens that the fetus has inherited from the father. The maternal blood develops antibodies against the fetal red cell antigens. Usually this process, called **isoimmunization,** does not affect the fetus of a first pregnancy, because the initial sensitization generally does not occur until the onset of labor. During subsequent pregnancies with an Rh incompatible fetus, the maternal antibody crosses the placenta and reacts with the Rh antigen on the fetal red cells. The resulting antigen-antibody reaction causes hemolysis of fetal red cells. A transfusion with Rh-positive blood prior to pregnancy also may sensitize the mother.

ABO incompatibility occurs when the major blood group antigens of the fetus are different from those of the mother. (The major blood groups are A, B, AB, and O.) An example of this incompatibility is a mother with O blood and an infant with A blood. Although ABO incompatibilities are more likely to occur than Rh incompatibilities, the effects of ABO incompatibilities are far less severe, often remaining subclinical.

SIGNS AND SYMPTOMS The severity of the disease ranges from mild anemia with jaundice to death of

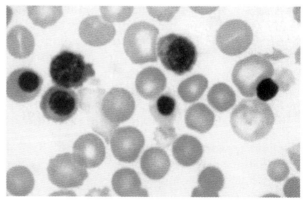

Figure 4–2 Erythroblastosis fetalis. The peripheral blood contains numerous erythroid precursors normally confined to the bone marrow. (From Rubin, E, and Farber, JL [eds]: Pathology, ed 3. Lippincott-Raven, Philadelphia, 1999, p 1085, with permission.)

the fetus. Jaundice may appear within 3 to 24 hours after birth. The jaundice is the result of high levels of **bilirubin** that accumulate because of the increased red cell destruction (hemolysis). The spleen and liver may be enlarged. In severely affected infants, **pallor,** anemia, edema, **petechiae,** lethargy, and convulsions may result.

DIAGNOSTIC PROCEDURES A maternal history and blood typing of both mother and father are essential. A history of blood transfusions may be indicative of potential problems. **Amniotic fluid** analysis may be completed to determine bilirubin levels (elevated levels indicate possible hemolysis) and Rh titers. A direct Coomb's test, bilirubin test, and hematocrit of the infant's blood may be done for diagnosis.

TREATMENT An intrauterine transfusion may be done on the fetus if the amniotic fluid analysis indicates a need. The goal of treatment is to stop the hemolytic process. An **exchange transfusion** is frequently the treatment of choice. Albumin infusions, to aid in the binding of bilirubin, and **phototherapy** may be used. If severe hemolysis is detected in utero, the delivery may be advanced 2 to 4 weeks, or an intrauterine peritoneal transfusion may be tried and repeated until the fetus can be safely delivered.

PROGNOSIS The prognosis for an infant with ABO incompatibility is generally good. The prognosis for an infant with an Rh incompatibility is always guarded, with the outcome depending on the exact nature of the Rh incompatibility and the degree of damage done to other body tissues.

PREVENTION Prevention includes early prenatal care with blood typing. In the event of Rh incompatibility, Rh immune globulin (RhIg) may be given to the mother within 24 hours of delivery or abortion to prevent isoimmunization to Rh positive antigens. This treatment is effective only if the mother is not already immune to the Rh factor.

■ CONGENITAL HEART DEFECTS

DESCRIPTION *Congenital heart defects* can be broadly classified according to whether or not poorly oxygenated blood entering from the veins mixes in the heart with the freshly oxygenated blood reentering the systemic circulation. *Acyanotic defects* are those in which there is no mixing of poorly oxygenated blood with the blood reentering the systemic circulation. *Cyanotic defects* are those in which poorly oxygenated blood mixes with the blood reentering the systemic circulation.

Acyanotic defects include:

- *Ventricular septal defect* (VSD), a congenital heart defect in which there is an abnormal opening between the right and left ventricle (Fig. 4–3). The extent of the opening may vary from pin size to complete absence of the ventricular **septum,** creating one common ventricle. This defect typically accompanies other congenital anomalies, especially Down syndrome, or renal and other cardiac defects. VSD is the most commonly occurring congenital heart defect.
- *Atrial septal defect* (ASD), an abnormal opening between the right and left atria. The size and location of the opening determines the severity of the defect. ASD occurs twice as often in girls and boys.
- *Coarctation of the aorta,* a malformation in a portion of the wall of the aorta that causes narrowing of the aortal **lumen** at the point of the defect (Fig. 4–4). Consequently, blood pressure is increased proximal to the defect and decreased distal to it.
- *Patent ductus arteriosus* (PDA), a defect resulting from the failure of the **ductus arteriosus** to close after birth. During the prenatal period, much of the fetal circulation bypasses the lungs through this blood vessel, which connects the pulmonary artery to the aorta. When this fetal structure fails to close after birth, blood from the aorta flows back into the pulmonary artery.

Cyanotic defects include:

- *Tetralogy of Fallot,* a combination of four congenital heart defects, including (1) pulmonary **stenosis,** a narrowing of the opening into the pulmonary artery from the right ventricle; (2) ventricular septal defect, an abnormal opening in the septum between the left and right ventricles; (3) dextroposition of the aorta, in which the opening of the aorta bridges the ventricular septum, receiving blood from both the left and right ventricles; and (4) right ven-

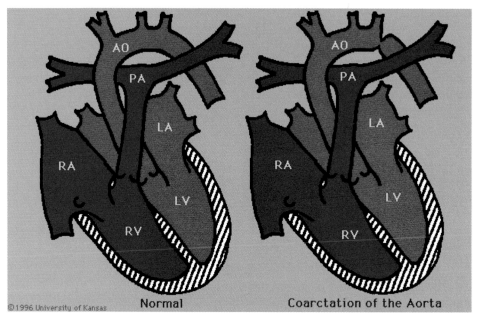

Figure 4–3 Ventricular septal defect. (From *http://www.kumc.edu/instruction/medicine/pedcard/cardiology/pedcardio/vsddiagram.gif,* courtesy of The University of Kansas Medical Center © 1996.)

tricular **hypertrophy.** Tetralogy of Fallot is the most common cyanotic heart defect.

- *Transposition of the great vessels,* a condition in which the two major arteries of the heart are reversed, with the aorta arising from the right ventricle and the pulmonary artery from the left ventricle. The result is two noncommunicating circulatory systems—one circulating blood in a closed loop between the heart and lungs and the other, between the heart and systemic circulation.

ETIOLOGY The etiology of congenital heart defects is unknown, but genetic anomalies are strongly suspected. Predisposing factors may include maternal **rubella,** diabetes, alcoholism, and poor maternal nutrition.

Clinical features vary with age and seriousness of the defect.

SIGNS AND SYMPTOMS OF ACYANOTIC DEFECTS

- *VSD:* The classic clinical feature is a loud, early systolic murmur heard during **auscultation.** The typical murmur is described as blowing or rumbling.
- *ASD:* The classic clinical feature is a crescendo-decrescendo type of systolic ejection murmur.

- *Coarctation of the aorta:* The clinical features vary with age. A murmur may or may not be present. An infant may exhibit **dyspnea,** pulmonary edema, **tachypnea,** and failure to thrive. Symptoms appearing after adolescence may include dyspnea, **claudication,** headache, **epistaxis,** and hypertension.
- *PDA:* The clinical feature is a "machinery" murmur usually associated with a **thrill,** and often accompanied by a widened pulse pressure. Respiratory distress is common.

SIGNS AND SYMPTOMS OF CYANOTIC DEFECTS

- *Tetralogy of Fallot:* **Cyanosis** is often evident at birth or within several months of birth and is considered the hallmark of the disorder. The child may exhibit other signs of poor oxygenation, such as increasing dyspnea on exertion, diminished exercise tolerance, and delayed physical growth and development.
- *Transposition of the great vessels:* The infant is typically severely cyanotic at birth and has tachypnea. Signs of congestive heart failure and **cardiomegaly** follow.

DIAGNOSTIC PROCEDURES A history and physical examination are essential and may be all that is

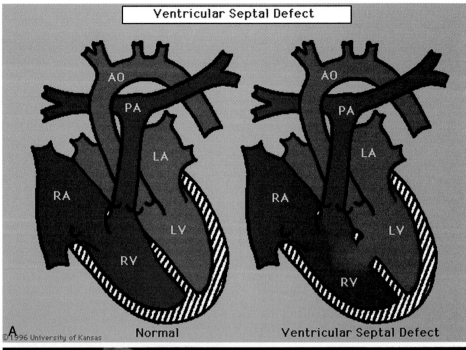

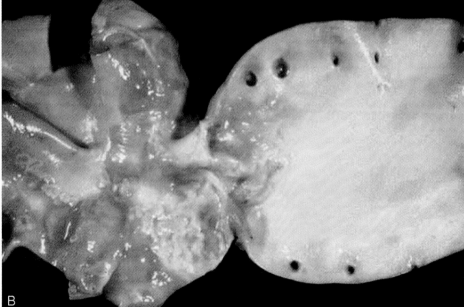

Figure 4–4 (*A*) Illustration of a normal aorta and coarctation of the aorta. (From *http://www.kumc.edu/instruction/medicine/pedcard/cardiology/pedcardio/coarctationdiagram.gif,* courtesy of The University of Kansas Medical Center © 1996). (*B*) The aorta is opened longitudinally to reveal a coarctation. In the region of narrowing, there was increased turbulence that led to increased atherosclerosis. (From The Internet Pathology Laboratory for Medical Education, *http://www-medlib.med.utah.edu/WebPath/CVHTML/CV082.html,* courtesy of Edward C. Klatt, MD.)

necessary to diagnose tetralogy of Fallot. Other diagnostic procedures may include x-rays, electrocardiogram (ECG), echocardiogram, and heart catheterization. Laboratory studies may be ordered for determining the degree of cyanosis and for detecting possible acidosis.

TREATMENT Surgery is usually the treatment of choice for a congenital heart defect. Surgery may be performed soon after birth, or it may be delayed until the child is old enough to withstand corrective surgery.

PROGNOSIS The prognosis is dependent on the type of defect, its location, and its severity. If the defect is small and surgery is successful, the prognosis is often good; otherwise, the prognosis is guarded.

PREVENTION There is no known prevention other than proper prenatal care and minimizing suspected risk factors.

Genitourinary Diseases

■ UNDESCENDED TESTES
(Cryptorchidism)

DESCRIPTION This congenital condition is the failure of the testes to descend into the scrotal sac from the abdominal cavity. The condition may be unilateral or bilateral. It more commonly affects the right testis.

ETIOLOGY The cause is unknown, but it may be linked to inadequate or improper hormone levels in the fetus. The testes normally descend into the scrotal sac during the eighth month of gestation, so the condition is most often seen in premature births.

SIGNS AND SYMPTOMS When the condition is unilateral, the testis on the affected side is not palpable in the scrotum. In bilateral cryptorchidism, the scrotum will appear underdeveloped.

DIAGNOSTIC PROCEDURES Physical examination reveals cryptorchidism. A serum gonadotropin test will confirm the presence of testes, because it assesses the level of circulating hormone produced by the testes.

TREATMENT In many cases, the testes will descend during the infant's first year. Otherwise, the treatment of choice is surgical correction before age 4. Rarely, human chorionic gonadotropin is tried to stimulate descent.

PROGNOSIS The prognosis is good with proper attention. Corrected cryptorchidism does not cause sexual dysfunction later. Testes that have not descended by the time of adolescence will atrophy, causing sterility, but testosterone levels remain normal.

PREVENTION Because the cause is essentially unknown, prevention also is unknown.

■ CONGENITAL DEFECTS OF THE URETER, BLADDER, AND URETHRA

The causes of congenital defects of the ureter, bladder, and urethra are unknown. Some of the problems are obvious at birth; others are not apparent until later, when they produce symptoms. The following is a brief discussion of the most common congenital urinary tract anomalies, together with their symptoms and possible treatments. Diagnostic tests include excretory urography, voiding cystoscopy, cystourethrography, urethroscopy, and ultrasound.

Duplicated ureter means that each kidney has two ureters rather than one. Sometimes the two ureters join before they enter the urinary bladder. The common symptoms may include frequent urinary infections, urinary frequency and urgency, diminished urine output, and flank pain. Surgery is the treatment of choice.

Retrocaval ureter occurs when the right ureter passes behind the inferior vena cava before entering the urinary bladder. The symptoms may include **hydroureter,** right flank pain, urinary tract infection, **renal calculi,** and hematuria. Surgical **resection** and **anastomosis** of the ureter constitute the treatment of choice.

Ectopic orifice of the ureter occurs when the ureteral opening inserts into the vagina in females or in the prostate or vas deferens in males. The symptoms may include urinary obstruction, **reflux,** incontinence, flank pain, and urinary urgency. Resection and ureteral reimplantation into the bladder are necessary for correction.

Stricture or stenosis of the ureter means that one of the ureters is tightened or partially closed. The affected ureter may become enlarged, and **hydronephrosis** may result. Surgical repair is necessary. A **nephrectomy** may be required if severe renal damage has occurred as a result of hydronephrosis.

Ureterocele is the bulging of the ureter into the urinary bladder, sometimes almost filling the bladder. There will be urinary obstruction difficulties and recurrent urinary tract infections. Surgical repair or resection of the ureterocele is necessary.

Exstrophy of the bladder is a congenital malformation in which the lower portion of the abdominal wall and the anterior wall of the bladder are missing. Consequently, the inner surface of the posterior wall of the bladder is everted through the opening in the abdominal wall. In effect, the bladder appears turned inside out. The skin covering the hole in the abdominal wall is easily **excoriated** by accumulating urine, and infection typically results. Surgical closure of the defect is necessary. Reconstruction of the bladder and abdominal wall is required, and urinary diversion may be necessary.

Congenital bladder diverticulum is caused by a pouching out (diverticulum) of the bladder wall. Fever, urinary frequency, and pain on urination are common. Surgery is the treatment of choice to correct the herniation and reflux.

Hypospadias is an abnormal opening of the male urethra onto the undersurface of the penis, or of the female urethra into the vagina. *Epispadias* is an abnormal opening of the male urethra onto the upper surface of the penis, or of the female urethra through a fissure in the labia minora and clitoris. In all these instances, normal urination is difficult or impossible. Surgical repair is almost always necessary.

Musculoskeletal Diseases

▦ CLUBFOOT (Talipes)

DESCRIPTION *Clubfoot* is a nontraumatic, frequently occurring congenital deformity in which the foot is permanently bent. The four basic forms are (1) *talipes varus,* an inversion or inward bending of the foot; (2) *talipes valgus,* an eversion or outward bending of the foot; (3) *talipes equinus,* or plantar flexion, in which the toes are lower than the heel; and (4) *talipes calcaneus,* or dorsiflexion, in which the toes are higher than the heel. An individual also may have a combination of these basic forms: for example, talipes equinovarus, in which the toes point downward and the body of the foot bends inward.

ETIOLOGY The exact cause is unknown, but a combination of genetic and environmental factors in utero have been implicated. It is twice as common in boys as in girls.

DIAGNOSTIC PROCEDURES The deformity is usually obvious at birth.

SIGNS AND SYMPTOMS Clubfoot varies greatly in severity; however, in all cases the talus is deformed, the Achilles' bursa is shortened, and the calcaneus is flattened and shortened. It is painless.

TREATMENT Treatment is aimed at correcting the deformity and maintaining the corrected position. Simple manipulation and casting may be done and repeated several times. Corrective surgery may be required. Maintenance treatment includes special exercises, night splints, and orthopedic shoes. Close follow-up observation is essential.

PROGNOSIS The prognosis is good with prompt treatment.

PREVENTION There is no known prevention.

▦ CONGENITAL HIP DYSPLASIA

DESCRIPTION Hip **dysplasia** is an abnormality of the hip joint that may take three forms: (1) unstable hip dysplasia, in which the hip can be dislocated manually; (2) incomplete dislocation, in which the **femoral head** is on the edge of the **acetabulum;** and (3) complete dislocation, in which the femoral head is outside the acetabulum.

ETIOLOGY The cause is not known; however, two unproven etiologies have been proposed. First, hormones that relax the maternal ligaments during labor also may relax the hip ligaments of the infant. Second, hip dislocation may result if the fetus is not positioned correctly within the uterus prior to and during birth.

SIGNS AND SYMPTOMS The signs are typically quite obvious when children attempt to walk, if the condition has not been discovered prior to that time.

DIAGNOSTIC PROCEDURES Observations during physical examination may suggest the diagnosis, but a positive **Ortolani's sign** will confirm the diagnosis.

TREATMENT It is important for treatment to begin as soon as possible. Prior to 3 months of age, treatment requires closed reduction of the dislocation followed by the use of a splint-brace for 2 to 3 months. If the child is much older, open reduction followed by casting may be necessary.

PROGNOSIS When treatment occurs before age 5, the prognosis is excellent. If not treated promptly, abnormal development of the hip and permanent disability may result.

PREVENTION There is no known prevention.

Metabolic Factors

CYSTIC FIBROSIS

DESCRIPTION *Cystic fibrosis* is a congenital disorder of the **exocrine** glands characterized by the production of copious amounts of abnormally thick mucus, especially in the lungs and pancreas.

ETIOLOGY The disease is caused by an underlying biochemical defect transmitted as an **autosomal recessive trait** (see Chapter 1, Hereditary Diseases). If both parents are carriers of the recessive gene, the offspring have a 25 percent chance of having the disease.

SIGNS AND SYMPTOMS The signs of cystic fibrosis may appear soon after birth or take some time to develop. Because all exocrine glands can be affected, the symptoms can be quite numerous. The sweat glands and respiratory and gastrointestinal functions are those most commonly affected. The sweat glands typically express increased concentrations of salt in sweat. Respiratory symptoms may include wheeze respirations, a dry cough, dyspnea, and tachypnea, all stemming from accumulations of thick secretions in the **bronchioles** and **alveoli** of the lungs. Gastrointestinal symptoms may include intestinal obstruction, vomiting, constipation, electrolyte imbalance, and the inability to absorb fats. Fibrous tissue and fat slowly replace the normal saclike swellings found in the pancreas, resulting in pancreatic insufficiency characterized by insufficient insulin production.

DIAGNOSTIC PROCEDURES The presence of abnormal quantities of salt in a child's sweat, accompanied by pulmonary and pancreatic insufficiencies, confirms the diagnosis. Family history may show siblings or other relatives with cystic fibrosis. DNA testing may be done prenatally to diagnose the disease. Chest x-rays and pulmonary function tests may be ordered to diagnose and evaluate respiratory function.

TREATMENT The treatment for cystic fibrosis is largely supportive. Client management includes generous salting of food to replace salt lost in sweat, physical therapy to combat pulmonary dysfunction, loosening and removal of mucopurulent secretions, and oxygen therapy. Vitamin and oral pancreatic supplements may be given. Both the family and the client require emotional support. A referral to the Cystic Fibrosis Foundation may be helpful.

PROGNOSIS The prognosis is poor. There is no cure for cystic fibrosis, but the average life expectancy is 28 years of age or older. Cystic fibrosis is the most common fatal genetic disease. Death is usually due to such complications as shock and **arrhythmias** that may occur during hot weather due to profuse sweating. Serious, often fatal respiratory complications include pneumonia, emphysema, and **atelectasis.** Gastrointestinal complications include rectal prolapse and malnutrition.

PREVENTION There is no known prevention. Genetic counseling may be advisable in families known to be at risk.

PHENYLKETONURIA (PKU)

DESCRIPTION *Phenylketonuria* is an autosomal recessive defect resulting in an error in phenylalanine metabolism.

ETIOLOGY During normal metabolic processes, the enzyme phenylalanine hydroxylase converts the amino acid phenylalanine to tyrosine, another amino acid. In PKU, this enzyme is not produced by the body, so that phenylalanine accumulates in the blood and urine. Mental retardation will result if the condition is not quickly corrected. The full extent of cerebral damage is complete by 2 or 3 years of age and is irreversible.

SIGNS AND SYMPTOMS The infant is typically asymptomatic until about 4 months of age, when signs and symptoms of mental retardation, such as hyperactivity, personality disorders, **macrocephaly,** and irritability, begin to appear. There is often a characteristic musty odor to the child's perspiration and urine due to the presence of phenylacetic acid, a metabolite of phenylalanine.

DIAGNOSTIC PROCEDURES An elevated blood phenylalanine level and urine phenylpyruvic acid level present at birth will confirm the diagnosis. Repeated testing may need to be done.

TREATMENT Treatment consists of following a protein-restrictive diet for 3 to 6 years or, some authorities maintain, for life. Most natural proteins need to be restricted, because phenylalanine is a component of most proteins. Serum phenylalanine levels need to be monitored to determine the efficacy of the diet.

PROGNOSIS The sooner the protein-restrictive diet is started, the better is the prognosis. If the disease is detected and treated before 2 years of age, the chances of the child achieving normal intelligence are good. The protein-restrictive diet will not reverse any existing mental retardation, but it will prevent further progression.

PREVENTION Prevention includes genetic counseling and PKU testing at birth.

BIBLIOGRAPHY

Burns, MV: Pathophysiology: A Self-Instructional Program. Appleton & Lange, Stamford, Conn., 1998.
Fauci, AS, et al: Harrison's Principles of Internal Medicine, ed 4. McGraw-Hill, New York, 1998.
Kent, TH, and Hart, N: Introduction to Human Disease. Appleton & Lange, Stamford, Conn., 1998.
Mulvihill, ML: Human Diseases: A Systemic Approach. Appleton & Lange, Stamford, Conn., 1995.
Professional Guide to Diseases, ed 6. Springhouse Corporation, Springhouse, Pa., 1998.

REVIEW QUESTIONS

MULTIPLE CHOICE

1. Select all the correct statements concerning cerebral palsy:
   a. It is caused by central nervous system damage prior to birth.
   b. It may be spastic, athetoid, and ataxic.
   c. A neurological assessment is the most common diagnostic tool.
   d. The condition is curable.
   e. There is no known prevention.

2. Select all the correct signs and symptoms of cystic fibrosis:
   a. Intestinal obstruction
   b. Vomiting
   c. Constipation
   d. Wheezy respirations
   e. Dry cough
   f. Dyspnea

g. Tachypnea

h. Electrolyte imbalance

i. Inability to absorb fats

j. Deficient insulin

3. Select all the correct answers from the following statements concerning erythroblastosis fetalis:

a. It is a hemolytic disease of the newborn.

b. The fetal blood cells build antibodies against maternal cells.

c. It affects the fetus in the first pregnancy.

d. ABO incompatibility is more common than an Rh type.

e. Jaundice is a common symptom.

f. Phototherapy is the treatment of choice.

MATCHING

1. Select the correct definition for these spinal cord defects:

_____ Incomplete closure of one or more vertebrae

_____ Incomplete closure of vertebrae with protrusion of spinal fluid and meninges into sac

_____ External sac contains meninges, cerebrospinal fluid, and a portion of the cord and nerve roots

a. Meningomyelocele

b. Meningocele

c. Spina bifida occulta

2. Match the following congenital defects of the heart with their definitions:

_____ Abnormal opening between the two atria

_____ Failure of the fetal ductus arteriosus to completely close

_____ Abnormal opening between the right and left ventricles

_____ Localized narrowing of the aorta

a. Ventricular septal defect

b. Atrial septal defect

c. Coarctation of the aorta

d. Patent ductus arteriosus

e. Tetralogy of Fallot

SHORT ANSWER

1. The two different types of hydrocephalus are _____ and

_____ .

2. The characteristic symptom in pyloric stenosis is _____ .

3. Another name for undescended testes is _____ .

4. What does PKU stand for? Describe it.

5. Name at least three congenital defects of the ureter, bladder, and urethra:

a.

b.

c.

6. List the four most common forms of clubfoot or talipes:

a.

b.

c.

d.

7. List the three forms of congenital hip dysplasia:

a.

b.

c.

ANSWERS

MULTIPLE CHOICE

1. a, b, c, and e
2. All of these symptoms are possible in cystic fibrosis.
3. a and e

MATCHING

1. c, b, and a
2. b, d, a, and c

SHORT ANSWER

1. Noncommunicating (where there is an obstruction in cerebrospinal fluid flow); communicating (where there is faulty absorption of cerebrospinal fluid)
2. Projectile vomiting (due to increased size of the pyloric muscle)
3. Cryptorchidism
4. Phenylketonuria. It is an inherited genetic defect due to an error in phenylalanine metabolism. Phenylalanine hydroxylase, an enzyme, is needed to convert phenylalanine to tyrosine. In PKU, this enzyme is absent, so phenylalanine accumulates in the blood and urine.
5. Duplicated ureter, retrocaval ureter, ectopic orifice of ureter, stricture or stenosis of ureter, ureterocele, exstrophy of the bladder, congenital bladder diverticulum, hypospadias, and epispadias
6. a. Talipes varus
   b. Talipes valgus
   c. Talipes equinus
   d. Talipes calcaneus or dorsiflexion
7. a. Unstable hip dysplasia (where the hip can be dislocated manually)
   b. Incomplete dislocation (where the femoral head is on the edge of the acetabulum)
   c. Complete dislocation (where the femoral head is outside the acetabulum)

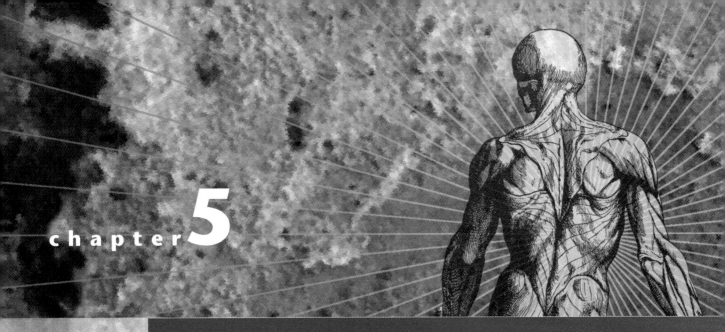

chapter 5

Urinary System Diseases

CHAPTER OUTLINE

Kidney Diseases
Polycystic Kidney Disease
Pyelonephritis (Acute)
Glomerulonephritis (Acute)
Nephrotic Syndrome
Chronic Renal Failure (Uremia)
Acute Tubular Necrosis (ATN)
Renal Calculi (Uroliths or Kidney Stones)
Hydronephrosis

Lower Urinary Tract Diseases
Cystitis and Urethritis
Neurogenic Bladder

Tumors of the Urinary System
*Adenocarcinoma of the Kidney
  (Hypernephroma)*

Tumors of the Bladder

**Special Focus: Treatment of Renal
  Failure**
Dialysis
Kidney Transplantation

**Common Symptoms of Urinary System
  Diseases**

References

Bibliography

Case Studies

Review Questions

LEARNING OBJECTIVES

Upon successful completion of this chapter, you will:

- Identify the major diseases of the kidney.
- Name the most common diagnostic procedures used to detect kidney and kidney-related diseases.
- List at least three characteristics common to polycystic kidney disease.
- Identify complications of kidney-related diseases.
- Compare and contrast pyelonephritis and glomerulonephritis.
- Recall infectious precursors to kidney-related diseases.
- Explain why women are more prone to urinary tract infections.
- List the characteristics unique to nephrotic syndrome.
- Name at least three causes of uremia.
- Describe how acute tubular necrosis occurs.
- Discuss the complications of renal calculi.
- Identify possible treatments for renal calculi.
- Repeat the common signs and symptoms of urinary tract diseases.
- Describe the prognosis of lower urinary tract infections.
- Define neurogenic bladder.
- Compare and contrast the malignant tumors of the bladder and of the kidney.
- Distinguish between the two types of kidney dialysis.
- List at least four common complaints of the urinary system.

KEY WORDS

Anorexia (ăn•ō•rĕk′sē•ă)
Antiemetic (ăn•tĭ•ē•mĕt′ĭk)
Antipyretic (ăn•tĭ•pī•rĕt′ĭk)
Ascites (ă•sī′tēz)
Autosomal dominant defect
 (aw•tō•sō′mal)
Autosomal recessive defect
Calyx (pl. *calyces*) (kā′lĭks) (kā′lĭ•sēz)
Cast (kăst)
Creatinine (krē•ăt′ĭn•ĭn)
Cystectomy (sĭs•tĕk′tō•mē)
Dementia (dē•mĕn′shē•ă)
Dysuria (dĭs•ū′rē•ă)
Edema (ě•dē′mă)
Electrolyte (ē•lĕk′trō•līt)
Hematuria (hē•mă•tū′rē•ă)
Hydronephrosis (hī•drō•něf•rō′sĭs)
Hyperkalemia (hī•pěr•kă•lē′mē•ă)
Hyperlipemia (hī•pěr•lĭp•ē′mē•ă)
Hyperparathyroidism
 (hī•pěr•păr•ă•thī′roy•dĭzm)
Hypertension (hī•pěr•těn′shun)
Hypoalbuminemia
 (hī•pō•ăl•bū•mĭn•ē′mē•ă)

Incontinence (ĭn•kŏn′tĭ•nĭnts)
Insidious (ĭn•sĭd′ē•ŭs)
Ischemia (ĭs•kē′mē•ă)
Lipiduria (lĭp•ĭ•dū′rē•ă)
Lumbar (lŭm′băr)
Malaise (mă•lāz′)
Metastasis (mě•tăs′tă•sĭs)
Micturition (mĭk•tū•rĭ′shŭn)
Nephrectomy (ně•frěk′tō•mē)
Nephrosclerosis (něf•rō•sklě•rō′sĭs)
Nocturia (nŏk•tū′rē•ă)
Oliguria (ŏl•ĭg•ū′rē•ă)
Pallor (păl′ŏr)
Polyuria (pŏl•ē•ū′rē•ă)
Proteinuria (prō•tē•ĭn•ū′rē•ă)
Pruritis (proo•rī′tŭs)
Pyuria (pī•ū′rē•ă)
Renal calculi (sing. *calculus*) (rē′năl
 kăl′kū•lī)
Transurethral resection (trăns•ū•rē′thrăl
 rē•sěk′shŭn)
Urea (ū•rē′ă)
Uremia (ū•rē′mē•ă)
Urolith (ū′rō•lĭth)

The urinary system is responsible for the production and elimination of urine. The organs of this system include two kidneys, two ureters, the urinary bladder, and the urethra. Figure 5–1 illustrates the urinary system in relationship to the body, and Figure 5–2 illustrates the interior and exterior features of the urinary system organs.

The kidneys help to regulate the water, **electrolyte,** and acid-base content of the blood and selectively filter out the waste products of metabolism. They also play an important role in regulating blood pressure. Each kidney contains over 1 million nephrons (Fig. 5–3), which are the principal functional units of the kidney. It is here that the three-part process of selective filtration of wastes, reabsorption of vital minerals and fluid, and secretion of waste products and other substances takes place.

It is worth emphasizing the reabsorption process of the kidneys' nephrons. Were it not for this process, the body would rapidly be depleted of its fluid. Typically, only 1 percent of the fluid passing through a nephron is excreted as urine.

A routine diagnostic test for suspected urinary disease is a urinalysis, which includes testing the specific gravity, pH, presence of protein, blood, sugar, and ketones. It includes a microscopic examination for the presence of white and red blood cells, casts, bacteria, and crystals. Normal urine is amber-colored with a slightly acid reaction, has a peculiar odor with a bitter saline taste and frequently deposits a precipitate of phosphates when fresh. The specific gravity varies from 1.005 to 1.030. The greater the rate of urine excretion, the lower the specific gravity. Refer to Table 5–1, Significance of Changes in Urine, as you read the chapter, noting possible abnormalities and their significance to the disease in question.

Kidney Diseases

◼ POLYCYSTIC KIDNEY DISEASE

DESCRIPTION *Polycystic kidney disease* is a developmental defect of the collecting tubules in the cortex of the kidneys. Groups of tubules that fail to empty properly into the renal pelvis slowly swell into multiple, grapelike, fluid-filled sacs or cysts. The pressure from the expanding cysts slowly destroys adjacent normal tissue, progressively impairing kidney function. Both kidneys are usually affected and are grossly enlarged.

ETIOLOGY There are two forms of the disease, each due to a genetic defect. The more common adult form, usually manifested during midlife, is an **autosomal dominant defect.** The much less common infant and childhood forms, manifested at birth or during childhood, are **autosomal recessive defects.** The following discussion pertains to the more frequently occurring adult form. The majority of the adult cases are inherited as an autosomal dominant trait, and the remainder are spontaneous mutations.

SIGNS AND SYMPTOMS The disease is usually asymptomatic until midlife. Then the patient may complain of colic and **lumbar** pain, or mention seeing blood in the urine or passing **renal calculi.** The onset is **insidious.**

DIAGNOSTIC PROCEDURES The history may reveal a family tendency toward renal disease. The physical examination may reveal palpably enlarged kidneys and **hypertension.** The physician may order an excretory urography, ultrasound examination, or computed tomography (CT) scan to detect enlarged kidneys and the presence of cysts. Urinalysis may be ordered to evaluate renal function and to detect **hematuria.**

TREATMENT No treatment will stop the course of the disease; however, treatment attempts to minimize the symptoms. Treatment goals include guarding against or managing urinary tract infections and controlling secondary hypertension. Urine cultures should be performed at regular intervals to detect infection. In the event of renal failure, renal dialysis or kidney transplantation may be attempted to prolong life.

PROGNOSIS The prognosis is variable yet poor. Kidney function is progressively impaired, leading to

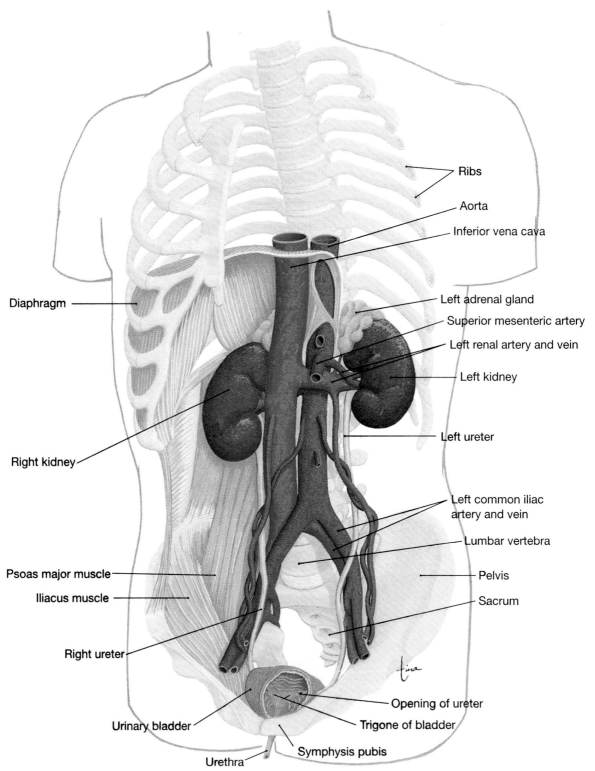

Figure 5–1 The urinary system. (From Scanlon, VC, and Sanders, T: Essentials of Anatomy and Physiology, ed 3. FA Davis, Philadelphia, 1999, p 403, with permission.)

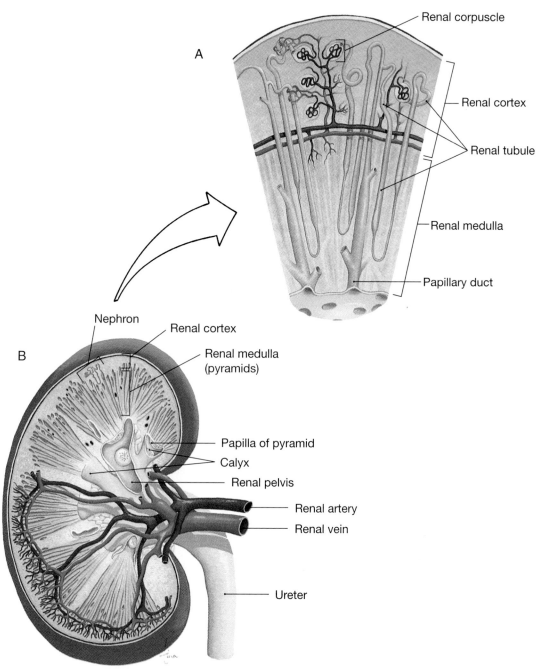

Figure 5–2 (*A*) Frontal section of the right kidney showing internal structures and blood vessels. (*B*) The magnified section of the kidney shows several nephrons. (From Scanlon, VC, and Sanders, T: Essentials of Anatomy and Physiology, ed 3. FA Davis, Philadelphia, 1999, p 405, with permission.)

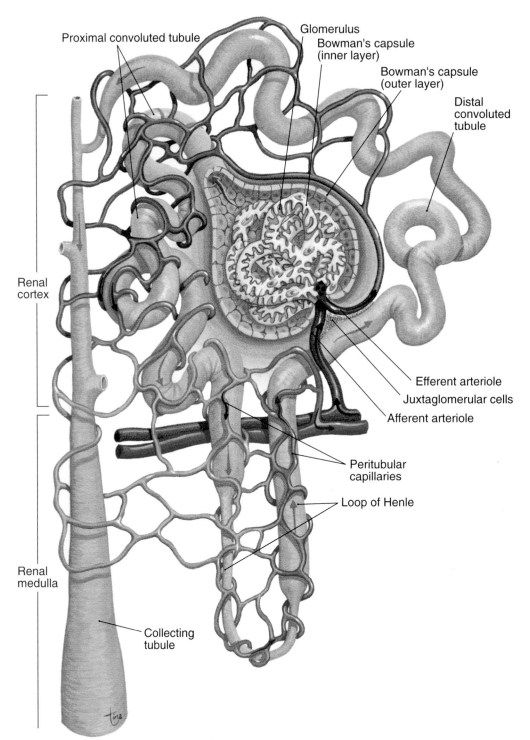

Figure 5–3 A nephron with its associated blood vessels. The arrows indicate the direction of blood flow and the flow of renal filtrate. (From Scanlon, VC, and Sanders, T: Essentials of Anatomy and Physiology, ed 3. FA Davis, Philadelphia, 1999, p 406, with permission.)

Table 5–1 Significance of Changes in Urine

Quantity		
Normal	**Abnormal**	**Significance**
1000–1500 ml (approx. 95% H_2O)		Depends on water and fluid, foods consumed, exercise, temperature, kidney function
	High (polyuria)	Diabetes mellitus, diabetes insipidus, nervous diseases, certain types of chronic nephritis (kidney disorder), diuretics (e.g., caffeine, digitalis) causing increased urinary excretion
	Low (oliguria)	Acute nephritis, heart disease, fevers, eclampsia, diarrhea, vomiting, inadequate fluid intake
	None (anuria)	Uremia (nitrogenous wastes in blood), acute nephritis, metal poisoning (e.g., due to bichloride of mercury), complete obstruction of urinary tract

Color		
Normal	**Abnormal**	**Significance**
Yellow to amber		Depends on concentration of pigment (urochrome)
	Pale	Diabetes insipidus; due to a very dilute urine
	Milky	Fat globules, pus in genitourinary infections
	Reddish	Blood pigments, drugs, or food pigments
	Greenish	Bile pigment, associated with jaundice
	Brown-black	Poisoning (mercury, lead, phenol), hemorrhage

Transparency		
Normal	**Abnormal**	**Significance**
Clear		Normal
Cloudy on standing		Precipitation of mucin from urinary tract; not pathological
Turbid		Precipitation of calcium phosphate; not pathological
	Milky	Presence of fat globules; pathological
	Turbid	Presence of pus due to inflammation of urinary tract; pathological

Odor		
Normal	**Abnormal**	**Significance**
Faintly aromatic		Normal
	Pleasant (sweet)	Acetone, associated with diabetes mellitus
	Unpleasant	Decomposition or ingestion of certain drugs or foods
Peppermint		Menthol ingestion
Acrid		Asparagus in diet
Spicy		Ingestion of sandalwood oil or saffron

Proteinuria		
Normal	**Abnormal**	**Significance**
Albumin and globulin		Excretion of 10–100 mg each 24 hr is normal but this amount is not detected by usual tests
	Albumin	Evidence of altered renal function; may be due to renal pathology or a systemic disease such as diabetes mellitus
	Globulin	Bence Jones proteins associated with multiple myeloma and diseases of globulin metabolism. Other types of globulins may be present in acute and chronic pyelonephritis

Table continued on following page

Table 5–1 Significance of Changes in Urine (*Continued*)

Specific Gravity		
Normal	**Abnormal**	**Significance**
1.010–1.025 specific gravity; can vary in the absence of pathology		Ordinary; specific gravity inversely proportional to volume
	Low (chronic)	Dilution if volume is large; otherwise nephritis
	High (chronic)	Acute nephritis; concentrated if volume is small; otherwise, if light colored and volume is large, diabetes mellitus

Acidity		
Normal	**Abnormal**	**Significance**
Acid (slight)		Diet of acid-forming foods (meats, eggs, prunes, wheat) overbalances the base-forming foods (vegetables and fruits)
	High acidity	Acidosis, diabetes mellitus, many pathological disorders (fevers, starvation)
	Alkaline	Vegetarian diet changes urea into ammonium carbonate; infection or ingestion of alkaline compounds

Source: Thomas, CL (ed): Taber's Cyclopedic Medical Dictionary, ed 18. FA Davis, Philadelphia, 1997, pp 2039–2040, with permission.

renal failure, **uremia,** and eventual death, usually within 10 years.

PREVENTION No prevention is known. Genetic counseling may be indicated for families at risk.

◼ PYELONEPHRITIS (Acute)

DESCRIPTION *Pyelonephritis,* also called *infective tubulointerstitial nephritis,* is inflammation of the kidney and renal pelvis due to infection. One or both kidneys may be affected. The infection can result in the destruction or scarring of renal tissue, impairing kidney function. It is the most common type of kidney disease and is far more common in women than in men. The higher incidence of acute pyelonephritis in women may be due in part to the anatomic difference between men and women. Because the female urethra is shorter and the urinary meatus is closer to the rectum in women, bacteria have less distance to travel to reach the bladder.

ETIOLOGY Pyelonephritis is most commonly due to infection by the bacteria *Escherichia coli. E. coli* is a normal intestinal bacteria that grows rapidly. It is found in fecal matter. Staphylococcal and streptococcal bacteria are less frequent agents of infection.

The bacteria typically ascend to the kidneys from the lower urinary tract, but they also may enter the kidneys through the blood or lymph.

Women are most at risk, particularly, those who are pregnant or practice poor genital hygiene. In men, pyelonephritis may arise as a complication of prostate enlargement. Any catheterization of the urinary tract also increases the likelihood of infection.

SIGNS AND SYMPTOMS The individual experiencing acute pyelonephritis may complain of nausea, vomiting, diarrhea, chills, fever, and lumbar pain. These symptoms may be accompanied by **pyuria, dysuria,** and **nocturia.** The patient often looks quite ill and reports that the symptoms appeared rapidly.

DIAGNOSTIC PROCEDURES The physical examination may reveal tenderness during palpation of abdominal or lumbar areas. Culture and sensitivity tests are performed on a clean-catch urine specimen, which may appear cloudy and have a "fishy" odor. Urinalysis also may reveal **casts,** white blood cells, bacteria, and hematuria. X-ray studies, such as of kidney, ureter, and bladder (KUB), and excretory urography may be necessary.

TREATMENT Antibiotic therapy, appropriate to the infecting organism, is the treatment of choice. **Antipyretics** may be ordered for fever. An increase in liquids is helpful.

PROGNOSIS The prognosis is variable but usually good with proper treatment and follow-up care. Acute pyelonephritis frequently subsides in a few days, even without treatment with antibiotics. Reinfection is likely, however, for persons of high risk, such as those with prolonged use of an indwelling catheter. Repeated infection may lead to a chronic form of the disease, causing enough destruction of kidney tissue to produce renal failure.

PREVENTION Individuals should practice proper genital hygiene to avoid introducing bacteria into the urinary tract. If the disease recurs, it would be helpful to determine any factor that might predispose a person to recurrent infection.

■ GLOMERULONEPHRITIS (Acute)

DESCRIPTION *Glomerulonephritis,* which is the allergic inflammation of the glomeruli in the kidney's nephrons, is also known as *acute poststreptococcal glomerulonephritis* (APSGN). It usually follows a streptococcal infection of the respiratory tract. The rate of filtration of the blood is reduced, causing retention of water and salts. Resulting injury to the glomeruli may allow red blood cells and serum protein to pass into the urine. Both kidneys are affected.

ETIOLOGY The disease is caused by circulating antigen-antibody complexes that become trapped within the network of the capillaries of a glomerulus. The complexes are produced as a consequence of an infection elsewhere in the body, most frequently following an infection of the upper respiratory tract or the middle ear by streptococcal bacteria. The interval between the original infection and the glomerulonephritis may be 2 weeks or more. Other bacteria, however, and certain viruses and parasites, also may induce glomerulonephritis. This suggests that it is an immunologic inflammatory response, as described in Chapter 1. The disease also may arise as a consequence of various multisystem diseases such as lupus erythematosus. (See Chapter 12.)

SIGNS AND SYMPTOMS There may be headaches from secondary hypertension, puffy eyes due to **edema** from leaky, inflamed capillaries; pain in the lumbar region from swollen kidneys, and **oliguria** due to the nephron damage. There also may be **malaise, anorexia,** and a low-grade fever.

DIAGNOSTIC PROCEDURES A detailed medical history is important and may reveal a recent streptococcal infection of the upper respiratory tract. Blood tests may show elevated blood urea nitrogen, creatinine, and a rapid sedimentation rate. The nitrogen and creatinine are present in the blood because these final products of decomposition cannot be excreted in normal amounts. Urine may be described as "bloody," "coffee-colored," or "smoky." Urinalysis will show hematuria and proteinuria. KUB x-rays may reveal bilateral kidney enlargement. A renal biopsy may be necessary to confirm the diagnosis. New methods of fluorescent and electron microscopy have been helpful in distinguishing between different forms of glomerulonephritis.

TREATMENT Treatment goals are generally supportive. The physician may prescribe diuretics to control edema and hypertension. Bed rest is usually indicated. Dietary restrictions on salt, protein, and fluid intake may be advised. If an underlying streptococcal infection can be confirmed, antibiotics may be prescribed.

PROGNOSIS The prognosis is generally good. Most patients with acute glomerulonephritis experience a resolution of symptoms within a few weeks of onset. Children generally recover more rapidly than adults. A few cases, though, may progress into a chronic form of the disease. Repeated acute attacks also may induce the onset of chronic glomerulonephritis.

PREVENTION Prompt treatment of any streptococcal pharyngitis or other upper respiratory tract infection is important.

■ NEPHROTIC SYNDROME

DESCRIPTION *Nephrotic syndrome* is a condition or a complex of signs and symptoms (syndrome) of the basement membrane of the glomerulus. (The basement membrane surrounds each of the many fine capillaries comprising a glomerulus.) The disease is characterized by severe **proteinuria,** often to the extent that the body cannot keep up with the protein loss (**hypoalbuminemia**). The disease is further characterized by **hyperlipemia, lipiduria,** and generalized edema.

ETIOLOGY Nephrotic syndrome may result from a variety of disease processes having the capacity to damage the basement membrane of the glomerulus. Between 70 and 75 percent of the cases of nephrotic syndrome result from some form of glomerulonephritis. The syndrome also may arise as a consequence of diabetes mellitus, systemic lupus erythematosus, neoplasms, or reactions to drugs or toxins. The disease is occasionally idiopathic in origin.

SIGNS AND SYMPTOMS Edema is the most common symptom, and it may be either slow in onset or sudden. As body fluid accumulates, the patient may experience shortness of breath and anorexia. **Ascites,** hypertension, **pallor,** and fatigue may result.

DIAGNOSTIC PROCEDURES Nephrotic syndrome may be difficult to diagnose. Urinalysis may reveal proteinuria and increased waxy, fatty, granular casts. Blood serum tests may show decreased albumin levels and increased cholesterol. Renal biopsy is important in reaching a definitive diagnosis.

TREATMENT Treatment is symptomatic and supportive. The physician will attempt to manage the edema and hyperlipemia. High-protein diets, vitamin supplementation, and salt restriction may be prescribed. Any underlying disease or condition determined to be responsible for the nephrotic syndrome must be treated as well. Corticosteroids may be prescribed. Some people will recover spontaneously.

PROGNOSIS The prognosis varies according to the underlying cause and the age of the client. The prognosis is good for children. With adults, nephrotic syndrome is frequently a manifestation of a serious, progressive kidney disorder or of a disorder elsewhere in the body leading to renal failure. Renal vein thrombosis is a complication that significantly worsens the prognosis.

PREVENTION Nephrotic syndrome·may sometimes be avoided through prompt diagnosis and treatment of underlying disorders with the capacity to produce this syndrome.

■ CHRONIC RENAL FAILURE (Uremia)

DESCRIPTION *Chronic renal failure* (CRF) is the gradual, progressive deterioration of kidney function. As the kidney tissue is progressively destroyed, the kidney loses its ability to excrete the nitrogenous end products of metabolism such as **urea** and **creatinine,** which accumulate in the blood, eventually reaching toxic levels (thus the alternate name *uremia*). As kidney function diminishes, every organ in the body is affected, accounting for the loss of symptoms presented by an individual with CRF.

ETIOLOGY Diabetes mellitus and hypertensive renal disease are the leading causes of CRF. Chronic glomerulonephritis, which was previously the leading cause of CRF, is now usually controlled with aggressive treatment.

SIGNS AND SYMPTOMS The patient may complain of progressive weakness and lethargy, weight loss, anorexia, diarrhea, hiccups, **pruritus,** and **polyuria.** The individual with CRF also may appear mentally confused and have skin that is pallid and scaly. The severity of signs and symptoms varies depending on the extent of the renal damage and remaining function.

DIAGNOSTIC PROCEDURES The history may reveal a previous renal disease or other predisposing disorder. The physical examination may reveal one or more of the presenting signs and symptoms, along with hypertension. Blood testing typically reveals elevated serum creatinine, blood urea nitrogen, and potassium levels, along with decreased hemoglobin and hematocrit. Urinalysis may reveal proteinuria and urine that is highly diluted. X-rays such as KUB, intravenous pyelogram (IVP), and renal scintiscans may be done to determine the extent of renal damage.

TREATMENT Treatment is generally directed at relieving symptoms and guarding against complications. Dietary restrictions of protein, sodium, and potassium intake may be attempted. **Antiemetics** may be prescribed for nausea. Hypertension must be controlled. Dialysis or kidney transplantation may be attempted to prolong life.

PROGNOSIS The prognosis is poor, with an alteration in function of virtually every organ system in the body. A variety of complications often cause death before complete kidney failure occurs. Chief among these are infections; others include a spectrum of cardiovascular, blood, and gastrointestinal abnormalities.

PREVENTION No prevention is known, other than prompt treatment of underlying disorders that may eventually lead to chronic renal failure.

◼ ACUTE TUBULAR NECROSIS (ATN)

DESCRIPTION *Acute tubular necrosis* is the rapid destruction or degeneration of the tubular segments of nephrons in the kidneys. ATN is characterized by a sudden deterioration in renal function, with resulting accumulation of nitrogenous wastes in the body. Impaired or interrupted renal function from ATN is considered reversible.

ETIOLOGY The majority of cases of ATN are due to renal **ischemia,** the interruption or impairment of blood flow in and out of the kidneys. ATN is the most common cause of acute renal failure in critically ill persons. Although there can be numerous causes for such impairment, renal ischemia leading to ATN is most frequently produced by severe bodily trauma or as a complication following surgery. The renal tubules also can be damaged in other ways. ATN may be toxin-induced (as a result of exposure to solvents, heavy metals, or certain antibiotics). It also may be caused by transfusion reactions or arise as a complication of pregnancy.

SIGNS AND SYMPTOMS Because renal failure affects the function of nearly every organ in the body, the individual with ATN may have a host of widely distributed symptoms. Principal symptoms include oliguria and **hyperkalemia.** Other generalized symptoms include weakness, mental confusion, and edema.

DIAGNOSTIC PROCEDURES A history of chronic and debilitating illness, trauma, surgery, transfusion, or pregnancy complications may indicate a risk for ATN. The clinician also may seek to determine if the individual could have been exposed to any toxins or was taking certain antibiotics. The clinician will attempt to eliminate any underlying kidney diseases or urinary tract obstructions as possible causes for the renal failure. Diagnostic tests ordered may include urinalysis, which for ATN reveals dilute urine with red blood cells and casts. Blood tests will often indicate increased blood urea nitrogen and creatinine, or reveal disturbances in the electrolyte balance of the blood. Most of the time, diagnosis occurs when the disease is more advanced.

TREATMENT The clinician will generally attempt to promote proper renal circulation if the ATN is due to ischemia. If the ATN is toxin-induced, dialysis may be attempted to cleanse the blood. Otherwise, treatment is largely supportive until kidney function increases. Supportive treatment may include dietary modifications and careful control of fluid intake. Dialysis may be indicated to allow the kidneys to rest and to improve conditions for regeneration.

PROGNOSIS The prognosis is guarded. Before adequate renal function resumes (highly variable period), many individuals with ATN die from complications. These may include cardiovascular complications, gastrointestinal disorders, blood abnormalities, and infections.

PREVENTION Prevention includes avoiding exposure to toxins and careful monitoring of individuals known to be at risk.

◼ RENAL CALCULI (Uroliths or Kidney Stones)

DESCRIPTION A *renal calculus* is a concentration of various mineral salts in the renal pelvis or **calyces** of the kidney or elsewhere in the urinary tract (Fig. 5–4). Most stones are from calcium salts, uric acid, cystine, and struvite, in descending order of frequency.

ETIOLOGY Renal calculi form as a result of a disturbance in the kidney's delicate balancing act of preventing water loss while at the same time eliminating water-soluble mineral wastes. Many factors, such as prolonged dehydration or immobilization, can upset this balance. The balance also may be upset by underlying diseases such as gout, **hyperparathyroidism,** Cushing's syndrome, or urinary tract infections and neoplasms. A person may develop renal calculi because of an excessive intake of vitamin D or dietary calcium. The condition appears to be hereditary for certain types of stones, with men much more commonly affected than women. In many instances, no specific cause can be pinpointed.

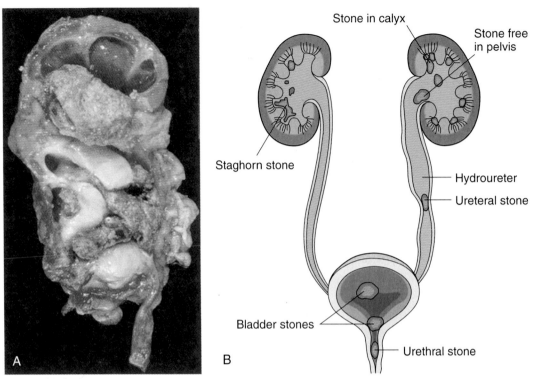

Figure 5–4 (*A*) Staghorn calculi, the kidney shows hydronephrosis and stones that are casts of the dilated calyces. (From Rubin, E, and Farber, JL [eds]: Pathology, ed 3. Lippincott-Raven, Philadelphia, 1999, p 909, with permission.) (*B*) Location of calculi in the urinary tract. (From Williams, LS, and Hopper, PD [eds]: Understanding Medical-Surgical Nursing. FA Davis, Philadelphia, 1999, p 691, with permission.)

SIGNS AND SYMPTOMS A person having renal calculi may remain asymptomatic for long periods. If a stone or calculus fragment lodges in a ureter, however, the individual may complain of intense flank pain and urinary urgency. If calculi are in the renal pelvis and calyces, the pain is duller and more constant. Back pain and severe abdominal pain may occur. Other presenting symptoms include nausea, vomiting, chills and fever, hematuria, and abdominal distention.

DIAGNOSTIC PROCEDURES The history may reveal a familial tendency toward the formation of kidney stones. A urinalysis may be ordered to detect elevated levels of red or white blood cells in the urine or to check for the presence of protein, pus, and bacteria. A KUB x-ray or IVP may be ordered to determine the locations of calculus formation. Blood testing may be helpful in confirming imbalances of minerals in the blood or the existence of other metabolic disorders.

TREATMENT Treatment is directed at clearing obstructive stones and preventing the formation of new ones. Increased fluid intake (more than 3 liters per day) may enhance elimination of stones in some cases, but large stones may require surgical intervention, especially if renal function is threatened. Techniques such as ultrasonic percutaneous lithotripsy and extracorporeal shock wave lithotripsy pulverize stones in place, allow them to be passed in the urine or removed by suction. Lithotripsy via a ureteroscope can also be used to remove urethral stones. Antibiotics may be prescribed if it is determined that the calculus buildup is due to bacterial infection. Analgesics may be necessary for relief of intense pain.

PROGNOSIS The prognosis is good if urinary tract obstruction is prevented, and underlying disorders are promptly treated. However, about 60 percent of people who have a calcium stone have further stone formation later.

PREVENTION An adequate daily fluid intake is the best way to minimize the chance of stone formation, especially among individuals at risk. Fruit juices, especially cranberry juice, help acidify urine and may help prevent the formation of renal calculi.

HYDRONEPHROSIS

DESCRIPTION **Hydronephrosis** is the distension of the renal pelvis and calyces of a kidney due to pressure from accumulating urine. The pressure impairs, and may eventually interrupt, kidney function. One or both kidneys may be affected.

ETIOLOGY Hydronephrosis is caused by a urinary tract obstruction. The ureters and renal pelvis dilate proximal to, or behind, the obstruction. This swelling causes the hydronephrosis with resultant destruction of functional tissue. In children, the obstruction is usually the result of some congenital defect in urinary tract structure. In adults, the obstruction is more often acquired, resulting from blockage by **uroliths** or neoplasms. Urinary tract obstruction in men may be produced by benign or malignant enlargement of the prostate. Women may experience urinary tract obstruction as a complication of pregnancy. Underlying disorders, such as neurogenic bladder, also may allow urine to accumulate to the extent that it produces hydronephrosis.

SIGNS AND SYMPTOMS If the obstruction is above the opening of the bladder, only one kidney may be affected and the person may be asymptomatic for a prolonged period ("silent" hydronephrosis). Symptoms may be severe, however, especially if both kidneys are affected. The person may complain of intense flank pain, nausea, vomiting, oliguria or anuria, and hematuria.

DIAGNOSTIC PROCEDURES A thorough physical examination of all urogenital structures will be performed. Palpation and percussion of the abdomen may reveal distention of the kidney or urinary bladder. A history of changes in urinary volume, difficulty in voiding, and pain may be found. Ultrasound may be ordered to visualize obstructions. An excretory urogram may be ordered to further define the site of obstruction. If necessary, a retrograde or antegrade urography may be attempted. Urinalysis may reveal hematuria, pus, and bacteria, and may be helpful in determining the extent of any impairment of renal function.

TREATMENT Treatment goals include removing the obstruction, preventing complications, and treating underlying disorders. Catheterization may be attempted for the immediate relief of urinary pressure. Analgesics may be prescribed. Antibiotics are required if infection occurs. Surgery is sometimes required to dilate a ureteral stricture. Treatment procedures for renal stones were discussed in the preceding section.

PROGNOSIS The prognosis is variable, depending on whether one or both kidneys are affected, whether the obstruction can be removed, and whether permanent renal damage has occurred.

PREVENTION There are no specific preventative measures.

Lower Urinary Tract Diseases

CYSTITIS AND URETHRITIS

DESCRIPTION *Cystitis,* inflammation of the bladder, and *urethritis,* inflammation of the urethra, are common lower urinary tract infections (UTIs). Together these diseases account for the majority of physician visits by individuals experiencing urinary tract problems.

ETIOLOGY Infection by the bacteria *Escherichia coli* accounts for most cases of cystitis and urethritis. Other causative organisms may include *Proteus, Klebsiella, Enterobacter,* and *Pseudomonas* bacteria. These organisms typically ascend the urinary tract from the opening of the urethra, but they also may be introduced as a result of urinary tract catheterization. Urethritis also may be caused by sexually transmitted organisms such as *Chlamydia trachomatis* and *Neisseria gonorrhoeae* (the agents of chlamydia and gonorrhea, respectively).

Women are 10 times more susceptible to ascending urinary tract infections than men (except for men older than 50 years of age). This is due in part to a shorter urethra in women and the comparative ease with which fecal contaminants can be spread from the anus to the opening of the vagina. Women who are sexually active are more predisposed to cystitis, because sexual intercourse enhances the bacterial transfer from the urethra into the bladder. Finally, both women and men are more at risk of contracting a lower urinary tract infection as a complication of any disorder that obstructs normal urinary flow.

SIGNS AND SYMPTOMS Signs and symptoms cannot be relied upon for the diagnosis or localization of a urinary tract infection. Some individuals may present with few symptoms, yet have significant bacteriuria. The person presenting with cystitis may complain of dysuria, urinary frequency and urgency, and pain above the pubic region. Cloudy, bloody, or foul-smelling urine also may be noted. The individual with urethritis will typically present similar symptoms, with the exception that the quality of the urine is often not affected. Any other symptoms, such as fever, nausea, vomiting, and low back pain, may indicate a simultaneous upper UTI such as pyelonephritis.

DIAGNOSTIC PROCEDURES The medical history may reveal past urinary tract infections, recent catheterization, or a change in sexual partners. A urine culture is necessary to identify the organism responsible for the infection. The presence of red and white blood cells in the urine sample is also an indicator. Sensitivity tests are necessary to prescribe the appropriate antimicrobial agent.

TREATMENT Antibiotics or sulfa drugs appropriate to combat the particular causative organisms may be prescribed. Fluid intake may be increased to promote urinary outflow. Analgesics may be prescribed for short-term pain relief. The physician may also prescribe urinary antiseptics and antispasmodics for the relief of bladder spasms.

PROGNOSIS If no complications arise, the prognosis for complete recovery from cystitis and urethritis is quite good. If the disease is uncomplicated, infections of the lower urinary tract usually respond to short courses of therapy, whereas those of the upper urinary tract require a longer course of treatment. Reinfection in susceptible individuals is likely, however.

PREVENTION Preventive measures include maintaining adequate fluid intake, complete emptying of the bladder, and avoiding "holding urine." Proper feminine hygiene, including wiping the perineum from front to back and cleansing well after a bowel movement, will lessen the chance of introducing disease-causing microorganisms into the urethra. Women with a history of lower UTI also may be placed on a long-term course of antibiotics. Fruit juices, especially cranberry juice, may help acidify urine. Most bacteria grow poorly in an acid environment.

■ NEUROGENIC BLADDER

DESCRIPTION *Neurogenic bladder* is any loss or impairment of bladder function caused by central nervous system injury or by damage to nerves supplying the bladder. Impaired bladder function may be manifested as either loss of voluntary control of **micturition** or loss of the autonomic reflex, producing the sensation that the bladder is full.

ETIOLOGY Physical trauma to the spinal cord is a frequent cause of neurogenic bladder. Other causes may include nerve damage as a consequence of chronic alcoholism or heavy-metal poisoning. Metabolic disorders (such as diabetes mellitus or hypothyroidism) and collagen diseases (such as systemic lupus erythematosus) may cause this disorder. Neurogenic bladder may arise as a consequence of multiple sclerosis, **dementia,** and Parkinson's disease.

SIGNS AND SYMPTOMS An individual with neurogenic bladder may complain of mild to severe urinary **incontinence,** inability to empty the bladder completely, difficulty in starting or stopping voiding, and bladder spasms.

DIAGNOSTIC PROCEDURES Neurogenic bladder often is difficult to diagnose. A detailed history and a physical examination that includes a neurological evaluation are essential. Special tests that may be ordered include a cystourethrograph to evaluate bladder function; a urine flow study to assess urine flow; and a sphincter electromyelograph to evaluate how well the bladder and urinary sphincter muscles work together.

TREATMENT Treatment goals include preventing complications from urinary tract infection and controlling incontinence through learning special bladder evacuation techniques. The physician may recommend one of two common methods of evacuation to patients who are unable to empty the bladder completely. In *Credé's method,* the patient presses on the lower abdomen while voiding. The second method, *intermittent self-catheterization,* requires the patient to insert a catheter into his or her bladder through the urethra.

Any underlying diseases that are detected will be treated. Various forms of drug therapy or surgery may be attempted to restore bladder function.

PROGNOSIS The prognosis depends on whether the damage to the nerves supplying the bladder is reversible. Such complications as urinary tract infections and the formation of renal calculi worsen the prognosis. If the disorder is of the form in which sensation of a full bladder is lost, urine may back up, causing **hydronephrosis** and possible renal failure.

PREVENTION There is no specific prevention other than prompt treatment of diseases that may produce the nerve damage that leads to neurogenic bladder.

Tumors of the Urinary System

Tumors of the urinary tract may be benign or malignant; however, small benign adenomas or fibromas are not clinically significant. The most common malignant tumor of the kidney is adenocarcinoma. Tumors of the lower urinary tract are more common than those of the kidney and will be discussed after adenocarcinoma.

ADENOCARCINOMA OF THE KIDNEY
(Hypernephroma)

DESCRIPTION *Adenocarcinoma of the kidney,* or *hypernephroma,* is an uncommon malignant neoplasm of the epithelium of a nephron's proximal convoluted tubule. The disease frequently metastasizes to the lungs, liver, brain, and bone marrow.

ETIOLOGY The cause of hypernephroma is not known, but there appears to be a genetic predisposition to the disease. Other risk factors may include exposure to smoke or heavy metals. Adenocarcinoma tends to occur more frequently in men than in women, especially in later midlife.

SIGNS AND SYMPTOMS An affected individual typically remains asymptomatic until later stages of the disease. Gross, painless hematuria is the most common presenting symptom. Later on, the individual may report intermittent fever and flank pain.

DIAGNOSTIC PROCEDURES Physical examination may reveal a palpably enlarged kidney in later stages of the disease; x-ray examination may confirm this.

IVP and CT scan of the kidney may be employed to confirm the presence of a renal tumor.

TREATMENT **Nephrectomy** is a common treatment procedure, whether or not the tumor has metastasized. If it is determined that **metastasis** has occurred, radiation therapy may be attempted and various palliative measures, such as analgesia, will be undertaken.

PROGNOSIS The prognosis varies, depending on the staging of the tumor. The 5-year survival rate is about 59 percent, but the 10-year survival rate is lower.[1]

PREVENTION No prevention is known.

TUMORS OF THE BLADDER

DESCRIPTION *Tumors of the bladder* arise from the epithelial cell membrane lining the bladder interior. These neoplasms are almost always malignant, and they metastasize readily. Bladder tumors are staged according to their depth of penetration.

ETIOLOGY The cause of bladder tumors is unknown. Predisposing factors may include exposure to certain types of industrial chemicals, and there is an association with cigarette smoking. Individuals with chronic cystitis also seem prone to develop bladder tumors. The disease affects men three times more frequently than women and generally appears after the age of 50. Bladder cancer is the fourth most common cancer in men.

SIGNS AND SYMPTOMS Many persons are asymptomatic until advanced stages of the disease. For those presenting with symptoms, however, painless, gross hematuria is the most common indicator. Less frequently, the individual may complain of dysuria, urinary frequency and urgency, or nocturia.

DIAGNOSTIC PROCEDURES The history may reveal occupational exposure to certain industrial chemicals. A complete physical examination and a urinalysis to detect hematuria will be performed. Cystoscopy and biopsy of the suspected lesions are usually required to reach a definite diagnosis. A bone scan will help determine possible metastases. A CT scan may be ordered to help diagnose the tumor.

TREATMENT The choice of treatment is based on the extent of the disease. If the disease is superficial, an endoscopic resection may be all that is necessary. If it is invasive, further surgery is required. The tumor may be surgically removed by **transurethral resection** or fulguration (electrical destruction). For advanced cases, radical **cystectomy** may be required, followed by radiation or chemotherapy treatment.

PROGNOSIS The prognosis varies, depending on the depth of penetration of the tumor. Although the immediate prognosis for an individual with a superficial bladder tumor may be good, there is still a great likelihood of recurrence within 3 years. When the tumor penetrates the bladder more deeply or has metastasized, the prognosis is poor, with a low 5-year survival rate.

PREVENTION The best prevention is to minimize risk factors by protecting oneself from exposure to industrial chemicals and by not smoking.

SPECIAL FOCUS TREATMENT OF RENAL FAILURE

Whether or not to begin or continue dialysis or use transplantation is debated among medical professionals. Most agree, however, that persons with acute renal failure should have dialysis to allow renal function to return. Transplantation should be considered only when less conservative treatment has not succeeded and the person's renal failure is nonreversible. The transplantation, however, must be done before the person is critically ill or death is imminent.

Dialysis

The blood of an individual experiencing acute or chronic renal failure typically contains high concentrations of metabolic waste products. Dialysis may be attempted to remove these wastes. In its broadest sense, *dialysis* is a process in which water-soluble substances diffuse across a semipermeable membrane. Renal dialysis involves diffusing dissolved substances in the blood across such a semipermeable membrane to remove toxic materials and to maintain proper fluid, electrolyte, and acid-base balances. Most patients have 9 to 12 hours of dialysis per week, equally divided between several sessions. Factors determining the amount of dialysis include the patient's size, dietary intake, illnesses, and remaining renal function.[2] Two methods are currently used to dialyze the blood: *peritoneal dialysis* and *hemodialysis*.

Peritoneal Dialysis

This process uses a person's own peritoneum as the dialyzing membrane. A plastic tube is inserted through the patient's abdomen into the peritoneal cavity and sutured in place. A dialyzing fluid is passed through the tube into the person's peritoneal cavity and left there for a prescribed period. During this time, wastes diffuse across the peritoneal membrane into the fluid. The contaminated fluid is then drained and replaced with fresh solution (Fig. 5–5). This process can be performed manually or automatically by machine; generally, it is repeated three times a week or as often as required. This type of dialysis may be continuous or intermittent and is easier than hemodialysis for individuals to perform on themselves.

Hemodialysis (Extracorporeal Hemodialysis)

In this process, blood is drawn outside the person's body for dialysis in an artificial kidney, or *dialyzer,* and then returned to the individual by means of tubes connected to the person's circulatory system (Fig. 5–6). This form of dialysis treatment takes from 3 to 5 hours, about half the time of peritoneal dialysis. It is the pre-

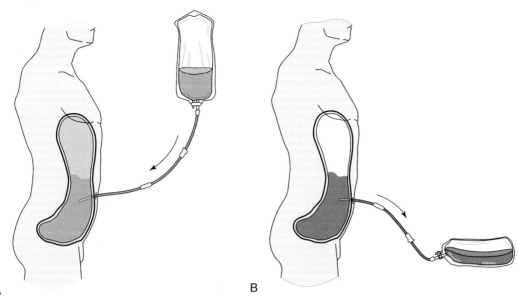

A   B

Figure 5–5 (*A*) Peritoneal dialysis works inside the body. Dialysis solution flows through a tube into the abdominal cavity, where it collects waste products from the blood. (*B*) Periodically, the used dialysis solution is drained from the abdominal cavity, carrying away waste products and excess water from the blood. (From Williams, LS, and Hopper, PD [eds]: Understanding Medical-Surgical Nursing. FA Davis, Philadelphia, 1999, p 707, with permission.)

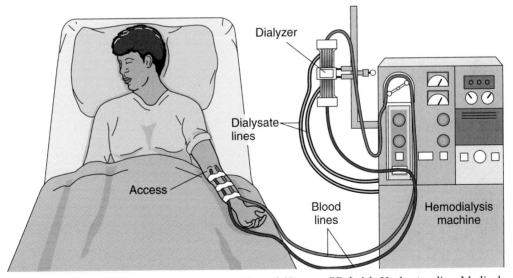

Figure 5–6 Hemodialysis. (From Williams, LS, and Hopper, PD [eds]: Understanding Medical-Surgical Nursing. FA Davis, Philadelphia, 1999, p 705, with permission.)

ferred dialysis method in cases of acute renal failure.

Kidney Transplantation

At times, physicians approach treatment of serious kidney disease with a combination of dialysis and transplantation. The results, in many instances, have been promising. Kidney transplantation is being used increasingly, despite the technical and immunologic risks associated with the procedure.

The donor of a kidney can be either a close relative of the person receiving the kidney or a recently deceased person (cadaver donor). If the donor and recipient are related, the graft has a better chance of survival.

Every transplanted kidney contains antigens foreign to the recipient, unless it is donated by an identical twin. Once the donor antigens are in the recipient, a rejection process begins, in which the recipient's immune system produces antibodies that lead to the destruction of the tissue of the transplanted kidney. Immunosuppressive drugs may be administered to combat this process. Still, some recipients may reject the kidney. Once rejection occurs, the donated kidney is removed, and the patient must resume dialysis.

For those persons who do not reject the donor kidney, life can seem relatively normal. Immunosuppressive drugs must be continued indefinitely, however, making the person more susceptible to infections and other diseases. Sometimes, too, the underlying disease process that destroyed the original kidney may destroy the donor kidney as well.

COMMON SYMPTOMS OF URINARY SYSTEM DISEASES

Individuals may present with the following common complaints, which deserve attention from health professionals:

- Any change in normal urinary patterns, such as nocturia, hematuria, pyuria, proteinuria, dysuria, or urgency and frequency
- Pain in the lumbar region or flank pain, varying from slight tenderness to intense pain
- Fever
- Nausea and vomiting or anorexia
- Malaise, fatigue, and lethargy

Serious urinary system diseases also may produce circulatory system and respiratory system symptoms. These symptoms might include hypertension, edema, ascites, and shortness of breath.

REFERENCES

1. Professional Guide to Diseases, ed 6. Springhouse Corporation, Springhouse, Pa., 1998, p 90.
2. Fauci, AS, et al: Harrison's Principles of Internal Medicine, ed 14. McGraw-Hill, New York, 1998, p 1521.

BIBLIOGRAPHY

Crowley, LV: Introduction to Human Diseases, ed 3. Jones & Bartlett, Boston, 1992.
Walter, JB: An Introduction to the Principles of Disease. WB Saunders, Philadelphia, 1992.

CASE STUDIES

I A 27-year-old man comes into an ambulatory care facility complaining of extreme flank pain and frequent urination. The physician asks if he has noted any difference in the color or appearance of his urine, and the client reports that he has noted some bits that look like sand in his urine. He also says he recently was treated for a urinary tract infection.

1. What diagnostic tests might the physician order?
2. What are some effective preventative measures for urinary disease?

II A 35-year-old woman reports pain upon urination, pain in the pubic area, and the need for frequent urination. She also says that the need to urinate is urgent, and that her urine is foul-smelling.

1. When this person comes to the ambulatory care setting, what questions will you ask?
2. What tests do you think the physician will order for this person?
3. What preventative measure could this person take in the future?

REVIEW QUESTIONS

MULTIPLE CHOICE

Select the best answer:

1. The kidney is responsible for:

    a. Regulation of body fluids

    b. Filtration of wastes from blood

    c. Regulation of blood pressure

    d. All of the above

    e. Only a and b

2. Of the fluid that passes through the nephron, _____ percent becomes urine.

    a. 1

    b. 5

    c. 10

    d. 50

    e. 98

3. Urinary tract infections:

    a. Are more common in males

    b. Usually exhibit dysuria, urgency, and frequency

   c. Commonly are caused by a virus

   d. Do not respond to antibiotic therapy

   e. Have a poor prognosis

4. The two forms of dialysis are:

   a. Peritoneal and hemodialysis

   b. Perineal and hemodialysis

   c. Peritoneal and extracorpeal

   d. Perineal and extracorpeal

   e. a and c

5. The inability to control urine excretion is called:

   a. Incontinence

   b. Micturition

   c. Ischemia

   d. Anuria

   e. Nocturia

MATCHING

_____ 1. Nocturia

_____ 2. APSGN

_____ 3. KUB

_____ 4. Ascites

_____ 5. Uremia

_____ 6. Micturition

_____ 7. Pruritus

_____ 8. Pyuria

_____ 9. Oliguria

_____ 10. Hematuria

a. Acute poststreptotocccal glomerulonephritis
b. Accumulation of serous fluid in abdominal cavity
c. Blood in urine
d. Urination
e. Excessive urination at night
f. Kidneys, ureters, and bladder
g. Scanty urine
h. Urine in blood
i. Pus in urine
j. Itching

FILL IN THE BLANKS

Select from the following:

nephrotic syndrome
pyelonephritis
renal calculi
polycystic kidney
uremia

acute tubular necrosis (ATN)
neurogenic bladder
glomerulonephritis
urinary tract infection

1. A disease that exhibits multiple, grapelike, fluid-filled sacs or cysts in the kidney cortex is _____ .

2. When the body cannot keep up with the loss of protein in the urine, the result is _____ .

3. Chronic renal failure is referred to as _____ .

4. The most common cause of acute renal failure is _____ .

5. Intense pain with urinary frequency, nausea, vomiting, fever, hematuria, and flank pain may indicate _____ .

6. A disorder, often difficult to diagnose, that is related to some kind of nerve dysfunction of the bladder is _____ .

7. A procedure in which contrast medium is used and x-rays are taken as the medium from the blood is _____ .

8. The most common type of kidney disease is _____ .

9. Headaches from secondary hypertension and puffy eyes due to edema from leaky capillaries may indicate _____ .

10. UTI refers to _____ .

ANSWERS

MULTIPLE CHOICE

1. d
2. a
3. b

4. e
5. a

MATCHING

1. e
2. a
3. f

4. b
5. h
6. d

7. j
8. i

9. g
10. c

FILL IN THE BLANKS

1. polycystic kidney
2. nephrotic syndrome
3. uremia
4. acute tubular necrosis (ATN)
5. renal calculi

6. neurogenic bladder
7. pyelonephritis
8. glomerulonephritis
9. urinary tract infection

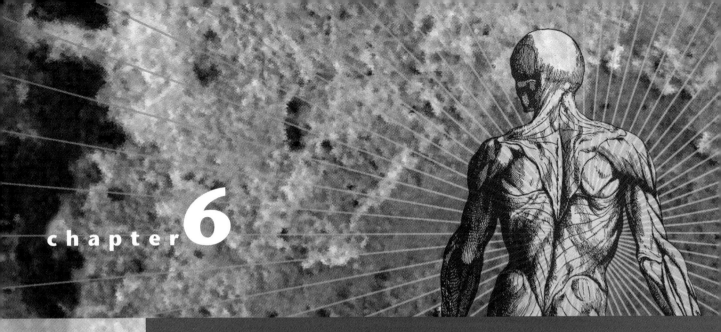

chapter 6

Reproductive System Diseases

CHAPTER OUTLINE

Sexual Dysfunction
Dyspareunia (Painful Intercourse)
Erectile Dysfunction (Impotence)
Arousal and Orgasmic Dysfunction in
    Women
Premature Ejaculation
Male and Female Infertility

Sexually Transmitted Diseases (STDs)
Gonorrhea
Genital Herpes
Genital Warts
Syphilis
Trichomoniasis
Chlamydial Infections
Common Symptoms of STDs

Male Reproductive Diseases
Prostatitis
Epididymitis
Orchitis
Benign Prostatic Hyperplasia (BPH)
Prostatic Cancer
Testicular Cancer
Common Symptoms of Male Reproductive
    Diseases

Female Reproductive Diseases
Premenstrual Syndrome (PMS)

Amenorrhea
Dysmenorrhea
Ovarian Cysts and Tumors
Endometriosis
Uterine Leiomyomas
Pelvic Inflammatory Disease (PID)
Menopause
Abnormal Premenopausal and
    Postmenopausal Bleeding
Common Symptoms of Female Reproductive
    System Diseases

Diseases of the Breasts
Mammary Dysplasia or Fibrocystic Disease
Benign Fibroadenoma
Carcinoma of the Breast

Special Focus: Breast Reconstruction

Disorders of Pregnancy and Delivery
Spontaneous Abortion
Ectopic Pregnancy
Toxemias of Pregnancy (Preeclampsia and
    Eclampsia)
Placenta Previa
Abruptio Placentae
Premature Labor/Premature Rupture of
    Membranes (PROM)
Common Symptoms and Disorders of
    Pregnancy and Delivery

Special Focus: Cesarean Birth

References

Bibliography

Case Studies

Review Questions

LEARNING OBJECTIVES

Upon successful completion of this chapter, you will:

- Describe the twofold function of human sexuality.
- List the three components of sexual health identified by the World Health Organization.
- Discuss the three factors that cause dyspareunia.
- Compare erectile dysfunction (impotence) in males to arousal and to orgasmic dysfunction in females.
- Identify the possible causes of premature ejaculation.
- List the factors that contribute to both female and male fertility.
- Identify the classic symptoms of infertility.
- Discuss diagnostic procedures used to identify infertility in men and women.
- Describe the necessity for a complete sexual history when obtaining a client's medical history.
- List seven sexually transmitted diseases (STDs).
- Contrast the causes of STDs.
- Identify the diseases related to the prostate gland.
- Discuss the complications of prostate-related disorders.
- Restate the common causes of epididymitis and orchitis.
- Compare the diseases related to a woman's menses.
- List the characteristic signs and symptoms of ovarian cysts or tumors.
- Define endometriosis.
- Identify a primary complication of endometriosis.
- Describe the most common tumor in women.
- List the causes of pelvic inflammatory disease.
- Discuss the signs and symptoms of menopause.
- Identify the diagnostic procedures used for diagnosing breast-related diseases.
- List the three reasons for breast reconstruction.
- Recall the possible causes of spontaneous abortion.
- Define ectopic pregnancy.
- Compare preeclampsia to eclampsia.
- Compare placenta previa and abruptio placentae.
- Define PROM.
- List the most common reasons for cesarean birth.
- Recall at least six common complaints of the reproductive system.

KEY WORDS

Alopecia (ăl•ō•pē′shē•ă)
Analgesic (ăn•ăl•jē′sĭk)
Antipyretic (ăn•tĭ•pī•rĕt′ĭk)
Anuria (ăn•ū′rē•ă)
Azoospermia (ă•zō•ō•spēr′mē•ă)
Cervicitis (sĕr•vĭ•sī′tĭs)
Chancre (shăng′kĕr)
Coitus (kō•ī′tŭs)

Conceptus (kŏn•sĕp′tus)
Conization (kŏn•ĭ•zā′shŭn)
Corpus luteum (kŏr′pŭs lū′tē•ŭm)
Cryosurgery (krī•ō•sĕr′jĕr•ē)
Cryptorchidism (krĭpt•ŏr′kĭd•ĭzm)
Débridement (dā•brēd•mĕnt′)
Disseminated intravascular coagulation (dĭs•ĕm′ĭn•ā•tĕd ĭn•tră•văs′kū•lŏr kō•ăg•ū•lā′shŭn)

Dysplasia (dĭs•plā′zē•ă)
Dysuria (dĭs•ū′rē•ă)
Ectopic (ĕk•tŏp′ĭk)
Edema (ĕ•dē′mă)
Effacement (ē•fās′mĕnt)
Electrocautery (ē•lĕk•trō•kăw′tĕr•ē)
Endometrium (ĕn•dō•mē′trē•ŭm)
Erythematous (ĕr•ĭ•thĕm′ă•tŭs)
Follicle-stimulating hormone (fŏl′ĭk•l
    stĭm′ū•lā•tĭng hŏr′mōn)
Gonorrheal ophthalmia neonatorum
    (gŏn•ŏ•rē′ăl ŏf•thăl′mē•ă
    nē•ō•nă•tŏr′ŭm)
Hematuria (hĕm•ă•tū′rē•ă)
Hydrocele (hī′drō•sēl)
Hyperplasia (hī•pĕr•plā′zē•ă)
Hypothyroidism (hī•pō•thī′royd•ĭzm)
Hypovolemic shock (hī•pō•vō•lē′mĭk
    shŏk)
Hysterosalpingography
    (hĭs•tĕr•ō•săl•pĭn•gŏg′ră•fē)
Iatrogenic (ē•ăt•rō•jĕn′ĭk)
Intromission (ĭn•trō•mĭ′shŭn)
Leiomyoma (lī•ō•mī•ō′mă)
Lesion (lē′zhŭn)
Leukorrhea (loo•kō•rē′ă)
Luteinizing hormone (loo•tē′ĭn•ī•zĭng
    hŏr′mōn)
Lymphadenopathy (lĭm•făd•ĕ•nŏp′ă•thē)
Macular (măk′ū•lăr)
Menarche (mĕn•ăr′kē)
Menorrhagia (mĕn•ō•rā′jē•ă)

Metastasize (mĕ•tăs′tă•sīz)
Metrorrhagia (mĕt•rō•rā′jē•ă)
Myalgia (mī•ăl′jē•ă)
Myotonia (mī•ō•tō′nē•ă)
Nystagmus (nĭs•tăg′mŭs)
Oligomenorrhea (ŏl•ĭ•gō•mĕn•ō•rē′ă)
Oligospermia (ŏl•ĭ•gō•spĕr′mē•ă)
Oliguria (ŏl•ĭg•ū′rē•ă)
Orchidectomy (ŏr•kĭ•dĕk′tō•mē)
Panhysterosalpingo-oophorectomy
    (păn•hĭs•tĕr•ō•săl•pĭng•gō•ō•ŏf•ĕr•
    ek′tō•mē)
Papilloma (păp•ĭ•lō′mă)
Papillomatosis (păp•ĭ•lō•mă•tō′sis)
Papillomavirus (păp•ĭ•lō•mă•vī′rus)
Papular (păp′ū•lĕr)
Parity (păr′ĭ•tē)
Parturition (păr•tū•rĭsh′ŭn)
Primigravida (pl. *primigravidae*)
    (prī•mĭ•grăv′ĭ•dă)
Prostaglandins (prŏs′tă•glăn•dĭns)
Prosthesis (prŏs•thē′sĭs)
Purulent (pūr′ū•lĕnt)
Pustule (pŭs′tūl)
Rhonchus (pl. *rhonchi*) (rŏng′kŭs)
Septicemia (sĕp•tĭ•sē′mē•ă)
Stenosis (stĕ•nō′sĭs)
Tachycardia (tăk•ē•kăr′dē•ă)
Teratoma (tĕr•ă•tō′mă)
Varicocele (văr′ĭ•kō•sēl)
Vasoconstriction (văs•ō•kŏn•strĭk′shŭn)
Vesicle (vĕs′ĭ•kl)

The only mammals known to express caring and loving in the sexual act are human beings. For men and women, the function of sexuality is twofold—reproduction and the enhancement of caring and pleasure.

The World Health Organization identifies the following as components of sexual health:[1]

- The enjoyment and control of sexual and reproductive behavior according to personal and social ethics.
- Freedom from fear, shame, guilt, misconceptions, and other psychological factors that inhibit sexual response and can impair sexual relationships.
- Freedom from organic disorders, diseases, and deficiencies that may interfere with either sexual or reproductive functions.

Experiences of arousal, plateau, orgasm, and resolution characterize the stages of the human sexual response cycle. *Arousal,* or excitement, is psychologically determined, whereas the remaining stages have both psychological and physiological components. The major physiological processes of the sexual response cycle include **vasoconstriction** and **myotonia.** Sexual dysfunction may result if some physical or mental condition arises that interferes with any of these stages.

Sexual Dysfunction

An important consideration in the treatment of any sexual dysfunction is a sensitivity to open communication about the problem. Both the client and the physician may have difficulty raising questions regarding sexual functions. If this occurs, dysfunctions may go undetected and untreated.

All health-care professionals need to be alert to individuals' signals and questions that may indicate a sexual concern. Clients often feel more comfortable raising a question with someone other than the physician; therefore, it is important that the physician include a detailed sexual history as part of the medical history. All health professionals need to feel comfortable initiating questions about sexual function. Health care that treats the total person cannot ignore the human sexual response and its function or dysfunction.

■ DYSPAREUNIA (Painful Intercourse)

DESCRIPTION *Dyspareunia* is the occurrence of pain in women during sexual intercourse.

ETIOLOGY Painful intercourse may result from any of the following causes:

- *Anatomic:* Deformities or lesions of the vagina, an intact hymen, or retroversion of the uterus.
- *Pathological:* Scar tissue, genitourinary tract infections, pelvic inflammatory disease, abnormal growths, endometriosis, or allergic reactions to contraceptive materials.
- *Psychosomatic:* Fear of pain or injury, feelings of guilt or shame, lack of arousal resulting in insufficient lubrication, ignorance of sexual anatomy and physiology, or fear of pregnancy.

SIGNS AND SYMPTOMS The individual may experience mild to severe discomfort during or after intercourse. Vaginal itching or burning also may occur.

DIAGNOSTIC PROCEDURES A physical examination will be performed and diagnostic tests ordered to detect any underlying anatomic or pathological causes of the dyspareunia. A detailed sexual history is important to help reveal any psychological factors that may be causing the disorder.

TREATMENT Individuals may be instructed to use creams or water-soluble jellies for lubrication prior to intercourse. Medications may be prescribed if any infections are detected. Excision of any scars and gentle stretching of the vaginal orifice may be needed. Education about the sexual response and counseling or psychotherapy may be indicated.

PROGNOSIS The prognosis is good with adequate treatment, proper education, and sensitivity on the part of the woman's sexual partner.

PREVENTION Preventive measures include prompt treatment of any infections or inflammatory diseases of the genitourinary tract.

■ ERECTILE DYSFUNCTION (Impotence)

DESCRIPTION *Erectile dysfunction,* now the preferred term, is the inability of a man to achieve or sustain an erection sufficient to complete sexual intercourse.

ETIOLOGY Erectile dysfunction may be psychological or physiological in cause. Psychological causes include anxiety or depression and feelings of inadequacy. Physiological causes include certain pharmacological agents, drug and alcohol abuse, diabetes mellitus, surgical complications, spinal cord and disk injuries, and neurological, endocrine, or urologic disorders.

SIGNS AND SYMPTOMS Erectile dysfunction may be *partial,* when the patient is unable to achieve full erection, or intermittent, when the patient is sometimes potent with the same partner. Erectile dysfunction is selective if the patient is potent only with certain women.

DIAGNOSTIC PROCEDURES The diagnostic procedures will help to differentiate between physiological and psychological causes of the impotence. They will typically include a physical examination, medical history, and detailed sexual history.

TREATMENT Treatment of erectile dysfunction may include therapy to correct any underlying physiological disorders and counseling or psychotherapy to alleviate psychological problems. The surgical implantation of a penile **prosthesis** is a treatment option for individuals when erectile dysfunction is due to untreatable neurological or vascular disorders. Most recently, the drug sildenafil (Viagra) has proved successful at a rate of about 70 percent in men with erectile dysfunction. The drug enhances the effect of nitric oxide, the chemical released into the penis during sexual arousal, allowing the increased blood circulation necessary for an erection.

PROGNOSIS The prognosis is variable, depending on how long the patient has suffered from the dysfunction and how severe it is. Sildenafil should be taken while the patient is in the care of a physician, who will need to determine the appropriate dosage.

PREVENTION Prompt treatment of any physiological cause is important.

AROUSAL AND ORGASMIC DYSFUNCTION IN WOMEN

DESCRIPTION *Orgasmic dysfunction* is an inability to achieve orgasm. *Arousal dysfunction* is characterized by the lack of desire for sexual activity and arousal.

ETIOLOGY Arousal or orgasmic dysfunction may be caused by physiological factors, especially diseases that produce nerve damage, such as diabetes mellitus or multiple sclerosis. Drug reactions, pelvic infections, and vascular disease also may be the cause. More commonly, however, arousal dysfunction is due to psychological factors such as anxiety, depression, stress and fatigue, sexual misinformation, inadequate or ineffective stimulation, and early traumatic sexual experiences.

SIGNS AND SYMPTOMS A woman with arousal dysfunction may express a loss of sexual desire or report slow sexual arousal. She may lack the vaginal lubrication and vasocongestive response of sexual arousal. The woman with orgasmic dysfunction has an inability to achieve orgasm totally or under some circumstances.

DIAGNOSTIC PROCEDURES A physical examination, a medical history, and a detailed sexual history are needed to differentiate physiological causes from psychological causes.

TREATMENT The treatment of arousal dysfunction is directed toward correcting underlying physiological disorders or alleviating any psychological problems. The latter may involve sex therapy for both partners. The goal of treatment for orgasmic disorder is to eliminate involuntary inhibition of the orgasmic reflex. Treatment may include experiential therapy, psychoanalysis, or behavior modification.

PROGNOSIS In the absence of nerve damage, the prognosis is good if the woman has had some pleasurable sexual arousal previously. Psychological causes may require lengthy treatment.

PREVENTION Early treatment of any physiological or psychological problem is the best prevention.

PREMATURE EJACULATION

DESCRIPTION *Premature ejaculation* is the expulsion of seminal fluid prior to complete erection of the penis or immediately following the beginning of sexual intercourse.

ETIOLOGY Psychological factors of premature ejaculation include anxiety or guilt feelings about sex. Negative sexual relationships, such as may exist when a man unconsciously dislikes women or seeks to deny his partner's need for sexual gratification, also may induce premature ejaculation. Pathological factors are rare, but they may be linked to degenerative neurological disorders, urethritis, or prostatitis.

SIGNS AND SYMPTOMS Ejaculation during foreplay, prior to complete erection of the penis, or as soon as **intromission** occurs are the classic symptoms.

DIAGNOSTIC PROCEDURES Physical examination and laboratory tests may be ordered to rule out any pathological causes. A detailed sexual history is important to adequately assess this dysfunction.

TREATMENT An intensive program of sex therapy may be necessary. It is important that both partners be involved in the treatment to learn the technique of delaying ejaculation, and that they understand that the condition is reversible.

PROGNOSIS The prognosis is excellent with proper treatment and understanding on the part of both partners. A positive self-image should be encouraged by explaining that premature ejaculation is a disorder that does not reflect on one's masculinity.

PREVENTION No prevention is known.

MALE AND FEMALE INFERTILITY

DESCRIPTION *Infertility* is diagnosed as the failure to become pregnant after 1 year of regular, unprotected intercourse. About 10 percent of couples are infertile. Female fertility normally peaks at 24 years of age and diminishes after 30, with pregnancy occurring rarely after the age of 50. Hormonal balances, the ovulation cycle, and vaginal secretions determine female fertility. A woman is most fertile within 24 hours of ovulation.

Male fertility peaks usually at age 25 and declines after age 40. Sperm count, semen composition, and bodily hormonal changes affect male fertility. The greatest fertility for a man occurs when he has sexual intercourse four times a week.

ETIOLOGY Causes of infertility in women include hormonal problems, nutritional deficiencies, infections, tumors, and anomalies of the reproductive organs. In men, persistent infertility may be caused by sperm deficiencies, congenital abnormalities, endocrine imbalances, and chronic inflammation of the testes, epididymis, or vas deferens.

SIGNS AND SYMPTOMS There is typically no obvious sexual dysfunction in either the man or woman other than the woman's inability to conceive.

DIAGNOSTIC PROCEDURES In a woman, a complete medical, surgical, and gynecologic history and examination are essential. The laboratory studies ordered may include urinalysis, complete blood count, blood hormone levels, and the serology test for syphilis. **Hysterosalpingography** may be necessary to detect uterine abnormalities. One test that may be done is an analysis of cervical mucus within 1 hour after **coitus** to check for motile sperm cells. This test is called the *Huhner test*. Vaginal smears or an endometrial biopsy may be required. A laparoscopy may be ordered to detect abnormalities of the abdominal and pelvic areas.

In a man, a complete ejaculate following sexual abstinence for 4 days should be examined within 1 to 2 hours of collection. A complete physical examination including rectal and genital palpation is essential. The laboratory studies ordered may include a sperm count, complete blood count, and the serology test for syphilis. A testicular biopsy may be performed if **azoospermia** or **oligospermia** is determined. Cystoscopy and catheterization of ejaculatory ducts may be ordered to detect any occlusion or stenosis of the tubes.

TREATMENT The treatment of infertility is dependent on the cause. In a woman, treatment may include any of the following:

- Salpingostomy
- Lysis of adhesions
- Removal of ovarian abnormalities
- Correction of endocrine imbalance
- Alleviation of **cervicitis**
- Hormone therapy
- Microsurgical excision of tubal obstructions

In a man, treatment may include any of the following:

- Surgical correction of any abnormality
- Correction of testicular hypofunction secondary to **hypothyroidism**
- Surgical correction of **varicocele** or **hydrocele**
- Hormone therapy

PROGNOSIS About 50 percent of the couples who are treated for infertility achieve pregnancy. The remainder of the cases are untreatable and complicated.

PREVENTION Prevention of infertility in women and men generally involves avoiding the causative factors leading to acquired infertility, such as infections, drugs and alcohol, trauma, and environmental agents.

Infertile couples may suffer loss, and they may experience guilt and anger. They need emotional support and information.

Sexually Transmitted Diseases (STDs)

■ GONORRHEA

DESCRIPTION *Gonorrhea* is a contagious bacterial infection of the epithelial surfaces of the genitourinary tract in men and women. It is currently one of the most prevalent sexually transmitted (venereal) diseases in the United States.

ETIOLOGY Gonorrhea is caused by the bacterium *Neisseria gonorrhoeae.* The disease is transmitted during sexual intercourse with an infected partner or by other forms of intimate sexual contact. Infants born of infected mothers can contract gonorrhea during vaginal delivery, and the bacteria may infect the conjunctivae, respiratory tract, or anal canal.

SIGNS AND SYMPTOMS The signs and symptoms of gonorrhea vary according to the site and duration of the infection, the particular characteristics of the infecting strain, and whether the infection remains localized or becomes systemic. It is worth emphasizing, however, that many cases of gonorrhea, especially in women, are asymptomatic or produce symptoms that are so slight that they are ignored by the infected individual.

The presenting symptoms of an infected man are typically those of acute urethritis: **purulent** urethral discharge, **dysuria,** and urinary frequency. A purulent discharge from the pharynx or rectum with accompanying pain may be the presenting symptoms among infected homosexual men.

The symptoms of an infected woman are typically those of acute cervicitis: purulent greenish-yellow discharge from the cervix, dysuria, urinary frequency, and itching and burning pain. Other symptoms may include pelvic pain with muscular rigidity or abdominal tenderness and distension.

In the newborn, **gonorrheal ophthalmia neonatorum** may produce a purulent discharge from the eyes 2 to 3 days after birth. Eyelid **edema** may be evident as well.

DIAGNOSTIC PROCEDURES Bacterial cultures from the site of infection will generally establish the diagnosis.

TREATMENT Antibiotics will be given, with various penicillins or tetracycline being the drugs of choice. Clients are advised to have a second culture 1 to 2 weeks after the first, and a further culture in about 6 months, to ensure that they no longer have the disease.

PROGNOSIS The prognosis is good with prompt diagnosis and treatment of localized gonorrheal infections. Systemic gonorrheal infections may produce joint destruction or potentially life-threatening complications such as meningitis or endocarditis. Pelvic inflammatory disease is a serious complication of gonorrheal infection among women, producing fever, nausea, vomiting, and tachycardia.

PREVENTION The use of condoms, avoidance of multiple partners, and the tracing of the sexual contacts of an infected individual can prevent the spread of gonorrhea. Instillation of a 1 percent silver nitrate solution in the eyes of the newborn has reduced the incidence of gonococcal ophthalmia neonatorum.

■ GENITAL HERPES

DESCRIPTION *Genital,* or *venereal, herpes* is a highly contagious viral infection of the male and female genitalia. Unlike other sexually transmitted diseases, genital herpes tends to recur spontaneously. The disease has two stages. During the active stage, characteristic skin lesions and other accompanying symptoms may occur. During the latent stage, the individual is asymptomatic. The incidence of genital herpes is steadily increasing in the United States.

ETIOLOGY Genital herpes is caused by the herpes simplex virus (HSV). Two strains of the virus—designated HSV-1 and HSV-2—may produce the disease. Most cases of genital herpes, however, are attributable to HSV-2. The disease is transmitted by direct contact with infected bodily secretions. Infection typically occurs during sexual intercourse, oral-genital sexual activity, kissing, and hand-to-body contact. A particularly life-threatening form of the disease can occur in infants infected by the virus during vaginal birth.

SIGNS AND SYMPTOMS During the active phase of the disease, males and females may present with characteristic skin **lesions** on their genitals, mouth, and/or anus. These appear as multiple, shallow ulcerations, **pustules,** or **erythematous vesicles** (Fig. 6–1). The vesicles tend to rupture, causing acute pain and consequent itching. Other generalized symptoms may include fever, headache, malaise, muscle pain, anorexia, and dysuria. **Leukorrhea** may be a further symptom in women.

DIAGNOSTIC PROCEDURES Physical examination for evidence of the characteristic lesions is usually suf-ficient for diagnosis. Scraping and biopsy of the ulceration with evidence of HSV-2 may be required to confirm the diagnosis.

TREATMENT Treatment of genital herpes is generally symptomatic. Topical medications may be ordered to reduce edema and pain. The individual should be encouraged to keep any lesions clean and dry. Treatment with new classes of antiviral drugs, such as acyclovir, has shown promise in reducing the active phase of the disease, although these will not eradicate the virus. Secondary infections need to be prevented or speedily managed.

PROGNOSIS Genital herpes cannot be cured. The prognosis varies according to the individual's age,

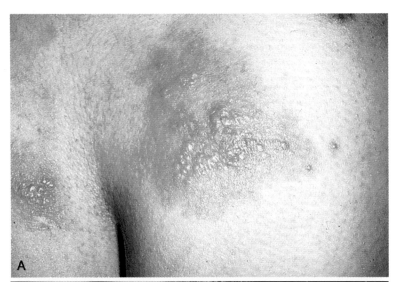

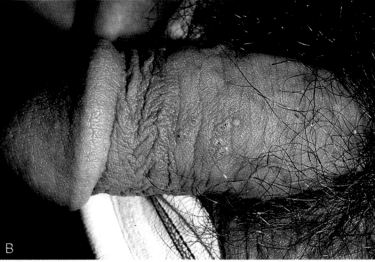

Figure 6–1 (*A*) Herpes simplex of the sacral area, often bilateral. (*B*) Typical mild eruption of small cluster vesicles in recurrent herpes on the penis. (From Reeves, JRT, and Maibach, H: Clinical Dermatology Illustrated: A Regional Approach. FA Davis, Philadelphia, 1991, p 79, with permission.)

the severity of the infection, and the individual's immunologic response. It is estimated that as many as 80 percent of individuals with primary genital herpes infections will experience a recurrence within 12 months. Very serious complications can result if the virus spreads systemically. The virus is also associated with cervical cancer.

PREVENTION No proven method of prevention among adults has been established other than avoiding sexual intercourse with infected individuals and using condoms during all sexual exposure. Transmission of the disease to infants can be minimized through cesarean delivery when it is known that the mother is infected.

GENITAL WARTS

DESCRIPTION *Genital warts* are circumscribed, elevated skin lesions, usually seen on the external genitalia or near the anus. These **papillomas** have fibrous tissue overgrowth from the dermis and a thickened epithelium.

ETIOLOGY Genital warts are caused by several types of human **papillomaviruses** (HPV). They are typically spread from person to person during intimate sexual contact. These warts have a prolonged incubation period of 1 to 6 months and grow rapidly in the presence of heavy perspiration, poor hygiene, or pregnancy.

SIGNS AND SYMPTOMS The patient may be asymptomatic or experience tenderness in the area of the wart. Genital warts appear as solitary or clustered lesions. In males, the warts typically occur at the end of the penis, but they may appear anywhere along the penis as well (Fig. 6–2). They also may appear in the perianal area, especially among homosexual males. In women, the warts typically appear near the opening of the vagina, and they commonly spread to the perianal area. The warts may vary in size from tiny to 3 or 4 inches in diameter.

DIAGNOSTIC PROCEDURES The characteristic appearance and location of the lesions are usually sufficient for diagnosis. Scrapings from wart cells may help in confirming the diagnosis.

TREATMENT The goal of treatment is to eradicate genital infections. Topical medication may be applied or surgery, **cryosurgery, electrocautery,**

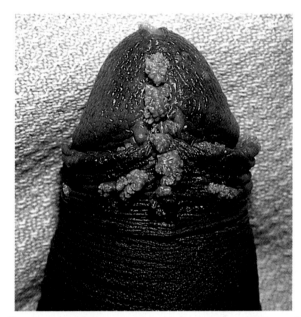

Figure 6–2 Penile warts. (From Reeves, JRT, and Maibach, H: Clinical Dermatology Illustrated: A Regional Approach. FA Davis, Philadelphia, 1991, p 83, with permission.)

or **débridement** may be attempted. Small warts may require no treatment.

PROGNOSIS The prognosis is variable. Spontaneous "cures" are rare, and the remainder may be unresponsive to any form of treatment.

PREVENTION There is no known prevention other than avoiding sexual intercourse with infected individuals and regularly washing the genitalia with soap and water.

SYPHILIS

DESCRIPTION *Syphilis* is a highly infectious, chronic, sexually transmitted disease characterized by lesions that may involve any organ or tissue.

ETIOLOGY Syphilis is caused by the bacterium *Treponema pallidum*. The bacteria are transmitted by direct contact with infected lesions, typically through sexual intercourse or through contact with infected bodily fluids. Syphilis also may be contracted as a consequence of transfusion with infected blood (a rare occurrence). In pregnant women, *T. pallidum* can cross the placenta and infect the fetus, causing serious fetal damage.

The bacteria rapidly penetrate skin or mucous membrane. From the point of infection, they spread into the lymphatic system and the blood, producing a systemic infection. Typically, the bacteria will have been carried throughout the body long before the first clinical symptoms appear.

SIGNS AND SYMPTOMS When untreated, syphilis typically progresses through three clinical stages, each with characteristic signs and symptoms. Note, however, that some infected individuals will be asymptomatic or present with symptoms that are not readily evident upon casual inspection.

Primary syphilis, which has an incubation period of about 3 weeks, is characterized by the appearance of a distinctive, painless lesion, called a **chancre,** at the point of infection. In men, the chancre typically appears on the penis (Fig. 6–3). The chan-

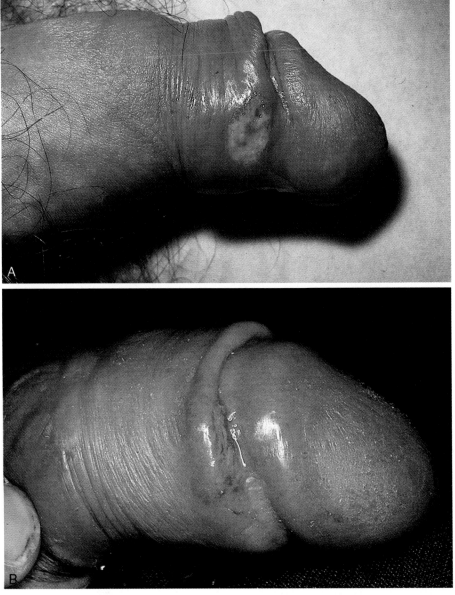

Figure 6–3 (*A*) Typical single punched-out ulcer of primary syphilis. (*B*) Commonly the chancre is not ulcerated but is only an area of induration. (From Reeves, JRT, and Maibach, H: Clinical Dermatology Illustrated: A Regional Approach. FA Davis, Philadelphia, 1991, p 88, with permission.)

cre also may appear on the anus or within the rectum of homosexual males. Among women, the lesion typically appears on the labia of the vagina or within the vagina or cervix. Among both men and women, chancres also may appear on the lips, tongue, fingers, or nipples. The appearance of the chancre also may be accompanied by regional **lymphadenopathy.** It must be emphasized that the chancres are *highly contagious.*

Secondary syphilis can produce a host of symptoms, many of which may be mistaken for other diseases. Most frequently, though, individuals at this stage of the disease will present with a rash characterized by uniform **macular, papular,** pustular, or nodular lesions. These typically, but not exclusively, appear on the palms or soles. In moist areas of the body, these lesions may erode and become contagious. Various general or systemic manifestations may accompany the rash, including headache, malaise, gastrointestinal upset, sore throat, fever, **alopecia,** and brittle nails.

After the manifestations of secondary syphilis subside, a *latent* stage of the disease begins in which the infected individual is generally asymptomatic. The bacteria may remain latent indefinitely. But in roughly half of untreated individuals with latent syphilis, manifestations of the final, or *tertiary,* stage of the disease begin to appear 2 to 7 years after the initial infection. In tertiary syphilis, the *Treponema* bacteria may cause life-threatening damage to the aorta of the heart, the central nervous system, or the musculoskeletal system. No organ system is immune from damage, however. Consequently, the symptoms of tertiary syphilis mimic the symptoms of other organ system diseases, making diagnosis difficult.

DIAGNOSTIC PROCEDURES The most sensitive test available for detecting syphilis is the *fluorescent treponemal antibody-absorption (FTA-ABS) test.* A Venereal Disease Research Laboratories (VDRL) and cerebrospinal fluid (CSF) examination also may be performed.

TREATMENT Penicillin, intramuscularly, is the antibiotic of choice for treatment of all stages of syphilis. Tetracycline or erythromycin may be used in the event of allergic reaction to penicillin. Any lesions should be kept as dry and clean as possible. Regular VDRL testing typically accompanies the drug therapy in order to be certain that the *Treponema* bacteria have been eradicated.

PROGNOSIS The prognosis varies with the age of the affected individual and with the stage at which the disease is detected and treated. The prognosis for complete recovery is very good for adults treated for primary and secondary syphilis. Although tertiary syphilis also can be successfully treated, any organ system damage that may have occurred to that point is generally irreversible. Untreated, the disease may lead to life-threatening heart, central nervous system, or musculoskeletal disorders. The prognosis is poor for a fetus infected with syphilis, with spontaneous abortion or stillbirth occurring in nearly 20 percent of cases.

PREVENTION The use of condoms during sexual intercourse can reduce the possibility of transmitting or acquiring syphilis, but contact tracing of intimate partners and serological screening remain the most important methods in limiting the spread of this disease.

■ TRICHOMONIASIS

DESCRIPTION *Trichomoniasis* is a protozoal infestation of the vagina, urethra, or prostate.

ETIOLOGY *Trichomonas vaginalis,* a motile protozoan, is the cause of trichomoniasis. The disease usually is transmitted by sexual intercourse and affects 10 to 15 percent of sexually active persons. Women may increase their susceptibility to *Trichomonas* infection by using vaginal sprays and over-the-counter douches. These preparations may change the natural flora of the vagina enough that a more hospitable environment for the parasite is created.

SIGNS AND SYMPTOMS Nearly half the women with trichomoniasis are asymptomatic for the first 6 months. When symptoms occur, they are usually those of acute vaginitis: a strong-smelling, greenish yellow, frothy vaginal discharge, possibly accompanied by itching, swelling, dyspareunia, and dysuria. Symptoms may persist for several months if untreated.

In most men, the disease is asymptomatic. When symptoms are present, they are typically those of urethritis, such as dysuria and urinary frequency.

DIAGNOSTIC PROCEDURES Diagnosis of trichomoniasis is facilitated by microscopic examination of vaginal or seminal discharges. The disease also may be detected through urinalysis.

TREATMENT Treatment of both partners with antiparasitic drugs usually cures trichomoniasis. After treatment, both sexual partners should have a follow-up examination.

PROGNOSIS The prognosis is good with proper treatment. Reinfection may occur, however.

PREVENTION Over-the-counter douches and vaginal sprays should be avoided; abstinence from intercourse or the use of condoms is recommended. Persons can reduce the risk of infection by wearing cotton and loose-fitting underwear that allows ventilation, because protozoa grow in warm, dark, and moist places. Cleanliness is also important.

CHLAMYDIAL INFECTIONS

DESCRIPTION *Chlamydial infection* is a sexually transmitted infection that causes inflammation of the urethra and epididymis in men and inflammation of the cervix in women. Chlamydial infections are now highly prevalent and among the most potentially damaging of all the sexually transmitted diseases in the United States.

ETIOLOGY Chlamydial infection is caused by the bacterium *Chlamydia trachomatis*. Transmission is usually through sexual intercourse, rectal intercourse, or genital-oral contact with an infected person.

SIGNS AND SYMPTOMS An individual may be asymptomatic or present with very mild symptoms. Thus this disease is sometimes called the "silent" STD. Clinical manifestations in many women may resemble those of gonorrhea. These include itching and burning in the genital area, mucopurulent vaginal discharge, and cervicitis. In men, urethritis and epididymitis may result.

DIAGNOSTIC PROCEDURES Diagnosis can be confirmed by cytological and serological studies, which reveal *C. trachomatis* in infected body fluids.

TREATMENT The recommended treatment is an antibiotic such as tetracycline or erythromycin. Both partners should be treated simultaneously.

PROGNOSIS The prognosis is good if treatment is instituted early. If left untreated, complications include disease of the fallopian tubes, pelvic inflammatory disease, and infertility in women. Men may suffer from epididymitis and become sterile.

PREVENTION The use of condoms during sexual intercourse can reduce the possibility of transmitting or acquiring chlamydial infection, but contact tracing of intimate partners and serological screening remain the most important methods of limiting the spread of this disease.

Common Symptoms of STDs

Individuals with STDs may present with the following common symptoms, which deserve attention from health professionals:

- Dysuria, **hematuria,** urinary frequency or incontinence, purulent discharge, or burning and itching upon urination
- Pelvic or genital pain
- Any skin ulcerations, especially in the genital area
- Fever and malaise
- Dyspareunia

Male Reproductive Diseases

PROSTATITIS

DESCRIPTION *Prostatitis* is inflammation of the prostate gland (Fig. 6–4). The condition may be acute or chronic, the latter being more common in men older than 50 years of age.

ETIOLOGY Prostatitis may be either bacterial or nonbacterial in origin. Bacterial causes of the disease include *E. coli, Klebsiella, Enterobacter, Proteus, Staphylococcus, Streptococcus,* or *Pseudomonas.* Routes of infection can be either via the urethra or bloodstream. In nonbacterial prostatitis, no infectious agent is detectable.

SIGNS AND SYMPTOMS Low back pain, **myalgia,** perineal fullness or pain, fever, dysuria, urethral discharge, and urinary frequency and urgency are

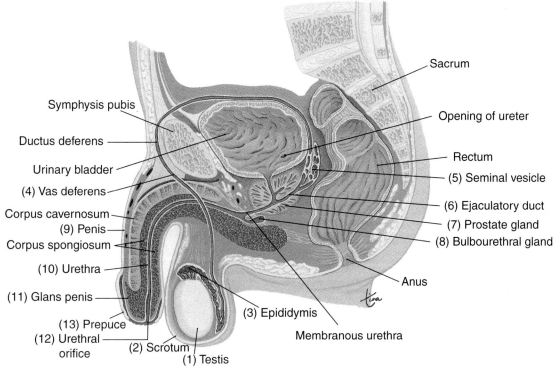

Symphysis pubis

Ductus deferens

Urinary bladder

(4) Vas deferens

Corpus cavernosum

(9) Penis

Corpus spongiosum

(10) Urethra

(11) Glans penis

(13) Prepuce

(12) Urethral orifice

(2) Scrotum

(1) Testis

(3) Epididymis

Sacrum

Opening of ureter

Rectum

(5) Seminal vesicle

(6) Ejaculatory duct

(7) Prostate gland

(8) Bulbourethral gland

Anus

Membranous urethra

Figure 6–4 Male reproductive system. (From Scanlon, VC, and Sanders, T: Essentials of Anatomy and Physiology, ed 3. FA Davis, Philadelphia, 1999, p 442, with permission.)

common symptoms of acute prostatitis. The prostate, when palpated, may be enlarged, tender, and boggy. An individual with chronic prostatitis may be asymptomatic or experience sporadic, mild forms of acute symptoms.

DIAGNOSTIC PROCEDURES Urinalysis, urine culture, and a rectal examination help in diagnosing prostatitis. Abnormally high urine leukocyte counts in the absence of detectable bacteria are indicative of nonbacterial prostatitis.

TREATMENT Antimicrobial therapy is initiated, and the client is usually advised to rest and increase fluid intake. **Analgesics, antipyretics,** and stool softeners also may be ordered. Sitz baths may be recommended. If drug therapy is not effective, transurethral resection of the prostate may be necessary.

PROGNOSIS Acute prostatitis responds well to treatment; however, chronic prostatitis does not. Complications may include epididymitis, cystitis, and urethritis. Chronic prostatitis predisposes to recur-

rent urinary tract infections, urethral obstruction, and acute urinary retention.

PREVENTION Early treatment of urinary tract infections is the best prevention.

■ EPIDIDYMITIS

DESCRIPTION *Epididymitis* is inflammation of the epididymis due to infection (Fig. 6–5). The condition is typically unilateral and is one of the most common infections of the male reproductive system.

ETIOLOGY *Chlamydia trachomatis* and *Neisseria gonorrhoeae* are the most common infectious agents causing epididymitis among sexually active men. Other bacterial causes of this condition include *E. coli, Staphylococcus,* and *Streptococcus.* Epididymitis can occur as a result of prostatitis, a urinary tract infection, mumps, tuberculosis, or sexually transmitted diseases such as gonorrhea and syphilis. Trauma, prostatectomy, or the prolonged use of

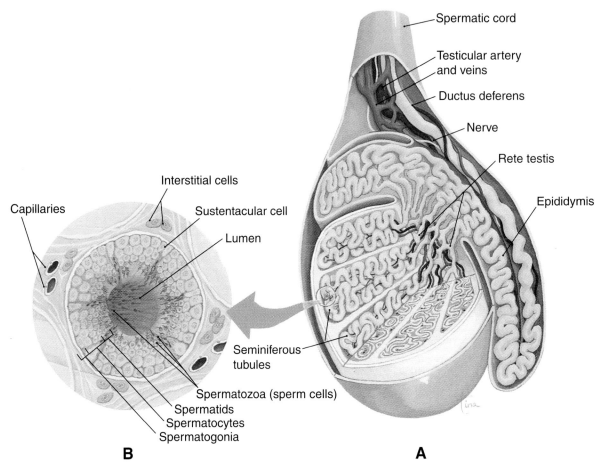

Figure 6–5 (*A*) Midsagittal section of portion of a testis; the epididymis is on the posterior side of the testis. (*B*) Cross-section through a seminiferous tubule showing development of sperm. (From Scanlon, VS, and Sanders, T: Essentials of Anatomy and Physiology, ed 3. FA Davis, Philadelphia, 1999, p 443, with permission.)

an indwelling catheter may predispose to epididymitis.

SIGNS AND SYMPTOMS The epididymis may become enlarged, hard, and tender, causing pain. Scrotal and groin tenderness, fever, and malaise also may occur. Groin tenderness is the result of enlarged lymph nodes in the groin. Patients may "waddle" as they walk, trying to protect the scrotal area.

DIAGNOSTIC PROCEDURES Urinalysis and urine cultures help in the diagnosis. An increased leukocyte count is common.

TREATMENT Antimicrobial therapy appropriate for the particular causative agent will be initiated. A scrotal support and analgesics may be helpful. Bed rest may be necessary in the acute phase.

PROGNOSIS The inflammation generally responds well to therapy, but portions of the epididymis may be scarred. Consequently, sterility may result if treatment is delayed, especially if the disease is bilateral. Orchitis may develop as a further complication.

PREVENTION Early treatment of urinary tract infection is the best prevention. The use of a condom during sexual intercourse is recommended.

ORCHITIS

DESCRIPTION *Orchitis* is inflammation of the testes due to infection and is a serious complication of epididymitis. The condition may be either bilateral or unilateral.

ETIOLOGY Orchitis may also arise as a consequence of infection from the mumps virus. Other viruses and bacteria also can produce this condition. Scrotal trauma may predispose an individual to orchitis.

SIGNS AND SYMPTOMS Testicular swelling or tenderness with acute pain, either unilateral or bilateral, are the common presenting symptoms of orchitis. These symptoms are typically accompanied by chills, fever, malaise, nausea, and vomiting.

DIAGNOSTIC PROCEDURES The individual's clinical history may reveal a recent or ongoing case of mumps or other related disease. Testicular examination will suggest the diagnosis. Serology, urinalysis, or throat cultures may be used to isolate mumps virus or identify other causative agents.

TREATMENT No specific treatment is effective against orchitis induced by the mumps virus. Treatment is typically supportive. Analgesics and antipyretics may be prescribed. Certain adrenal steroid drugs may be used to reduce swelling and fever in severe cases. Bed rest is generally indicated, and the wearing of a scrotal support may be helpful. If the orchitis is bacterial in origin, the appropriate antibiotic therapy should be instituted.

PROGNOSIS The prognosis is good. Atrophy of the affected testicle occurs in half the cases, but complete sterility is unusual.

PREVENTION To prevent mumps orchitis, the mumps vaccine is recommended for prepubertal boys and all adult men who have not had clinical mumps.

■ BENIGN PROSTATIC HYPERPLASIA (BPH)

DESCRIPTION *Benign prostatic hyperplasia* is the overproliferation of cells within the inner portion of the prostate. The condition is common in men older than 50 years of age and the incidence increases with age. It is only clinically significant if the enlarging, hyperplastic portion of the prostate obstructs urinary outflow.

ETIOLOGY The etiology of BPH is not well understood, but it seems to be due to metabolic and hormonal changes associated with aging. In clinically significant BPH, the gland compresses the urethra or the neck of the bladder, obstructing urinary flow. Less frequently, the enlarged portion of the prostate may press against the rectum, causing constipation.

SIGNS AND SYMPTOMS The individual may report symptoms of urinary obstruction, such as difficulty in initiating urination or in completely emptying the bladder. Other symptoms may include dysuria, nocturia, dribbling, urinary frequency, weak urine stream, or urinary or fecal incontinence. In severe cases of urinary obstruction due to BPH, the individual may present with symptoms of hydronephrosis or pyelonephritis.

DIAGNOSTIC PROCEDURES Symptomatology of the individual and a rectal examination may be sufficient for diagnosis, but urinalysis, urine culture, intravenous pyelogram (IVP), and cystoscopy may be ordered for confirmation. Prostatic biopsy may be required to ensure that prostatic carcinoma is not causing the enlargement. The distended bladder may be palpable.

TREATMENT Symptomatic treatment may include prostatic massage, catheterization, and sitz baths. Various medications that act to shrink the prostate or relax the muscles in the prostate show moderate success. More recently, a new treatment is under study. This nonsurgical option is called *transurethral thermo-ablation therapy* (T3). T3 uses microwave energy to heat and destroy the constricting tissue while preserving the urethra and nonprostatic tissues. Various surgical procedures, such as transurethral prostate resection (TURP), may be done to remove urinary tract obstruction.

PROGNOSIS Prognosis is good with proper intervention, and the mortality rate is low. If untreated, infections may ascend to the kidney, or various urinary obstructive disorders may result. Complications include cystitis, dilation of the ureters, hydronephrosis, pyelonephritis, and uremia.

PREVENTION No specific prevention is known, but older men should be encouraged to have a regular prostate examination in order to detect any enlargement.

■ PROSTATIC CANCER

DESCRIPTION *Prostatic cancer* is a malignant neoplasm of the prostate tissue. The majority of these neoplasms are classified as adenocarcinomas. Prostatic cancer is the third leading cause of cancer deaths in men (after lung and colon cancers). Prostate cancer tends to **metastasize,** often spreading to the bones of the spine or pelvis before it is detected. The disease is rare before the age of 50.

ETIOLOGY The cause of prostatic cancer is not known. No specific risk factors, other than the increasing incidence with age, have been identified. There may be a familial association.

SIGNS AND SYMPTOMS Most individuals with prostatic cancer are asymptomatic on diagnosis. When symptoms are present, they are typically those of urinary obstruction, such as dysuria, difficulty in voiding, urinary frequency, or urinary retention. Hip or back pain may be present in advanced stages of the disease.

DIAGNOSTIC PROCEDURES A rectal examination will help in diagnosing the tumor. A biopsy is essential for confirmation of the diagnosis. A computed tomography (CT) scan or ultrasonography may be useful in localizing and gauging the extent of the tumor.

A prostate-specific antigen (PSA) blood test is used to detect prostate cancer. It detects prostatic cancer when the levels of prostatic antigens are elevated.

TREATMENT The course of treatment selected will depend on the stage of the disease and the patient's physical condition and age. Surgery may be performed to remove the prostate and adjacent affected tissues. Various hormonal therapies also may be attempted to limit prostatic cell growth, including **orchidectomy** and estrogen therapy. Radiation therapy may be tried in some cases, and this further helps to relieve bone pain. Chemotherapy may be used in treating advanced stages of the disease.

PROGNOSIS The earlier the cancer is detected, the better is the prognosis. Survival rates for all stages combined have steadily increased from 50 to 76 percent.

■ TESTICULAR CANCER

DESCRIPTION *Testicular cancer* is a malignant neoplasm of a testis. There are various forms of the disease, classified according to the type of testicular tissue from which the malignancy originates. The disease primarily affects young to middle-aged men and is rare in men older than the age of 40.

ETIOLOGY The cause of cancer of the testes is essentially unknown. Predisposing factors include **cryptorchidism,** even after this condition has been surgically corrected. Other risk factors include a prior history of mumps or an inguinal hernia during childhood.

SIGNS AND SYMPTOMS The first sign often is a smooth, firm, painless mass in the testicles. Later symptoms may include breast enlargement and nipple tenderness.

DIAGNOSTIC PROCEDURES Diagnosis generally is through palpation of the testes. Further tests such as the CT scan or magnetic resonance imaging (MRI) may be necessary to differentiate the cell type of the mass.

TREATMENT Treatment may include any combination of surgery (orchidectomy), radiation, and chemotherapy, as determined by the tumor-cell type and staging.

PROGNOSIS The prognosis varies according to the cancer's type and staging. Cure rates of roughly 90 percent can be expected following the successful treatment of early-stage testicular cancers.

PREVENTION Although no specific prevention is known, early detection is crucial to successful treatment. Young men should be encouraged to perform monthly testicular self-examination.

Common Symptoms of Male Reproductive Diseases

Men may present with the following common complaints, which deserve attention from health professionals:

- Any urinary complaints such as frequency, urgency, incontinence, dysuria, and so on
- Pain in any of the reproductive organs
- Swelling or enlargement of any of the reproductive organs
- Any sexual dysfunction, such as erectile dysfunction

Female Reproductive Diseases

◾ **PREMENSTRUAL SYNDROME** (PMS)

DESCRIPTION *Premenstrual syndrome* is a cluster of symptoms that regularly recur several days prior to the onset of menstruation. PMS appears more frequently in women in their thirties and forties. (Refer to Figs. 6–6 and 6–7 to review the structure of the female reproductive system.)

ETIOLOGY The cause of PMS is not clearly understood. Some theories suggest that the condition may be attributable to water retention, estrogen-progesterone imbalance, psychological factors, or dietary deficiencies. Some believe there is a relationship between PMS and changes in the endorphin levels.

SIGNS AND SYMPTOMS The particular assortment of symptoms and their severity vary from woman to woman. Symptoms associated with PMS include:

- Irritability
- Sleeplessness
- Fatigue
- Depression
- Headaches
- Vertigo

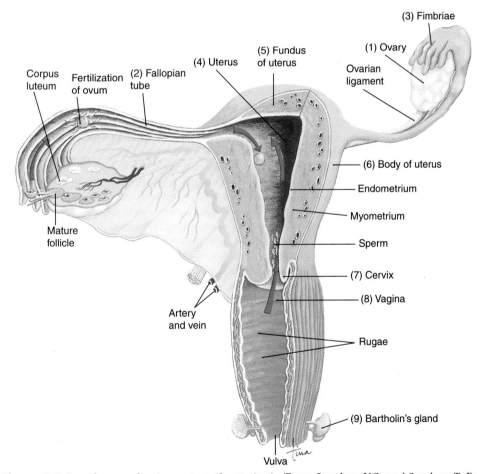

Figure 6–6 Female reproductive system (front view). (From Scanlon, VC, and Sanders, T: Essentials of Anatomy and Physiology, ed 3. FA Davis, Philadelphia, 1999, p 447, with permission.)

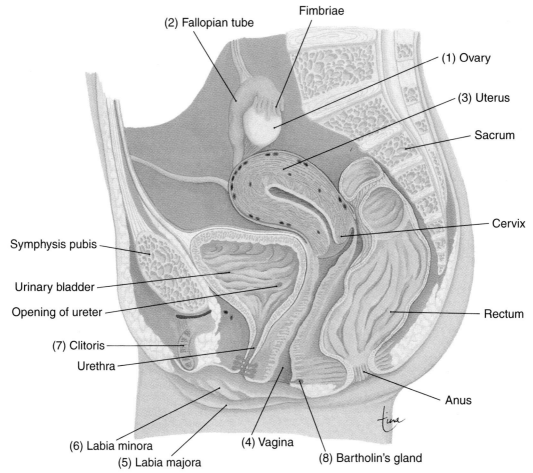

Figure 6–7 Female reproductive system (side view). (From Scanlon, VC, and Sanders, T: Essentials of Anatomy and Physiology, ed 3. FA Davis, Philadelphia, 1999, p 446, with permission.)

- Syncope
- Lowered resistance to infections
- Personality changes
- Nervousness
- Arthralgia
- Abdominal bloating and weight gain
- Palpitations
- Acne
- Swollen and tender breasts
- Easily bruised skin
- Alterations in appetite (e.g., cravings for sweet or salty foods)

DIAGNOSTIC PROCEDURES Diagnosis depends on the timing of the symptoms rather than on the appearance of any specific set of symptoms. Conse-

quently, the affected individual should be encouraged to keep a journal recording the onset, duration, and intensity of all symptoms. Evaluation of estrogen and progesterone levels in the blood to check for imbalances should be performed. Blood tests may be done to rule out other hormonal imbalances or anemia.

TREATMENT There is no one effective treatment for PMS. A reduction of salt intake for 2 weeks prior to menses will minimize water retention. Avoidance of stimulants (coffee, nicotine, and alcohol) is beneficial for some. Proper diet, exercise, and sufficient amounts of rest are important. Reduction of stress, relaxation techniques, and medication may be ordered to relieve the symptoms.

PROGNOSIS The prognosis is variable. The disorder is considered chronic but will cease at menopause and does not have long-term effects.

PREVENTION There is no known prevention.

AMENORRHEA

DESCRIPTION
Amenorrhea is the absence of **menarche** beyond age 16 (*primary* amenorrhea) or the absence of menstruation for 6 months in a woman who has previously had regular, periodic menses (*secondary* amenorrhea).

ETIOLOGY Medically significant primary or secondary amenorrhea may be caused by a variety of hormonal imbalances capable of preventing ovulation. Several forms of congenital anatomic defects, such as the absence of a uterus, also may cause amenorrhea. The condition is also associated with endometrial problems, ovarian or pituitary tumors, malnutrition, psychological stress, or too much physical exercise.

SIGNS AND SYMPTOMS A young woman reporting delayed menarche or a woman reporting skipped periods should be carefully assessed for amenorrhea.

DIAGNOSTIC PROCEDURES A thorough pelvic examination will rule out pregnancy and anatomic abnormalities. Analysis of blood and urine samples may reveal hormonal difficulties. X-rays and laparoscopy with an endometrial biopsy may be necessary to detect tumors.

TREATMENT Hormone therapy usually starts the menstrual cycle, but some cases of this disorder may require more aggressive treatment, such as surgery.

PROGNOSIS Prognosis is good when the underlying cause can be determined and corrected. It is important that an accurate record of the menstrual cycle be kept to aid in the detection of amenorrhea.

PREVENTION Preventive measures include adequate diet, reduction of psychological stress, and a balanced physical exercise program.

DYSMENORRHEA

DESCRIPTION *Dysmenorrhea* is pain associated with menstruation. It is one of the most frequent gynecologic disorders. Dysmenorrhea is divided into primary and secondary categories. *Primary* dysmenorrhea is not associated with any identifiable pathological disorder, whereas *secondary* dysmenorrhea accompanies some underlying disease condition.

ETIOLOGY A specific cause of primary dysmenorrhea is difficult to pinpoint. Hormonal imbalances such as increased **prostaglandin** secretions may be the cause. Secondary dysmenorrhea arises as a consequence of some other problem, such as endometriosis, cervical **stenosis,** or pelvic inflammatory disease. Secondary dysmenorrhea is occasionally associated with the presence of uterine polyps or benign tumors.

SIGNS AND SYMPTOMS Sharp, cramping pains in the lower abdominal area are the classic symptoms. The pain may radiate to the thighs, back, and genitalia. These symptoms usually start just prior to or immediately after menses and subside within 18 to 24 hours.

DIAGNOSTIC PROCEDURES A detailed history and pelvic examination will be performed to determine the cause. Laparoscopy and dilation and curettage (D&C) may be attempted.

TREATMENT Analgesics and nonsteroid anti-inflammatory drugs usually are sufficient for relieving the pain of this disorder. Aspirin, moreover, when taken prior to menses, is an inhibitor of prostaglandins. Heat applied to the abdomen may provide comfort. Sometimes sex steroid therapy (oral contraceptives) may be prescribed to relieve pain by suppressing ovulation. Uterine **leiomyomas** may require surgery.

PROGNOSIS The prognosis is good. Primary dysmenorrhea may disappear after a female becomes sexually active or gives birth to a child.

PREVENTION Correction of any hormonal imbalance may be helpful in prevention.

OVARIAN CYSTS AND TUMORS

DESCRIPTION Benign *cysts* of the ovary are derived from ovarian follicles and the **corpus luteum.** These cysts may occur anytime from puberty to menopause. Nonneoplastic cysts (*tumors*) usually are small and produce few symptoms. True ovarian neoplasms may be benign, malignant, cystic, or solid. Dermoid or benign cystic **teratomas** also are common in the ovary.

ETIOLOGY The etiology of ovarian cysts and tumors is not known.

SIGNS AND SYMPTOMS Large cysts may produce pelvic pain, low back pain, and dyspareunia. Cysts that are mobile and can twist may produce acute spasmodic abdominal pain. Urinary retention can result if a large fluid-filled cyst presses on the area near the bladder.

DIAGNOSTIC PROCEDURES Visualization of the ovaries through laparoscopy or sonography may indicate ovarian cysts.

TREATMENT Cysts may disappear spontaneously by reabsorption or silent rupture or may require drug-induced ovulation therapy or surgical resection. If any question exists regarding malignancy, surgery may be necessary for diagnosis as well as treatment.

PROGNOSIS Prognosis varies according to whether the diagnosis indicates nonneoplastic cysts or a true ovarian neoplasm, either benign or malignant.

PREVENTION There is no known prevention.

■ ENDOMETRIOSIS

DESCRIPTION *Endometriosis* is the appearance and growth of endometrial tissue in areas outside the **endometrium,** the uterine cavity's lining. The misplaced endometrial tissue generally is found within the pelvic area, but it can appear anywhere in the body (Fig. 6–8). Despite its location at an **ectopic** site, the tissue still responds to the hormonal signals of the woman's menstrual cycle, but the "menstruating" tissue cannot be sloughed off through the vagina. This situation gives rise to a variety of symptoms and may lead to scarring of the ectopic site. Endometriosis is a disease of women during their active reproductive years.

ETIOLOGY The cause of endometriosis is still not known, although various theories have been proposed, such as a familial susceptibility. One suspected cause is surgery (such as cesarean section) in which the uterus is opened.

SIGNS AND SYMPTOMS Dysmenorrhea occurs, with pain in the lower back and the vagina. The severity of the pain does not necessarily indicate the extent of the disease. There will be pain at the ectopic site during menses. The client may report profuse

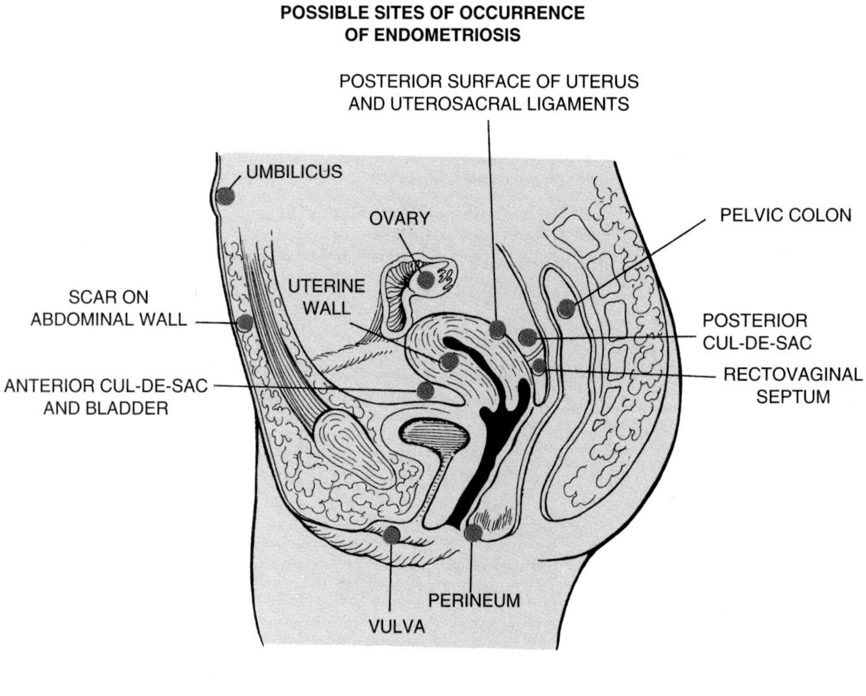

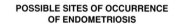

POSSIBLE SITES OF OCCURRENCE OF ENDOMETRIOSIS

POSTERIOR SURFACE OF UTERUS AND UTEROSACRAL LIGAMENTS

UMBILICUS

OVARY

PELVIC COLON

SCAR ON ABDOMINAL WALL

UTERINE WALL

POSTERIOR CUL-DE-SAC

ANTERIOR CUL-DE-SAC AND BLADDER

RECTOVAGINAL SEPTUM

PERINEUM

VULVA

Figure 6–8 Possible sites of endometriosis. (From Thomas, CL [ed]: Taber's Cyclopedic Medical Dictionary, ed 18. FA Davis, Philadelphia, 1997, p 639, with permission.)

menses and infertility. She may experience dyspareunia, dysuria, and even painful defecation.

DIAGNOSTIC PROCEDURES Diagnosis is usually made by visualizing the ectopic deposits within the pelvis through laparoscopy. Palpation may detect tender nodules or areas of the pelvis. These nodules become more tender during menses.

TREATMENT Hormone therapy that will completely suppress the menstrual cycle may be recommended. Birth-control pills will suppress endometriosis as well. Young women may be put on androgens, which may produce a temporary remission. Laparoscopy may be used to lyse adhesions. Surgery, which may involve a **panhysterosalpingo-oophorectomy,** may be indicated.

PROGNOSIS The prognosis varies according to the location of the ectopic sites and the intensity of symptoms experienced by each affected individual. A primary complication of endometriosis is infertility. Females who have not had a child may be advised not to postpone pregnancy.

PREVENTION It may be best for adolescents to use sanitary napkins rather than tampons to prevent displacement of the endometrial lining.

■ UTERINE LEIOMYOMAS

DESCRIPTION *Uterine leiomyomas* are often mislabeled as fibroids or fibroid tumors. They are not composed of fibrous tissue, however. Rather, they are composed of smooth muscle tissue. These benign tumors may vary in size, number, and location within the uterine muscle. They are the most common tumors in females, but they tend to calcify after menopause.

ETIOLOGY The etiology of leiomyomas is not known, but their development is stimulated by estrogen.

SIGNS AND SYMPTOMS Frequently, leiomyomas are asymptomatic. If symptoms do occur, they may include pelvic pressure, urinary frequency, constipation, and **menorrhagia.** A palpable mass may be detected.

DIAGNOSTIC PROCEDURES The client's symptoms and a thorough history and physical examination, including palpation of the tumor, are essential for di-

agnosis. Other possible tests are ultrasonography and D&C to detect submucosal leiomyomas in the endometrial cavity, and laparoscopy, to visualize leiomyomas on the surface of the uterus.

TREATMENT Treatment is dependent on the woman's age, **parity,** desire to have children, tumor status, and the severity of symptoms. If the tumors are small, no treatment may be necessary, other than periodic monitoring of the leiomyomas' growth. A pelvic examination every 6 to 12 months may then be advised. Surgical removal of the tumors may be done, or a hysterectomy may be performed.

PROGNOSIS The prognosis is good. Only a very small percentage of leiomyomas develop into a malignancy. The leiomyomas may cause infertility or, if the client is pregnant, spontaneous abortion or premature labor.

PREVENTION No prevention is known.

■ PELVIC INFLAMMATORY DISEASE (PID)

DESCRIPTION *Pelvic inflammatory disease* is an acute or a subacute, or a recurrent or chronic infection of the fallopian tubes, ovaries, and adjacent tissues. There may be inflammation of the cervix (cervicitis), uterus (endometritis), fallopian tubes (salpingitis), and ovaries (oophritis).

ETIOLOGY The causes of PID include (1) infections following **parturition;** (2) infections from *N. gonorrhoeae, C. trachomatis, Pseudomonas,* and *E. coli;* and (3) **iatrogenic** causes—for instance, PID may follow **conization,** cervical cauterization, or insertion of an intrauterine device (IUD) or biopsy curet. PID is most common in young nulliparous women, but it can also occur after childbirth, abortion, or miscarriage.

SIGNS AND SYMPTOMS This disease may exhibit both acute and chronic symptoms. Acute symptoms include sudden pelvic pain, a purulent and foul-smelling vaginal discharge, fever, sexual dysfunction, **metrorrhagia,** and rebound pain. Chronic symptoms such as cervical **dysplasia** and laceration may go undetected for an indefinite period of time.

DIAGNOSTIC PROCEDURES Diagnosis includes taking a smear of uterine secretions for culture. Ultrasonography may be used to identify a uterine mass.

TREATMENT Appropriate antibiotics are the best treatment for PID. Supplemental therapy may include analgesics and bed rest. Surgery may be necessary to prevent **septicemia.**

PROGNOSIS The prognosis of PID is good when treatment is instituted early, and few complications such as septicemia, infertility, or shock occur. If treatment is delayed, scar tissue and adhesions can form.

PREVENTION There is no known prevention.

■ MENOPAUSE

DESCRIPTION *Menopause* (not a disease) is the cessation of menses and ovarian function, with a resultant decrease in estrogen levels.

ETIOLOGY Menopause occurs naturally in women between the ages of 40 and 50. It also can be surgically induced by oophorectomy or can result from malnutrition, severe stress, or a disease that has an adverse effect on hormone balance.

SIGNS AND SYMPTOMS Menstrual irregularities, a decrease in the amount of menstrual flow, and finally, cessation of menses are the common symptoms. These occur over a period of months or years. Other changes can occur in the body systems as well, producing hot flashes, night sweats, syncope, **tachycardia,** loss of elasticity in the skin, reduction of size and firmness of breast tissue, some atrophy of the genitalia, and a decrease in secretion from Bartholin's gland. Some women experience transient psychological symptoms such as depression, poor memory, and loss of interest in sex.

DIAGNOSTIC PROCEDURES A careful history usually will suggest menopause. Blood serum levels will be checked for increased production of **follicle-stimulating hormone** (FSH) and **luteinizing hormone** (LH).

TREATMENT Some individuals need no treatment; others may require hormone replacement therapy, counseling, or both. A woman requiring hormone replacement therapy should be informed of the possible increased risks of endometrial cancer and should be monitored carefully.

PROGNOSIS The prognosis is generally good.

PREVENTION Menopause cannot be prevented, but it is important to recognize that emotional swings may occur.

Abnormal Premenopausal and Postmenopausal Bleeding

Premenopausal or *postmenopausal bleeding* is bleeding occurring at times other than during the normal menstrual flow. Whether these conditions are troublesome or cause few problems, they should be investigated to determine the underlying cause. **Oligomenorrhea,** menorrhagia, metrorrhagia, or a brownish spotting from the vagina are the most common signs. To help assess the problem, it is important to monitor the dates of abnormal bleeding and the number of tampons or pads used per day. D&C may be necessary to relieve bleeding.

Common Symptoms of Female Reproductive System Diseases

Women may present with the following common symptoms, which deserve attention from health professionals:

- Pre- and postmenstrual complaints such as amenorrhea, dysmenorrhea, oligomenorrhea, and metrorrhagia; skin changes; and psychological reactions to hormonal changes
- Lower abdominal or pelvic pain
- Any abnormal vaginal discharge or itching
- Fever
- Dyspareunia or any sexual dysfunction
- Breast changes, such as unusual swelling, lumpiness, mass formation, pain, or nipple abnormalities

Diseases of the Breasts

■ MAMMARY DYSPLASIA OR FIBROCYSTIC DISEASE

DESCRIPTION *Fibrocystic disease of the breast* is a generalized diagnosis for a condition in which there are palpable lumps or cysts in the breasts that fluctuate in size with the menstrual cycle. Other benign changes in the breast epithelium include **papillomatosis,** fibrosis, and **hyperplasia.** The condition is sometimes known as *chronic cystic mastitis.* The disease is seen more frequently in women 30 to 50 years old and rarely after menopause. It is the most common disease of the breast. Refer to Figure 6–9 for a review of the structure of the breast.

ETIOLOGY The causes of fibrocystic disease are not well understood, but they are linked to the hormonal changes associated with ovarian activity.

SIGNS AND SYMPTOMS The upper, outer quadrant of the breast is the most frequent segment involved. There may be widespread lumpiness or a localized

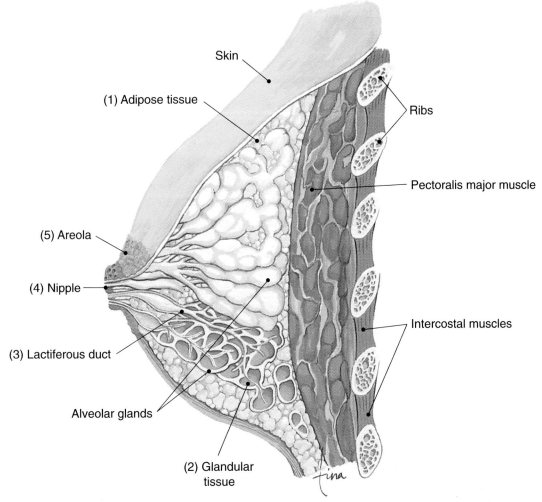

Figure 6–9 The breast. (From Scanlon, VC, and Sanders, T: Essentials of Anatomy and Physiology, ed 3. FA Davis, Philadelphia, 1999, p 451, with permission.)

mass. Pain, tenderness, and a nipple discharge may be present. The mass tends to grow in size and becomes tender just before the menstrual period.

DIAGNOSTIC PROCEDURES Palpation is essential. A mammogram may be a useful aid, but biopsy is essential to confirm the diagnosis. The clinical picture of pain, fluctuation in size, and lumpiness help to differentiate mammary dysplasia from breast cancer.

TREATMENT Breast aspiration may be attempted to remove the watery fluid typically contained in most lesions. Breast pain may be alleviated with a good supportive bra worn both day and night. Caffeine intake may be restricted, because some studies indicate that its elimination aids in reducing dysplasia.

PROGNOSIS The prognosis is good, although exacerbations may continue until menopause, after which they subside. Cancer of the breast is more common in women who also have mammary dysplasia.

PREVENTION There is no known prevention. Monthly self-examination of the breast is advised.

■ BENIGN FIBROADENOMA

DESCRIPTION A *fibroadenoma* is a benign, well-circumscribed tumor of fibrous and glandular breast tissue. It is a common tumor occurring in women 20 years after puberty.

ETIOLOGY The cause is unknown.

SIGNS AND SYMPTOMS The breast mass is typically round, firm, discrete, and relatively movable. It is nontender and usually discovered by accident.

DIAGNOSTIC PROCEDURES Palpation, followed by a mammogram, is essential for diagnosis. Because of its distinctive characteristics, the tumor is not difficult to diagnose, but it must be differentiated from a cyst or carcinoma through biopsy.

TREATMENT The mass is excised under local anesthesia.

PROGNOSIS The prognosis is good following excision of the tumor.

PREVENTION There is no known prevention.

■ CARCINOMA OF THE BREAST

DESCRIPTION *Breast cancer* encompasses a variety of malignant neoplasms of the breast. It is the most common site of cancer in women and until recently was the leading cause of cancer deaths among women in the United States, a position that is now occupied by lung cancer.

ETIOLOGY The exact causes of breast cancer are unknown, although hereditary patterns to the disease are quite obvious. Women who have a family history of breast cancer have an increased risk. Those at greatest risk of developing breast cancer include women over the age of 40 who have not had children, or women who have not had children until after age 35. Other risk factors include a history of chronic breast disease, obesity, and exposure to high doses of radiation, especially during adolescence. The risk of breast cancer increases with age.

SIGNS AND SYMPTOMS Breast changes such as a lump, thickening, dimpling, swelling, skin irritation, distortion, retraction or scaliness of the nipple, nipple discharge, pain, or tenderness are the most common signs and symptoms. Advanced symptoms include edema, redness, nodularity, or ulceration of the skin, and enlargement or shrinkage of the breast. Generally, the lump is in the upper outer quadrant of the breast.

DIAGNOSTIC PROCEDURES The best method of early detection continues to be the monthly self-examination of the breast. Mammography and ultrasonography are also frequently used screening methods. Diagnosis, however, must be made without delay because of the possibility of metastasis. Biopsy is essential for definitive diagnosis. Diagnosed breast cancer will be staged and typed according to its pattern of growth.

TREATMENT Treatment may be curative or palliative. If the cancer is advanced, palliative treatment is indicated. Curative treatment nearly always involves surgical management of the cancer, but no single procedure is now recognized as ideal for all affected individuals. Surgical options range from removing the affected breast, underlying chest muscles, and associated lymphatics (called a *total radical mastectomy*) to removing only the tumor and immediately adjacent breast tissue (called a *lumpectomy*).

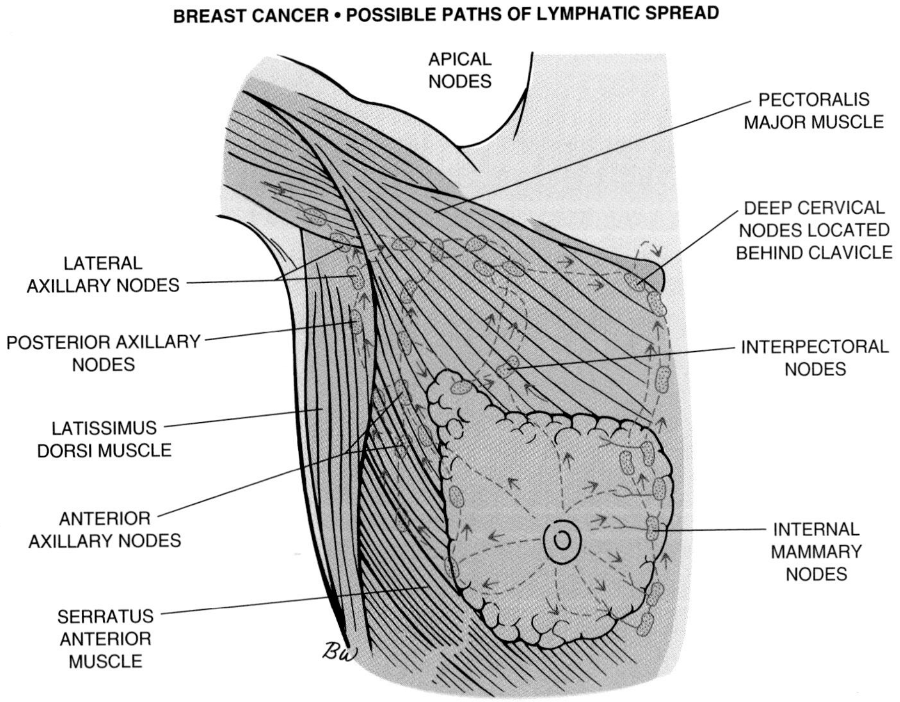

BREAST CANCER • POSSIBLE PATHS OF LYMPHATIC SPREAD

APICAL NODES

PECTORALIS MAJOR MUSCLE

DEEP CERVICAL NODES LOCATED BEHIND CLAVICLE

LATERAL AXILLARY NODES

POSTERIOR AXILLARY NODES

INTERPECTORAL NODES

LATISSIMUS DORSI MUSCLE

ANTERIOR AXILLARY NODES

INTERNAL MAMMARY NODES

SERRATUS ANTERIOR MUSCLE

Figure 6–10 Breast cancer: possible sites of lymphatic spread. (From Thomas, CL [ed]: Taber's Cyclopedic Medical Dictionary, ed 18. FA Davis, Philadelphia, 1997, p 263, with permission.)

Radiation may be done before surgery to shrink the tumor or postoperatively to destroy any remaining malignancy. Surgery will be followed by a course of radiation therapy and/or chemotherapy. If surgery is done, breast reconstruction may follow.

The tumor tissue will be tested for the presence of hormone receptors in order to determine if the tumor is estrogen- or progesterone-dependent. If this is the case, hormonal manipulation such as removal of the ovaries or adrenal glands and administration of testosterone may be attempted to halt tumor regrowth or to prevent its spread (Fig. 6–10).

PROGNOSIS The most reliable indicator of the prognosis is the stage of the breast cancer. In the early stages, the prognosis is good, especially if no metastasis has occurred. According to the American Cancer Society, the 5-year survival rate for localized breast cancer has risen to 97 percent. If the cancer has spread regionally, however, the survival rate is reduced to 76 percent.

PREVENTION There is no known prevention of breast cancer.

SPECIAL FOCUS BREAST RECONSTRUCTION

Breast reconstruction may be performed to augment, reduce, or repair the breast. New developments in plastic surgery have greatly reduced the risks of the procedure and provide a woman with a choice about her body's appearance. Whatever the reason for the reconstruction, women need to be emotionally prepared for the surgery and especially well informed of its potential results.

Disorders of Pregnancy and Delivery

■ SPONTANEOUS ABORTION

DESCRIPTION *Spontaneous abortion,* or *miscarriage,* is the expulsion of the **conceptus** before viability. As many as 10 to 30 percent of pregnancies may end in spontaneous abortion. The incidence is higher in first pregnancies.

ETIOLOGY Spontaneous abortion may be a result of (1) defective development of the embryo (chromosomal abnormalities), (2) faulty implantation of the fertilized ovum, (3) placental problems, (4) maternal infections, (5) hormonal imbalances, (6) trauma, or (7) an unknown cause.

SIGNS AND SYMPTOMS A pink or brown discharge may precede the onset of cramping and increased vaginal bleeding. The cervix will dilate, and the uterine contents will be expelled. The discharge may appear as a clotty menstrual flow. Pulse rate is increased, and blood pressure is lowered.

DIAGNOSTIC PROCEDURES Evidence of the expelled uterine contents, pelvic examination, ultrasound, and laboratory studies will confirm the occurrence of a spontaneous abortion.

TREATMENT Bed rest may be required for as long as spotting continues. Hospitalization may be necessary to control hemorrhage. If remnants of the conceptus remain in the uterus, D&C should be performed.

PROGNOSIS The prognosis for full recovery is good, barring any complications such as hemorrhage, anemia, or infections.

PREVENTION The progression of a spontaneous abortion usually cannot be prevented.

■ ECTOPIC PREGNANCY

DESCRIPTION *Ectopic pregnancy* occurs when the fertilized ovum implants and grows somewhere other than the uterine cavity. The most common ectopic site is within one of the fallopian tubes. Less frequently, ectopic implantation may occur in an ovary or the abdominal cavity (Fig. 6–11).

ETIOLOGY Ectopic pregnancy is often due to scarring or inflammation of the fallopian tubes as a result of infection, or it may be due to congenital malformations of the tubes. In general, any factor that impedes the migration of the fertilized ovum into the uterus before attachment takes place increases the likelihood of an ectopic pregnancy.

SIGNS AND SYMPTOMS Signs of early pregnancy may be present. There also may be abdominal pain and tenderness, as well as slight vaginal bleeding. A rupture of a fallopian tube due to the development of the conceptus is life-threatening and will cause severe abdominal pain and intra-abdominal bleeding.

DIAGNOSTIC PROCEDURES A pelvic examination and a careful history may suggest ectopic pregnancy. A serum pregnancy test and an ultrasound examination likely will be used in this determination. Laparoscopy and exploratory laparotomy also may help in the diagnosis of this condition.

TREATMENT Laparotomy is frequently necessary. A ruptured fallopian tube may require removal. All attempts will be made to save the ovary. Transfusion of whole blood may be necessary in the event of severe intra-abdominal bleeding or **hypovolemic shock.**

PROGNOSIS The prognosis is good when emergency treatment is sought quickly. If rupture of the tube occurs, complications may be life-threatening. They include hemorrhage, shock, and peritonitis.

PREVENTION Prompt treatment of any genitourinary infection may help reduce the likelihood of ectopic pregnancy.

■ TOXEMIAS OF PREGNANCY
(Preeclampsia and Eclampsia)

DESCRIPTION *Toxemia of pregnancy* is a hypertensive disorder that may develop during the third trimester. Most health-care professionals prefer to use the more precise terms of *preeclampsia* and *eclampsia* to designate the condition. *Preeclampsia* is the initial cluster of symptoms, characterized by hyperten-

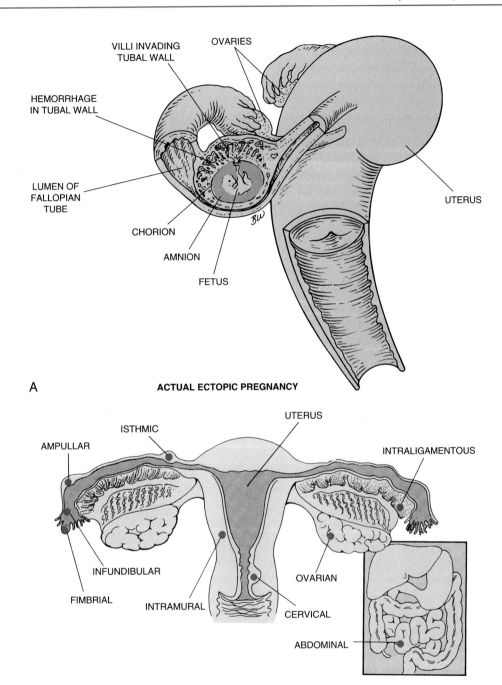

A   **ACTUAL ECTOPIC PREGNANCY**

B   **VARIOUS SITES OF ECTOPIC PREGNANCY**

Figure 6–11 Ectopic pregnancy. (*A*) Actual ectopic pregnancy. (*B*) Various sites of ectopic pregnancy. (From Thomas, CL [ed]: Taber's Cyclopedic Medical Dictionary, ed 18. FA Davis, Philadelphia, 1997, p 601, with permission.)

sion, edema, and proteinuria. *Eclampsia* is the subsequent group of symptoms, characterized by convulsions and coma. Eclampsia is a medical emergency. The condition is more likely to occur in **primigravidae** who are 12 to 18 years old or older, or in women older than 35 who have had multiple pregnancies.

ETIOLOGY The cause of preeclampsia and eclampsia is not known, but it may be related to malnutrition, especially a lack of protein in the diet. Predisposing factors include preexisting vascular and renal disease, age (adolescents and primiparas older than 35 years are at higher risk), and familial factors.

SIGNS AND SYMPTOMS Hypertension, generalized edema, proteinuria, and sudden weight gain are the classic symptoms of preeclampsia. High sodium ingestion may be a contributing factor. Headache, vertigo, malaise, irritability, epigastric pain, and nausea also may occur. Eclampsia symptoms may include tonoclonic convulsions, coma, **rhonchi, nystagmus,** and **oliguria** or **anuria.**

DIAGNOSTIC PROCEDURES Elevated—especially steadily rising—blood pressure, proteinuria, and oliguria are suggestive of preeclampsia. The clinical picture of convulsions confirms a diagnosis of eclampsia.

TREATMENT In preeclampsia, the goal of treatment is to prevent eclampsia and to deliver a normal baby. Bed rest is advised, with sedatives prescribed. Antihypertensives may be necessary. The fetus will be delivered as soon as it is judged viable, possibly be cesarean section. With the onset of eclampsia, the patient will be hospitalized and intensive treatment instituted. Immediate termination of the pregnancy is indicated, whether or not the fetus is judged viable.

PROGNOSIS The prognosis is good for preeclampsia. In eclampsia, the maternal mortality rate is about 15 percent.

PREVENTION Adequate nutrition, good prenatal care, and control of high blood pressure during pregnancy are important. Early treatment of preeclampsia can prevent eclampsia.

■ PLACENTA PREVIA

DESCRIPTION In *placenta previa,* the placenta is implanted abnormally low in the uterus so that it covers all or part of the internal cervical os, or opening (Fig. 6–12). This condition is dangerous because the placenta may prematurely separate from the

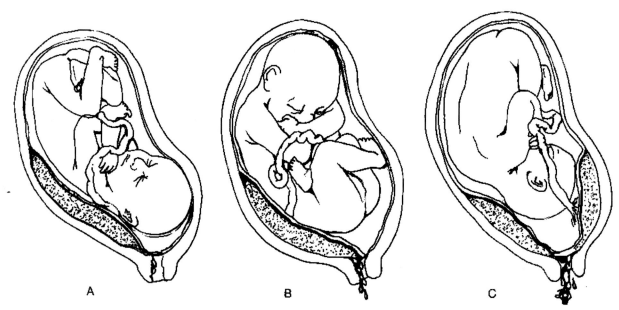

Figure 6–12 Placenta previa. (*A*) Low implantation. (*B*) Partial placenta previa. (*C*) Central (total) placenta previa. (From Beare, PG: Davis's NCLEX-RN Review, ed 2. FA Davis, Philadelphia, 1966, p 61, with permission.)

uterus, causing maternal hemorrhaging and interrupting oxygen flow to the fetus.

ETIOLOGY The cause is unknown, but predisposing factors include multiparity, advanced maternal age, previous uterine surgery, and early or late fertilization.

SIGNS AND SYMPTOMS A typical symptom is slight, painless bleeding, generally occurring in the third trimester, that may become more severe. The fetus may present in a variety of positions, but the situation is not critical as long as fetal heart tones remain strong. Vital signs may indicate shock.

DIAGNOSTIC PROCEDURES Ultrasonography will help in the diagnosis.

TREATMENT Hospital treatment is aimed at controlling and treating any blood loss, delivering a healthy infant, and preventing complications. A cesarean section may be necessary.

PROGNOSIS The maternal prognosis depends on the amount of bleeding; the fetal prognosis depends on gestational age, blood loss, and consequences of possible anorexia. Complications include shock and maternal or fetal death. With prompt and effective treatment, however, both mother and child usually survive.

PREVENTION There is no known prevention.

ABRUPTIO PLACENTAE

DESCRIPTION *Abruptio placentae* is the premature separation of a normally implanted placenta from the uterine wall about the 20th week of gestation. The condition is most common in multigravidae.

ETIOLOGY The cause is unknown, but predisposing factors include trauma, chronic hypertension, and preeclampsia or eclampsia.

SIGNS AND SYMPTOMS Abruptio placentae is characterized by sudden, severe abdominal pain with boardlike rigidity, tenderness of the uterus, hemorrhage, and the onset of shock.

DIAGNOSTIC PROCEDURES Ultrasonography, pelvic examination, and history will help confirm the diagnosis.

TREATMENT The goals of treatment are to control the bleeding, deliver a healthy infant, and to prevent complications. Hospitalization is required, and a cesarean section is typically performed. Blood replacement may be necessary.

PROGNOSIS The maternal prognosis is good if the bleeding can be controlled. The fetal prognosis depends on gestational age and the amount of blood loss. Complications include **disseminated intravascular coagulation** (DIC) and renal failure.

PREVENTION There is no known prevention.

PREMATURE LABOR/PREMATURE RUPTURE OF MEMBRANES (PROM)

DESCRIPTION *Premature rupture of membranes* is early rupture of the amniotic sac. *Premature labor* is the early onset of rhythmic uterine contractions after fetal viability but before fetal maturity.

ETIOLOGY These conditions may be caused by "incompetent cervix," preeclampsia, multiple pregnancy, abruptio placentae, anatomic malformations, infections, or fetal death. A predisposing factor may be poor prenatal care.

SIGNS AND SYMPTOMS There may be a blood-tinged flow from the vagina, with uterine contractions and cervical dilation and **effacement.** Premature rupture of the membranes is marked by the flow of amniotic fluid from the vagina.

DIAGNOSTIC PROCEDURES Diagnosis is confirmed by prenatal history, and vaginal and physical examination. Ultrasonography also may be used. Electronic fetal monitoring is used to confirm the fetal condition.

TREATMENT Attempts will be made to suppress premature labor by bed rest and appropriate drug therapy. PROM typically requires induction of labor or cesarean delivery.

PROGNOSIS The maternal prognosis is good with proper attention and care. The fetal prognosis depends on gestational age.

PREVENTION The best prevention is good prenatal care.

Common Symptoms of Disorders of Pregnancy and Delivery

Pregnant women may present with the following common complaints, any of which deserve attention from health professionals:

- Abdominal pain, tenderness, or cramping
- Unusual discharge, pink or brown in color, or clotted
- Hypertension, rapid weight gain, edema, and malaise, which indicate possible toxemia

SPECIAL FOCUS CESAREAN BIRTH

In a *cesarean birth,* an incision is made through the abdomen and uterus to remove the fetus and placenta. The most common situations requiring cesarean birth include malpresentation of the fetus, fetal distress, a maternal pelvis too small to accommodate the fetal head, the presence of sexually transmitted disease organisms in the birth canal, preeclampsia or eclampsia, and previous cesarean births. Prolonged labor, abnormal fetal heart actions, and maternal distress are also indicators for a possible cesarean birth.

Ultrasound, auscultation of the fetal heart rate, and x-ray pelvimetry may be helpful in making a decision about cesarean delivery. Amniocentesis also may be used. Maternal complications of the procedure may include cardiovascular and pulmonary difficulties and urinary tract infections.

REFERENCES

1. World Health Organization: Education and Treatment in Human Sexuality: The Training of Health Professionals (Technical Report Series No. 572). WHO, Geneva, 1975.

BIBLIOGRAPHY

Alternative Medicine: The Definitive Guide. Burton Goldberg Group, Future Medicine Publishing, Fife, Wash., 1995.

Burns, MV: Pathophysiology: A Self-Instructional Program. Appleton & Lange, Stamford, Conn., 1998.

Comarow, A: Viagra tale. U.S. News and World Report 124(17):64–66.

Fauci, AS, et al: Harrison's Principles of Internal Medicine, ed 14. McGraw-Hill, New York, 1998.

Frazier, MS, Drzymkowski, JA, and Doty, SJ: Essentials of Human Disease and Conditions. WB Saunders, Philadelphia, 1996.

Kent, TH, and Hart, MN: Introduction to Human Disease. Appleton & Lange, Stamford, Conn., 1998.

Professional Guide to Diseases, ed 6. Springhouse Corporation, Springhouse, Pa., 1998.

CASE STUDIES

I   A 15-year-old girl who has been sexually active is informed by her boyfriend that he has gonorrhea. She had noted a slight vaginal discharge and some urinary difficulties, but thought that these were just symptoms of a urinary tract infection, because she has had a UTI twice before.

1. If this girl called the physician's office and told you, a medical assistant, these facts, what would you advise her to do?

2. Could the girl's symptoms be those of a urinary tract infection? Could they be symptoms of gonorrhea? Explain.

3. Based on the assumption that the symptoms were those of a UTI, what diagnostic tests would the physician order? What if the physician suspected gonorrhea?

II   A 51-year-old woman notices that her menstrual cycle is irregular and occurs less frequently, with decreased flow. She has severe hot flashes and mood swings and experiences pain from vaginal dryness during intercourse.

1. What are the implications of the patient's age in regard to these symptoms?

2. If the physician suspected the onset of menopause, what tests would she order?

3. What might be the cause of the hot flashes?

III   A 38-year-old woman visits the physician because she has been experiencing pain in her left breast. The pain appears to be localized. In reply to the physician's question, she reports that she has been examining her breasts monthly and has not noted any lumps or abnormalities. After asking her to describe the pain and indicate its location, the physician examines the patient and finds no abnormalities. The physician advises the patient to return in 6 months; if the pain is still present, he tells her, he will order a mammogram.

1. What are the recommendations of the American Cancer Society that apply to this situation?

2. Is pain an early symptom of cancer?

3. What would you suggest to this woman?

REVIEW QUESTIONS

SHORT ANSWER

1. List the two functions of sexuality in humans:

   a.

   b.

2. Name three inflammatory diseases of the male reproductive system and distinguish between them:

a.

b.

c.

3. List two common diagnostic procedures for prostatic cancer:

a.

b.

4. What is the difference between amenorrhea and dysmenorrhea?

5. Spell out the following abbreviations:

a. BPH:

b. PMS:

c. PID:

MATCHING

Match the definitions with the correct sexual dysfunction:

_____ 1. Erectile dysfunction in males

_____ 2. Sexual dysfunction in females

_____ 3. Ejaculation immediately on, or prior to, intromission

a. Dyspareunia

b. Impotence

c. Premature ejaculation

d. Alopecia

e. Coitus

f. Arousal and orgasmic dysfunction

Match the causes with the corresponding sexually transmitted diseases:

_____ 4. Disease caused by various types of papillomavirus

_____ 5. Disease caused by a motile protozoan

_____ 6. Disease caused by bacteria

_____ 7. Disease caused by the simplex virus

a. Herpes, type 2

b. Genital warts

c. Gonorrhea

d. Chlamydial infection

e. Syphilis

f. Trichomoniasis

Match the three disorders of the breast with the correct signs and symptoms:

_____ 8. Breast mass is round, firm, discrete, and relatively movable; nontender

_____ 9. Widespread lumpiness in the upper, outer quadrant of the breast

_____ 10. Breast dimpling, swelling, skin irritation, nipple discharge

a. Mammary dysplasia

b. Benign fibroadenoma

c. Carcinoma of the breast

Match the following diseases or conditions with their common diagnostic procedures:

_____ 11. Ultrasound and x-ray

_____ 12. Pelvic exam, lab studies, and evidence of expelled uterine contents

_____ 13. Prenatal history, physical examinations, and ultrasound

_____ 14. Pelvic exam, patient history, serum pregnancy test, and ultrasound

_____ 15. Proteinuria, oliguria, and high blood-pressure readings

a. Abortion

b. Toxemias

c. Cesarean birth

d. PROM

e. Ectopic pregnancy

TRUE/FALSE

T   F   1. Benign cysts of the ovary are derived from ovarian follicles and the corpus luteum.

T   F   2. Large ovarian cysts may produce pelvic pain and dyspareunia.

T   F   3. The cause of endometriosis is bacterial in nature.

T   F   4. Endometriosis most frequently occurs postmenopausally.

T   F   5. Uterine leiomyomas are composed of fibrous tissue.

T   F   6. Frequently leiomyomas are asymptomatic.

T   F   7. Menopause is the cessation of ovarian function with an increase in estrogen.

ANSWERS

SHORT ANSWER

1. Reproduction and enhancement of caring and pleasure.
2. Prostatitis, epididymitis, and orchitis. Prostatitis is inflammation of the prostate that may result from urethritis or directly from the bloodstream. Epididymitis is an inflammation of the epididymis that results from prostatitis, UTI, or trauma or that is secondary to an infection elsewhere in the body. Orchitis is inflammation of the testes caused by injury or mumps.
3. Prostate-specific antigen (PSA) test and a rectal examination. Biopsy is essential for confirmation.
4. Amenorrhea, the absence of menstruation, is an abnormal condition that occurs in women at any time other than before puberty, after menopause, or during pregnancy. Dysmenorrhea is painful menstruation or cramps.
5. a. Benign prostatic hyperplasia
   b. Premenstrual syndrome
   c. Pelvic inflammatory disease

MATCHING

1. b	5. f	9. a	13. d
2. f	6. c, d, and e	10. c	14. e
3. c	7. a	11. c	15. b
4. b	8. b	12. a	

TRUE/FALSE

1. T	5. F
2. T	6. T
3. F	7. F
4. F	

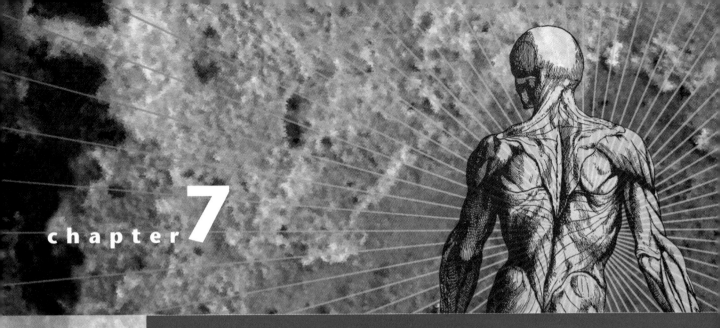

chapter 7

Digestive System Diseases

CHAPTER OUTLINE

Upper Gastrointestinal Tract
Stomatitis
Gastritis
Gastroenteritis
Gastric Ulcer (Peptic Ulcer of the Stomach)
Hiatal Hernia

Lower Gastrointestinal Tract
Malabsorption Syndrome
Celiac Sprue (Gluten-Induced Enteropathy)
*Duodenal Ulcer (Peptic Ulcer of the
    Duodenum)*
Acute Appendicitis
Irritable Bowel Syndrome (IBS)
*Crohn's Disease (Regional Enteritis,
    Granulomatous Colitis)*
Ulcerative Colitis
Diverticulitis
Hemorrhoids
Abdominal Hernias
Colorectal Cancer
Diarrhea

**Accessory Organs of Digestion:
    Pancreas, Gallbladder, and Liver**
Acute Pancreatitis
Chronic Pancreatitis

Pancreatic Cancer
Cholelithiasis
Acute Cholecystitis
Cirrhosis
Acute Viral Hepatitis

Special Focus: Eating Disorders
Anorexia Nervosa
Bulimia

**Special Focus: Digestive Diseases
    Common in Children**
Infantile Colic
Diarrhea
Vomiting
Food Allergies
Helminths (Worms)

**Common Symptoms of Digestive System
    Diseases**
□ ALTERNATIVE MEDICINE

References

Bibliography

Case Studies

Review Questions

LEARNING OBJECTIVES

Upon successful completion of this chapter, you will:

- Define stomatitis.
- List the three types of hiatal hernias.
- Identify at least four causes of gastritis.
- Discuss the signs and symptoms of gastroenteritis.
- Describe the destructive process that causes gastric ulcers.
- Describe the steps to be taken for prevention of *E. coli* infections.
- Describe the symptoms for appendicitis.
- Discuss the inflammatory pattern of Crohn's disease.
- List at least three predisposing factors of ulcerative colitis.
- Restate the cause of, and treatment for, abdominal hernias.
- Identify populations at risk for colorectal cancer.
- Describe the condition of hemorrhoids.
- Compare and contrast anorexia nervosa and bulimia.
- Explain the symptoms of malabsorption syndrome.
- Define duodenal ulcer.
- Discuss the treatment of duodenal ulcers.
- Review causes of irritable bowel syndrome.
- Define diarrhea as a symptom.
- Explain the implications of pancreatitis.
- Recall the incidence of pancreatic cancer.
- Discuss the relationship between cholecystitis and cholelithiasis.
- Describe cirrhosis and its treatment.
- Name two complications of cirrhosis.
- Define the different types of hepatitis.
- Discuss the etiology of colic
- Compare and contrast acute and chronic diarrhea.
- List the most common nutritional allergens.
- Compare and contrast roundworm and pinworm infestations.
- List at least three common complaints of the digestive system.

KEY WORDS

Alkalosis (ăl•kă•lō′sĭs)
Anorexia (ăn•ō•rĕk′sē•ă)
Anticholinergic (ăn•tĭ•kō•lĭn•ĕr′jĭk)
Antidiarrheal (ăn•tĭ•dī•ă•rē′ăl)
Antiemetic (ăn•tĭ•ē•mĕt′ĭk)
Ascites (ă•sī′tēz)
Bile (bīl)
Bilirubin (bĭl•ĭ•roo′bĭn)
Bilirubinuria (bĭl•ĭ•roo•bĭn•ū′rē•ă)
Cachexia (kă•kĕks′ē•ă)
Cholestasis (kō•lē•stā′sĭs)
Colectomy (kō•lĕk′tō•mē)
Coryza (kŏ•rī′ză)
Diaphoresis (dī•ă•fō•rē′sĭs)
Dysphagia (dĭs•fā′jē•ă)
Electrolyte (ē•lĕk′trō•līt)
Enteropathy (ĕn•tĕr•ŏp′ă•thē)
Epigastric (ĕp•ĭ•găs′trĭk)
Fecalith (fē′kă•lĭth)

Fistula (fĭs′tū•lă)
Gamma globulin (găm′ă glŏb′ū•lĭn)
Hematemesis (hĕm•ăt•ĕm′ĕ•sis)
Hemolysis (hē•mŏl′ĭ•sĭs)
Hepatomegaly (hĕp•ă•tō•mĕg′ă•lē)
Hyperglycemia (hī•pĕr•glī•sē′mē•ă)
Hypokalemia (hī•pō•kă•lē′mē•ă)
Ileostomy (ĭl•ē•ŏs′tō•mē)
Jaundice (jawn′dĭs)
Lassitude (lăs′ĭ•tūd)
Leukocytosis (loo•kō•sī•tō′sĭs)
Lymphadenopathy (lĭm•făd•ĕ•nŏp′ă•thē)
Malaise (mă•lāz′)
McBurney's point
Myalgia (mī•ăl′jē•ă)
Occult blood (ŭ•kŭlt′)
Pallor (păl′or)
Parenteral (păr•ĕn′tĕr•ăl)
Polyposis (pŏl•ē•pō′sĭs)
Proteinuria (prō•tē•ĭn•ūr′ē•ă)

Pruritus (proo•rī′tŭs)
Pyuria (pī•ū′rē•ă)
Rauwolfia (serpentina) (raw•wŏlf′ē•ă)
Reflux (rē′flŭks)
Salicylate (săl•ĭs′ĭl•āt)

Splenomegaly (splē•nō•mĕg′ă•lē)
Tetany (tĕt′ă•nē)
Toxemia (tŏks•ē′mē•ă)
Varices (văr′ĭ•sēz)
Villi (intestinal) (vĭl′ī)

The digestive system consists of the set of organs and glands associated with the ingestion and digestion of food and the absorption of nutrients (Fig. 7–1). This system also eliminates solid wastes from the body. It may be the system most abused. Whether a person is eating foods of little value or a well-balanced diet, the task of the digestive system is the same—to nourish the cells of the body.

Upper Gastrointestinal Tract

STOMATITIS

DESCRIPTION Stomatitis or inflammation of the oral mucosa comes in two forms: *acute herpetic stomatitis* (cold sore) and *aphthous stomatitis* (canker sores). Painful blisters or ulcers characterize both.

ETIOLOGY Acute herpetic stomatitis is caused by herpes simplex type 1. The cause of aphthous stomatitis is unknown. Acute herpetic stomatitis lies dormant in nervous tissue with recurring lesions appearing throughout life. Aphthous stomatitis is activated periodically. Stress, fatigue, anxiety, and immunosuppression exacerbate both.

DIAGNOSTIC PROCEDURES Diagnosis is based on physical examination. The herpetic form of stomatitis is characterized by blisters and ulcerating and crusting inflammatory lesions that heal in less than 2 weeks. The ulcers in aphthous stomatitis are discrete and shallow and gradually heal in 7 to 10 days.

TREATMENT Supportive measures such as warm-water mouth rinses and topical anesthetics to relieve the pain are recommended.

PROGNOSIS Both forms are self-limiting.

PREVENTION Alleviation of precipitating factors can be helpful. Recurrence is likely for both forms.

GASTRITIS

DESCRIPTION *Gastritis,* the most common stomach ailment, consists of the inflammation and erosion of the gastric mucosa.

ETIOLOGY The etiology of gastritis is varied and complex. Irritating foods, alcoholic beverages, caffeine, aspirin, and ingested poisons can cause gastritis. It can be secondary to elevated blood pressure in the portal vein, sprue, and influenza. In many cases, though, gastritis is idiopathic.

SIGNS AND SYMPTOMS After exposure to the offending substances, the acute form of gastritis may feature gastrointestinal (GI) bleeding, belching, **epigastric** pain, and vomiting, including **hematemesis.** A client with the chronic form of gastritis may exhibit similar symptoms, mild discomfort, or no symptoms. When symptoms do develop, they may be hard to pinpoint. A person may experience a loss of appetite, a "full" feeling in the stomach, or have vague epigastric pain.

DIAGNOSTIC PROCEDURES A medical history that reveals exposure to a GI irritant may suggest this disorder. Gastroscopy (with biopsy) will help confirm the diagnosis. Laboratory analysis to detect blood in vomitus or stool may be performed.

TREATMENT Symptoms will be relieved by eliminating the irritant or cause. In the event of ingestion of toxic substances, an antidote or **antiemetic**

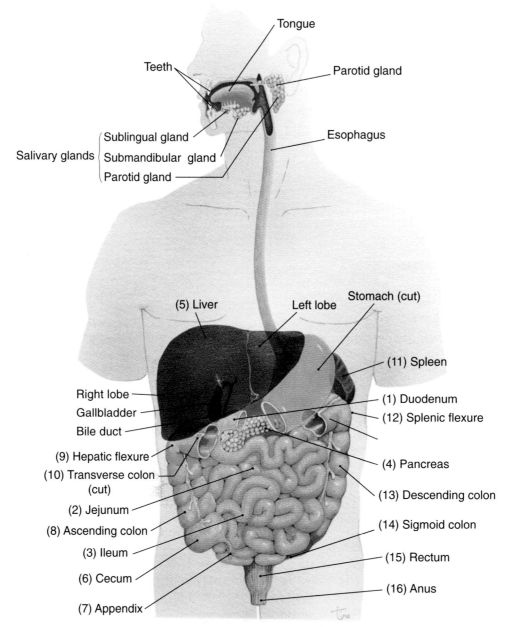

Figure 7–1 The digestive system. (Modified from Scanlon, VC, and Sanders, T: Essentials of Anatomy and Physiology, ed 3. FA Davis, Philadelphia, 1999, p 353, with permission.)

may be prescribed. **Anticholinergics** and antacids may relieve distress, too. If there is severe bleeding, blood replacement may be necessary.

PROGNOSIS The prognosis is good with proper treatment.

PREVENTION Prevention includes avoiding gastric irritants. Taking prescribed medications with milk or food and avoiding aspirin-containing substances will be helpful. Spicy foods, alcohol, caffeine, and tobacco should be avoided.

■ GASTROENTERITIS

DESCRIPTION *Gastroenteritis* is the inflammation of the stomach and small intestine; it may also be called intestinal flu, traveler's diarrhea, or food poisoning.

ETIOLOGY Causes of gastroenteritis include infection from bacteria, amebae, parasites, and viruses. The ingestion of toxins, allergic reactions to certain foods, and drug reactions also may produce this disease.

SIGNS AND SYMPTOMS The etiology of the particular case will determine, in part, the signs and symptoms, which may include diarrhea, cramping, nausea, vomiting, **malaise,** fever, and rumbling stomach sounds.

DIAGNOSTIC PROCEDURES The medical history may suggest gastroenteritis. A stool and/or blood culture will identify any bacteria or parasite. An endoscopy may be performed.

TREATMENT Treatment is symptomatic and supportive. Fluid and nutritional support are important to minimize electrolyte and fluid imbalances. **Antidiarrheals** and antiemetics may be prescribed. Children and elderly persons must be carefully monitored for fluid and electrolyte imbalance.

PROGNOSIS The prognosis varies with the etiology, but is generally good once the cause has been isolated and treatment has begun. Gastroenteritis occurs in persons of all ages.

PREVENTION All perishable food should be properly refrigerated, and hands should be washed thoroughly before handling food. Cook all foods thoroughly. Eliminate flies and roaches in the home. People traveling in underdeveloped countries should be especially careful of contaminated water or food.

■ GASTRIC ULCER (Peptic Ulcer of the Stomach)

DESCRIPTION A *gastric ulcer* is a lesion in the musocal lining of the stomach. In this disease, a patch of mucosal tissue becomes necrotic and is subsequently eroded by the acids and pepsins released within the stomach. Put simply, the stomach begins digesting itself (Fig. 7–2).

ETIOLOGY Gastric ulcers represent a breakdown in the balance between acid-pepsin secretion and mucosal defense in the stomach. The causes of this breakdown are not clear, but they seem related to chronic oversecretion of gastric juices, stress, and hereditary factors. Reactions to drugs such as **sali-**

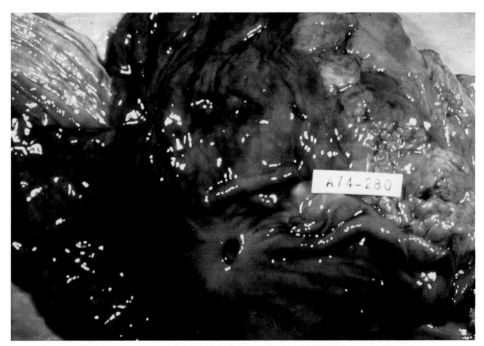

Figure 7–2 Gastric ulcer. (From Gylys, BA, and Wedding, MA: Medical Terminology: A Systems Approach, ed 4. FA Davis, Philadelphia, 1999, p 94, with permission from WRS Group.)

cylates, and smoking and alcohol, may be contributing factors. The disease is more common in middle-aged to elderly men.

Recently, researchers have found some support for the theory that gastric ulcers are caused by bacterial infection.

SIGNS AND SYMPTOMS Persistent "heartburn" and indigestion are the classic symptoms. There may be nagging stomach pain as well. Gastrointestinal bleeding, nausea, vomiting, and weight loss may be additional symptoms. The onset of symptoms is more common about 2 hours after meals and after the consumption of orange juice, coffee, aspirin, or alcohol.

DIAGNOSTIC PROCEDURES A barium x-ray and an upper gastrointestinal endoscopy are the most frequent methods used to diagnose a gastric ulcer. Biopsy will rule out malignancy.

TREATMENT Treatment of gastric ulcers is aimed at reduction of acid secretions, healing of the mucosal lining, and relief of symptoms. Treatment may consist of the use of antacids or the prescription of a class of drugs known as H_2 receptor antagonists, which inhibit the release of stomach acid. Bland diets may have some limited benefit, but affected in-

dividuals should be advised to avoid alcohol, caffeine, and smoking. Surgical management of a gastric ulcer is generally avoided unless it proves malignant or perforation occurs.

PROGNOSIS The prognosis varies. Gastric ulcers are frequently chronic, tending to heal and then reform in the same location. Complications of gastric ulcers include hemorrhage and perforation, both potentially life-threatening situations. Gastric ulcers must be carefully monitored for signs of malignancy.

PREVENTION There is no known prevention, although carefully following a treatment protocol may prevent recurrence.

■ HIATAL HERNIA

DESCRIPTION A *hiatal hernia* is the protrusion of some portion of the stomach into the thoracic cavity through the opening in the diaphragm through which the esophagus passes (the esophageal hiatus) (Fig. 7–3). There are three varieties of hiatal hernia: (1) in *sliding hernias* (most common), the gastroesophageal junction and the upper portion of the stomach slide upward through the esophageal hia-

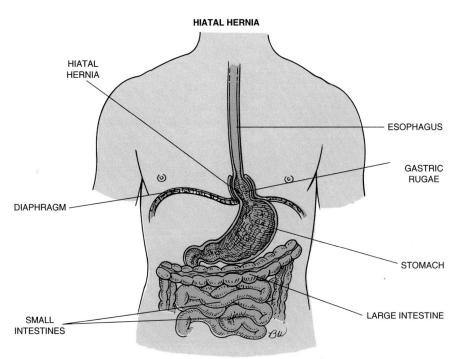

HIATAL HERNIA

HIATAL HERNIA

ESOPHAGUS

GASTRIC RUGAE

DIAPHRAGM

STOMACH

SMALL INTESTINES

LARGE INTESTINE

Figure 7–3 Hiatal hernia. (From Thomas, CL [ed]: Taber's Cyclopedic Medical Dictionary, ed 18. FA Davis, Philadelphia, 1997, p 890, with permission.)

tus; (2) in *paraesophageal,* or *"rolling,"* hernias, the gastroesophageal junction remains fixed, but some portion of the stomach passes through the esophageal hiatus; and (3) in *mixed hernias,* the characteristics of sliding and paraesophageal hernias are combined. Figure 7–4 illustrates the configuration of hiatal hernias.

ETIOLOGY The cause of hiatal hernias is unclear. They may be due to intra-abdominal pressure, or weakening of the gastroesophageal junction caused by trauma or the loss of muscle tone. The incidence of hiatal hernia increases with age, and sliding hernias are far more common than paraesophageal and mixed hernias combined.

SIGNS AND SYMPTOMS Over half of those having hiatal hernias may remain asymptomatic. If symptoms are present, they commonly include heartburn—aggravated by reclining—chest pain, **dysphagia,** esophageal **reflux;** or severe pain if a large portion of the stomach is caught above the diaphragm.

DIAGNOSTIC PROCEDURES Diagnosis of hiatal hernias will be made by chest x-ray, barium x-ray, endoscopy and biopsy, and pH studies of any reflux (to eliminate the possibility of gastric ulcer).

TREATMENT The goal in treatment is to alleviate symptoms. Surgery is not the first choice of treatment unless strangulation of the hernia is evident or symptoms cannot be controlled. An attempt is made to reduce episodes of reflux through dietary modification or by strengthening the lower esophageal sphincter with medication. Activity restrictions may be indicated, and the person may be advised to avoid tight or restrictive clothing. Stool softeners and laxatives, to prevent straining at stool, and antacids may be prescribed. Avoiding food intake before sleep and elevating the heat of the bed may be advised.

PROGNOSIS The prognosis is good with proper treatment. Complications including stricture, significant bleeding, pulmonary aspiration, or strangulation require surgical repair.

PREVENTION No prevention is known.

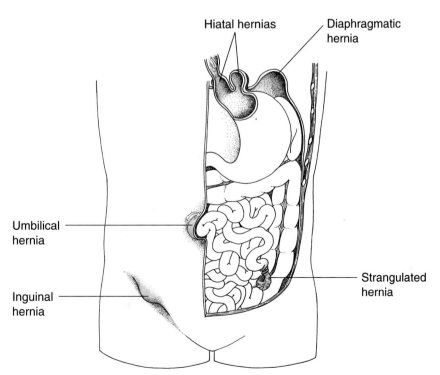

Figure 7–4 Hernias and their locations. (From Gylys, BA, and Wedding, ME: Medical Terminology: A Systems Approach, ed 4. FA Davis, Philadelphia, 1999, p 95, with permission.)

Lower Gastrointestinal Tract

MALABSORPTION SYNDROME

Malabsorption syndrome encompasses a host of diseases of the small intestine, characterized by the impaired passage of nutrients, minerals, or fluids through intestinal tissue into the blood or lymph. Possible causes of malabsorption syndrome include:

- Inadequate digestion caused by gastrectomy or pancreatic deficiencies.
- Inadequate absorptive surface as a result of intestinal resection or bypass.
- Mucosal absorptive defects caused by various inflammatory disorders or biochemical or genetic defects.
- Reduced concentrations of **bile** as a result of liver disease, bile duct obstruction, bacterial reduction of bile salts, or drug reactions.
- Endocrine or metabolic disorders such as diabetes mellitus or hyperparathyroidism.
- Lymphatic disorders.
- Cardiovascular disorders.

The signs and symptoms of malabsorption syndrome are legion and vary with the specific pathophysiology of the case, but typically they include chronic diarrhea and abnormal bowel movements. The treatment of and prognosis for malabsorption syndrome also vary with etiology. A common malabsorption disorder, celiac sprue, is discussed in the following section.

CELIAC SPRUE (Gluten-Induced Enteropathy)

DESCRIPTION *Celiac sprue* is a disease of the small intestine marked by malabsorption, gluten intolerance (gluten is a protein found in wheat and wheat products), and damage to, and characteristic changes in, the mucosal lining of the intestine. Because of the gluten intolerance characterizing celiac sprue, the disease is sometimes referred to as *gluten-induced* **enteropathy.**

ETIOLOGY The cause of celiac sprue is not clearly understood. The gluten-induced damage to the intestine's mucosal lining may result from either a toxic or immunologic reaction to this protein. The disease may be inherited because the incidence is high among siblings. Women are affected twice as frequently as men.

SIGNS AND SYMPTOMS Symptoms of celiac sprue may include weight loss, **anorexia,** abdominal distension, flatulence, intestinal bleeding, peripheral neuritis, dermatitis, and muscle wasting. The condition is also marked by the passage of diarrheal, abnormally large stools that are characteristically light yellow to gray, greasy, and foul-smelling. The resultant chronic malnutrition may cause mineral depletion that may be revealed as bone pain, tenderness, compression deformities, and **tetany.**

DIAGNOSTIC PROCEDURES The disease often is difficult to diagnose and differentiate from other intestinal disorders. If malabsorption is indicated, two criteria must be met for a definitive diagnosis of celiac sprue: (1) biopsy of the small intestine indicating destruction of **villi** and (2) remission of symptoms and improvement in the condition of the villi after institution of a gluten-free diet.

Currently, an initial serological test followed by biopsy is recommended. The serology includes testing for antigliadin antibodies (IgA and IgG) and antiendomysium antibodies. If these antibody tests are positive, there is a 99.6 percent chance that the individual has celiac sprue, and a biopsy is ordered to confirm the diagnosis.

Laboratory tests may show a decrease in minerals and a deficiency of vitamins B, D, and K. A D-xylose test may indicate a decrease in intestinal absorption. X-rays may reveal demineralization of bone, collapsed vertebrae, and osteoid seams.

TREATMENT Treatment consists of strict adherence to a gluten-free diet. A few persons who do not experience improved small bowel function after instituting a gluten-free diet may be treated with corticosteroid drugs.

PROGNOSIS With proper treatment and a lifelong gluten-free diet, the prognosis is good. Symptomatic relief often occurs within a few weeks, but improvement in tests of absorption function and small bowel tissue characteristics may not occur for months, sometimes years. Antibody testing can be used to check on compliance with the gluten-free diet. If the antibody test is negative it means the individual is complying with the diet. If positive, there is gluten ingestion. If persons go on and off the diet, tissue regeneration may no longer be possible. Persons with celiac sprue have an increased incidence of abdominal lymphoma and carcinomas later in life. Individuals who develop gastrointestinal symptoms while in remission and on a gluten-free diet should be carefully evaluated for malignancy.

PREVENTION There is no known prevention of the disease.

◼ DUODENAL ULCER (Peptic Ulcer of the Duodenum)

DESCRIPTION A *duodenal ulcer* is a circumscribed, craterlike lesion in the mucous membrane of the short, wide segment of the small intestine called the *duodenum*. Duodenal ulcers tend to be chronic and recurrent; they are a major health problem in the United States, but have been declining in frequency. More common in men, they can occur at any time from infancy to later life. The majority of these ulcers appear in the first few inches of the duodenum.

ETIOLOGY The cause is obscure, but it is most likely due to infection with *Helicobacter pylori,* use of salicylates, hypersecretion of stomach acids, damage to duodenal tissue, or critical illness. Genetic factors and smoking are associated with the likelihood of developing the disease. Precipitating factors include trauma, infections, and physical or emotional stress.

SIGNS AND SYMPTOMS Typical symptoms include chronic, periodic heartburn pain that may radiate into the back region. Often, there is a peculiar sensation of hot water bubbling in the back of the throat. Usually the symptoms appear about 2 hours after eating, or consuming orange juice, caffeine, alcohol, or aspirin.

DIAGNOSTIC PROCEDURES Diagnosis is difficult, since duodenal ulcers may be confused with gastric ulcers, gastritis, or irritable bowel syndrome, especially if the symptoms are atypical. Laboratory findings may reveal anemia, **occult blood** in stools, and hypersecretion of stomach acids. X-rays are essential to differentiate the disease from other disorders, but they may not always show an ulcer. Endoscopy will be used if x-rays do not confirm the diagnosis.

TREATMENT General rest is advised, with alleviation of as much anxiety as possible. Restriction of alcohol, smoking, and some medications, such as salicylates and **rauwolfia,** is recommended. Dietary measures include a well-balanced diet and restriction of coffee, tea, colas, orange juice, and other foods known to aggravate symptoms. Prescribed medications may include antacids; antihistamine drugs, especially H_2 blocking agents that reduce stomach acid secretions; prostaglandins; and anticholinergic drugs. Vagotomy, severing one or more branches of the vagus nerve to reduce hydrochloric acid secretion, may be helpful.

PROGNOSIS Duodenal ulcers generally have a chronic course. Many can be controlled, however, by medical treatment. Complications that may worsen the prognosis include hemorrhage, perforation, and bowel obstruction.

PREVENTION There is no specific prevention. Changing to a less stressful lifestyle and following treatment protocols are beneficial.

◼ ACUTE APPENDICITIS

DESCRIPTION *Acute appendicitis* is an inflammation of the vermiform appendix.

ETIOLOGY Appendicitis may be initiated by obstruction of the interior of the appendix by a **fecalith,** neoplasm, foreign body, or worms (Fig. 7–5). In many cases, though, ulceration of the mucosal lining of the appendix appears to be the causative factor. Regardless of the etiology, the course of the disease is the same. Bacteria multiply and invade the appendix wall, compromising circulation to the organ. Necrosis of appendiceal tissue, gangrene, and eventually perforation occur. Perforation of the appendix is life-threatening because the infection is then able to spread into the peritoneal cavity.

SIGNS AND SYMPTOMS The classic symptoms are generalized abdominal pain followed by pain localized in the lower right quadrant (Fig. 7–6). Nausea, vomiting, and anorexia will likely occur. Fever,

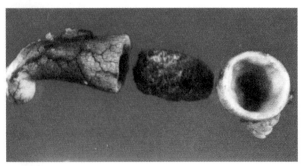

Figure 7–5 Acute appendicitis. The lumen of this acutely inflamed appendix is dilated and contains a large fecalith. (From Rubin, E, and Farber, JL [eds]: Pathology, ed 3. Lippincott-Raven, Philadelphia, 1999, p 749, with permission.)

malaise, diarrhea, or constipation are among the later symptoms.

DIAGNOSTIC PROCEDURES Physical examination and the characteristic symptomatology generally indicate appendicitis. Tenderness upon pressure on **McBurney's point,** and the patient's ability to pinpoint the area of maximum tenderness are the strongest diagnostic indicators of appendicitis. Laboratory findings may reveal **leukocytosis** and **pyuria.** Hospitalization and observation may be necessary to differentiate appendicitis from other abdominal disorders. Abdominal and rectal examinations and complete blood counts may need to be repeated.

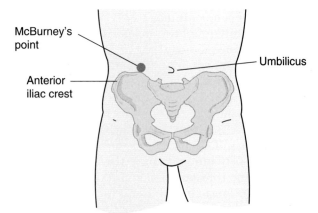

Figure 7–6 Pain at McBurney's point is a symptom of appendicitis. (From Williams, LS, and Hopper, PD [eds]: Understanding Medical-Surgical Nursing. FA Davis, Philadelphia, 1999, p 599, with permission.)

TREATMENT Appendectomy is the recommended treatment.

PROGNOSIS With early diagnosis and treatment, the prognosis is good. If the appendix ruptures, however, peritonitis may ensue, greatly increasing the likelihood of death.

PREVENTION No prevention is known.

◼ IRRITABLE BOWEL SYNDROME (IBS)

DESCRIPTION *Irritable bowel syndrome* is a symptom complex marked by abdominal pain and altered bowel function—typically constipation, diarrhea, or alternating constipation and diarrhea—for which no organic cause can be determined. The disease is chronic, with the onset of symptoms usually occurring in early adulthood and lasting intermittently for years. IBS is the most frequently occurring gastrointestinal disorder in the United States. Its management often proves frustrating to client and physician alike. IBS is sometimes incorrectly referred to as "spastic colon."

ETIOLOGY The cause of IBS is unknown, but it is suspected that the disease may arise from a number of underlying disorders. What is known is that IBS is associated with a change in colonic motility, either decreased motility or increased motility. The disease also has a strong psychological component, with certain personality types more frequently affected than others.

SIGNS AND SYMPTOMS The hallmark of IBS is abdominal pain with constipation, or constipation alternating with diarrhea. The totally diarrheal form of IBS is often painless. Heartburn, abdominal distension, back pain, weakness, and faintness also may accompany the primary symptoms. Stool may be reported as mucus-covered. Symptoms usually are experienced as acute attacks that subside within 1 day, but recurrent exacerbations are likely.

DIAGNOSTIC PROCEDURES The chronic, intermittent nature of the symptoms without obvious cause suggests the diagnosis; however, irritable bowel syndrome must be differentiated from other gastrointestinal diseases. A careful client history, especially of psychological factors, is essential. A complete blood count and stool examination for occult blood, ova, parasites, and pathogenic bacteria will help rule out closely related conditions. Sigmoidoscopy, colonoscopy, barium enema, and rectal biopsy may provide similarly useful information.

TREATMENT There is no one successful treatment for controlling IBS. Dietary modification may be attempted, such as avoiding irritating foods or adding fiber if constipation is a symptom. The client is advised to get adequate sleep and exercise and alleviate as much stress as possible. A sedative or antispasmodic drug may be ordered. Educating the patient about the chronic but benign nature of the disease is an essential part of the treatment process.

PROGNOSIS Because IBS cannot be cured, the prognosis varies according to how successfully the symptoms can be controlled. There is a higher incidence of diverticulitis and colon cancer in individuals with irritable bowel syndrome. Accordingly, regular checkups including sigmoidoscopy and rectal examination are important.

PREVENTION There is no known prevention.

CROHN'S DISEASE (Regional Enteritis, Granulomatous Colitis)

DESCRIPTION *Crohn's disease* is a serious, chronic inflammation, usually of the ileum, although it may affect any portion of the intestinal tract. Crohn's disease is distinguished from closely related bowel disorders by its inflammatory pattern. The inflammation extending through all layers of the intestinal wall results in a characteristic thickening or toughening of the wall and narrowing of the intestinal lumen. The inflammation tends to be patchy or segmented (compare with ulcerative colitis).

ETIOLOGY The cause of Crohn's disease is unknown. Researchers do not believe this disease is caused by emotional stress or irritating foods. Research is under way in the fields of immunology and microbiology. Many scientists now believe that the interaction of a virus or bacterium with the body's immune system may trigger the disease, or that such an agent may cause damage to the intestinal wall, initiating or accelerating the disease process.[1]

SIGNS AND SYMPTOMS Signs and symptoms include colicky or steady abdominal pain in the right lower quadrant, diarrhea, lack of appetite, and weight loss. A variety of sores, fissures, or **fistulas** may appear in the anal area.

DIAGNOSTIC PROCEDURES Crohn's disease is diagnosed by differentiating its characteristic pattern of inflammation from those of other bowel disorders. A thorough medical history is essential. Barium enema, sigmoidoscopy, and colonoscopy may be necessary. Only a biopsy provides a definitive diagnosis.

TREATMENT Treatment of Crohn's disease is symptomatic and supportive. Oral forms of mesalamine (the generic name for 5-aminosalicylic acid [5-ASA]), the active component of sulfasalazine, have been found beneficial in treating Crohn's disease and in preventing relapses. Corticosteroids (given orally, rectally, or by injection) are given when symptoms are more severe. Surgical treatment of the disease is usually reserved for managing complications, but **colectomy** or **ileostomy** may be necessary in persons with extensive disease.

PROGNOSIS The prognosis depends on the severity of the initial onset of the disease and its clinical history. The prognosis worsens over time. Complications may include intestinal obstruction and fistula formation, resulting in peritonitis and sepsis.

PREVENTION There is no known prevention or cure.

ULCERATIVE COLITIS

DESCRIPTION *Ulcerative colitis* is a chronic inflammation and ulceration of the colon, often beginning in the rectum or sigmoid colon and extending upward into the entire colon. Ulcerative colitis is distinguished from closely related bowel disorders by its characteristic inflammatory pattern. The inflammation involves only the mucosal lining of the colon, which exhibits erythema and numerous hemorrhagic ulcerations. In addition, the affected portion of the colon is uniformly involved, with no patches of healthy mucosal tissue evident (compare with Crohn's disease).

ETIOLOGY The etiology for ulcerative colitis is the same as for Crohn's disease. Researchers believe that the body's defenses are operating against some substance in the body, perhaps even the digestive tract, which is recognized as foreign. These foreign substances or antigens may stimulate the body's defenses to produce an inflammation.[2]

SIGNS AND SYMPTOMS The classic symptom is recurrent bloody diarrhea, often containing pus and mucus, accompanied by abdominal pain and severe urgency to move the bowels. Other symptoms may include fever, weight loss, and signs of dehydration. There is a tendency toward periodic exacerbation and remission of symptoms.

DIAGNOSTIC PROCEDURES The disease is diagnosed by the characteristics of the inflammatory process. Sigmoidoscopy may reveal the mucosal lining to be friable (easily broken or pulverized). Colonoscopy may be necessary to determine the extent of the disease. A biopsy may be done at the same time to rule out carcinoma.

TREATMENT The treatment program generally includes measures to suppress the inflammatory response, permit healing, and relieve the symptoms. Sulfasalazine (a compound derived from sulfapyridine and 5-ASA) is an effective treatment for mild to moderate episodes of ulcerative colitis. Oral forms of 5-ASA appear to be effective in treating active ulcerative colitis and in preventing relapses. Corticosteroid treatment, as described in the section on Crohn's disease, is also effective against ulcerative colitis. Surgical excision and resection of the entire colon and rectum are reserved for management of serious complications. This procedure necessitates an ileostomy.

PROGNOSIS The prognosis for an individual with ulcerative colitis depends on the severity of the acute episodes of the disease. Complications may be life-threatening and include anemia and perforated colon with resulting **toxemia.** Persons with ulcerative colitis involving the whole colon for 8 to 10 years run an above-average risk of developing colorectal cancer.

PREVENTION There is no known prevention and no known cure.

■ DIVERTICULITIS

DESCRIPTION *Diverticulitis* is the acute inflammation of small, pouchlike herniations in the intestinal wall called *diverticula* (Fig. 7–7). The diverticula may form anywhere along the intestinal tract but most commonly develop in the sigmoid colon. The presence of diverticula (diverticulosis) usually does not produce symptoms; rather, it is the infection of the diverticula that produces the clinically significant condition.

ETIOLOGY The cause of diverticulitis is not clearly understood, but it probably involves the accumulation of intestinal matter within a diverticulum to form a small fecalith. Bacteria multiply around the fecalith, attacking the inner surface of the diverticulum; the resulting inflammation may lead to perforation. The formation of diverticula and, hence, the incidence of diverticulitis may be due in part to a diet of highly refined, low-residue foods.

SIGNS AND SYMPTOMS The symptoms of diverticulitis vary from case to case in both intensity and duration. Typically, though, an acute attack is characterized by fever; pain in the left lower abdomen that is relieved following a bowel movement; and abdominal muscle spasms, guarding, and tenderness. The person usually experiences constipation, but diarrhea may sometimes occur instead.

DIAGNOSTIC PROCEDURES Sigmoidoscopy and colonoscopy are useful in the diagnosis of diverticulitis. A barium enema or a biopsy of the diverticula may be attempted, but not if the disease is in the active phase because of the possibility of perforation and hemorrhage. Blood testing may reveal an elevated erythrocyte sedimentation rate (ESR), leukocytosis, and the presence of occult blood.

TREATMENT Treatment of uncomplicated diverticular disease consists of a high-residue diet that includes bran, bulk additives, and stool softeners. Anticholinergic drugs or antibiotics may be ordered. If perforation or hemorrhage occur, hospitalization, surgery, and blood transfusions may be necessary.

PROGNOSIS The prognosis becomes less favorable with advancing age. Proper dietary measures and antibiotics can generally forestall acute episodes of the disease. Perforation of the intestinal wall in diverticulitis can lead to acute peritonitis, sepsis, and shock.

PREVENTION There is no known prevention.

MULTIPLE DIVERTICULA OF THE COLON

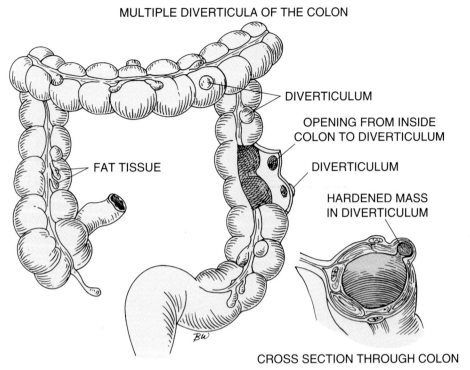

DIVERTICULUM

OPENING FROM INSIDE
COLON TO DIVERTICULUM

DIVERTICULUM

HARDENED MASS
IN DIVERTICULUM

FAT TISSUE

CROSS SECTION THROUGH COLON

Figure 7–7 Multiple diverticula of the colon. (From Thomas, CL [ed]. Taber's Cyclopedic Medical Dictionary, ed 18. FA Davis, Philadelphia, 1997, p 565, with permission.)

HEMORRHOIDS

DESCRIPTION *Hemorrhoids* are dilated, tortuous veins in the mucous membrane of the anus or rectum. There are two kinds: *external hemorrhoids,* those involving veins below the anorectal line; and *internal hemorrhoids,* those involving veins above or along the anorectal line (Fig. 7–8).

ETIOLOGY Straining at stool, constipation, prolonged sitting, and anorectal infections are factors that contribute to the development of hemorrhoids. Other factors may be loss of muscle tone due to old age, pregnancy, and anal intercourse.

SIGNS AND SYMPTOMS There may be rectal bleeding and vague discomfort. In some cases, the hemorrhoids may protrude from the anus. There may be a discharge of mucus from the rectum, too.

DIAGNOSTIC PROCEDURES Physical examination will reveal external hemorrhoids. Proctoscopy will reveal internal hemorrhoids and rule out rectal

polyps. If there is significant bleeding, red blood cell and hemoglobin levels may be low.

TREATMENT Treatment generally includes measures to ease pain and discomfort, such as taking warm sitz baths. A high-roughage diet and using stool softeners also may be recommended. Protruding hemorrhoids may be reduced manually with a lubricated gloved finger, by ligation, or by cryo-surgery. In the event of severe complications or chronic discomfort, complete internal or external hemorrhoidectomy may be advised.

PROGNOSIS With proper treatment, the prognosis is good. Complications may include **pruritus,** fecal incontinence, anorectal infections, prolapse and strangulation of the hemorrhoidal vein, and secondary anemia due to chronic blood loss.

PREVENTION Prevention includes avoiding straining at stool and adherence to a proper diet and exercise regime.

HEMORRHOIDS

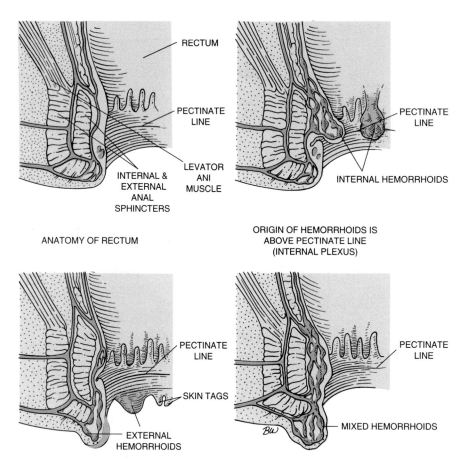

ANATOMY OF RECTUM

ORIGIN OF HEMORRHOIDS IS
ABOVE PECTINATE LINE
(INTERNAL PLEXUS)

ORIGIN OF HEMORRHOIDS IS
BELOW PECTINATE LINE
(EXTERNAL PLEXUS)

ORIGIN OF HEMORRHOIDS IS
ABOVE AND BELOW PECTINATE LINE
(INTERNAL AND EXTERNAL PLEXUS)

Figure 7–8 Hemorrhoids. (From Thomas, CL [ed]: Taber's Cyclopedic Medical Dictionary, ed 18. FA Davis, Philadelphia, 1997, p 881, with permission.)

◼ ABDOMINAL HERNIAS

DESCRIPTION An *abdominal hernia* is the protrusion of an internal organ, typically a portion of the intestine, through an abnormal opening in the musculature of the abdominal wall. Abdominal hernias are categorized according to the location of the herniation and include umbilical, inguinal, and femoral hernias (see Fig. 7–4). Inguinal hernias are the most common.

ETIOLOGY Hernias may result from a congenital weakness in the abdominal wall or muscle. Heavy

lifting, pregnancy, obesity, and straining at stool are predisposing factors.

SIGNS AND SYMPTOMS Inguinal and umbilical hernias are evidenced by the appearance, over the herniated area, of a lump that tends to disappear when the person is supine. Sharp, steady, accompanying pain may be present in the groin. Strangulation of a herniated portion of the intestine will cause severe pain and can cause bowel obstruction (see Fig. 7–4).

DIAGNOSTIC PROCEDURES Physical examination will reveal the herniated area. A medical history of sharp abdominal pain when lifting or straining also may help confirm the diagnosis. An x-ray will be ordered if bowel obstruction is suspected.

TREATMENT Umbilical hernias may require only taping or binding the affected area until the hernia closes. Femoral and inguinal hernias require reduction of the hernia and trussing the weakened portion of the abdominal wall. Herniorrhaphy is the corrective surgery indicated.

PROGNOSIS The prognosis is excellent with proper treatment and care.

PREVENTION Preventive measures include following recommended guidelines for lifting heavy objects, maintaining a soft stool consistency, and practicing moderate exercise.

■ COLORECTAL CANCER

DESCRIPTION *Colorectal cancer,* almost always adenocarcinoma, is the collective designation for a variety of malignant neoplasms that may arise in either the colon or rectum (Fig. 7–9).

ETIOLOGY The cause of colorectal cancer is unknown, but there is a higher incidence in societies that have a diet high in red meat and low in fiber. Other predisposing factors include diseases of the digestive tract, a history of irritable bowel syndrome, and familial **polyposis.** The incidence of colorectal cancer increases after the age of 40.

SIGNS AND SYMPTOMS Symptoms are vague in the early stages. Rectal bleeding and blood in the stool may occur. Later symptoms may include **pallor, ascites, cachexia, lymphadenopathy,** and **hepatomegaly.** Any significant change in bowel habits should be regarded as suspicious. This may include alternating states of diarrhea and constipation and the presence of blood in the stool.

DIAGNOSTIC PROCEDURES Digital examination of the rectum may be sufficient to detect rectal tumors. Testing for occult blood in the stool is the most effective diagnostic indicator of colorectal cancer. Sigmoidoscopy and colonoscopy are also helpful in detection. Barium x-ray can locate lesions that are manually or otherwise visually undetectable.

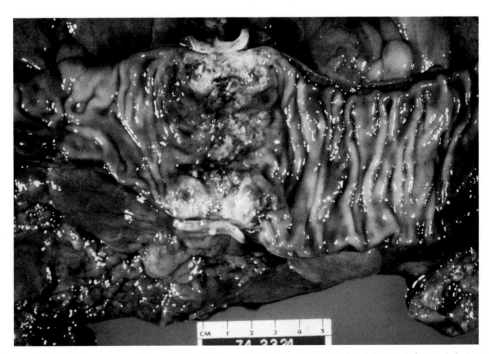

Figure 7–9 Colon cancer. (From Gylys, BA, and Wedding, ME: Medical Terminology: A Systems Approach, ed 4. FA Davis, Philadelphia, 1999, p 97, with permission from WRS Group.)

TREATMENT Surgery to remove the tumor and adjacent tissues and any affected lymph nodes is the treatment of choice. Chemotherapy and radiation therapy also may be used if the cancer has deeply perforated the bowel wall or metastasized.

PROGNOSIS The prognosis varies. This cancer tends to progress slowly and remains localized for a fair length of time. If diagnosed early and localized, colorectal cancer is potentially curable in about 92 percent of cases.

PREVENTION A high-fiber, low-fat diet may reduce the risk of colorectal cancer for some individuals. The American Cancer Society reports that recent studies suggest that estrogen replacement therapy and nonsteroidal anti-inflammatory drugs such as aspirin may reduce colorectal cancer risk.

DIARRHEA

DESCRIPTION *Diarrhea* is the frequent passage of feces, with an accompanying increase in fluidity and volume. Diarrhea is not a disease; it is, rather, a symptom of another underlying condition. "Normal" bowel habits vary widely; consequently, what is considered diarrhea in some individuals may be normal in others.

ETIOLOGY Diarrhea is the result of an abrupt increase in intestinal motility. The highly liquid content of the small intestine is rushed through the colon without sufficient time for fluid reabsorption, resulting in the watery stools characteristic of diarrhea. Numerous diseases and conditions can cause such an increase in intestinal motility. Childhood diarrhea may be an inflammatory process of infectious origin or a toxic reaction to dietary indiscretions. Adult diarrhea may result from malabsorption syndrome, gastritis, lactose intolerance, irritable bowel syndrome, Crohn's disease, ulcerative colitis, gastrointestinal tumors, diverticular disease, viral and bacterial infections of the intestine, parasitic infections, psychogenic disorders, food allergies, and a variety of medications.

SIGNS AND SYMPTOMS The diarrhea may vary in fluidity and volume. It may be accompanied by flatulence, abdominal distension, fever, headache, anorexia, vomiting, malaise, and **myalgia.**

DIAGNOSTIC PROCEDURES The clinical history of the diarrhea involves determining whether its onset was abrupt or gradual, and whether it is acute or chronic. The characteristics of the diarrheal stools also will be evaluated. To help determine underlying causes, bacterial cultures and microscopic examination of the stools may be performed. Additional tests include proctoscopy, radiological studies, and tests for occult blood.

TREATMENT Treatment goals in diarrhea include relief of symptoms and correction of underlying disorders. Clear liquids may be prescribed for children.

PROGNOSIS The prognosis depends on the cause. Possible complications include dehydration and **electrolyte** imbalances. Severe childhood diarrhea may require hospitalization.

PREVENTION Cases of diarrhea due to infectious agents can often be prevented by following proper hygiene and sanitation procedures. Cases due to allergic reactions can be prevented by avoiding known allergens.

Accessory Organs of Digestion: Pancreas, Gallbladder, and Liver

ACUTE PANCREATITIS

DESCRIPTION *Acute pancreatitis* is a severe, often life-threatening inflammation of the pancreas (Fig. 7–10). In this disease, pancreatic enzymes that normally remain inactive until reaching the duodenum begin digesting pancreatic tissue, causing varying degrees of edema, swelling, tissue necrosis, and hemorrhage. The pancreas is both an exocrine and endocrine organ, thus the pancreas becomes inflamed, hemorrhagic, and necrotic. The disease can be mild and self-limiting or chronic and fatal.

ETIOLOGY The causes of this autodigestive process in acute pancreatitis are not well understood, although a number of conditions are known to lead

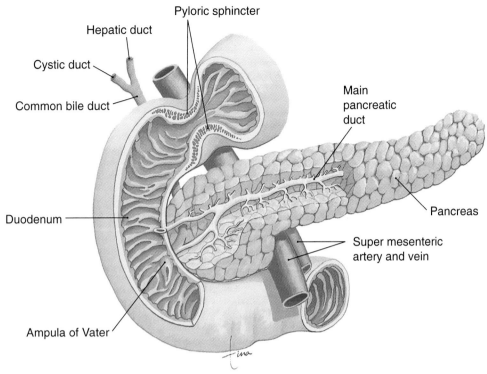

Figure 7–10 The pancreas, sectioned to show the pancreatic ducts. The main pancreatic duct joins the bile duct. (From Scanlon, VC, and Sanders, T: Essentials of Anatomy and Physiology, ed 3. FA Davis, Philadelphia, 1999, p 364, with permission.)

to the disease. Chief among these is alcoholism. Other conditions include gallstones, trauma to the abdomen, viral infections, drug reactions, systemic immunologic disorders, pancreatic cancer, or complications from a duodenal ulcer. Acute pancreatitis is on occasion idiopathic.

SIGNS AND SYMPTOMS The most important symptom of acute pancreatitis is the sudden onset of severe, persistent abdominal pain that is centered over the epigastric region and that may radiate toward the back. The abdomen is tender. Severe attacks of acute pancreatitis also may cause abdominal distension, persistent vomiting, fever, and tachycardia. Vital signs show rapid, shallow respirations, a fall in blood pressure, and an elevated temperature.

DIAGNOSTIC PROCEDURES A clinical history of acute onset of the characteristic abdominal pain may suggest the diagnosis. A blood test revealing an elevated level of the enzyme amylase in the serum generally confirms the diagnosis. Ultrasonography and abdominal CT scans may reveal pancreatic enlargement. Leukocytosis may be an additional finding.

TREATMENT Treatment is largely symptomatic. The aim is to maintain circulation and fluid volume, decrease pain and pancreatic secretions, and control any complications. Analgesic drugs, intravenous administration of fluids, and fasting with **parenteral** hyperalimentation may be necessary.

PROGNOSIS The prognosis is guarded. Acute pancreatitis is usually self-limiting, and pancreatic function is eventually restored. A host of possible complications, however, may worsen the prognosis. The prognosis is poor and the mortality rate high when acute pancreatitis follows alcoholism.

PREVENTION There is no known prevention.

■ CHRONIC PANCREATITIS

DESCRIPTION *Chronic pancreatitis* is the slow, progressive destruction of pancreatic tissue, accompanied by variable amounts of inflammation, fibrosis, and dilation of the pancreatic ducts. As with acute pancreatitis, the damage to the pancreas is thought to result from autodigestion by pancreatic enzymes (see Acute Pancreatitis).

ETIOLOGY Although the exact cause is unclear, the leading etiologic factor in chronic pancreatitis in adults appears to be alcoholism. The etiologic factors implicated in acute pancreatitis also may play a limited role. In contrast to the acute form of the disease, however, many cases of chronic pancreatitis are idiopathic.

SIGNS AND SYMPTOMS Severe, persistent, dull abdominal pain, often worsening following a meal, is the primary symptom of chronic pancreatitis, although this pain may be less specifically focused than in acute pancreatitis. Other symptoms may include weight loss, malabsorption, and hyperglycemia.

DIAGNOSTIC PROCEDURES Extensive history, x-rays revealing pancreatic calcification, elevated ESR, and stool examination for steatorrhea are relevant.

TREATMENT Treatment is generally directed at pain management and correcting any nutritional disorders resulting from malabsorption. A low-fat diet is often prescribed. Pain relief may be accomplished either through drug therapy or various surgical procedures. Pancreatic enzyme replacement therapy helps to correct malabsorption problems and also may provide additional pain relief.

PROGNOSIS The prognosis is poor for individuals with chronic pancreatitis caused by alcoholism, with a mortality rate approaching 50 percent. Others may do well, although therapy must be maintained indefinitely. Diabetes mellitus is a possible complication of chronic pancreatitis (see Diabetes Mellitus in Chapter 11).

PREVENTION There is no known prevention other than alcohol avoidance.

PANCREATIC CANCER

DESCRIPTION *Pancreatic cancer* is a neoplasm, usually an adenocarcinoma, which occurs most frequently in the head of the pancreas. Pancreatic cancer is the fifth leading cause of cancer deaths in the United States. The highest incidence is among people 60 to 70 years of age.

ETIOLOGY The etiology is not known, but is linked to inhalation or absorption of carcinogens that are excreted by the pancreas. Cigarette smoking, exposure to occupational chemicals, and a diet high in fats and protein are associated with an increased incidence of pancreatic cancer.

SIGNS AND SYMPTOMS The classic symptoms are abdominal pain, anorexia, jaundice, and weight loss. Other symptoms include weakness, fatigue, diarrhea, nausea and vomiting, and boring pain in the midback. If the disease affects the islets of Langerhans, symptoms of insulin deficiency appear. These symptoms include glucosuria, **hyperglycemia,** and glucose intolerance.

DIAGNOSTIC PROCEDURES Blood tests include hematocrit and hemoglobin, which will indicate bleeding. A gastrointestinal x-ray series may be ordered. Ultrasonography, computed tomography (CT) scanning, and endoscopic retrograde cholangeopancreatography (ERCP) are useful in establishing a diagnosis. Percutaneous needle aspiration biopsy of the affected portion of the pancreas is used to confirm the diagnosis.

TREATMENT Treatment usually is palliative because most pancreatic cancers are diagnosed after they have metastasized to the lungs, liver, and bones. If surgical resection is possible, localized tumors will be removed. Radiation therapy and multidrug chemotherapy may be given, but pancreatic carcinomas usually respond poorly. It is important to manage the pain and to correct any nutritional defects.

PROGNOSIS The prognosis is poor because 80 to 85 percent of individuals have advanced disease at first diagnosis.

PREVENTION There is no known prevention.

CHOLELITHIASIS

DESCRIPTION *Cholelithiasis* is the formation or presence of stonelike masses called gallstones within the gallbladder or bile ducts (Fig. 7–11). These stones may be formed of either cholesterol or calcium-based compounds and range from a few millimeters to a few centimeters in size. Cholelithiasis

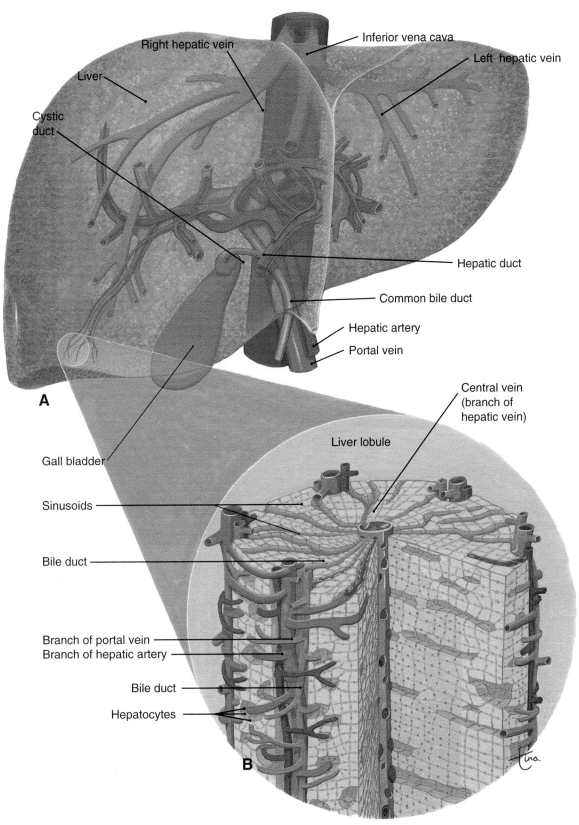

Figure 7–11 (*A*) The liver and gallbladder with blood vessels and bile ducts. (*B*) Magnified view of one liver lobule. (From Scanlon, VC, and Sanders, T: Essentials of Anatomy and Physiology, ed 3. FA Davis, Philadelphia, 1999, p 362, with permission.)

is a common condition in the United States, with women affected more than twice as frequently as men. Most individuals with gallstones remain asymptomatic. Clinically significant symptoms result when a gallstone obstructs a biliary duct.

ETIOLOGY The cause of cholelithiasis is not well understood. Any factors that cause the bile to become overladen with cholesterol may increase the likelihood of the formation of cholesterol-based gallstones. Such factors include obesity, high-calorie diets, certain drugs, oral contraceptives, multiple pregnancies, and increasing age. The production of calcium-based (pigmented) gallstones is even less well understood, but it may be related to genetic factors, hemolytic disease, alcoholic cirrhosis, or persistent biliary tract infections.

SIGNS AND SYMPTOMS As mentioned previously, many individuals with gallstones remain asymptomatic. If bile ducts are obstructed, though, a classic "gallbladder attack," more properly referred to as biliary colic, may result. The telltale symptom is the acute onset of upper right quadrant abdominal pain radiating to the shoulder and back. Nausea and vomiting may accompany the attack. Flatulence, belching, and heartburn also may occur at intervals. Gallbladder attacks typically tend to follow ingestion of large meals or fatty foods. The pain and other symptoms of an attack gradually subside on their own over a period of several hours.

DIAGNOSTIC PROCEDURES A clinical history of the characteristic pain of biliary colic suggests a diagnosis of gallstones. Various methods of visualizing the stones are employed for a definitive diagnosis. These typically include a gallbladder ultrasound, oral cholecystogram, intravenous cholangiogram, or a plain abdominal x-ray. If the common bile duct is obstructed, the serum **bilirubin** is elevated.

TREATMENT If the condition is asymptomatic, treatment will be nonsurgical, unless the symptoms reappear or unless there is a history of previous gallstones with complications. In elective surgery, a laparoscopic cholecystectomy will be performed. Cholecystectomy is the treatment of choice for symptomatic cholelithiasis. A new form of cholecystectomy consists of removal of the gallbladder through a small incision in the navel. The procedure is called laparoscopic cholecystectomy and drastically reduces the length of the hospital stay.

Surgical treatment for asymptomatic individuals remains controversial.

A nonsurgical treatment requires the insertion of a flexible catheter, guided by fluoroscopy, directly to the stone. A Dormia (stone) basket is threaded through the catheter, opened, and twirled to entrap the stone. It is then closed and withdrawn.

Another nonsurgical option is extracorporeal shock wave lithotripsy with litholytic therapy.

Still another nonsurgical approach involves dissolving cholesterol-based stones through bile acid therapy. This therapy inhibits the synthesis and secretion of cholesterol within the liver, altering the composition of the bile. Existing stones may be decreased in size or dissolved entirely.

PROGNOSIS The prognosis is generally good with prompt treatment. Complications may include cholecystitis (see Acute Cholecystitis) and pancreatitis.

PREVENTION No prevention is known.

ACUTE CHOLECYSTITIS

DESCRIPTION *Acute cholecystitis* is a severe inflammation of the interior wall the gallbladder.

ETIOLOGY Most cases of acute cholecystitis are a consequence of the obstruction of bile ducts by gallstones. The resulting inflammation may result from the increased pressure of accumulating bile within the gallbladder, chemical changes in the bile that erode the gallbladder tissue, or secondary infection from multiplying bacteria. Some forms of the disease are not caused by obstructing gallstones. These cases may be due to obstruction of bile ducts by neoplasms or to vascular disease, diabetes mellitus, parasitic infections, and various systemic diseases. The risk of nonobstructive, acalculous forms of acute cholecystitis is increased in burn patients and following trauma or surgery.

SIGNS AND SYMPTOMS A characteristic symptom of acute cholecystitis is the gradual onset of upper right quadrant pain that usually remains localized over the area of the gallbladder. Unlike the pain of biliary colic, which ceases once the gallstones are passed, the pain of acute cholecystitis does not tend to subside after a few hours. Anorexia, nausea, vomiting, and a low-grade fever and chills also may accompany the pain.

DIAGNOSTIC PROCEDURES Diagnosis of acute cholecystitis is usually suggested on the basis of the characteristic pain. In most cases, gallbladder enlargement is palpable. Laboratory findings typically reveal leukocytosis and elevated serum bilirubin and serum aminotransferase levels. Visualization of obstructing gallstones in suspected cases of acute cholecystitis is typically performed through radioisotope scintiscans, cholecystogram, gallbladder ultrasound, or abdominal x-ray.

TREATMENT Dietary modifications are recommended in uncomplicated cases, or if the pain persists, surgery will be performed. Cholecystectomy is the treatment of choice.

PROGNOSIS The prognosis is generally good with prompt treatment. Complications from perforation of the gallbladder include the possibility of peritonitis.

PREVENTION There is no known prevention.

CIRRHOSIS

DESCRIPTION *Cirrhosis* is a chronic, irreversible, degenerative disease of the liver characterized by the replacement of normal liver cells with fibrous scar tissue and other alterations in liver structure. Cirrhosis is the consequence of the repeated traumatizing of hepatic tissue by toxins, infectious agents, metabolic diseases, and circulatory disorders. The hepatic cells become necrotic, causing a change in liver structure that impairs the flow of blood and lymph. Hepatic insufficiency results.

ETIOLOGY Cirrhosis has a diverse set of etiologies. The most common cause of cirrhosis is chronic alcoholism. Other forms of cirrhosis, classified by their pathogenesis, include biliary cirrhosis, which is manifested by **cholestasis;** postnecrotic cirrhosis, resulting from hepatitis; pigment cirrhosis (hemochromatosis), which is due to a genetic disorder of iron metabolism; and cardiac cirrhosis, caused by congestive heart failure. Cirrhosis also may be idiopathic in origin. A genetic factor tends to be important. It is more common in men than in women.

SIGNS AND SYMPTOMS The person may be asymptomatic for a prolonged period, or symptoms may be vague or unspecific. Symptoms may include nausea, vomiting, anorexia, dull abdominal ache, weakness, fatigability, weight loss, pruritus, peripheral neuritis, bleeding tendencies, **jaundice,** and edema of the legs.

DIAGNOSTIC PROCEDURES Palpation will reveal the liver to be enlarged and firm—if not hard—with a blunt edge. Plain abdominal x-rays also may show an enlarged liver. A liver scan and biopsy are essential for diagnosis. Laboratory findings may reveal anemia, folate deficiency, **hemolysis,** and blood loss. Liver enzymes (alanine aminotransferase [ALT], formerly called serum glutamic pyruvic transaminase [SGPT]; and aspartate aminotransferase [AST], formerly called serum glutamic-oxaloacetic transaminase [SGOT]) are assayed to check for elevated enzyme levels. Bilirubin will be increased, too.

TREATMENT Treatment is aimed at the cause of the cirrhosis in an attempt to prevent further liver damage. Adequate rest and diet are essential, as is restriction of alcohol. Vitamin and mineral supplements may be prescribed. In the event of gastric upset or internal bleeding, antacids may be given. If the patient has ascites, the fluid will be removed by paracentesis.

PROGNOSIS The prognosis is poor in advanced cirrhosis, especially for alcoholic cirrhosis should the person continue drinking. Hematemesis, jaundice, and ascites are unfavorable signs. Elevated blood pressure in the portal vein, called *portal hypertension,* is a common complication of cirrhosis. As a consequence, blood pressure increases within the spleen, causing **splenomegaly,** and blood bypasses the liver, producing ascites or esophageal **varices.** Hemorrhage of esophageal varices often requires emergency treatment. If cirrhosis is not treated, hepatic failure and death result.

PREVENTION There is no known prevention unless alcohol is a contributing factor.

ACUTE VIRAL HEPATITIS

DESCRIPTION *Acute viral hepatitis* is the infection and subsequent inflammation of the liver caused by any one of several viruses. Most acute cases of hepatitis are caused by one of five viral agents: hepatitis A virus (HAV), hepatitis B virus (HBV), hepatitis C virus (HCV), hepatitis D virus (HDV) and hepatitis E virus (HEV). A sixth virus, hepatitis G (HGV) has been discovered, but little is known. Both the hepatitis type (e.g., hepatitis A) and the viral type (e.g., HAV) will be used interchangeably in text. The hepatic cells are destroyed and become necrotic. If the client is generally healthy, the hepatic cells will regenerate unless the person is elderly.

ETIOLOGY   There are six types of viral hepatitis:

1. Hepatitis A (HAV) was formerly known as infectious hepatitis. It has an incubation period of 4 weeks. It is caused by a ribonucleic acid (RNA) virus. It is highly contagious through the fecal-oral routes or parenterally. It is rarely fatal and does not become chronic.

2. Hepatitis B (HBV) is a serum hepatitis caused by a DNA virus. It has a long incubation period of 4 to 12 weeks, and is transmitted by contaminated blood or through human secretions or feces. Health professionals are frequently exposed to type B hepatitis, which is potentially more serious than type A. Hepatitis B may become chronic but will usually resolve.

3. Hepatitis C (HCV) is rare and is transmitted through transfusions from asymptomatic individuals or through contaminated needles. It is spread similarly to B and is due to an RNA virus. Its incubation period is 7 weeks. This disease insidiously damages the liver for up to 20 years before symptoms emerge. Therefore, the incidence of hepatitis C has greatly increased. The Centers for Disease Control predict that deaths from the disease will triple in the next decade.

4. Hepatitis D (HDV) is also called *delta hepatitis*. Its incubation period is 4 to 12 weeks. It occurs in persons frequently exposed to blood, such as hemophiliacs or intravenous drug users. Hepatitis D requires infection with hepatitis B in order to occur. If types B and D occur together, pulmonary complications are likely.

5. Hepatitis E (HEV) was formerly grouped as type C under non-A and non-B hepatitis. It occurs in people who have been to an area such as India or Asia where it is endemic. Fecal-contaminated water is the mode of transmission. Its incubation period is 5 to 6 weeks.

6. Hepatitis G (HGV) has been discovered, but little is known about it. It is a blood-borne RNA virus.

SIGNS AND SYMPTOMS   Initial symptoms are flulike, vague, and include malaise, fatigue, anorexia, myalgia, **lassitude,** fever, dark-colored urine, clay-colored stools, rashes, hives, abdominal pain or tenderness, pruritus, and jaundice. Nausea, vomiting, headache, photophobia, cough, and **coryza** may precede jaundice. An aversion to smoking and certain foods is common.

DIAGNOSTIC PROCEDURES   The specific type of hepatitis has to be established. Specific blood tests will show the antibody-antigen type. A clinical history of exposure to jaundiced persons, recent blood transfusions, or intravenous drug use may suggest a diagnosis of hepatitis. The liver may be enlarged and tender. Splenomegaly may occur. Laboratory findings in most forms of hepatitis will include **proteinuria** and **bilirubinuria.** Increased levels of liver enzymes, alkaline phosphatase, and **gamma globulin** may also be evident. Liver biopsy helps to confirm the diagnosis.

TREATMENT   There is no specific treatment for hepatitis, with the exception of type C, which is treated with alpha interferon. Rather, the client is treated with general supportive measures. Bed rest, adequate diet, and fluid intake are advised. Antiemetics may be ordered. In the recovery phase the symptoms subside but the liver enlargement and abnormalities are evident. Recovery may take 1 to 4 months, depending on the individual and the type of hepatitis. The disease needs to be reported to the public health department for proper follow-up because of the possibility of contagion.

PROGNOSIS   The extent of liver damage, especially in HCV, will determine the prognosis. A serious consequence is that chronic active hepatitis may occur. Any type of hepatitis can recur.

PREVENTION   Prevention for all forms of hepatitis includes proper hygienic practices, especially when using needles for injections and when handling human secretions. When individuals are exposed to type A hepatitis, immune globulin (IgG) may be administered as a preventive measure. The best protection against type B hepatitis is provided by a type B vaccine. Its use is recommended for those in high-risk groups, such as health-care professionals. Pediatricians are vaccinating infants against hepatitis B before the age of 1 year.

SPECIAL FOCUS — EATING DISORDERS

ANOREXIA NERVOSA

DESCRIPTION *Anorexia nervosa* is a complex psychogenic eating disorder characterized by an all-consuming desire to remain thin. It is also marked by weight loss, clinical evidence of semistarvation, amenorrhea, and an alteration in body image. Anorexia nervosa should not be confused with simple anorexia, a loss of appetite symptomatic of one of many possible underlying physical diseases. On the contrary, most individuals with anorexia nervosa never suffer a loss of appetite. The disorder primarily affects young women around the age of puberty. White women from middle-class backgrounds are affected most frequently. The reported incidence of anorexia in men is low.

ETIOLOGY The cause of anorexia nervosa is not known, although most health professionals believe it is essentially a psychiatric disorder. A client's socioeconomic status, family background, and cultural conditioning may be predisposing factors in development of the condition.

SIGNS AND SYMPTOMS A loss of at least 25 percent of original body weight, in the absence of any detectable underlying medical disorder, may suggest a diagnosis of anorexia nervosa. Evidence of food avoidance, vomiting, and excessive exercise also suggest the diagnosis. In severe cases, a host of secondary symptoms may be evident as a result of metabolic and hormonal disturbances resulting from malnutrition. The affected individual also may tend to deny feelings of hunger and will typically claim to be overweight despite physical evidence to the contrary.

DIAGNOSTIC PROCEDURES Careful interpretation of clinical data is important to rule out other disorders that cause physical wasting. No specific diagnostic tests exist for anorexia nervosa, but blood testing may reveal associated nutritional anemia and vitamin or mineral deficiencies.

TREATMENT Medical treatment of anorexia nervosa generally involves reversing the effects of malnutrition. Noncooperation on the part of the affected individual, however, typically makes treatment of this disorder a difficult, uncertain matter. Intensive individual or family psychotherapy may be recommended. Hospitalization may be required in the event of severe weight loss and malnutrition. Providing the individual with nutritional guidelines and information about proper eating habits also may be useful in the recovery process. Therapy must address the patient's underlying problems of low self-esteem, anxiety, anger, guilt, and feelings of hopelessness and depression.

PROGNOSIS The prognosis varies. Relapses are frequent. Death may occur from malnutrition and complications such as hypothermia and cardiac disturbances in as many as a quarter of diagnosed cases, especially when the person is not anxious to overcome the disorder.

PREVENTION No specific prevention is known, but it seems helpful that an individual develop a sense of self-esteem that is not dependent on the thin, "model-like" body image so prized in today's society.

BULIMIA

DESCRIPTION *Bulimia* is a psychogenic eating disorder characterized by repetitive gorging with food, followed by self-induced vomiting. The condition also may involve laxative abuse. Whereas the individual with anorexia nervosa seems obsessed with becoming even thinner, the person with bulimia has a morbid fear of becoming fat. Other behavioral abnormalities include obsessive secrecy about the condition and may involve food stealing. The disorder principally affects young women.

ETIOLOGY The cause of bulimia is not known. As is the case with anorexia nervosa, most health professionals believe bulimia is essentially a psychiatric disorder. There may be a struggle for self-identity and a history of depression.

SIGNS AND SYMPTOMS Most persons with bulimia hide the behavioral evidence of their condition, and they are often of normal weight or even slightly overweight upon diagnosis. They may still exhibit signs of malnutrition, however, since the "binge" diet of a bulimic individual is often wildly unbalanced, usually consisting of "junk" foods such as donuts, ice cream, and candy. Owing to the high sugar content of the binge diet and the subsequent reflux of gastric juices during vomiting, the bulimic person typically has a high incidence of dental caries. Reflux of gastric secretions also may produce a chronic sore throat. Menstrual irregularities are much less common in bulimia than in anorexia nervosa.

DIAGNOSTIC PROCEDURES Blood testing may reveal **hypokalemia** and **alkalosis** as a consequence of vomiting and laxative abuse. Other tests may reveal cardiac arrhythmias or evidence of renal dysfunction.

TREATMENT Long-term psychotherapy is usually indicated. The bulimic person knows that the eating patterns are abnormal but is unable to control them. As with the anorexic person, noncooperation on the part of the bulimic client generally makes treatment difficult and frustrating. Depression and obsessive-compulsive behavior frequently accompany this disorder.

PROGNOSIS The prognosis is guarded unless the client responds to therapy. Bulimic persons have twice as high an incidence of suicide as anorexics. Other complications may include pneumonia, rupturing of the esophagus or stomach, and pancreatitis.

PREVENTION There is no specific prevention for bulimia.

SPECIAL FOCUS: DIGESTIVE DISEASES COMMON IN CHILDREN

INFANTILE COLIC

DESCRIPTION *Infantile colic* is paroxysmal abdominal pain or cramping. The condition usually occurs during the first few months of life.

ETIOLOGY Excessive fermentation and gas production in the intestines are thought to be the cause of colic. Other factors include too rapid feeding, overeating, swallowing air, or poor burping techniques. Many times the cause cannot be determined.

SIGNS AND SYMPTOMS Loud crying and drawing of the legs up to the abdomen are behaviors typically of an infant experiencing colic. The symptoms are more apt to occur late in the afternoon or in early evening.

DIAGNOSTIC PROCEDURES There is no specific diagnostic test for this disorder. Observing the parent and infant interacting may help in the diagnosis.

TREATMENT The best treatment may be the availability of a calm setting for feeding time for both parent and child, and gentle burping midway through the feeding and again at the end. Support of the parent is necessary too. A vicious circle can occur if the parent's anxiety about the problem is sensed by the infant. At times, no form of treatment is effective.

PROGNOSIS The prognosis is good. The infant will continue to thrive and develop even with colic. Colic usually disappears spontaneously after 3 months of age.

PREVENTION The best prevention includes frequent and smaller feedings and relaxation on the part of the parents.

Note: Diarrhea and vomiting are not disease entities; rather, they are symptoms of a problem. Because they are so common in infants and children, the following material is provided.

DIARRHEA

Acute diarrhea is a sudden change in the frequency and liquid content of the stool. *Chronic diarrhea* is the passage of loose stools with increased frequency for 2 weeks or more. The latter may be caused by anatomic defects, allergic reactions, or disorders of malabsorption. A variety of factors can cause either type of diarrhea in the infant and child. Diarrhea may be caused by an inflammatory process of infectious origin, a toxic reaction to "dietary indiscretions," or ingestion of poisons. Diarrhea can cause dehydration and electrolyte imbalance if fluid loss continues.

Treatment of diarrhea is dependent on its cause and severity. Treatment includes reducing the child's activities and encouraging a diet of clear liquids for a few days. Severe diarrhea may require hospitalization to prevent dehydration.

VOMITING

Vomiting may be caused by overfeeding, gastrointestinal disorders, infections, increased intracranial pressure, and ingestion of toxic substances. The signs and symptoms range from mild regurgitation to projectile vomiting, such as occurs with pyloric stenosis. In diagnosis, the frequency and duration of vomiting will be considered as well as the character of the vomitus.

Treatment is dependent on the cause and severity of the vomiting and includes taking the child off solid foods and allowing the gastrointestinal tract to rest. Feeding smaller amounts more frequently may be helpful.

FOOD ALLERGIES

DESCRIPTION A *food allergy* is a hypersensitivity reaction to certain foods.

ETIOLOGY Some of the more common food allergens are milk products, eggs, wheat, nuts, legumes, fish, chocolate, berries, citrus fruits, and nitrate-containing products such as weiners and bacon.

SIGNS AND SYMPTOMS Symptoms may include inflammation and swelling of the face or around the lip, gastrointestinal disturbances, vomiting, and diarrhea.

DIAGNOSTIC PROCEDURES If food allergies are suspected, the child may be taken off the regular diet. Foods may then be added gradually, one at a time, until a reaction occurs. This may pinpoint an allergen.

TREATMENT Once the identity of the allergen is determined, it should be avoided and not reintroduced into the diet for 6 months. It may be necessary to find alternatives for those foods that must be avoided yet are necessary to a balanced diet.

PROGNOSIS The prognosis is good with proper dietary management. Many children "outgrow" their food allergies.

PREVENTION Food allergies sometimes can be prevented. If there is a strong family history of allergy to certain foods, these should be avoided during the child's first year.

HELMINTHS (Worms)

ETIOLOGY *Toxocariasis* is caused by the ingestion of roundworm larvae, often deposited by family dogs and cats. It is likely to occur when children eat dirt or sand that contains the ova of roundworms. The ova hatch in the intestine, mature, and migrate to the lymph vessels and other parts of the body.

Enterobiasis, infestation by pinworms, is caused by *Enterobius vermicularis,* which lives in the lower gut. The female worms deposit their eggs around the anus during the night and then die. Severe pruritus ani occurs, which causes children to scratch. The ova then are deposited on the hands and under the nails. The children put their fingers into their mouths, then swallow the ova, which develop into more mature worms in the intestine.

SIGNS AND SYMPTOMS Roundworm infestation produces symptoms that correspond to the affected body part. General symptoms may include fever, cough, hepatomegaly, nausea, vomiting, and weight loss. Pruritus ani is the classic symptom of enterobiasis.

DIAGNOSTIC PROCEDURES Toxocariasis is diagnosed through a clinical history and blood testing. Enterobiasis is diagnosed by a history of pruritus ani and the recovery of *Enterobius* ova from the perianal area.

TREATMENT Treatment for toxocariasis usually is symptomatic. Enterobiasis requires drugs to destroy the parasites. Daily bathing of children (showers preferred) and regular changes of bed linens and nightclothes are necessary in the proper management of enterobiasis. It is important in both conditions to test and treat the entire family.

PROGNOSIS The prognosis for both conditions is good no matter how unpleasant either may sound.

PREVENTION The best prevention is to teach children proper personal hygiene, such as hand washing and keeping fingers out of the mouth. Worming of pets and proper disposal of animal feces are important in preventing toxocariasis.

COMMON SYMPTOMS OF DIGESTIVE SYSTEM DISEASES

Individuals may present with the following common symptoms, which deserve attention from health professionals:

- Loss of appetite and weight loss
- Nausea and vomiting
- Any change in bowel habits, such as diarrhea, constipation, and flatulence
- Blood or mucus in the stool
- Fever
- Pain in the area of the gastrointestinal tract
- Heartburn, indigestion, dysphagia, and any discomfort after eating certain foods
- Malaise, loss of strength, and fatigability
- **Diaphoresis**

 ## ALTERNATIVE MEDICINE

Disorders of the gastrointestinal tract are quite common and lead to inadequate digestion. A number of factors to consider are:

- The typical Western diet is high in carbohydrates and highly processed foods with many additives. Lack of fiber can lead to a sluggish digestive system. A high complex carbohydrate, high-fiber, low-fat, and moderate protein diet can be beneficial.
- Common culprits in digestive disorders are milk, dairy products, and wheat, and they should be avoided by some individuals.
- Several digestive disorders involve the immune system. If IgA, an antibody normally present in the intestine, is lacking or deficient, increased infections occur. Techniques that may enhance the immune system can be very helpful.
- Bacterial, viral, and parasitic infections can be harmful to the digestive system and cause an imbalance of the normal flora of the GI tract. Vitamins A and C, zinc, and beta-carotene are infection fighters.
- Too much or too little hydrochloric acid secreted by the stomach is problematic. The use of herbs, lemon juice, or black pepper can aid in digestion.
- Psychological stress affects the digestive system; therefore, methods to reduce stress and enhance relaxation are beneficial.
- Insufficient exercise leads to a decrease in the enzyme secretion necessary for proper digestion. Ten to 15 minutes of exercise or a daily brisk walk can reduce the incidence of GI disorders.

REFERENCES

1. Questions and Answers about Crohn's Disease and Ulcerative Colitis. CCFA Crohn's and Colitis Foundation of America, 1993, New York, p 4.
2. Ibid, p 3.

BIBLIOGRAPHY

Alternative Medicine: The Definitive Guide. Burton Goldberg Group, Future Medicine Publishing, Fife, Wash., 1995.
Burns, MV: Pathophysiology: A Self-Instructional Program. Appleton & Lange, Stamford, Conn., 1998.

Crowley, LV: Introduction to Human Diseases, ed 3. Jones & Bartlett, Boston, 1992.

Diseases. Springhouse Corporation, Springhouse, Pa., 1993.

Fauci, AS, et al: Harrison's Principles of Internal Medicine, ed 14. McGraw-Hill, New York, 1998.

Frazier, MS, Drzymkowski, JA, and Doty, SJ: Essentials of Human Disease and Conditions. WB Saunders, Philadelphia, 1996.

Kent, TH, and Hart, MN: Introduction to Human Disease. Appleton & Lange, Stamford, Conn., 1998.

Mulvihill, ML: Human Diseases: A Systemic Approach. Appleton & Lange, Stamford, Conn., 1995.

Professional Guide to Disease, ed 6. Springhouse Corporation, Springhouse, Pa., 1998.

Sheldon, H: Boyd's Introduction to the Study of Disease, ed 11. Lea & Febiger, Philadelphia, 1992.

Shute, N: Hepatitis C: A Silent Killer. US News and World Report, 124(24):60–66, 1998.

Walter, JB: An Introduction to the Principles of Disease, ed 3. WB Saunders, Philadelphia, 1992.

CASE STUDIES

I A 52-year-old man, who has in the past been diagnosed as having irritable bowel syndrome, reports that he is having three to five bowel movements per day. The movements are runny, loose, and filled with red blood. The patient has not experienced any constipation. The patient's family practitioner refers him to a gastroenterologist.

1. Describe irritable bowel syndrome.

2. Are the reported symptoms compatible with IBS?

3. Of these symptoms, which is most significant?

4. What tests is the gastroenterologist likely to order?

II A 35-year-old woman experiences flatus, weight loss, abdominal distension, and loss of appetite. She has complained of these symptoms on several previous occasions. In response to her physician's question, she reports that her stool floats in the toilet bowl and is foul-smelling.

1. What steps do you think the physician might take?

2. How would a complete physical help in the diagnosis of this case?

REVIEW QUESTIONS

SHORT ANSWER

1. Identify three functions of the gastrointestinal tract:

   a.

   b.

   c.

2. Name an upper gastrointestinal tract disease related to the mouth: _____

3. Common diagnostic procedures used to diagnose disease of the upper gastrointestinal tract include:

   a.

   b.

c.

4. Common symptoms of gastric and duodenal ulcers include:

    a.

    b.

5. Name and define three childhood GI disorders:

    a.

    b.

    c.

6. Name four of the more common food allergens:

    a.

    b.

    c.

    d.

7. Define:

    a. Toxicariasis

    b. Enterobiasis

MATCHING

Match the following terms and definitions:

_____ 1. Most common malabsorption disorder

_____ 2. Examination of colon using fiberoptic endoscope

_____ 3. Disorder whose symptoms include pain in the lower right quadrant of the abdomen

_____ 4. Chronic hepatic disease

_____ 5. Disorder whose symptoms include an abnormal fear of becoming fat

_____ 6. Inflammation of the gallbladder

_____ 7. Acute infection and inflammation of the liver

_____ 8. Inflammation of the stomach and bowel

_____ 9. Disorder associated with a change in colonic motility

a. Gastroenteritis
b. Celiac sprue
c. Appendicitis
d. Irritable bowel syndrome
e. Colonoscopy
f. Cholecystitis
g. Cirrhosis
h. Viral hepatitis
i. Bulimia
j. Duodenal ulcer
k. Hemorrhoids

DISCUSSION/FURTHER STUDY

Compare and contrast irritable bowel syndrome, Crohn's disease, and ulcerative colitis.

ANSWERS

SHORT ANSWER

1. a. Digestion
   b. Absorption
   c. Elimination of solid wastes
2. Stomatitis
3. a. X-ray
   b. Endoscopy
   c. pH studies or analysis
4. a. Indigestion
   b. Heartburn
5. a. Colic: Paroxysmal abdominal cramping accompanied by loud crying and drawing the legs up to the abdomen.
   b. Diarrhea: Change in frequency and liquid content of stool. May be acute or chronic.
   c. Vomiting: Spitting up; regurgitation; may be projectile.
6. Any four of the following:

Milk products	Fish
Eggs	Chocolate
Wheat	Berries
Nuts	Nitrate-containing products such as sausage and bacon
Legumes	

7. a. Toxocariasis: Caused by ingestion of roundworm larvae; ova hatch in intestine, mature, and migrate to lymph vessels. Symptoms correspond to body part affected.
   b. Enterobiasis: Caused by pinworm ingestion; worms live in lower gut. The female deposits eggs around anus; child itches; child puts fingers in mouth and the cycle begins again. Pruritus ani is classic symptom.

MATCHING

1. b.	4. g	6. f	8. a
2. e	5. i	7. h	9. d
3. c			

DISCUSSION/FURTHER STUDY

Irritable bowel syndrome: Chronic bowel disease; unknown etiology; abdominal pain; diarrhea; biopsy may be done; stool may contain mucus. ***Crohn's disease:*** Chronic bowel disease; inflammation; unknown etiology; abdominal pain; diarrhea; biopsy necessary for diagnosis. ***Ulcerative colitis:*** Chronic bowel disease; inflammation; unknown etiology; abdominal pain; diarrhea; biopsy may be done; bloody stool; rectum and sigmoid colon are primary sites.

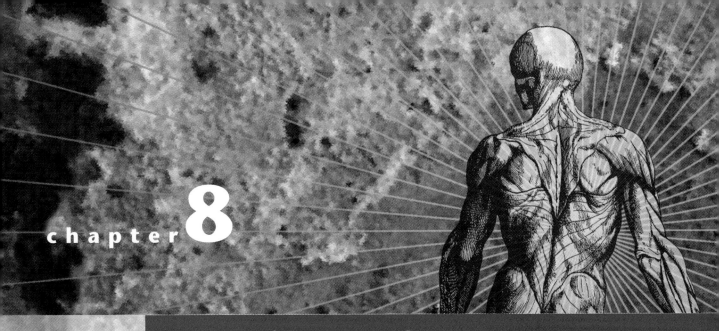

chapter 8

Respiratory System Diseases

CHAPTER OUTLINE

Epistaxis (Nosebleed)

Sinusitis

Acute and Chronic Pharyngitis

Acute and Chronic Laryngitis

Infectious Mononucleosis

Pneumonia

Legionella **Infections (Legionnaire's Disease)**

Lung Abscess

Pneumothorax

Pleurisy (Pleuritis)

Pleural Effusion

Chronic Obstructive Pulmonary Disease (COPD)

Chronic Bronchitis

Chronic Pulmonary Emphysema

Asthma

Pulmonary Tuberculosis (TB)

Pneumoconiosis
Silicosis
Asbestosis

Berylliosis
Anthracosis

Respiratory Mycoses

Pulmonary Edema

Cor Pulmonale

Pulmonary Embolism

Respiratory Acidosis (Hypercapnia)

Respiratory Alkalosis (Hypocapnia)

Atelectasis

Bronchiectasis

Lung Cancer

Special Focus: Respiratory Diseases of Childhood
Sudden Infant Death Syndrome (SIDS)
Acute Tonsillitis
Adenoid Hyperplasia
Croup
Acute Epiglottitis

Common Symptoms of Lung Diseases

References

Bibliography

Case Studies

Review Questions

157

LEARNING OBJECTIVES

Upon successful completion of this chapter, you will:
- Define epistaxis.
- List the causes of sinusitis.
- Describe the treatment for laryngitis.
- Identify the confirming diagnosis of mononucleosis.
- Contrast the three types of pneumonia.
- Describe the conditions under which a lung abscess may occur.
- Explain treatment modalities for pneumothorax.
- Define pleurisy.
- Differentiate between transudate and exudate fluid.
- Name the most common chronic lung disease.
- List the predisposing factors of chronic bronchitis.
- Recall the signs and symptoms of emphysema.
- Discuss the prognosis for asthma.
- Explain the growth of the tuberculosis bacteria.
- Compare the four pneumoconioses.
- Review the etiology of SIDS.
- Report the treatment of choice for chronic tonsillitis and adenoid hyperplasia.
- Describe the signs and symptoms of croup.
- Identify the etiology of epiglottitis.

KEY WORDS

Alveoli (pulmonary) (ăl•vē′ō•lī)
Analgesic (ăn•ăl•jē′sĭk)
Antipyretic (ăn•tĭ•pī•rĕt′ĭk)
Apnea (ăp•nē′ă)
Atelectasis (ăt•ĕ•lĕk′tă•sĭs)
Auscultation (aws•kŭl•tā′shŭn)
Biotin (bī′ō•tĭn)
Bleb (blĕb)
Bronchodilator (brŏng•kō•dī′lā•tŏr)
Cilia (sĭl′ē•ă)
Clubbing (klŭb′ĭng)
Cyanosis (sī•ă•nō′sĭs)
Diaphoresis (dī•ă•fō•rē′sĭs)
Diuretic (dī•ū•rĕt′ĭk)
Dyspnea (dĭsp•nē′ă)
Edema (ĕ•dē′mă)
Exudate (ĕks′ū•dāt)
Granuloma (grăn•ū•lō′mă)
Hemoptysis (hē•mŏp′tĭ•sĭs)
Hyperplasia (hī•pĕr•plā′zē•ă)
Hypertrophy (hī•pĕr′trō•fē)
Hypoxia (hī•pŏks′ē•ă)
Kyphoscoliosis (kī•fō•skō•lē•ō′sĭs)
Ligation (lī•gā′shŭn)
Malaise (mă•lāz′)
Orthopnea (ŏr•thŏp′nē•ă)
Pallor (păl′or)

Percussion (pĕr•kŭsh′ŭn)
pH (pē′aitch′)
Phagocytosis (fā•gō•sī•tō′sĭs)
Pleura (ploo′ră)
Pleurectomy (ploo•rĕk′tō•mē)
Plication (plī•kā′shŭn)
Polycythemia vera (pŏl•ē•sī•thē′mē•a vē′ră)
Postural drainage
Pulmonary infarction (pŭl′mō•nĕ•rē ĭn•fark′shŭn)
Purulent (pūr′ū•lĕnt)
Rales (rālz)
Rhinitis (rī•nī′tĭs)
Rhonchus (pl. *rhonchi*) (rŏng′kus)
Septic (sĕp′tĭk)
Sputum (spū′tŭm)
Stenosis (stĕn•ō′sĭs)
Stridor (strī′dor)
Tachycardia (tăk•ē•kăr′dē•ă)
Tachypnea (tăk•ĭp•nē′ă)
Thoracentesis (thō•ră•sĕn•tē′sĭs)
Thoracotomy (thō•răk•ŏt′ō•mē)
Thready pulse
Thrombocytosis (thrŏm•bō•sī•tō′sĭs)
Transillumination (trăns•ĭl•lū•mĭ•nā′shŭn)
Transudate (trăns′ū•dāt)

espiration is essential for life. The body can survive a fair length of time without food, a few days without water, but only minutes without air. Refer to Figure 8–1 for a review of the structure of the respiratory system.

There are two levels involved in the respiratory process—external and internal respiration. *External*

respiration is the exchange of two gases within the lungs. Oxygen that is present in inhaled air is exchanged for carbon dioxide that diffuses from the blood, across cell walls, into the airspaces of the lungs. The carbon dioxide is then exhaled from the lungs. *Internal respiration* is the exchange of oxygen and carbon dioxide at the cellular level within the

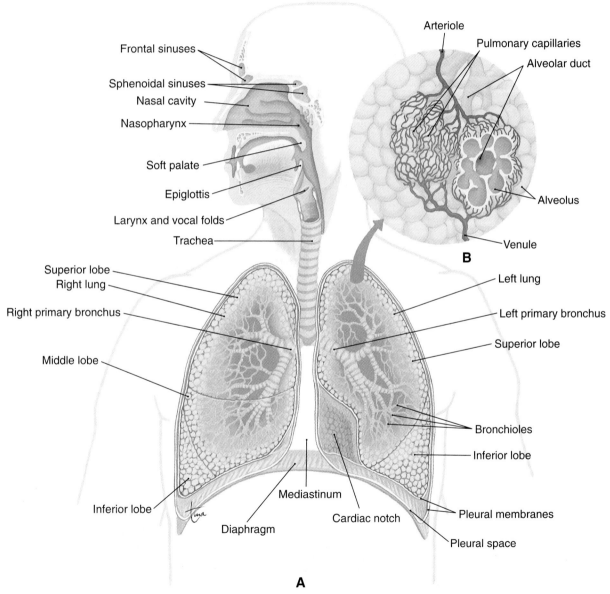

A

Figure 8–1 The respiratory system. (*A*) Anterior view of the upper and lower respiratory tracts. (*B*) Microscopic view of alveoli and pulmonary capillaries. (From Scanlon, VC, and Sanders, T: Understanding Human Structure and Function. FA Davis, Philadelphia, 1997, p 268, with permission.)

organs of the body. Carbon dioxide is a waste product when oxygen and nutrients are metabolized within body cells.

EPISTAXIS (Nosebleed)

DESCRIPTION *Epistaxis* is hemorrhage from the nose. This condition is more common in children than adults.

ETIOLOGY Primary epistaxis is caused by trauma to the nose (including nose-picking). The condition may occur secondary to sinusitis, **rhinitis,** inhalation of irritating chemicals, hypertension, and various systemic infections or blood disorders. High altitudes or dry climates also may cause epistaxis.

SIGNS AND SYMPTOMS Bright red blood oozing from one or both nostrils is the common sign. If the blood is swallowed through the pharynx, the person may appear asymptomatic unless blood vomitus is evident. Bleeding is considered severe if it persists longer than 10 minutes after pressure is applied. Prolonged epistaxis may cause significant blood loss.

DIAGNOSTIC PROCEDURES Casual observation may reveal epistaxis, but a more careful examination is necessary to locate the bleeding site. Any underlying causes of epistaxis require diagnosis and treatment.

TREATMENT The person's head should be elevated, and the soft portion of the nostrils should be pressed against the septum. Cold wet compresses also can be applied. A vasoconstricting agent such as epinephrine may be applied to the bleeding site on a cotton ball. Cauterization or petrolatum gauze nasal packing may be needed. The patient may require antibiotics to prevent secondary infection.

PROGNOSIS The prognosis for most individuals with a nosebleed is good.

PREVENTION Prevention includes keeping foreign objects out of the nose and refraining from picking the nose. The use of a humidifier may help persons living in dry climates or at high altitudes.

SINUSITIS

DESCRIPTION *Sinusitis* is inflammation of the paranasal sinus. The condition may be acute or chronic.

ETIOLOGY Acute sinusitis is usually caused by pneumococcal, streptococcal, or staphylococcal bacterial infections. The infection may spread to the sinuses when an individual has a cold, usually because of excessive nose blowing. Sinusitis also can result from swimming or diving, dental abscess or tooth extractions, or nasal allergies. Chronic sinusitis may be caused by the same etiologic factors as acute sinusitis, but more frequently its etiology cannot be determined.

SIGNS AND SYMPTOMS An individual with acute or chronic sinusitis may exhibit the following symptoms: nasal congestion; pain; tenderness, redness, and swelling over the involved sinus; **purulent** nasal discharge; headache; **malaise;** and a nonproductive cough. A low-grade fever also may be present. Allergic sinusitis may be accompanied by watering eyes and sneezing.

DIAGNOSTIC PROCEDURES A nasal examination is commonly performed. A specimen of nasal secretions may be taken for culture in order to identify any infectious agent. X-rays and **transillumination** may show clouding of the involved sinus.

TREATMENT **Analgesics** for pain relief, vasoconstrictors to decrease nasal secretions, and antibiotics for control of infection are typically the treatments of choice. Bed rest may be recommended. Patients are to be encouraged to drink plenty of fluids to help liquefy secretions. The application of heat over the affected sinus may be helpful.

PROGNOSIS The prognosis is good. Sinusitis is an uncomfortable condition, but usually it does not last long with proper care.

PREVENTION Prevention involves prompt treatment of any respiratory tract infection.

ACUTE AND CHRONIC PHARYNGITIS

DESCRIPTION *Pharyngitis,* inflammation of the pharynx, is the most common throat disorder.

ETIOLOGY Acute pharyngitis can be caused by any of a number of bacterial or viral infections. *Streptococcus pyogenes* is the most common of many possible bacterial pathogens, whereas the influenza virus and common cold viruses are the most common viral pathogens causing the condition. Acute pharyngitis also may arise secondary to systemic viral infections such as measles or chickenpox. Noninfectious causes of the disease include trauma to the mucosa of the pharynx from heat, sharp objects, or chemical irritants. Chronic pharyngitis is more likely to have a noninfectious origin and is often associated with a practice such as mouth-breathing.

SIGNS AND SYMPTOMS The hallmark of acute pharyngitis is sore throat. The pain may be mild, or of such severity that swallowing becomes difficult. Accompanying symptoms may include malaise, fever, headache, and muscle and joint pain.

DIAGNOSTIC PROCEDURES Physical examination of the pharynx will typically reveal red, swollen mucous membranes. In severe cases, pustular ulcerations of the pharyngeal wall may be evident. A throat culture is usually performed in order to identify the infecting organism.

TREATMENT Antibiotics are generally prescribed if the source of the infection is determined to be bacterial. Otherwise, treatment is symptomatic and may typically include the use of warm saline gargles, analgesics, and **antipyretics.** Bed rest and adequate fluid intake may be advised.

PROGNOSIS The prognosis for most forms of pharyngitis is generally good. Uncomplicated pharyngitis usually subsides in 3 to 10 days. Serious complications may result from streptococcal acute pharyngitis; these include rheumatic fever and glomerulonephritis.

PREVENTION There are no specific preventive measures for pharyngitis.

ACUTE AND CHRONIC LARYNGITIS

DESCRIPTION *Laryngitis* is inflammation of the laryngeal mucosa and the vocal cords.

ETIOLOGY Acute laryngitis may result from bacterial or viral infections, excessive use of the voice, or the inhalation of dust or chemical irritants. Acute laryngitis also may occur as a complication of acute rhinitis, pharyngitis, or influenza. Chronic laryngitis may arise secondary to other nose and throat diseases and may be a symptom of various benign or malignant neoplasms of the vocal cords.

SIGNS AND SYMPTOMS Hoarseness or a complete lack of normal voice are the common signs. Also, there may be pain, dry cough, and malaise.

DIAGNOSTIC PROCEDURES Laryngoscopy will typically reveal red, inflamed, and possibly hemorrhagic vocal cords.

TREATMENT Resting the voice is necessary for successful treatment. Any underlying pathology must be diagnosed and treated. Antibiotic therapy may be necessary if a bacterial infection is causing the condition. Analgesics and cough suppressants may provide symptomatic relief.

PROGNOSIS The prognosis for acute laryngitis is good with proper treatment. The prognosis for chronic laryngitis varies according to the underlying cause.

PREVENTION Preventive measures for acute or chronic laryngitis include avoiding misuse or overuse of the voice and avoiding irritants, such as cigarette smoke, alcohol, and extremes of air temperature.

INFECTIOUS MONONUCLEOSIS

DESCRIPTION *Infectious mononucleosis* is an acute upper respiratory tract infection characterized by sore throat, fever, and swollen cervical lymph glands. The disease primarily affects adolescents and young adults.

ETIOLOGY Infectious mononucleosis is caused by the Epstein-Barr virus (EBV). This virus is shed in the saliva of infected individuals and is usually spread through the oral-pharyngeal route. Once in the body, EBV infects B lymphocytes, which are a type of white cell found in the lymph, blood, and connective tissue and which constitute one component of the body's immune system. The virus has an incubation period of 4 to 8 weeks.

SIGNS AND SYMPTOMS Initial symptoms are usually vague, but they may include malaise, anorexia, and chills. Later symptoms include sore throat, fever, and swollen lymph glands in the throat and neck.

DIAGNOSTIC PROCEDURES A thorough patient history and physical examination are essential to rule out closely related disorders. A blood test is necessary for confirming the diagnosis and will show increased numbers of atypical lymphocytes and antibodies to EBV.

TREATMENT Treatment is supportive because mononucleosis resists prevention and antimicrobial treatment. Bed rest may be indicated during the acute phase, and patients may still need to lessen their activities and get adequate rest until the disease completely subsides. Aspirin may be recommended for headache and sore throat. Warm saline gargles are also helpful.

PROGNOSIS The prognosis is good, but recovery may take several weeks or months.

PREVENTION The best prevention is to avoid oropharyngeal contact with a known EBV-infected person.

▉ PNEUMONIA

DESCRIPTION *Pneumonia* is an acute inflammation of the respiratory bronchioles, alveolar ducts, alveolar sacs, and **alveoli** of the lung. The inflammation may be either unilateral or bilateral and involve all or a portion of the affected lung. Pneumonia is the sixth leading cause of death in the United States. Pneumonia in childhood occurs more frequently in infants and young children.

ETIOLOGY As Table 8–1 illustrates, pneumonia may be caused by microorganisms such as bacteria, viruses, fungi, protozoans, or rickettsiae. The disease also may arise secondary to other systemic diseases or be induced by a variety of noninfectious agents such as chemicals and dusts. Most of the mi-

Table 8–1 Pneumonias

Specific Microbial Causes	Diseases That May Be Accompanied by Pneumonia	Pneumonia Not Caused by Infection
Viruses	Tularemia	Oil aspiration
Adenoviruses	Brucellosis	Radiation
Influenza	Rheumatic fever	Chemicals
Rhinoviruses	Syphilis	Vegetable dusts
Respiratory syncytial	Typhus	Silo-filler's disease
Coxsackieviruses	Typhoid	
Coronaviruses	Rocky Mountain fever	
Mycoplasmas	Q fever	
Mycoplasma pneumoniae	Acute viral respiratory disease	
Cocci	Infectious mononucleosis	
Pneumococcus	Trichiniasis	
Staphyloccus	Acquired immunodeficiency syndrome	
Hemolytic *Streptoccus*	(AIDS)	
Protozoan (probable)	Psittacosis	
Pneumocystis carinii	Plague	
Bacilli	Legionnaires' disease	
Hemophilus influenzae	Rickettsial diseases	
Mycobacterium tuberculosis		
Klebsiella pneumoniae		
(Friedländer's bacillus)		
Gram-negative bacilli		
Chlamydiae		
Chlamydia trachomatis		
C. psittaci		
Fungi		
Histoplasma capsulatum		
Coccidioides immitis		
Rickettsiae		
Rickettsia reckettsii		
R. burnettii		

Source: Thomas, CL (ed): Taber's Cyclopedic Dictionary, ed 17. FA Davis, Philadelphia, 1993, p. 1536.

crobial and noninfectious agents that cause pneumonia are either inhaled from the air or aspirated from the naso- and oropharynx. The term *aspiration pneumonia*, however, is usually reserved for pneumonia caused by irritation from large quantities of foreign matter, especially gastric contents, drawn into the lungs. In children, viral pneumonias occur more frequently than bacterial pneumonias and often follow a viral upper respiratory infection.

The pneumococcus bacterium and the influenza viruses are the leading causes of pneumonia. The likelihood of contracting any form of pneumonia, however, is greatly influenced by one's age, immunologic status, and environment. Certain pneumonias, for example, are far more likely to be acquired during hospitalization, whereas others occur more frequently in school environments, and still others in military settings.

SIGNS AND SYMPTOMS The main symptoms are coughing, **sputum** production, pleuritic chest pain, shaking chills, and high- or low-grade fever. Accompanying symptoms may include **rales, dyspnea, cyanosis,** and generalized weakness.

DIAGNOSTIC PROCEDURES A chest x-ray, taken in most suspected cases of pneumonia, will typically indicate the presence of infiltrates, the extent of lung involvement, and any complications present (Fig. 8–2). Sputum smears and blood cultures will usually be made to isolate the suspected microorganism.

TREATMENT The treatment procedure followed will necessarily vary with the etiology. Antibiotics will be prescribed for bacterial pneumonia. Supporting therapy for most types of pneumonia may include oxygen therapy, mechanical ventilation, a high-calorie diet, increased fluid intake, bed rest, analgesics, and **postural drainage.**

PROGNOSIS The prognosis varies with etiology. If the pneumonia is secondary to another disease or if the patient is already debilitated, the prognosis may be poor. A similar prognosis exists for influenza-caused pneumonia, especially among elderly persons. A frequent complication of influenza-caused pneumonia is lung abscess.

PREVENTION Those who are at higher-than-normal risk, such as elderly persons, should have annual influenza inoculations.

Figure 8–2 Viral pneumonia as seen on posterior-anterior chest radiograph. Viral pneumonia most often causes interstitial infiltration in both lungs. (From Wilkins, RL, and Dexter, JR: Respiratory Disease: A Case Study Approach to Patient Care, ed 2. FA Davis, Philadelphia, 1998, p 328, with permission.)

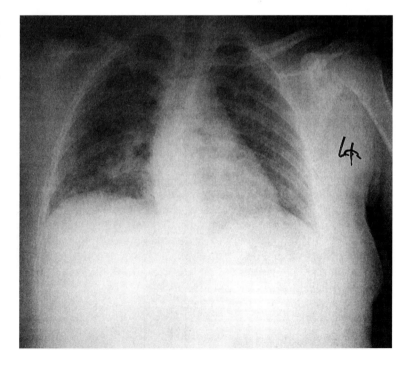

▪ *LEGIONELLA* INFECTIONS (Legionnaires' Disease)

DESCRIPTION A *Legionella* infection is an acute respiratory disease producing severe pneumonia-like symptoms. The disease is commonly called *Legionnaires' disease,* named after an epidemic outbreak of the illness that killed 34 people and sickened more than 200 attending an American Legion convention in Philadelphia in July of 1976. The disease may be mild and self-limiting or produce a pneumonia severe enough to be fatal.

ETIOLOGY Legionnaires' disease is caused by the gram-negative bacillus *Legionella pneumophilia.* Other closely related bacteria within the genus *Legionella* also can produce outbreaks of the disease that are clinically indistinguishable from classic Legionnaires' disease. The *Legionella* bacteria thrive in warm aquatic environments. They become problematic when they infect the cooling towers of air-conditioning systems and the hot-water plumbing of buildings. The bacteria are then inhaled into the lungs from aerosol water droplets. Legionnaires' disease has an incubation period of about 1 week. Predisposing factors include smoking and prior physical debilitation, especially among those with chronic obstructive pulmonary disease or alcoholism.

SIGNS AND SYMPTOMS The early symptoms of Legionnaires' disease are nonspecific and may include malaise, diarrhea, anorexia, and chills. A nonproductive cough develops, which later produces grayish and nonpurulent sputum.

DIAGNOSTIC PROCEDURES Laboratory studies may show elevated leukocytes, erythrocyte sedimentation rate (ESR), and liver enzyme activity. Bronchial washings, and blood and pleural fluid cultures, rule out other pulmonary infections. Special tests to isolate *Legionella* bacilli from respiratory secretions are necessary for confirmation of the diagnosis.

TREATMENT Antibiotic therapy is typically started even before the disease is definitely diagnosed. Antipyretics, fluid replacement, and oxygen may be used.

PROGNOSIS The prognosis is usually good if treatment is initiated early in the course of the disease. Even so, response to treatment is usually slow.

Complications may include pneumonia, hypoxia, delirium, heart failure, and shock. Shock usually is fatal.

PREVENTION Prevention includes detecting and eradicating *Legionella* bacteria from environments in which they may potentially infect people.

▪ LUNG ABSCESS

DESCRIPTION A *lung abscess* is an area of necrotized lung tissue containing purulent material (Fig. 8–3). Abscesses are more frequent in the lower dependent portions of the lungs, and in the right lung, which has a more vertical bronchus.

ETIOLOGY Lung abscesses caused by infectious organisms frequently arise as a complication of pneumonia. The major determinant in developing a

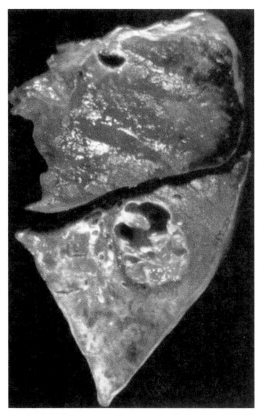

Figure 8–3 Pulmonary abscess. A large, cystic abscess that contains a purulent exudate and is contained by a fibrous wall. Pneumonia is present in the surrounding pulmonary parenchyma. (From Rubin, E, and Farber, JL [eds]: Pathology, ed 3. Lippincott-Raven, Philadelphia, 1999, p 614, with permission.)

lung abscess, as opposed to developing pneumonia only, is the causative microorganism's ability to necrotize lung tissue. A lung abscess also may be produced by a **septic** embolism being carried to the lung in the pulmonary circulation. Neoplasms, trauma from foreign objects lodged in lung tissue, or bronchial **stenosis** also may cause formation of lung abscesses.

SIGNS AND SYMPTOMS Lung abscesses produce a cough accompanied by bloody, purulent, or foul-smelling sputum and breath. Chest pain, sweating, chills, headache, fever, and dyspnea often are present.

DIAGNOSTIC PROCEDURES Chest **auscultation** reveals decreased breath sounds. A chest x-ray is necessary to localize the affected portions of the lung. Sputum culture also is used to detect possible infectious microorganisms. Blood culture may be used to assist in the diagnosis.

TREATMENT Antibiotic therapy of fairly long duration is the treatment of choice until the abscess is gone. Surgical resection of the lesion may be required if antibiotic therapy is unsuccessful.

PROGNOSIS The prognosis is good with proper care and follow-up. A complication may be the develop-ment of a brain abscess if infected materials are carried by the blood into the brain.

PREVENTION Postoperative patients should be monitored carefully to guard against aspiration of infected materials.

■ PNEUMOTHORAX

DESCRIPTION A *pneumothorax* is a collection of air in the pleural cavity. It typically results in the complete or partial collapse of the lung (**atelectasis**) (Fig. 8–4). One or both lungs may be affected. The condition is characterized as either spontaneous or secondary.

ETIOLOGY Spontaneous pneumothorax is caused by the rupturing of small **blebs** along the surface of the lung. What causes these blebs to form is not known, but they tend to form near the apex (bottom tip) of each lung. Pneumothorax also may be secondary to other lung diseases, such as asthma, emphysema, lung abscess, or lung cancer. Other secondary causes include chest trauma such as a knife wound or fractured rib. A perforated esophagus or use of mechanical ventilators also can cause pneumothorax.

Figure 8–4 Pneumothorax. (From Thomas, CL [ed]: Taber's Cyclopedic Medical Dictionary, ed 18. FA Davis, Philadelphia, 1997, p 1505, with permission.)

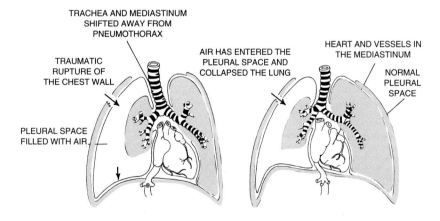

PNEUMOTHORAX
(OPEN—THE CHEST WALL INJURY PERMITS AIR TO FLOW IN AND OUT OF THE PLEURAL SPACE ON THE AFFECTED SIDE)

TRACHEA AND MEDIASTINUM SHIFTED AWAY FROM PNEUMOTHORAX

TRAUMATIC RUPTURE OF THE CHEST WALL

AIR HAS ENTERED THE PLEURAL SPACE AND COLLAPSED THE LUNG

HEART AND VESSELS IN THE MEDIASTINUM

NORMAL PLEURAL SPACE

PLEURAL SPACE FILLED WITH AIR

INHALATION: AIR ENTERS THE INJURED SIDE, CAUSING COLLAPSE OF THE LUNG AND SHIFT OF THE MEDIASTINUM AND HEART TOWARD THE UNAFFECTED SIDE

EXHALATION: THE AIR IS PARTIALLY FORCED FROM THE AFFECTED SIDE PLEURAL SPACE AND THE MEDIASTINUM SHIFTS TOWARD THE AFFECTED SIDE

SIGNS AND SYMPTOMS Classic symptoms are sudden, sharp pleuritic pain that worsens with chest movement, coughing, or breathing. There may be shortness of breath and cyanosis. In moderate to severe pneumothorax, there may also be profound respiratory distress accompanied by **pallor,** weak and rapid pulse, and anxiety.

DIAGNOSTIC PROCEDURES Physical examination may reveal asymmetric expansion of the chest during inspiration. Auscultation typically reveals diminished breathing sounds on the affected side. A chest x-ray will usually provide confirmation, showing air in the pleural space.

TREATMENT In spontaneous pneumothorax with no signs of increased pleural pressure or dyspnea, or where the lung collapse is less than 30 percent, the treatment of choice is bed rest and careful monitoring of vital signs. In traumatic pneumothorax, a medical emergency exists. A chest tube may be inserted for drainage and to allow the collapsed lung to expand. Recurring pneumothorax may require **thoracotomy** and **pleurectomy.**

PROGNOSIS The prognosis for pneumothorax is generally good with effective treatment. Spontaneous pneumothorax, however, tends to be a recurrent condition. A large pneumothorax can impair cardiac function.

PREVENTION Individuals with a history of spontaneous pneumothorax should not subject themselves to extremes of atmospheric pressure such as would be encountered by flying in an unpressurized aircraft or during scuba diving.

■ PLEURISY (Pleuritis)

DESCRIPTION *Pleurisy* is inflammation of the visceral (inner) and parietal (outer) pleural membranes that envelop each lung. The **pleura** of one or both lungs may be affected. The condition may be either primary or secondary.

ETIOLOGY Primary pleurisy is caused by infection of the pleura by bacteria or viruses. The condition is frequently secondary to pneumonia, tuberculosis, pulmonary infarction, neoplasm, systemic lupus erythematosus, and chest trauma.

SIGNS AND SYMPTOMS Symptoms may include coughing, fever and chills, and chest pain that is greater during inspiration. The sharp stabbing pain can be so severe that it limits movement on the affected side when breathing. Dyspnea also may occur.

DIAGNOSIS Chest auscultation reveals a pleural friction rub ("squeaky leather" or grating sounds) during respiration.

TREATMENT Treatment is aimed at the underlying cause but is otherwise symptomatic. Such treatment may include the use of strong analgesics, the application of heat, or taping the chest to restrict its movement. Bed rest is usually indicated. Severe pain may require the use of a regional anesthetic in a procedure called an *intercostal nerve block.*

PROGNOSIS Prognosis is dependent on etiology. Pleural effusion, a collection of fluid in the pleural space, may develop.

PREVENTION Early treatment of respiratory diseases is the best prevention.

■ PLEURAL EFFUSION

DESCRIPTION *Pleural effusion* is an excess of fluid between the parietal and visceral pleural membranes enveloping each lung. The accumulating fluid may be characterized as **transudate,** which has little or no protein, or **exudate,** which is protein-rich.

ETIOLOGY Pleural effusion may occur whether or not there is a pathological process affecting the pleurae themselves. Transudative pleural effusions frequently result from congestive heart failure. Exudative pleural effusions more often are seen with tuberculosis, rheumatoid arthritis, pancreatitis, respiratory neoplasms, and bacterial pneumonia.

SIGNS AND SYMPTOMS The person may be asymptomatic. When symptoms are manifested, they may include dyspnea and chest or pleuritic pain. The symptoms of pleural effusion will typically accompany those of any underlying condition.

DIAGNOSTIC PROCEDURES A chest x-ray may demonstrate pleural effusion. Auscultation of the chest reveals decreased breath sounds. **Percussion** elicits dull sounds over the effused area. **Thoracentesis** and analysis of the extracted fluid are necessary to distinguish transudative from exudative effusions.

TREATMENT Thoracentesis to alleviate fluid pressure may be necessary if the fluid is not reabsorbed. It is important, also, to treat the underlying cause of the pleural effusion.

PROGNOSIS The prognosis is dependent on the underlying disease.

PREVENTION There is no specific prevention for pleural effusion other than prompt treatment and management of disorders that may lead to the condition.

CHRONIC OBSTRUCTIVE PULMONARY DISEASE (COPD)

DESCRIPTION *Chronic obstructive pulmonary disease* is a functional diagnosis given to any pathological process that decreases the ability of the lungs and bronchi to perform their function of ventilation. It is characterized by permanent changes in the structure of the lungs and bronchi. COPD is a common cause of death and disability in the United States.

ETIOLOGY Diseases that may lead to COPD include emphysema, chronic bronchitis, chronic asthma, bronchiectasis, silicosis, and pulmonary tuberculosis. Smoking, prolonged exposure to polluted air, respiratory infections, and allergies are predisposing factors in this disease.

SIGNS AND SYMPTOMS COPD tends to develop insidiously, so no symptoms may be present initially. Later, a person may tire easily while exercising or doing strenuous work. A productive cough follows. Dyspnea upon minimal exertion then develops.

DIAGNOSTIC PROCEDURES A physical examination, chest x-ray, pulmonary function tests, arterial blood gases, and electrocardiogram (ECG) are the procedures used to diagnose COPD.

TREATMENT Treatment is aimed at preventing further lung damage, relieving symptoms, and preventing complications. Persons diagnosed with COPD should be advised not to smoke. **Bronchodilators** may be used, and antibiotics may be prescribed in the event of respiratory infections. Also, increasing fluid intake and maintaining a well-balanced diet can be helpful. Administration of oxygen may be necessary.

PROGNOSIS The prognosis for COPD is always guarded. The disease cannot be cured, nor can lost pulmonary function be restored. The degree of disability produced by COPD varies, but it tends to increase with time. COPD can cause disability, severe respiratory failure, and death.

PREVENTION Prevention includes not smoking, especially if family members have a history of the disease. Periodic physical examinations to evaluate chronic cough may be recommended.

CHRONIC BRONCHITIS

DESCRIPTION *Chronic bronchitis* is inflammation of the bronchial mucous membranes so that the patient has a chronically productive cough. It is characterized by **hypertrophy** and **hyperplasia** of bronchial mucous glands, damage to bronchial **cilia,** and narrowing of the bronchial airways.

ETIOLOGY Chronic bronchitis is strongly associated with long-term, heavy cigarette smoking. Occupational risk factors include exposure to textile dust fibers and certain petrochemicals. There is also evidence of a genetic predisposition to developing the disease.

SIGNS AND SYMPTOMS A chronic cough with sputum production is the classic symptom. A patient with chronic bronchitis may have only a minimal increase in airway resistance. As the disease progresses, the increase in airway resistance becomes greater. Weight gain due to **edema** and cyanosis, **tachypnea,** and wheezing may also be evident.

DIAGNOSTIC PROCEDURES A clinical diagnosis of chronic bronchitis requires that "productive cough be present for at least three months of the year over at least two consecutive years without other cause."[1]

TREATMENT Individuals diagnosed with chronic bronchitis must be encouraged not to smoke. All precautions should be taken to avoid respiratory infections. Bronchodilators and increased fluid intake may be of assistance. Diuretics may be prescribed for edema. Oxygen therapy may be necessary.

PROGNOSIS The prognosis is guarded. In the most serious cases, there typically is progressive deterioration of pulmonary function with increasing episodes of respiratory failure. Chronic bronchitis frequently leads to COPD (see COPD). There is a high mortality rate from complicating respiratory infections. Right ventricular failure also may develop as a complication of chronic bronchitis.

PREVENTION Avoiding known risk factors, such as smoking, is the best means of preventing chronic bronchitis.

CHRONIC PULMONARY EMPHYSEMA

DESCRIPTION *Chronic pulmonary emphysema* is the permanent enlargement of the air spaces beyond the terminal bronchioles resulting from destruction of alveolar walls (Fig. 8–5). As a consequence of this destruction, the lungs slowly lose their normal elasticity.

ETIOLOGY The exact cause of chronic pulmonary emphysema is not known. It is intimately associated with chronic bronchitis but does not necessarily result from that disorder. Known risk factors of emphysema include smoking and long-term exposure to air pollution and other respiratory tract irritants. Evidence suggests that some forms of the disease may be hereditary. In less common instances, the disease is associated with a deficiency of α_1-antitrypsin, a protein that plays a role in maintaining lung elasticity.

SIGNS AND SYMPTOMS The onset of the disease is insidious. Chronic pulmonary emphysema is generally characterized by progressive dyspnea on exertion. There may be a chronic cough. A characteristic "barrel chest" is often seen.

DIAGNOSTIC PROCEDURES A physical examination, chest x-ray, pulmonary function tests, arterial blood gases, ECG, and blood tests are used to diagnose emphysema. Technically, confirmation of the disease can be made only by a lung biopsy.

TREATMENT There is no effective treatment for emphysema other than management of the symptoms. Therapy during the acute phase should decrease the work of breathing and provide optimal oxygenation and ventilation. Long-term care should maximize patient autonomy and quality of life. Cigarette smoke and other toxic inhalants are to be avoided. Respiratory infections that do occur should be treated aggressively. Home oxygen and bronchodilators may be prescribed.

PROGNOSIS The prognosis is poor. Emphysema generally leads to COPD. Progressive diminution of pulmonary function and respiratory failure account for most deaths.

PREVENTION Although there is no specific prevention, avoiding smoking will certainly help.

ASTHMA

DESCRIPTION *Asthma* is a respiratory condition marked by recurrent attacks of labored breathing

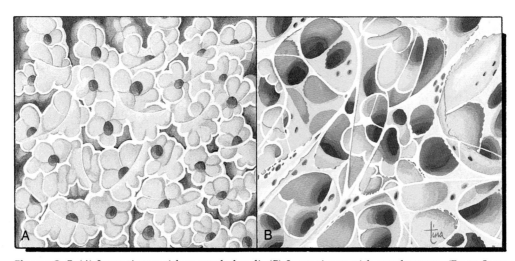

Figure 8–5 (*A*) Lung tissue with normal alveoli. (*B*) Lung tissue with emphysema. (From Scanlon, VC, and Sanders, T: Essentials of Anatomy and Physiology, ed 3. FA Davis, Philadelphia, 1999, p 335, with permission.)

accompanied by wheezing. Asthma is the consequence of spasms of the bronchial tubes or swelling of their mucous membranes. *Extrinsic* asthma occurs when the bronchospasm is the result of an allergic response to environmental irritants. *Intrinsic* asthma is present when the patient suffers attacks without evidence of allergic response. Extrinsic asthma is most common in childhood; intrinsic asthma more often begins in adulthood.

ETIOLOGY The etiology of asthma is uncertain. There is often a family history of allergy and an individual history of hypersensitivity. Upper respiratory infection, exercise, and anxiety can bring on an extrinsic attack.

SIGNS AND SYMPTOMS During an acute episode, there will be pronounced wheezing due to difficulty in exhaling air from the lungs. Dyspnea, tachypnea, and chest tightness also may occur. The person experiencing an asthmatic attack also may perspire profusely, exhibit pallor, and have difficulty speaking more than a few words. The person is usually anxious, exhausted, and complains of a "tight chest."

DIAGNOSTIC PROCEDURES A physical examination, chest x-ray during an attack, sputum analysis, pulmonary function tests, determination of arterial blood gases, and ECG may suggest the diagnosis. Skin tests may identify suspected allergens.

TREATMENT Treatment is directed toward achieving adequate oxygenation, providing bronchodilation, and decreasing airway inflammation. Aerosol or oral bronchodilators and nasal decongestants may be helpful for relief of symptoms. Metered-dose inhalers (MDI) are popular for administering the bronchodilator. Emergency treatment may include the administration of oxygen, bronchodilators, antibiotics, and intravenous corticosteroids.

PROGNOSIS Prognosis is good with proper attention and care. Many asthmatic children become asymptomatic after reaching adulthood, but children with onset of symptoms after age 15 typically have persistent disease in adulthood.

PREVENTION Among those with the condition, the frequency of asthmatic attacks may be reduced by avoiding known allergens as much as possible. Ed-

ucation about the use of medications and medication side effects is helpful in encouraging the person to lead an active, independent lifestyle.

■ PULMONARY TUBERCULOSIS (TB)

DESCRIPTION *Pulmonary tuberculosis* is a slowly developing bacterial lung infection characterized by progressive necrosis of lung tissue. An inflammatory response begins with **phagocytosis. Granulomas** form, and, when they calcify, leave lesions that may be visible on an x-ray. The lymph and blood generally are affected.

Since 1985 the downward trend in the incidence of tuberculosis has been interrupted by the advent of acquired immunodeficiency syndrome (AIDS). In general, tuberculosis is more common among elderly persons, the urban poor, members of minority groups, and patients with AIDS.

ETIOLOGY Pulmonary tuberculosis is caused by *Mycobacterium tuberculosis*. The infected individual's immune system usually is able to wall the bacteria into a tubercle or tiny nodule. The bacteria can lie dormant for years and then reactivate and spread when conditions are favorable. The disease is transmitted in aerosol droplets exhaled by infected individuals.

Note: Although the lungs are the organs most commonly infected, the bacteria can infect other parts of the body as well.

SIGNS AND SYMPTOMS Pulmonary tuberculosis may be asymptomatic. The onset generally is insidious. When symptoms are present, they are often vague and may include lassitude, malaise, fatigability, anorexia, afternoon fever, weight loss, cough, **hemoptysis,** and pleuritic chest pain. Advanced symptoms include wheezes, rales, and deviation of the trachea.

DIAGNOSTIC PROCEDURES A thorough physical examination, chest x-ray, and positive tuberculin test will confirm the diagnosis (Fig. 8–6). The tuberculin test of choice is the Mantoux test, which consists of an intradermal injection of a purified protein derivative (PPD) of the tuberculin bacillus. The bacteria may be identified in the sputum, urine, body fluids, or tissues of the patient. Sputum stud-

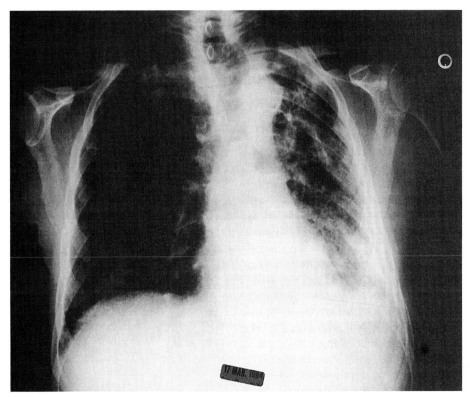

Figure 8–6 Typical chest radiograph for tuberculosis. Note the cavity lesion in the right upper lobe. (From Wilkins, RL, and Dexter, JR: Respiratory Disease: A Case Study Approach to Patient Care, ed 2. FA Davis, Philadelphia, 1998, with permission.)

ies are most helpful. Pulmonary and pleural biopsies may be ordered.

TREATMENT Drug therapy is indicated in every case of TB. There are many TB drugs, however, and these can be used in a number of different ways. To prevent the development of resistance, TB drugs are administered in combinations of two or more in most instances. Prolonged use is essential. Bed rest and isolation are indicated until the person is strong enough to resume activities or until the person is no longer deemed contagious. Surgery is recommended only in selected cases, such as in the event of bronchial stenosis or when drug therapy is not working.

PROGNOSIS The prognosis for an individual with active pulmonary tuberculosis is good if the disease is detected early and if the patient follows the prescribed regimen of drug therapy.

PREVENTION Preventive measures involve the isolation of infected persons, tuberculin testing of persons known to have been in close contact with infected persons, and treatment of tuberculin reactors. Generally, a person with a positive tuberculin reaction is put on a year of isoniazid prophylactically. Use of the bacille Calmette-Guérin (BCG) vaccination offers some protection for persons with a negative tuberculin test.

Pneumoconiosis

Pneumoconiosis is a disease of the respiratory tract caused by inhaling inorganic dust particles over a prolonged period. It is an occupational disorder associated with mining or stonecutting. Four of the most frequently seen varieties of pneumoconiosis are silicosis, asbestosis, berylliosis, and anthracosis.

■ SILICOSIS

DESCRIPTION *Silicosis* is a form of pneumoconiosis resulting from the inhalation of silica (quartz) dust. Silicosis is characterized by the formation of small, discrete, silicotic nodules in the lung tissue. As the disease advances, a dense fibrosis of the lungs develops and emphysema with respiratory impairment may result. The disease is chronic and progressive.

ETIOLOGY The occupations most prone to silica exposure are mining, drilling, blasting, grinding, and abrasive manufacturing. Required exposure varies from 2 to 30 years.

SIGNS AND SYMPTOMS The disease may be asymptomatic, even though x-rays exhibit evidence of nodule formation. Dyspnea on exertion generally is the first symptom. A dry cough that later turns productive, tachypnea, pulmonary hypertension, and malaise may result.

DIAGNOSTIC PROCEDURES A thorough medical history is essential. Chest x-rays are not always diagnostic but are used, especially in advanced silicosis. Arterial blood gases and pulmonary function tests confirm the diagnosis.

TREATMENT Treatment is symptomatic, especially for the cough and wheezing. A common complication, TB, must be aggressively treated.

PROGNOSIS The prognosis for an individual with silicosis is guarded if the disease has progressed to the fibrotic form. The disease can be rapidly fatal depending on the quantity and quality of the silica entering the lungs. Silicosis is always life-shortening.

PREVENTION Prevention involves minimizing exposure to silica dust in the work environment.

■ ASBESTOSIS

DESCRIPTION *Asbestosis* is a form of pneumoconiosis resulting from exposure to asbestos fibers. The disease is characterized by a slow, progressive, diffuse fibrosis of the lung tissue. Despite recent health and safety regulations limiting workplace exposure to asbestos, asbestosis remains the most frequently occurring form of pneumoconiosis.

ETIOLOGY Those at greatest risk of asbestosis include people who fabricate asbestos fibers, remove asbestos insulation from plumbing and buildings, or live within the area of an industry that discharges the fibers into the air. Family members of asbestos workers are also at risk of contracting the disease if they handle the worker's clothing. Ten years of moderate exposure to asbestos dust usually is required before the characteristic lesions of the disease become evident.

SIGNS AND SYMPTOMS The first symptom is dyspnea upon exertion, which worsens until dyspnea occurs even while at rest. Pleuritic chest pain, dry cough, and recurrent respiratory infections are common.

DIAGNOSTIC PROCEDURES A thorough medical history and physical examination are essential. Chest x-rays, pulmonary function studies, and arterial blood gases will confirm the diagnosis.

TREATMENT As with all pneumoconioses, treatment is symptomatic and supportive.

PROGNOSIS The prognosis is poor, especially if the affected person is a smoker. There is increased incidence of bronchogenic carcinoma even after brief exposure. If the person with asbestosis smokes, the incidence of cancer is about 90 percent.

PREVENTION Prevention involves avoidance of asbestos dust.

■ BERYLLIOSIS

DESCRIPTION *Berylliosis* is beryllium poisoning, usually of the lungs. The skin and other bodily organs also may be affected. The acute form of the disease is characterized by the onset of pneumonia-like symptoms and other respiratory tract disorders. The more common, chronic form is characterized by granuloma formation and diffuse interstitial pneumonitis.

ETIOLOGY Those at risk of contracting berylliosis include workers in the specialty metals, semiconductor, and ceramics industries. The metal may be either inhaled or directly absorbed through the skin in the form of dusts, salts, or fumes. As with asbestosis, berylliosis can affect family members who are exposed to dust in the worker's clothing.

SIGNS AND SYMPTOMS After exposure, nasal mucosal swelling and ulceration, and dry cough occur. As the condition worsens, substernal pain, tachycardia, dyspnea, weight loss, and pulmonary insufficiency result.

DIAGNOSTIC PROCEDURES A thorough medical history and physical examination are essential. Chest x-rays, pulmonary function studies, and arterial blood gas determination are ordered. A positive beryllium patch test establishes hypersensitivity to beryllium, not the disease. An in vitro lymphocyte transformation test diagnoses berylliosis.

TREATMENT Skin ulcers need to be excised. Corticosteroid therapy may be initiated. Oxygen, bronchodilators, and chest physical therapy methods may be required.

PROGNOSIS The prognosis is guarded. Individuals must modify their lifestyle. The disease is progressive.

PREVENTION The best prevention is avoidance of beryllium fumes or dusts.

ANTHRACOSIS

DESCRIPTION *Anthracosis*, also called *black lung disease* or *miner's asthma*, is a form of pneumoconiosis caused by the accumulation of carbon deposits in the lungs. The disease is characterized by symptoms resembling those of chronic bronchitis.

ETIOLOGY Anthracosis results from inhaling smoke or coal dust. Workers in the coal mining industry are those most likely to develop the disease. The effects of the disease are greatly compounded by smoking. Anthracosis frequently occurs with silico-

sis. Exposure of 15 years or longer is usually required before symptoms develop.

SIGNS AND SYMPTOMS Exertional dyspnea, productive cough with inky-black sputum, and recurrent respiratory infections are common symptoms.

DIAGNOSTIC PROCEDURES A thorough medical history and physical examination are essential and may reveal a barrel chest, rales, **rhonchi,** and wheezes. Chest x-rays, pulmonary function studies, and determination of blood gases will confirm the diagnosis.

TREATMENT Treatment is strictly symptomatic and typically includes the use of bronchodilating and corticosteroid drugs, chest physical therapy to help remove secretions, and the management of respiratory complications, such as TB or silicosis, that usually occur in association with anthracosis.

PROGNOSIS The prognosis is guarded. The disease is chronic and progressive. Complications worsen the prognosis.

PREVENTION Prevention involves avoidance of coal dust.

RESPIRATORY MYCOSES

DESCRIPTION *Mycoses* (fungal infections) are classified as either superficial or deep. Superficial mycoses affect only the skin and are considered in Chapter 13. Deep mycoses are systemic and may complicate other illnesses. The mycoses considered here are deep, systemic fungal infections that extensively affect the lungs: histoplasmosis, coccidioidomycosis, and blastomycosis.

ETIOLOGY *Histoplasmosis, Ohio Valley disease*, is caused by *Histoplasma capsulatum*. The fungus is found in soil, especially soil contaminated by bird and chicken droppings. The disease is transmitted by fungal spores that are inhaled or that penetrate the skin following injury. The primary lesion is in the lungs.

Coccidioidomycosis, valley fever, is caused by *Coccidioides immitis*, a fungus common in the dry desert soils of California and Arizona. The disease is transmitted by inhalation of fungal spores and commonly affects migrant farm laborers.

Blastomycosis, specifically *North American blastomycosis*, is caused by *Blastomyces dermatitidis*. It can cause a cutaneous infection, but usually it affects the lungs. In rare instances, a serious progressive systemic infection may occur.

SIGNS AND SYMPTOMS The symptoms of all three diseases may be mild and similar to those of a common cold. More severe symptoms include malaise, fever, myalgia, headache, cough, and chest pain. In coccidioidomycosis, however, the only symptom may be a persistent fever of several weeks' duration. In blastomycosis, nonpruritic and painless papules or macules may appear on exposed body surfaces.

DIAGNOSTIC PROCEDURES In histoplasmosis, a positive *Histoplasma* skin test, sputum culture, or special stainings of biopsied tissue confirm the diagnosis. In coccidioidomycosis, a positive coccidiodin skin test, chest x-ray, and special serologic tests are necessary for confirmation. In blastomycosis, cultures to isolate the fungus from sputum or skin lesions are necessary. Tissue biopsy from the skin or lungs may be ordered.

TREATMENT High-dose, long-term antifungal medications and supportive treatment for respiratory symptoms are used to treat histoplasmosis and blastomycosis. Coccidioidomycosis may heal spontaneously within a few weeks. Bed rest and symptomatic treatment may be all that are necessary. In some cases, surgery may be necessary to remove lung lesions.

PROGNOSIS The prognosis for an individual with histoplasmosis or coccidioidomycosis is usually excellent. Blastomycosis in its primary, acute form is self-limiting. If it progresses to a systemic infection, however, the prognosis is guarded.

PREVENTION Prevention includes following proper sanitary measures, wearing a face mask during exposure to potentially contaminated soil, and protecting exposed skin from invasion by the spores.

PULMONARY EDEMA

DESCRIPTION *Pulmonary edema* is a diffuse extravascular accumulation of fluid in the pulmonary tissues and air spaces. The condition is considered a medical emergency.

ETIOLOGY Most commonly, pulmonary edema represents the projection of cardiac disease processes such as atherosclerosis, hypertension, or valvular disease. The condition is usually a direct consequence of left ventricular failure. More blood is added to the pulmonary circulation than can be adequately removed. Noncardiogenic causes may include narcotic overdose, toxic inhalants, renal failure, cerebrovascular accident (CVA), skull fracture, and exposure to high altitudes.

SIGNS AND SYMPTOMS The onset of pulmonary edema frequently occurs at night after the person has been lying down for a while. Dyspnea, coughing, and **orthopnea** are common symptoms. **Tachycardia,** tachypnea, diffuse rales, and frothy bloody sputum also may occur. A decrease in blood pressure, **thready pulse,** and cold, clammy skin occur as cardiac output fails.

DIAGNOSTIC PROCEDURES Arterial blood gases and chest x-rays are useful in diagnosing this condition. Pulmonary artery catheterization may be used to confirm left ventricular failure.

TREATMENT Oxygen is typically administered along with bronchodilators and **diuretics.** Digitalis may be administered to stimulate heart action, and medication may also be prescribed to relieve anxiety. Fluid intake may be limited, and mechanical ventilation may be necessary.

PROGNOSIS The prognosis for an individual with pulmonary edema is guarded. When symptoms develop rapidly, the condition can be fatal.

PREVENTION There is no known prevention.

COR PULMONALE

DESCRIPTION *Cor pulmonale* is hypertrophy and failure of the right ventricle of the heart. Lung disease may cause pulmonary hypertension. As a result the heart's work load is increased, and the right ventricle hypertrophies in an effort to force blood into the lungs. Eventually the right ventricle is weakened by this effort, and blood pools in the right ventricle.

ETIOLOGY Cor pulmonale is caused by various disorders of the lungs, the pulmonary vessels, or the chest wall that impede pulmonary circulation. Disorders that may lead to cor pulmonale include COPD, chronic bronchitis, bronchiectasis, pulmonary hypertension, **kyphoscoliosis,** multiple pulmonary emboli, and living at high altitudes. The condition may be acute but is more commonly chronic.

SIGNS AND SYMPTOMS Symptoms include a productive, chronic cough, exertional dyspnea, fatigability, and wheezing respirations. Tachypnea, orthopnea, dependent edema, cyanosis, **clubbing,** and distended neck veins may occur as the condition worsens. The liver is enlarged and tender.

DIAGNOSTIC PROCEDURES Chest x-rays, an ECG, and pulmonary function studies are useful diagnostic tools. Echocardiography or angiography and determination of arterial blood gases confirm the diagnosis.

TREATMENT Cor pulmonale is frequently treated with medications such as digitalis to stimulate heart action; antibiotics for secondary respiratory infections; or pulmonary artery dilators, diuretics, anticoagulants, and bronchodilators. Oxygen may be necessary. Restriction of salt and fluids may be advised. The underlying cause needs to be treated, too.

PROGNOSIS The prognosis is typically poor for an individual with cor pulmonale, but it depends on the underlying cause of the condition.

PREVENTION There is no known prevention.

▪ PULMONARY EMBOLISM

DESCRIPTION A *pulmonary embolism* is a mass of undissolved matter in the pulmonary artery or one of its branches.

ETIOLOGY A pulmonary embolism generally originates in the pelvic veins or deep lower extremity veins and travels through the circulatory system until it blocks a pulmonary artery (Fig. 8–7). At high risk for pulmonary emboli are individuals immobilized with chronic diseases, those in body casts, persons with congestive heart failure or neoplasms, or postoperative patients. Also at risk are pregnant women; individuals with venous diseases such as **polycythemia vera, thrombocytosis,** or varicose veins; or women who are taking oral contraceptives.

SIGNS AND SYMPTOMS Signs and symptoms depend on the size and location of the embolus. Acute

symptoms may include dyspnea, anxiety, and substernal pain. Less severe symptoms are cough, pleuritic pain, and low-grade fever. Apprehension is common.

DIAGNOSTIC PROCEDURES Diagnosing this condition is frequently difficult, but an ECG may reveal tachycardia, and a chest x-ray may indicate the location of the embolus. Lung scintiscan, pulmonary angiography, or magnetic resonance imaging (MRI) may help in the diagnosis. Auscultation reveals rales and a pleural rub near the area of the embolism.

TREATMENT Treatment typically involves the use of anticoagulants such as heparin and warfarin to prevent clot formation and fibrinolytic therapy to dissolve the embolus. Surgical management may be indicated in exceptional cases. This involves removing the embolus or **ligation** or **plication** of the vena cava to prevent the migration of new emboli into the pulmonary circulation.

PROGNOSIS The prognosis is guarded if the embolism is massive enough to trigger a **pulmonary**

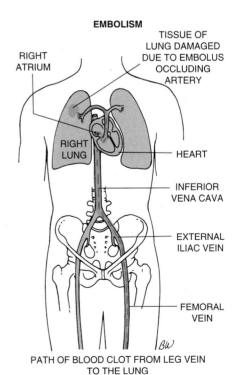

EMBOLISM

RIGHT ATRIUM

TISSUE OF LUNG DAMAGED DUE TO EMBOLUS OCCLUDING ARTERY

RIGHT LUNG

HEART

INFERIOR VENA CAVA

EXTERNAL ILIAC VEIN

FEMORAL VEIN

PATH OF BLOOD CLOT FROM LEG VEIN TO THE LUNG

Figure 8–7 Embolism. (From Thomas, CL [ed]: Taber's Cyclopedic Medical Dictionary, ed 18. FA Davis, Philadelphia, 1997, p 620, with permission.)

infarction (which occurs in about 10 percent of cases).

PREVENTION Prevention includes early postoperative ambulation or initiating prophylactic anticoagulant therapy for patients deemed to be at risk.

RESPIRATORY ACIDOSIS (Hypercapnia)

DESCRIPTION *Respiratory acidosis* is excessive acidity of body fluids attributable to inadequate removal of carbon dioxide (CO_2) by the lungs. Whenever CO_2 cannot be adequately ventilated, the CO_2 dissolved in the blood rapidly increases. As the level of CO_2—called the partial pressure of carbon dioxide, or PCO_2—rises, so does the amount of CO_2 that combines with water to form carbonic acid. Consequently, the **pH** of the blood decreases. The condition may be acute or chronic.

ETIOLOGY Acute respiratory acidosis occurs whenever there is a sudden impairment of ventilation resulting from airway obstruction. This may be due to causes such as a foreign object blocking the airway or to the effects of certain drugs, neuromuscular diseases, or cardiac arrest. Chronic respiratory acidosis is caused by pulmonary diseases that change the characteristics of lung tissue, impairing the ability to release CO_2. Examples of such diseases include emphysema, bronchitis, and chronic obstructive pulmonary disease. Chronic respiratory acidosis also may be a consequence of extreme obesity.

SIGNS AND SYMPTOMS Symptoms vary with the etiology, but typically they include weakness, shallow respirations, confusion, muscle tremors, and tachycardia.

DIAGNOSTIC PROCEDURES Diagnosis of respiratory acidosis is usually evident from the clinical situation. Arterial blood gas testing to confirm elevated PCO_2 levels is required to confirm the diagnosis.

TREATMENT The only useful treatment for respiratory acidosis involves measures to correct the underlying cause.

PROGNOSIS The prognosis for an individual with respiratory acidosis varies with the cause. Respiratory acidosis can cause shock or cardiac arrest.

PREVENTION There is no specific prevention other than treatment of the cause.

RESPIRATORY ALKALOSIS (Hypocapnia)

DESCRIPTION *Respiratory alkalosis* is excessive alkalinity of body fluids attributable to the excessive removal of CO_2 by the lungs. When excessive amounts of CO_2 are ventilated by the lungs, the PCO_2 in the blood decreases, initiating a series of chemical and metabolic changes that act to reduce the level of serum bicarbonate. Consequently, the pH of the blood increases. The condition may be acute or chronic.

ETIOLOGY Respiratory alkalosis is caused by acute or chronic hyperventilation. Acute respiratory alkalosis may result from hyperventilation induced by anxiety or psychological trauma, fever, pain, salicylate poisoning, excessive exercise, or excessive use of mechanical ventilators. It is also associated with **hypoxia** due to pneumonia, asthma, or pulmonary edema. Chronic respiratory alkalosis from hyperventilation is typically associated with hypoxia due to chronic cardiopulmonary diseases or high altitudes.

SIGNS AND SYMPTOMS Symptoms vary with etiology, but they may include numbness or tingling of the extremities, light-headedness, muscle spasms, and periods of apnea.

DIAGNOSTIC PROCEDURES Diagnosis of respiratory alkalosis usually is based on the clinical evidence presented, but it must be confirmed through a blood test revealing decreased levels of serum bicarbonate or decreased PCO_2 levels.

TREATMENT Treatment is aimed at correcting the underlying cause. Short-term measures may involve having the person breathe into a bag or administering a sedative to relieve hyperventilation in very anxious patients.

PROGNOSIS The prognosis of an individual with respiratory alkalosis varies with etiology but is generally good.

PREVENTION There are no specific preventive measures.

ATELECTASIS

DESCRIPTION *Atelectasis* is a collapsed or airless condition of all or part of a lung that allows unoxygenated blood to pass unchanged through the area, and this produces hypoxia. The condition may be acute or chronic.

ETIOLOGY The condition may be caused by obstruction of the lung by foreign matter, mucous plugs, or excessive secretion. Compression of the lung by tumors, aneurysms, enlarged lymph nodes, or pneumothorax also may cause lung collapse (see Pneumothorax). Atelectasis is sometimes a complication of abdominal surgery or a general consequence of postoperative immobilization.

SIGNS AND SYMPTOMS Symptoms of acute atelectasis typically include marked dyspnea, cyanosis, fever, tachycardia, anxiety, and **diaphoresis.** There may be a decrease in chest motion on the affected side. Chronic atelectasis may be marked only by the gradual onset of dyspnea.

DIAGNOSTIC PROCEDURES A thorough medical history, physical examination, and chest x-ray are essential for diagnosis. Sound on percussion may be dull, and auscultation will reveal decreased breath sounds. A bronchoscopy and arterial blood gases may be ordered.

TREATMENT Postural drainage, spirometry, chest percussion, and frequent coughing and deep breathing are advised. Early postoperative ambulation is recommended. Bronchodilators may be prescribed.

PROGNOSIS The prognosis in postoperative atelectasis usually is good, although death may result if the condition is untreated. In all other types of atelectasis, the prognosis is dependent on the cause.

PREVENTION Prevention includes postoperative exercise and prompt treatment of any pulmonary problems.

BRONCHIECTASIS

DESCRIPTION *Bronchiectasis* is the permanent abnormal dilation of small and medium-sized bronchi resulting from the destruction of muscular and elastic components of the bronchial walls. The condition usually is bilateral, involving the lower lobes of the lungs.

ETIOLOGY Bronchiectasis may be caused by pulmonary diseases such as pneumonia or tuberculosis, by bronchial obstruction, by inhalation of corrosive gas, or by heavy smoking. Bronchiectasis is also a frequent, life-threatening complication of cystic fibrosis.

SIGNS AND SYMPTOMS Affected individuals frequently have a chronic cough and expectorate large amounts of purulent, foul-smelling sputum, especially the first thing in the morning. Hemoptysis may occur to the extent that it frightens the patient. Dyspnea, wheezing, fever, and malaise may ensue as the condition progresses.

DIAGNOSTIC PROCEDURES Diagnosis of bronchiectasis may be difficult, especially initially, when symptoms are vague. Chest x-rays, bronchography, and CT scans are the most valuable tools for diagnosis. Sputum culture and pulmonary function studies are helpful.

TREATMENT Antibiotics are ordered. Environmental irritants such as smoke, dust, and fumes should be avoided. Postural drainage and bronchodilators may be ordered. Surgery may be performed if the condition is severe.

PROGNOSIS The condition is irreversible, and the prognosis is guarded.

PREVENTION Prevention includes avoiding pulmonary irritants and smoking, and seeking prompt treatment of any pulmonary ailments.

LUNG CANCER

DESCRIPTION *Lung cancer* comprises various malignant neoplasms that may appear in the trachea, bronchi, or air sacs of the lungs. For women over 40, it is the leading cause of cancer deaths, although recently the rate of increase in women has begun to slow. Its incidence has decreased in men since 1987.

ETIOLOGY Although the precise triggering mechanisms are not known, most lung cancers are caused either directly or indirectly by smoking. Tobacco smoke contains a number of chemicals known to be carcinogenic. Long-term exposure to atmospheric pollution and airborne pulmonary irritants is also associated with increased incidences of lung cancer. Other risk factors include radiation exposure from occupational, medical and environmental sources, and environmental tobacco smoke in nonsmokers.

SIGNS AND SYMPTOMS Early-stage lung cancer usually produces no symptoms and is difficult to detect. When symptoms appear, they may include smoker's cough, wheezing, chest pain, dyspnea, and hemoptysis.

DIAGNOSTIC PROCEDURES Chest x-ray, a sputum cytology test, and fiberoptic bronchoscopy are useful in diagnosing lung cancer. Tissue biopsy is required for definitive diagnosis.

TREATMENT Treatment most often involves a combination of surgery, radiation therapy, and chemotherapy, since lung cancer often metastasizes to other tissues by the time it is diagnosed. Metastasis to the brain, liver, and bone is common.

PROGNOSIS The prognosis is poor. According to the American Cancer Society, only 14 percent of lung cancer patients live more than 5 years. Despite advances in diagnosis, the overall survival rate for those with lung cancer has changed little over the past 30 years.

PREVENTION Lung cancer is largely preventable if individuals avoid smoking and toxic inhalants. If smokers stop at the time of early precancerous cellular changes, the damaged bronchial lining tissues often return to normal.[2]

SPECIAL FOCUS RESPIRATORY DISEASES OF CHILDHOOD

◼ SUDDEN INFANT DEATH SYNDROME (SIDS)

DESCRIPTION *Sudden infant death syndrome* is the completely unexpected and unexplained death of an apparently normal and healthy infant, usually 10 to 12 weeks old. Generally, the death occurs when the infant is sleeping. SIDS occurs more frequently in male than in female infants, in premature infants, and during the winter months. It is the number one cause of death in infants from 1 to 12 months of age.

ETIOLOGY The cause is unknown, but several possibilities have been suggested, including mechanical suffocation, prolonged **apnea,** lack of **biotin** in the diet, an unknown virus, immunoglobulin abnormalities, a defect in the respiratory mucosal defense, or an anatomically abnormal larynx.

SIGNS AND SYMPTOMS There are no premonitory signs and symptoms. The infant generally does not cry out or show evidence of distress or struggle. When found, the infant is dead and may have mottled skin indicating cyanosis. There may be blood-tinged sputum. The infant's diaper is likely to be wet or filled with stool.

DIAGNOSTIC PROCEDURES A diagnosis of SIDS is exclusionary, that is, made only after all other causes of death have been eliminated as possibilities.

TREATMENT There is no treatment. There are SIDS support groups for parents.

PROGNOSIS It is currently believed that children are no longer at risk of SIDS by 1 year of age.

PREVENTION Some home monitoring devices have been tried on infants who have experienced apneic periods, but their use remains controversial. Prevention of SIDS is largely aimed at trying to identify infants at risk.

◼ ACUTE TONSILLITIS

DESCRIPTION *Acute tonsillitis* is inflammation of a tonsil, especially one or both of the palatine tonsils that lie on either side of the opening of the throat.

ETIOLOGY Acute tonsillitis is most frequently caused by infection by the bacteria *Streptococcus pyogenes* or *Staphylococcus aureus,* although a variety of infectious agents may be involved. The condition is a common complication of pharyngitis.

SIGNS AND SYMPTOMS Tonsillitis is typically manifested by the sudden onset of chills and a high-grade fever. Additional symptoms may include malaise, headache, sore throat, and dysphagia.

DIAGNOSTIC PROCEDURES Upon physical examination, the tonsils will appear red and swollen. In severe cases, abscesses may be visible on the affected tonsil's surface. Blood tests may reveal leukocytosis. A throat culture to detect bacteria will typically be performed.

TREATMENT Antibiotic, especially penicillin, therapy is prescribed for bacterial tonsillitis in its early stages. Symptomatic relief includes saline gargles, analgesics, and antipyretics. Bed rest is usually indicated. Recurrent bouts of tonsillitis may require tonsillectomy.

PROGNOSIS The prognosis for acute tonsillitis is usually good. In severe cases, however, the tonsils may swell sufficiently to interfere with breathing. Serious complications include rheumatic fever, glomerulonephritis, and carditis. More localized complications may include otitis media, mastoiditis, and sinusitis.

PREVENTION There is no specific prevention for acute tonsillitis except for prompt treatment of any pharyngeal infection.

ADENOID HYPERPLASIA

DESCRIPTION *Adenoid hyperplasia* is the enlargement of the lymphoid tissue of the nasopharynx, causing partial breathing blockage.

ETIOLOGY The cause is essentially unknown. Circumstances that may cause the adenoids to continue to grow when they normally would atrophy (approximately ages 5 to 8) may include repeated infection and nasal congestion, chronic allergies, and heredity.

SIGNS AND SYMPTOMS The most common symptoms are chronic mouth-breathing, snoring, and frequent head colds. The child's speech has a nasal quality.

DIAGNOSTIC PROCEDURES Diagnosis is usually made by visualizing the hyperplastic adenoidal tissue or by lateral pharyngeal x-ray films.

TREATMENT The treatment of choice is adenoidectomy, often performed in conjunction with a tonsillectomy.

PROGNOSIS The prognosis is excellent with proper care and attention. If untreated, however, adenoid hyperplasia can lead to changes in facial features, and complications such as otitis media, which carries an accompanying risk of hearing loss.

PREVENTION There is no specific prevention for this condition.

CROUP

DESCRIPTION *Croup* is acute and severe inflammation and obstruction of the upper respiratory tract, occurring most frequently from 3 months to 3 years of age. It is more common in male infants and children.

ETIOLOGY The condition may be caused by parainfluenza virus, adenoviruses, respiratory syncytial viruses, and influenza and measles viruses. Croup generally follows an upper respiratory tract infection.

SIGNS AND SYMPTOMS Common symptoms include hoarseness, fever, a distinctive harsh, brassy, barklike cough, persistent stridor during inspiration, and respiratory distress. The infant or child may be anxious and frightened by the respiratory distress. The symptoms may last a few hours or persist for a day or two.

DIAGNOSTIC PROCEDURES Cultures of the causative organism are done. Neck x-ray and laryngoscopy may be performed, too.

TREATMENT Children are treated symptomatically at home in most cases with bed rest, liquids, and antipyretics. Cool humidification of the air is tried. If dehydration is suspected, hospitalization may be necessary and antibiotic therapy and oxygen therapy may be started.

PROGNOSIS The prognosis is good with treatment.

PREVENTION Prevention includes prompt treatment of any respiratory tract infections.

ACUTE EPIGLOTTITIS

DESCRIPTION *Acute epiglottitis* is severe inflammation of the epiglottis that tends to cause airway obstruction. It primarily affects children between the ages of 2 and 8 years.

ETIOLOGY The causative agent generally is *Haemophilus influenzae* type B. Pneumococci and group A streptococci also can cause epiglottitis.

SIGNS AND SYMPTOMS Common symptoms include fever, swollen and erythematous epiglottis, sore throat, **stridor,** and croupy cough. If the epiglottis is swollen and inflamed enough, there could be total obstruction of the larynx within 2 to 5 hours. The child may sit with the neck hyperextended and the mouth open and tongue protruding in an attempt to "get more air."

DIAGNOSTIC PROCEDURES Physical examination may be all that is necessary to reveal the inflamed large, bright-red epiglottis. Neck x-rays and laryngoscopy may be done, too.

TREATMENT The child will be hospitalized and possibly may require emergency tracheostomy or endotracheal intubation. Oxygen therapy, antibiotics, and close monitoring may be necessary.

PROGNOSIS The prognosis is good with prompt treatment.

PREVENTION The American Academy of Pediatrics recommends that children receive the *Haemophilus influenzae* 6 conjugate vaccine. Prevention includes prompt treatment of any respiratory illness.

COMMON SYMPTOMS OF LUNG DISEASES

Individuals may present with the following common symptoms, which deserve attention from health professionals:

- Pain anywhere in the respiratory tract, especially sore throat
- Cough, either productive or nonproductive, chronic or acute
- Breathing irregularities such as dyspnea, wheezing, tachypnea, or rales
- Fever
- Malaise
- Headache
- Cyanosis

REFERENCES

1. Sheldon, H: Boyd's Introduction to the Study of Disease, ed 11. Lea & Febiger, Philadelphia, 1992, p 346.
2. American Cancer Society: Cancer Facts and Figures— 1998, p 12.

BIBLIOGRAPHY

Diseases. Springhouse Corporation, Springhouse, Pa., 1993.
Fauci, AS, et al: Harrison's Principles of Internal Medicine, ed 14. McGraw-Hill, New York, 1998.
Frazier, MS, Drzymkowski, JA, and Doty, SJ: Essentials of Human Disease and Conditions. WB Saunders, Philadelphia, 1996.
Kent, TH, and Michael, NH: Introduction to Human Disease. Appleton & Lange, Stamford, Conn., 1998.
Professional Guide to Diseases, ed 6. Springhouse Corporation, Springhouse, Pa., 1998.

CASE STUDIES

I A 55-year-old naval shipyard worker begins to experience a slightly irritating cough. His wife tells him that it is probably the result of smoking three packs of cigarettes a day. She begs him to quit, as she did many years ago. He begins to experience trouble breathing (dyspnea) even when at rest. Soon, however, the man's wife also begins to experience symptoms of respiratory disease. The man visits his physician, who, based on the work and family history, suspects asbestosis. Because his wife has washed his work clothes for 26 years, she, too, is advised to see a physician.

1. What cause(s) or predisposing factor(s) is(are) apparent?
2. What are the pertinent symptoms of this case?
3. What could have prevented the wife's involvement in this case?
4. Comment on the role of smoking in this case.

II A 72-year-old man, despite a history of lung problems, has led an active life of working, hunting, and fishing. He has not yet retired.

As a child, he aspirated some peanut husks, with no obvious effects at the time. He and his wife of 51 years both smoked; he quit about 10 years ago. For the last 15 years, he has noted shortness of breath—at first after working in his garden, then after walking up an incline, lately after walking even a few steps. What takes him to the doctor is dyspnea and a chronic, productive, and painful cough.

1. Do the history and symptoms indicate a neoplasm? Explain.
2. What might be the contributing factors to illness in this case?
3. What implications does the person's age have in this case?

REVIEW QUESTIONS

MATCHING

Match the following terms with their correct definitions:

_____ 1. Air in pleural cavity

_____ 2. Chronic obstructive pulmonary disease

_____ 3. Sore throat

_____ 4. Caused by Epstein-Barr virus

_____ 5. Excess fluid in pleural space

_____ 6. Black lung disease

_____ 7. Nosebleed

_____ 8. Lungs lose normal elasticity

_____ 9. Inflammation of the pleura

a. Epistaxis
b. Pharyngitis
c. Adenoid hyperplasia
d. Infectious mononucleosis
e. Pneumothorax
f. SIDS
g. Pleural effusion
h. COPD
i. Emphysema
j. Anthracosis
k. Asthma
l. Cor pulmonale
m. Pleurisy
n. Laryngitis

_____ 10. Hoarseness or loss of voice

_____ 11. Unexplained sudden death of an infant

_____ 12. Enlargement of the lymphoid tissue of the nasopharynx

SHORT ANSWER

1. List the four major causes of sinusitis:

   a.

   b.

   c.

   d.

2. Treatment of acute tonsillitis and adenoid hyperplasia is apt to be _____ .

3. Identify the four causes of pneumonia:

   a.

   b.

   c.

   d.

4. From the preceding list, identify the most common form of pneumonia.

   _____

5. Identify a complication that may result from a lung abscess. _____

6. A diagnosis of chronic bronchitis requires _____ .

7. Identify the classic symptoms of asthma:

   a.

   b.

8. The diagnostic test of choice to confirm tuberculosis is _____ .

9. The best prevention for any of the four pneumoconioses is _____ .

10. Mycoses are _____ infections.

TRUE/FALSE

T F   1. Coccidioidomycosis is common in the Ohio Valley.

T F   2. Legionnaires' disease affects only members of the American Legion.

T F   3. Cor pulmonale is left atrial hypertrophy.

T F   4. Immobile patients may be at high risk for pulmonary embolism.

T F   5. Respiratory acidosis results from hypoventilation and CO_2 retention.

T F   6. Respiratory alkalosis results from hyperventilation and CO_2 elimination.

T F   7. Bronchiectasis is the collapse of part or all of a lung.

T F 8. Atelectasis is an abnormal dilation of bronchi.

T F 9. Early-stage lung cancer usually produces no symptoms.

T F 10. The body can survive only minutes without air.

ANSWERS

MATCHING

1. e	4. e	7. a	10. n
2. h	5. g	8. i	11. f
3. b	6. j	9. m	12. c

SHORT ANSWER

1. a. Bacterial infection
   b. Swimming or diving
   c. Dental abscess or extractions
   d. Nasal allergies
2. Tonsillectomy and adenoidectomy
3. a. Viral
   b. Bacterial
   c. Aspiration
   d. Viral and bacterial
4. Bacterial pneumonia
5. Development of brain abscess
6. Productive cough on most days for a minimum of 3 months of the year for at least 2 consecutive years
7. Marked wheezing and difficulty in expiration
8. Mantoux test
9. Avoidance of dust
10. Fungal

TRUE/FALSE

1. False	6. True
2. False	7. False
3. False	8. False
4. True	9. True
5. True	10. True

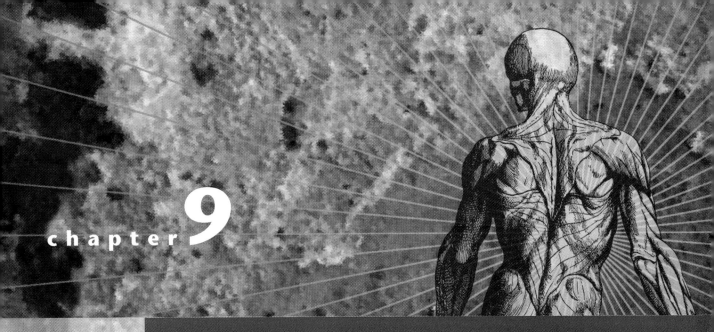

chapter 9

Circulatory System Diseases

CHAPTER OUTLINE

Rheumatic Fever and Rheumatic Heart Disease

Carditis
Pericarditis
Myocarditis
Endocarditis

Valvular Heart Disease
Mitral Insufficiency/Stenosis
Tricuspid Insufficiency/Stenosis
Pulmonic Insufficiency/Stenosis
Aortic Insufficiency/Stenosis

Hypertensive Heart Disease
Essential Hypertension

Coronary Diseases
Coronary Artery Disease
Angina Pectoris
Myocardial Infarction (Heart Attack)
Congestive Heart Failure (CHF)
Cardiac Arrest

Special Focus: Cardiac Advances

Blood Vessel Diseases
Aneurysms: Abdominal, Thoracic, and
* Peripheral Arteries*

Arteriosclerosis and Atherosclerosis
Thrombophlebitis
Varicose Veins

Anemias and Other Red Blood Cell Disorders
Iron Deficiency Anemia
Folic Acid Deficiency Anemia
Pernicious Anemia
Aplastic Anemia
Sickle Cell Anemia
Polycythemia Vera

Leukemias
Acute Myeloblastic (Myelogenous) Leukemia
* (AML)*
Acute Lymphoblastic (Lymphocytic)
* Leukemia (ALL)*
Acute Monoblastic (Monocytic) Leukemia
Chronic Myelocytic Leukemia (CML)
Chronic Lymphocytic Leukemia (CLL)

Lymphatic Diseases
Lymphedema
Hodgkin's Disease
Lymphosarcoma

Special Focus: Bone Marrow Transplantation

Special Focus: Circulatory Disease of Childhood
Reye's Syndrome

Common Symptoms of Circulatory System Diseases

☐ ALTERNATIVE MEDICINE

Bibliography

Case Studies

Review Questions

LEARNING OBJECTIVES

Upon successful completion of this chapter, you will:

- Describe the infectious heart diseases.
- Identify the valvular heart diseases.
- Identify individuals at high risk of developing hypertension.
- Recall the safe time duration of angina pectoris.
- List the classic signs and symptoms of myocardial infarction.
- Describe congestive heart failure.
- List the causes of heart murmurs.
- Contrast three types of aneurysms.
- Compare atherosclerosis to arteriosclerosis.
- Discuss the prevention of thrombophlebitis.
- Describe varicose veins.
- Recall the classic treatment protocol for polycythemia vera.
- Compare seven anemias.
- Discuss the various treatments of leukemia.
- Define lymphedema.
- Compare lymphosarcoma to Hodgkin's disease.
- Describe Reye's syndrome.
- List at least four common symptoms of cardiovascular disease.

KEY WORDS

Analgesic (ăn•ăl•jē′sĭk)
Aneurysm (ăn′ū•rĭzm)
Anorexia (ăn•ō•rĕk′sē•ă)
Antibodies (ăn′tĭ•bŏ•dēz)
Arrhythmia (ă•rĭth′mē•ă)
Ascites (ă•sī′tēz)
Blast (blăst)
Bradycardia (brăd•ē•kăr′dē•ă)
Bruit (brwē)
Cardiogenic shock (kăr•dē•ō•jĕn′ĭk shŏk)
Cellulitis (sĕl•ū•lī′tĭs)
Cholelithiasis (kō•lē•lĭ•thī′ă•sĭs)
Chorea (kō•rē′ă)
Claudication (klaw•dĭ•kā′shŭn)
Cyanosis (sī•ă•nō′sĭs)
Diaphoresis (dī•ă•fō•rē′sĭs)
Diastolic pressure (dī•ă•stŏl′ik prĕsh′ŭr)
Dilatation (dĭl•ă•tā′shŭn)
Diuretic (dī•ū•rĕt′ĭk)
Dyspnea (dĭsp•nē′ă)
Effusion (ĕ•fū′zhŭn)
Embolus (ĕm′bō•lŭs)

Fibrillation (fĭ•brĭl•ā′shŭn)
Gangrene (găng′grēn)
Hematopoietic (hē•mă•tō•poy•ĕt′ĭk)
Hemoglobin (hē•mō•glō′bĭn)
Hemoptysis (hē•mŏp′tĭ•sĭs)
Hepatomegaly (hĕp•ă•tō•mĕg′ă•lē)
Hypertrophy (hī•pĕr′trŏ•fē)
Hypoglycemia (hī•pĕr•glī•sē′mē•ă)
Hypoxia (hī•pŏks′ē•ă)
Idiopathic (ĭd•ē•ō•păth′ĭk)
Induration (ĭn•dū•rā′shŭn)
Ischemia (ĭs•kē′mē•ă)
Lumen (loo′mĕn)
Lymphangitis (lĭm•făn•jī′tĭs)
Lymphocytopenia (lĭm•fō•sīt•ō•pē′nē•ă)
Lysis (lī′sĭs)
Megakaryocyte (mĕg•ă•kăr′ē•ō•sīt)
Menorrhagia (mĕn•ō•rā′jē•ă)
Mitochondria (mī•tō•kŏn′drē•ă)
Mitral regurgitation (mī′trăl rē•gŭr•jĭ•tā′shŭn)
Myelosuppression (mī•ē•lō•sŭ•prĕ′shŭn)
Myocardium (mī•ō•kăr′dē•ŭm)

Nephrosclerosis (něf•rō•sklě•rō′sĭs)
Neuritis (nū•rī′tĭs)
Neutropenia (nū•trō•pē′nē•ǎ)
Orthopnea (ŏr•thŏp′nē•ǎ)
Parenteral (pǎr•ěn′těr•ǎl)
Percutaneous transluminal coronary
   angioplasty (pěr•kū•tā′nē•ŭs
   trǎns•loo′mĭn•ǎl kŏr′ō•nǎ•rē
   ǎn′jē•ō•plǎs•tē)
Pericardiocentesis
   (pěr•ĭ•kǎr•dē•ō•sěn•tē′sĭs)
Petechiae (plural) (pē•tē′kē•ē)
Pitting edema (pĭt′ing ě•dē′mǎ)
Plaque (plǎk)
Prolapse (prō′lǎps)
Pruritus (proo•rī′tŭs)
Purpura (pŭr′pū•rǎ)
Radioisotope (rā•dē•ō•ī′sō•tōp)
Rales (plural) (rǎls)

Reticulocyte (rě•tĭk′ū•lō•sīt)
Stasis pigmentation (stā′sĭs
   pĭg•měn•tā′shun)
Stenosis (stě•nō′sĭs)
Stridor (strī′dŏr)
Sympathectomy (sĭm•pǎ•thěk′tō•mē)
Syncope (sĭn′kō•pē)
Systolic pressure (sĭs•tŏl′ĭk prěsh′ŭr)
Tachycardia (tǎk•ē•kǎr′dē•ǎ)
Thrombocytopenia
   (thrŏm•bō•sī•tō•pē′nē•ǎ)
Thromboendarterectomy
   (thrŏm•bō•ěnd•ǎr•tě•rěk′tō•mē)
Thrombus (thrŏm′bŭs)
Tinnitus (tĭn•ī′tŭs)
Valvotomy (vǎl•vŏt′ō•mē)
Vasodilator (vǎs•ō•dī•lā′tŏr)
Ventricular septal rupture (věn•trĭk′ū•lǎr
   sěp′tal rŭp′chūr)

The circulatory system is composed of the heart and blood vessels (the cardiovascular system) and the lymphatic system. The heart and blood vessels function to transport oxygen, nutrients, and hormones to cells and to remove waste products and carbon dioxide from cells. The heart and blood vessels work together to pump and circulate the equivalent of 7200 quarts of blood through the heart every 24 hours. Blood transports hormones, nutrients, and waste products; it defends the body against infections; its ability to clot prevents blood loss. The heart, about the size of a human fist, is made of muscle and valves (Fig. 9–1). The blood vessel network of the body is composed of arteries, arterioles, veins, venules, and capillaries, the latter linking the arteries and veins. The lymphatic system is composed of lymph capillaries, lacteals, nodes, vessels, and ducts. The lymphatic system transports fluids, nutrients, and wastes exuded from tissues back to the bloodstream through connections with major veins.

■ RHEUMATIC FEVER AND RHEUMATIC HEART DISEASE

DESCRIPTION *Rheumatic fever* is a systemic inflammatory disease. It affects the joints, heart, central nervous system, skin, and other body tissues. The term *rheumatic* emphasizes the fact that the disease usually involves the joints, but the real importance of rheumatic fever lies in the danger it poses to the heart. If the inflammation occurs in the heart (*acute carditis*), the valves of the heart may be permanently scarred. This condition is called *rheumatic heart disease*. Rheumatic fever usually strikes children and adolescents from 5 to 15 years of age, although it may occur at other ages as well.

ETIOLOGY Rheumatic fever is a hypersensitivity reaction to a group A infection by hemolytic streptococci. The **antibodies** manufactured to combat the streptococci react to produce lesions at specific sites, especially in the heart and joints. Despite this association, the exact mechanism of the disease is not known. Indeed, the onset of rheumatic fever often occurs after group A streptococci are no longer detectable in the affected individual. The most popular theory of the etiology of rheumatic fever is that the disease is a bacterially induced autoimmune disorder: that is, one in which the antibodies produced to fight the initial streptococcal infection begin to attack body tissue. Genetic risk factors also may be involved in rheumatic fever, which may account for why only a small percentage of those individuals who experience a pharyn-

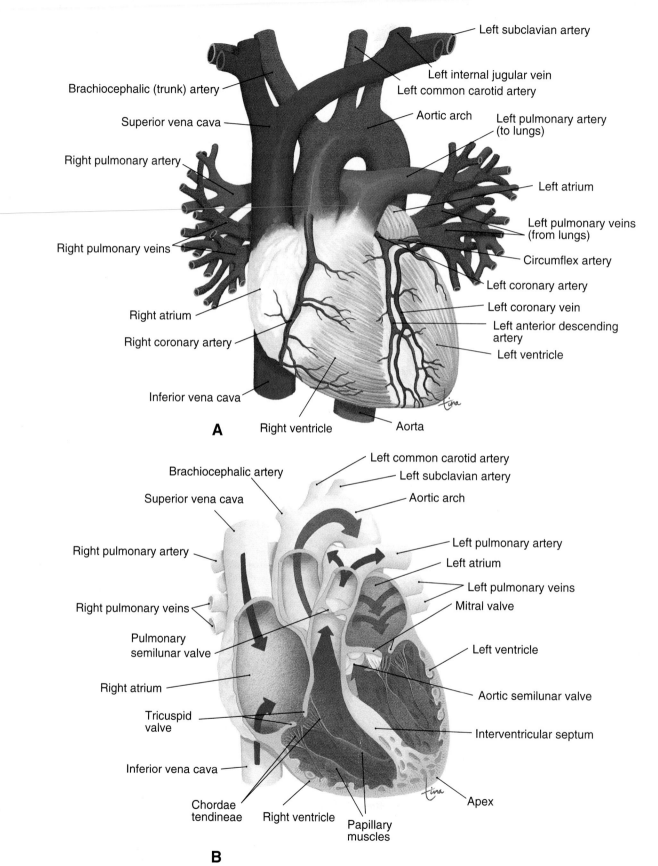

Figure 9–1 (*A*) Anterior view of the heart and major blood vessels. (*B*) Frontal section of the heart, anterior view, showing internal structures. (From Scanlon, VC, and Sanders, T: Essentials of Anatomy and Physiology, ed 3. FA Davis, Philadelphia, 1999, p 260, with permission.)

geal group A streptococcal infection ever actually contract the disease.

SIGNS AND SYMPTOMS Rheumatic fever is characterized by a specific cluster of symptoms that include fever, polyarthritis, carditis, **chorea,** subcutaneous nodules, and erythema. These characteristic symptoms may occur in any combination and with varying degrees of severity.

- *Polyarthritis.* This classic symptom of rheumatic fever is characterized by pain, redness, and swelling of the major joints of the extremities. The arthritic symptoms are often "migratory," in that as one joint begins to heal, another becomes inflamed.
- *Carditis.* Because any or all layers of the heart—endocardium, myocardium, and pericardium—may be involved, the symptoms of carditis associated with rheumatic fever may vary. Severe rheumatic carditis may cause significant mitral and aortic murmurs.
- *Chorea.* Usually a late symptom of rheumatic fever, chorea is characterized by sudden, jerking, involuntary movements accompanied by general muscle weakness. Agitation and emotional disturbance almost always accompany the muscular spasms. Chorea resolves without residual neurological damage.
- *Subcutaneous nodules.* These are painless, pea-sized swellings that form over bone surfaces, usually on the hands, elbows, and feet.
- *Erythema.* The erythema associated with rheumatic fever is mild and diffuse, rapidly forming and then subsiding over areas of the trunk and extremities.

DIAGNOSTIC PROCEDURES A medical history and a recognition of one or more of the classic symptoms is important for diagnosis. An antistreptolysin O (ASO) test will almost always be performed to detect the presence of streptococcal antibodies. Other laboratory data may show elevated white blood count (WBC), erythrocyte sedimentation rate (ESR), and cardiac enzymes levels.

TREATMENT The goal of treatment is to eradicate the streptococcal infection, relieve symptoms, and prevent recurrence so as to further reduce the chance of permanent cardiac complications. Treatment is largely symptomatic and supportive. In most cases, though, treatment with antibiotics is begun to ensure that group A streptococci are no longer present in the body. Salicylates are helpful in reducing fever and joint pain and swelling. Bed rest is required during an acute phase with active carditis. Because rheumatic fever may require long-term care, patient education is an important part of the treatment process.

PROGNOSIS The short-term prognosis for rheumatic fever varies according to the severity of the particular case. Most cases subside within 6 to 12 weeks. The long-term prognosis for the disease depends on the degree of scarring and deformity that involves the heart valves. Death may result from severe pancarditis. Rheumatic fever tends to be recurrent, especially within 5 years of the initial attack, and especially among those who experience heart damage.

PREVENTION Rheumatic fever is preventable through prompt treatment of any streptococcal infection. Recurrences are preventable through a continuous course of antibiotic therapy—a practice especially recommended for those who have suffered heart damage as a consequence of an initial case of the disease.

Carditis

■ PERICARDITIS

DESCRIPTION *Pericarditis* is inflammation of the pericardium, the saclike membrane that surrounds and protects the heart muscle (Fig. 9–2). The disease can be acute or chronic.

ETIOLOGY Pericarditis is usually caused by bacterial, fungal, or viral infection of the pericardium. The disease also may be caused by neoplasms metastasized from other organs, rheumatic fever, uremia, or a coronary thrombosis. Trauma or any injury that causes blood to leak into the pericardial sac

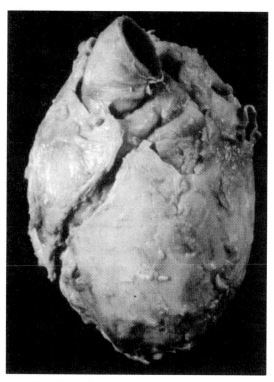

Figure 9–2 Constrictive pericarditis. The heart is encased in a fibrotic, thickened, and adherent pericardium. (From Rubin, E, and Farber, JL [eds]: Pathology, ed 3. Lippincott-Raven, Philadelphia, 1999, p 568, with permission.)

also may incite pericarditis. Chronic pericarditis may develop from the acute form of the disease, but it is often **idiopathic.**

SIGNS AND SYMPTOMS The classic symptom of pericarditis is a sharp and often sudden pleuritic pain that increases with deep inspiration. The fluctuating nature of pericardial pain clearly differentiates it from the pain produced by a myocardial infarction (heart attack). If pericardial **effusion** occurs in acute pericarditis, **orthopnea, dyspnea,** and **tachycardia** typically result. If the fluid accumulates rapidly, the pressure against the heart may result in clammy skin, pallor, and a decrease in blood pressure. This condition is then considered life threatening. **Hepatomegaly** and **ascites** may occur in chronic pericarditis.

DIAGNOSTIC PROCEDURES Auscultation may reveal pericardial friction rub (a grating sound heard as the heart beats), a classic symptom. Inflammation may be reflected in laboratory data showing elevated WBC, ESR, and cardiac enzyme levels. An electrocardiogram (ECG) may detect cardiac **arrhythmias.**

TREATMENT Underlying causes of the pericarditis must be treated and symptomatic relief provided. Bed rest, with the upper body elevated, may be prescribed, along with **analgesics.** If the case of pericarditis is bacterial in origin, antibiotic therapy may be started. **Pericardiocentesis** to promote drainage may also be part of the treatment course.

PROGNOSIS The prognosis is determined by the etiology of the particular case, but generally it is good.

PREVENTION The best—and only known—prevention is the avoidance of infections.

■ MYOCARDITIS

DESCRIPTION *Myocarditis* is inflammation of the cardiac muscle. The condition may be either acute or chronic.

ETIOLOGY Myocarditis may be caused by viral or bacterial infections or be a consequence of rheumatic fever. Myocardial inflammation also may be caused by chronic alcoholism, various toxins, or it may be a side effect of certain drugs or radiation therapy.

SIGNS AND SYMPTOMS The symptoms of myocarditis are often nonspecific, but they may include dyspnea, palpitations, fever, and fatigue.

DIAGNOSTIC PROCEDURES A medical history may reveal a recent upper respiratory infection. Laboratory tests confirming the diagnosis may show elevated cardiac enzyme levels, WBC, and ESR. An ECG typically shows diffuse ST-segment and T-wave abnormalities, conduction defects, and other supraventricular arrhythmias.

TREATMENT Bed rest is helpful, and antibiotics may be needed if a bacterial infection is determined to be the cause of the myocarditis. Oxygen therapy and sodium restriction may be recommended if congestive heart failure occurs. **Diuretics** and digitalis may be prescribed.

PROGNOSIS The prognosis for an individual with uncomplicated myocarditis is usually good. Complications may include left or right ventricular failure.

PREVENTION There is no specific prevention.

ENDOCARDITIS

DESCRIPTION *Endocarditis,* also known as *infective* or *bacterial endocarditis,* is inflammation of the membrane lining the valves and chambers of the heart. The disease is characterized by the formation of abnormal growths called *vegetations* on the heart valves in the endocardial lining, or in the endothelium of a blood vessel (Fig. 9–3). These vegetations may embolize to the spleen, kidneys, central nervous system, or lungs.

ETIOLOGY Endocarditis is most frequently caused by infection from group A nonhemolytic streptococcal bacteria following septic thrombophlebitis; open heart surgery for prosthetic valves; or bone, skin, and pulmonary infections. Increasingly it is seen in IV drug abusers where *Staphylococcus aureus* is the most common infecting organism. It also may arise as a consequence of rheumatic fever or systemic lupus erythematosus (see Chapter 12). Infecting organisms more readily establish themselves on the endocardium of a heart already damaged by congenital or acquired defects, although healthy endocardial tissue may be infected as well. A vegetation forms as the infected tissue is covered by a layer of platelets and fibrin.

SIGNS AND SYMPTOMS Symptoms vary according to etiology and the portion of the heart affected. There may be weakness and fatigue, night sweats, and an intermittent fever that persists for weeks. A loud regurgitant heart murmur may be heard that was not previously detected. Additional symptoms may arise if the vegetations break off into the bloodstream to form embolisms that lodge in other organs. Paralysis can occur if a large **embolus** lodges in the brain. If an embolus obstructs circulation in the kidney, there may be blood in the urine. If tiny vegetations lodge in the small vessels of the skin, subcutaneous ruptures called **petechiae** may appear.

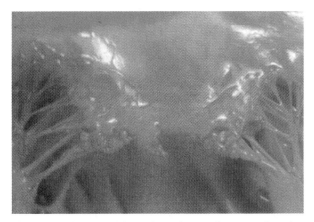

Figure 9–3 Bacterial endocarditis. The mitral valve shows destructive vegetations, which have eroded through the free margins of the valve leaflets. (From Rubin, E, and Farber, JL [eds]: Pathology, ed 3. Lippincott-Raven, Philadelphia, 1999, p 572, with permission.)

DIAGNOSTIC PROCEDURES The medical history may reveal predisposing factors of endocarditis. An *echocardiogram* may reveal the presence of vegetative growths. Blood testing typically reveals leukocytosis and high concentrations of bacterial antibodies. Repeated blood cultures will usually result in positive identification of the causative microorganism.

TREATMENT It is important to eliminate the infecting organism. Antibiotic therapy probably will continue over a number of weeks. Bed rest, analgesics, and increased fluid intake are helpful. Surgery may be necessary to repair severe valvular damage.

PROGNOSIS This disease is now curable when treated early with antibiotics. Before antibiotics became available, death was almost certain. Complications that may cause death include congestive heart failure and damage to vital organs as a result of embolism.

PREVENTION Individuals at high risk should receive antibiotic therapy prior to undergoing surgery or certain dental procedures.

Valvular Heart Disease

Figure 9–4 illustrates the heart valves. Refer to this figure throughout this section. Diseased heart valves may malfunction in two ways. The opening formed by a valve may be too large to close completely, so that blood leaks back past the valve into the heart chamber from which it was pumped. Or the valve opening may be too narrow (a condition called valvular **stenosis**), so that it impedes the flow of blood through the valve when it should be open and allows blood to leak back when it should be closed (Fig. 9–5). Either condition can cause heart failure.

Heart murmurs, periodic sounds heard during auscultation with a stethoscope, are generated by blood flow through the heart when there is an anomaly. Murmurs can be caused by blood leaking back through an incompetent or deformed valve, by blood forcing its way through a narrowed valve, by **dilatation** of the heart, or by a rapid diastolic

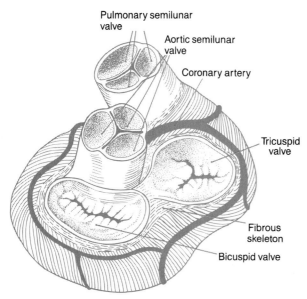

Figure 9–4 Heart valves in superior view. The atria have been removed. The fibrous skeleton of the heart is fibrous connective tissue that anchors the valve flaps and prevents enlargement of the valve opening. (From Scanlon, VC, and Sanders, T: Essentials of Anatomy and Physiology, ed 3. FA Davis, Philadelphia, 1999, p 261, with permission.)

flow. Exercise and tachycardia increase the intensity of any murmur.

Murmurs are graded on the basis of intensity, with grade 1 the least intense and grade 6 the most intense. Detecting and interpreting heart murmurs helps in diagnosing valvular heart disease and estimating its severity. Certain murmurs are consistently associated with severe heart dysfunctions. Conversely, other murmurs may be insignificant.

■ MITRAL INSUFFICIENCY/STENOSIS

DESCRIPTION In *mitral insufficiency,* blood from the left ventricle flows back into the left atrium. In *mitral stenosis,* blood flow is obstructed from the left atrium to the left ventricle. In both cases, the result is an enlarged left atrium.

ETIOLOGY Mitral insufficiency or stenosis results from rheumatic fever, mitral valve **prolapse,** myocardial infarction, or severe left-sided heart failure.

SIGNS AND SYMPTOMS In both conditions, there may be orthopnea, dyspnea, fatigue, palpitations, peripheral edema, hepatomegaly, **rales,** and distension of the jugular veins.

DIAGNOSTIC PROCEDURES In both conditions, cardiac catheterization, x-ray, echocardiography, and ECG may establish the diagnosis. The results of auscultation will be specific to each condition.

TREATMENT The treatment approach depends on the severity of the symptoms. Generally, the treatment of choice is **valvotomy** and valve reconstruction or valve replacement with an artificial valve.

PROGNOSIS The prognosis is good. The disease usually is not progressive, and many patients live a long time without surgery. Both mitral insufficiency and stenosis can lead to right ventricular **hypertrophy** and right ventricular failure.

PREVENTION There is no known prevention other than the prevention of rheumatic fever and its complications.

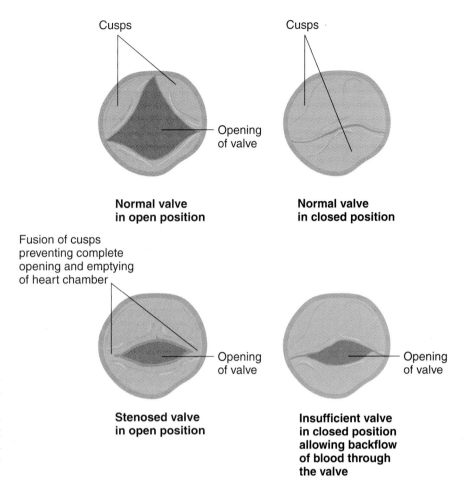

Figure 9–5 Openings of stenoses and insufficient valve compared with a normal valve. (From Williams, LS, and Hopper, PD [eds]: Understanding Medical-Surgical Nursing. FA Davis, Philadelphia, 1999, p 350, with permission.)

■ TRICUSPID INSUFFICIENCY/STENOSIS

DESCRIPTION In *tricuspid insufficiency,* blood flows back into the right atrium from the right ventricle, decreasing the blood flow to the left side of the heart. In *tricuspid stenosis,* the right atrium hypertrophies and increases pressure in the vena cava.

ETIOLOGY Tricuspid insufficiency or stenosis may be caused by rheumatic fever. Tricuspid stenosis often is associated with mitral valve disease. Tricuspid insufficiency results from right ventricular failure.

SIGNS AND SYMPTOMS In both tricuspid insufficiency and stenosis, the most common symptoms are dyspnea and fatigue. Peripheral edema, distended jugular veins, hepatomegaly, and ascites may occur. **Syncope** may occur in tricuspid stenosis. A systolic murmur often occurs in tricuspid insufficiency, whereas a diastolic murmur may indicate tricuspid stenosis.

DIAGNOSTIC PROCEDURES Cardiac catheterization, x-ray, echocardiography, and ECG may establish the diagnosis.

TREATMENT Treatment depends on the nature and severity of the condition. The condition may not be amenable to valvotomy. In some cases, the defective tricuspid valve may be replaced with a prosthetic valve (Fig. 9–6). The disease may regress if the mitral valve is replaced.

PROGNOSIS The prognosis is good. Complications in the presence of either tricuspid insufficiency or stenosis can lead to heart failure.

PREVENTION There is no known prevention.

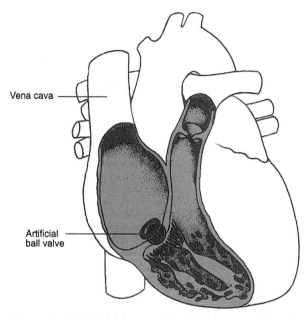

Figure 9–6 Artificial heart valve. In this example, a defective tricuspid valve has been replaced with an artificial ball valve. (From Gylys, BA, and Wedding, ME: Medical Terminology: A Systems Approach, ed 3. FA Davis, Philadelphia, 1995, p 155, with permission.)

▣ PULMONIC INSUFFICIENCY/STENOSIS

DESCRIPTION With *pulmonic insufficiency,* blood flows back into the right ventricle, causing right ventricular hypertrophy and eventual right ventricular failure. In *pulmonic stenosis,* blood flow is obstructed, causing dilation of the right atrium and eventual right ventricular failure.

ETIOLOGY Pulmonic insufficiency may result from pulmonary hypertension. Pulmonic stenosis may follow rheumatic heart disease. Both are often congenital in nature.

SIGNS AND SYMPTOMS Individuals with either condition may exhibit dyspnea, fatigue, syncope, and chest pain. Peripheral edema, distended jugular veins, and hepatomegaly also are possible. Pulmonic stenosis, however, may be asymptomatic. A diastolic murmur may be heard on auscultation in pulmonic insufficiency, whereas a systolic murmur may be heard in pulmonic stenosis.

DIAGNOSTIC PROCEDURES Cardiac catheterization and ECG are the most common diagnostic procedures

for both conditions; however, x-ray may be used to diagnose pulmonic insufficiency.

TREATMENT No treatment may be necessary if the person is able to live a normal life with the condition; if not, surgery is the treatment of choice.

PROGNOSIS With surgery, the prognosis generally is good. Infectious endocarditis is a possible complication.

PREVENTION There is no known prevention.

▣ AORTIC INSUFFICIENCY/STENOSIS

DESCRIPTION *Aortic insufficiency* results in blood flowing back into the left ventricle, eventually causing left ventricular hypertrophy and failure. *Aortic stenosis* causes increased ventricular pressure as a result of a greater cardiac workload. Left ventricular failure may result.

ETIOLOGY Either aortic insufficiency or stenosis can be caused by rheumatic fever. Syphilis, endocarditis, or hypertension can be the cause of aortic insufficiency. Congenital causes may give rise to aortic stenosis (Fig. 9–7).

SIGNS AND SYMPTOMS Dyspnea, fatigue, syncope, angina, and palpitations are the most common symptoms. Congestion in the pulmonary vein,

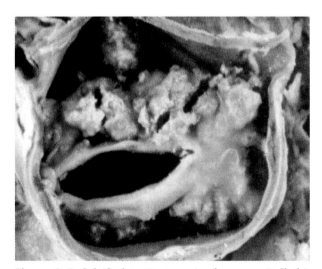

Figure 9–7 Calcified aortic stenosis of a congenitally bicuspid aortic semilunar valve. (From Rubin, E, and Farber, JL [eds]: Pathology, ed 3. Lippincott-Raven, Philadelphia, 1999, p 573, with permission.)

congestive heart failure, and pulmonary edema may occur upon failure of the left ventricle. Auscultation may reveal a characteristic diastolic murmur in aortic insufficiency and a systolic murmur in aortic stenosis.

DIAGNOSTIC PROCEDURES As in most of the valvular heart diseases, common diagnostic procedures include cardiac catheterization, x-ray, echocardiography, and ECG.

TREATMENT The person may need only to be assessed on a yearly basis by ECG, chest x-ray, and echocardiogram. Severe cases may require surgical replacement of the aortic valve.

PROGNOSIS The prognosis varies depending on the nature and severity of the disease. Complications include arrhythmias, ventricular **fibrillation,** and cardiac failure.

PREVENTION There is no known prevention.

Hypertensive Heart Disease

■ ESSENTIAL HYPERTENSION

When the heart must work against increased resistance in the form of high blood pressure, hypertensive heart disease often results. What constitutes hypertension—high blood pressure—may be different for each person, but the medical community generally agrees that the condition exists if **systolic pressure** persists over 140 mmHg and **diastolic pressure** persists over 90 mmHg. Many persons with hypertension live long, vigorous lives. Others do not respond well to treatment and eventually die of heart failure, a cerebral vascular accident (CVA), or kidney dysfunction.

DESCRIPTION *Essential hypertension* is persistently elevated blood pressure that develops without apparent cause.

ETIOLOGY Although essential hypertension is idiopathic, some persons are at a higher risk than others. They include African-Americans, chronically stressed individuals, the obese, and those who favor a diet high in salt and saturated fats. The disease may be familial. Older persons, those with sedentary lifestyles, smokers, and those taking oral contraceptives also have a higher risk of hypertension.

SIGNS AND SYMPTOMS Hypertension may remain asymptomatic for months or years or until vascular changes in the heart, brain, or kidneys occur. The person may exhibit vague symptoms, such as lightheadedness, **tinnitus,** a tendency to tire easily, and palpitations.

DIAGNOSTIC PROCEDURES Blood pressure readings taken on at least three separate occasions after the individual has rested will show pressure greater than 140/90 mmHg. It is important that a history of blood pressure readings be kept for comparison, because blood pressure can vary according to various situations. Auscultation may reveal **bruits.** ECG and chest x-ray will help detect cardiovascular damage.

TREATMENT Although there is no cure for essential hypertension, a change in lifestyle and diet, and the addition of antihypertensive drug therapy, can control the condition. A diet low in salt and fat, moderate exercise, and a reduction of stress are helpful. Diuretics or vasodilators also may be prescribed.

PROGNOSIS The prognosis is good if the disorder is detected early and if the person carefully follows the prescribed treatment regimen. Complications may include CVA, heart failure, and kidney failure.

PREVENTION Because the cause is idiopathic, there is no known prevention other than minimizing controllable risk factors.

Coronary Diseases

■ CORONARY ARTERY DISEASE

DESCRIPTION *Coronary artery disease* (CAD) is the narrowing of the coronary arteries to such an extent that there is an inadequate blood supply to portions of the myocardium, the heart muscle (Fig. 9–8). As the **lumen** of the coronary artery narrows, gradual **ischemia** causes cells in the **myocardium** to weaken and die. These are then replaced with scar tissue.

ETIOLOGY The leading cause of coronary artery disease is atherosclerosis, a condition in which the lumen of the coronary arteries is narrowed by fatty, fibrous plaques (see Atherosclerosis). Many factors seem to predispose individuals to this condition, including age, heredity, obesity, diabetes mellitus,

hypertension, smoking, and stress. The condition is more common in men, in whites, and in middle-aged and elderly persons.

SIGNS AND SYMPTOMS An immediate result of inadequate blood supply to the myocardium is *angina,* a burning, squeezing, tightness in the chest that may radiate to the neck, the shoulder blade, and the left arm. Nausea, vomiting, sweating, and a feeling of panic may accompany these symptoms. A complete discussion of angina pectoris follows.

DIAGNOSTIC PROCEDURES The medical history may reveal one or more of the risk factors for coronary artery disease and a pattern of angina. ECG changes during an angina attack may indicate the region of myocardial ischemia.

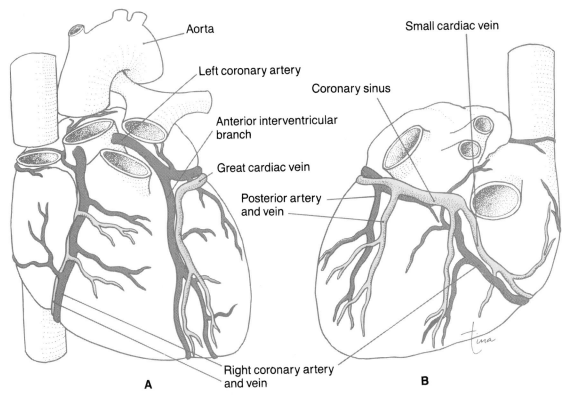

Figure 9–8 (*A*) Coronary vessels in anterior view. The pulmonary artery has been cut to show the left coronary artery emerging from the ascending aorta. (*B*) Coronary vessels in posterior view. The coronary sinus empties blood into the right atrium. (From Scanlon, VC, and Sanders, T: Essentials of Anatomy and Physiology, ed 3. FA Davis, Philadelphia, 1999, p 262, with permission.)

TREATMENT The goal of treatment is to reduce angina by reducing myocardial oxygen demand or increasing oxygen supply. Nitroglycerin preparations are helpful in increasing the oxygen supply to the heart by dilating the coronary arteries. Coronary artery bypass surgery may be necessary to bridge obstructive lesions (see Special Focus). There may be an attempt to compress the fatty **plaque** deposits in the coronary arteries by cardiac catheterization, or laser angioplasty, which corrects occlusion by vaporizing fatty deposits. Dietary restrictions may be necessary, and persons should be encouraged to refrain from smoking.

PROGNOSIS The prognosis varies greatly depending on the amount of arterial blockage and the extent of damage to the heart muscle.

PREVENTION The best way to prevent coronary artery disease is to minimize controllable risk factors.

ANGINA PECTORIS

DESCRIPTION *Angina pectoris* is chest pain resulting from ischemia to a part of the myocardium.

ETIOLOGY Angina pectoris is usually a clinical syndrome accompanying arteriosclerotic heart disease. Less frequently, it may be produced by a coronary spasm and severe aortic stenosis or aortic insufficiency. Angina attacks are frequently triggered in susceptible individuals by any condition that increases myocardial oxygen demand, such as stress, eating, exertion, or even extremes of temperature and humidity.

SIGNS AND SYMPTOMS The classic signs of an angina attack are burning, squeezing, and tightness in the chest; these may radiate to the neck and the left arm and shoulder blade. Sometimes there is nausea and vomiting. Acute anxiety may accompany angina, especially in the person who is already aware of having a heart problem and is worried about whether this episode of angina is a precursor to a myocardial infarction. An angina attack usually lasts less than 15 minutes and not more than 30 minutes; the average is 3 minutes.

DIAGNOSTIC PROCEDURES An ECG taken during the angina attack may indicate ischemia, and a medical history usually reveals a history of angina.

TREATMENT Nitroglycerin preparations taken either sublingually or applied topically usually relieve anginal pain. Sedatives or tranquilizers may be prescribed. Coronary diseases causing disabling angina pectoris that does not respond to treatment may require coronary bypass procedures or **percutaneous transluminal coronary angioplasty.** In coronary bypass procedures, one to five bypass grafts can be made in the patient. In angioplasty, a balloon-tipped catheter is passed through a systemic artery to the occluded coronary artery, where it is inflated to dilate the vessel. This procedure is performed under local anesthesia.

PROGNOSIS The prognosis depends on the severity of myocardial ischemia. Angina pectoris usually is considered a warning to the person to lessen exertion and stress that might bring on myocardial infarction and heart failure. If the pain persists longer than 30 minutes, the individual should see a physician immediately. Angina is classified as "unstable" when the pain is more frequent, lasts longer, and is less responsive to nitroglycerin than in a typical case. These more severe symptoms are a manifestation of more severe and progressive narrowing of the coronary arteries.

PREVENTION Prevention includes avoidance of precipitating factors in the presence of ongoing coronary artery disease.

MYOCARDIAL INFARCTION
(Heart Attack)

DESCRIPTION *Myocardial infarction* (MI) is a life-threatening condition caused by the occlusion of one or more coronary arteries and the subsequent necrosis of a section of the heart muscle tissue served by those arteries (Fig. 9–9). Myocardial infarction is a medical emergency requiring immediate attention.

ETIOLOGY The predisposing factors of MI are the same as those for many other cardiovascular diseases. They include heredity, obesity, aging, hypertension, elevated serum triglycerides, total cholesterol levels, and low-density lipoprotein (LDL) levels, smoking, diabetes mellitus, a sedentary lifestyle, chronic stress, and "type A" behavior. Men and postmenopausal women are more susceptible than premenopausal women; however, the in-

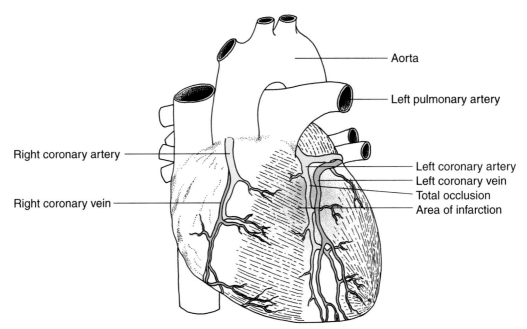

Figure 9–9 Myocardial infarction. The shaded area beneath the left coronary artery represents an area of necrotized myocardial tissue. (From Gylys, BA, and Wedding, ME: Medical Terminology: A Systems Approach, ed 3. FA Davis, Philadelphia, 1995, p 148, with permission.)

cidence of MI is rising, particularly among premenopausal women who smoke and use oral contraceptives.

SIGNS AND SYMPTOMS The classic symptom of MI is crushing chest pain that may radiate to the left arm, neck, and jaw. The pain may be similar to anginal pain but usually is severe and is not relieved by the same measures that relieve angina (see Angina). Some individuals, however, may exhibit few symptoms, or confuse the pain with indigestion. There is growing incidence showing that symptoms for women are fatigue, nausea, vomiting, and shortness of breath. Individuals with coronary heart disease should be suspicious if angina occurs with increasing frequency and duration. For some, an MI is preceded by vague feelings of discomfort, fear, nausea, and vomiting.

DIAGNOSTIC PROCEDURES A medical history revealing coronary artery disease and episodes of chest pain will help in the diagnosis. ECG and **radioisotope** studies may be performed. Blood tests for elevated cardiac enzyme levels—creatine phosphokinase (CPK and CPK-MB) levels—over a 72-hour period are useful in confirming MI.

TREATMENT Immediate hospitalization is important to relieve pain, stabilize heart rhythm, reduce cardiac workload, and preserve as much heart tissue as possible. Complete bed rest with sedation and analgesia is usually instituted. In many cases the affected individual is placed on a cardiac monitor to detect cardiac arrhythmias, a common problem during the first 48 hours following an attack. If cardiac arrest occurs, cardiopulmonary resuscitation (CPR) efforts are begun immediately.

PROGNOSIS The prognosis for an individual experiencing MI depends on the extent of damage to the myocardium. The prognosis is guarded at best. Mortality is high if treatment is delayed, and almost half of sudden deaths due to an MI occur before hospitalization, within 1 hour of symptoms. Complications of myocardial infarction include arrhythmias, congestive heart failure, **cardiogenic shock, mitral regurgitation, ventricular septal rupture,** pericarditis, and ventricular aneurysm.

PREVENTION Prevention includes avoidance of any predisposing factors such as diets high in cholesterol, smoking, obesity, and stress.

■ CONGESTIVE HEART FAILURE (CHF)

DESCRIPTION *Congestive heart failure* is a condition in which the pumping ability of the heart is progressively impaired to the point that it no longer meets bodily needs. Circulatory congestion may occur in the systemic venous circulation resulting in peripheral edema. Or the congestion may occur in the pulmonary circulation causing pulmonary edema, an acute, life-threatening condition (Fig. 9–10).

ETIOLOGY Either the left or right ventricles, alone or together, may be the sources of the inadequate pumping action. Chronic congestive heart failure is the product of many cardiac and pulmonary disease processes. Acute congestive heart failure most often results from a myocardial infarction.

SIGNS AND SYMPTOMS Left ventricular failure may be manifested as dyspnea and fatigue, and will result in primarily pulmonary symptoms. Right ventricu-

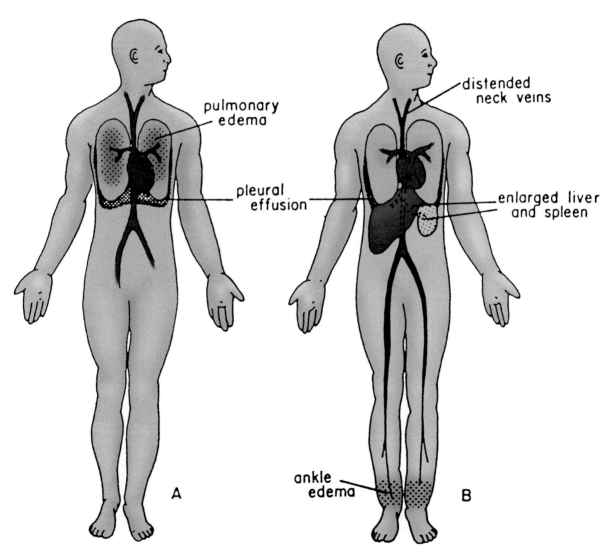

Figure 9–10 Effects of congestive heart failure. (*A*) Left-sided heart failure results primarily in pulmonary edema. (*B*) Right-sided heart failure results in peripheral edema (swollen ankles, enlarged organs). (From Kent, TH, and Hart, MN: Introduction to Human Diseases, ed 2. Appleton-Century-Crofts, Norwalk, 1987, p 141, with permission.)

lar failure may cause distended neck veins and hepatomegaly, and is more likely to result in systemic symptoms. Symptoms of advanced CHF may include tachypnea, palpitations, edema, **diaphoresis,** and **cyanosis.** As the disease progresses, there may be **hemoptysis,** cyanosis, and **pitting edema** of the ankle.

DIAGNOSTIC PROCEDURES An ECG, a chest x-ray, and an elevated central venous pressure will indicate the diagnosis.

TREATMENT The goal of treatment is to improve the heart's pumping function. Treatment may involve the use of diuretics to reduce circulatory congestion by reducing total blood volume. Bed rest may be recommended. Drug therapy may include the prescription of vasodilators and digitalis to strengthen heart action. Dietary sodium may be restricted to combat edema. A controversial treatment for an enlarged heart, which is the result of congestive heart failure, is receiving attention. A surgeon in Brazil, trained in Canada and the United States, cuts away a chunk of heart muscle to make the heart stronger. The prestigious Cleveland Clinic Foundation in Ohio has been performing the surgery since 1996 and has had a 72 percent success rate. This procedure is presently performed on only those patients for whom all other treatment modalities have failed and the possibility of a heart transplant is unlikely.

PROGNOSIS Acute congestive heart failure usually responds quickly to therapeutic measures. The prognosis is good, although it depends on the cause. If the congestion is severe and chronic, the prognosis is poor. The person usually must continue medication indefinitely and be carefully supervised by a physician.

PREVENTION Prevention consists of avoiding any predisposing factors.

◼ CARDIAC ARREST

DESCRIPTION *Cardiac arrest* is the sudden, unexpected interruption of heart function. It is a medical emergency.

ETIOLOGY Cardiac arrest may result from myocardial infarction, circulatory collapse due to various forms of shock, or ventricular fibrillation. Cardiac arrest also may result from drug reactions, electrocution, drowning, or other forms of accidental physical trauma.

SIGNS AND SYMPTOMS Prolonged angina, acute dyspnea or orthopnea, light-headedness, or sustained tachycardia may be characteristic of cardiac arrest. The onset is precipitous and without warning. Symptoms of impending cardiac arrest may include sudden tachycardia or **bradycardia,** a drop in blood pressure, respiratory failure, and changes in ECG patterns. An individual experiencing cardiac arrest usually loses consciousness and ceases to breathe.

DIAGNOSTIC PROCEDURES The diagnosis is based on the absence of respiration and pulse and accompanying loss of consciousness.

TREATMENT Emergency first aid treatment may include establishing an airway, ventilating through artificial means, and giving external cardiac massage until the person can be transported to a hospital to receive more advanced life support.

PROGNOSIS The prognosis is guarded at best. Persons may survive, however, especially if treatment begins within 3 minutes. Irreversible brain damage may occur after that time.

PREVENTION The best prevention is early treatment for cardiac symptoms, living a healthy lifestyle, and carefully monitoring any individual with heart disease.

SPECIAL FOCUS CARDIAC ADVANCES

Cardiac surgeons are inducing angiogenesis through gene therapy. The gene coding for a protein called *vascular endothelial growth factor* (VEGF) is injected into the heart to encourage new blood vessels to grow from existing ones. Sometimes a virus is the delivery vehicle used. The end result is that new vessels grow and restore circulation to the heart muscle within hours to a few days.

In another new form of cardiac therapy through the use of lasers a small incision is made into the chest through the left ventricle. The laser drills tiny holes through the muscle, and almost instantly, new vessels form around the injured area.

Both of these procedures are in the experimental stages. The potential, however, is that they may radically change treatment for coronary disease.

Blood Vessel Diseases

ANEURYSMS: ABDOMINAL, THORACIC, AND PERIPHERAL ARTERIES

DESCRIPTION An **aneurysm** (Fig. 9–11) is a local dilation of an artery or chamber of the heart due to weakening of its walls. Aneurysms may be *sacculated* (shaped like a sac), *fusiform* (a spindle-shaped enlargement), or *dissecting* (the layers of the vessel wall are separated). Aneurysms may cause **thrombus** formation, hemorrhage from rupture, or ischemia. Three common types of aneurysms discussed here are abdominal, thoracic, and peripheral artery aneurysms.

ETIOLOGY Aneurysms may be congenital, or result from trauma, arteriosclerosis, inflammation, infection, and degeneration produced by atherosclerosis.

SIGNS AND SYMPTOMS *Abdominal aneurysms* may be asymptomatic, but if the person is slender, a pulsating middle and upper abdominal mass may be detected on routine physical examination. Other symptoms may include mild to severe weakness, sweating, tachycardia, and hypotension.

Thoracic artery aneurysms may produce pain, they may be asymptomatic, or the affected individual may exhibit signs of pressure on the trachea or superior vena cava. These signs include dyspnea, **stridor,** or edema in the neck and arms with distended neck veins. Pain is likely in the neck, back, or substernal areas.

In *peripheral artery aneurysms,* there may be no symptoms or the person may have pain in the area of the aneurysm, edema, and venous distension. Severe ischemia caused by aneurysms in the foot or leg may result in **gangrene.**

DIAGNOSTIC PROCEDURES In abdominal aneurysms, an ECG and ultrasonography may be done. X-ray, ECG, aortography, and computed tomography (CT) scans may be performed to detect thoracic aneurysms. Palpation, ultrasonography, and angiography may be used to detect peripheral artery aneurysms.

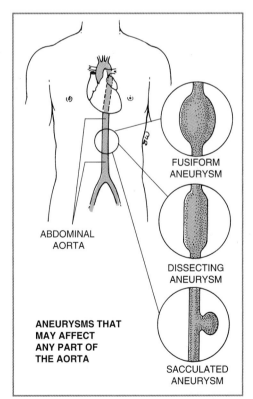

Figure 9–11 Aortic aneurysms. (From Thomas, CL [ed]: Taber's Cyclopedic Medical Dictionary, ed 18. FA Davis, Philadelphia, 1997, p 102, with permission.)

TREATMENT The course of treatment chosen for any form of aneurysm depends on the size and site of the affected artery, the size of the aneurysm and the likelihood of its rupturing, as well as the general physical status of the individual. Most aneurysms are treated surgically: In small arteries treatment may consist of clipping off the artery before the aneurysm. Larger arteries may require surgical excision of the weakened portion of the vessel, arterial grafting, or arterial bypass.

PROGNOSIS The prognosis is guarded for persons with most forms of aneurysm. Death may result from rupture of the aneurysm causing hemorrhage and shock. A possible complication includes formation of a thrombus along the wall of an aneurysm. A piece of the thrombus may break off, producing an embolus that may block the flow of blood to vital organs.

PREVENTION There is no known prevention.

ARTERIOSCLEROSIS AND ATHEROSCLEROSIS

DESCRIPTION *Arteriosclerosis* is widespread thickening of the walls of small arteries and arterioles with a resulting loss of elasticity. One type of arteriosclerosis is *atherosclerosis,* which is a condition characterized by the accumulation of yellowish plaques of cholesterol, lipids, and cellular debris on the inner layers of the walls of large and medium-sized arteries (Fig. 9–12). The vessel walls become thickened, fibrotic, and calcified, and the arterial lumen narrows. The most commonly affected vessels include the coronary and cerebral arteries. Circulatory impairment is the consequence of both diseases; however, in atherosclerosis, the arteries are major and supply vital tissues. These arterial diseases are responsible for about 40 percent of the deaths in the United States.

ETIOLOGY The etiology is unclear, but it may include trauma or the accumulation of lipids due to dietary excesses, faulty carbohydrate metabolism, or a genetic defect. Both diseases are seen with aging and are often associated with diabetes mellitus, hypertension, obesity, **nephrosclerosis,** and scleroderma.

SIGNS AND SYMPTOMS Typical signs and symptoms include intermittent **claudication,** changes in skin temperature and color, bruits over the involved artery, headache, dizziness, and memory defects. Pain may be present, especially at night, due to sepsis or ischemia. Muscle cramping may occur. The effects of atherosclerosis are gradual lumen obstruction, thrombosis, and subsequent weakening of the vessel with dilation.

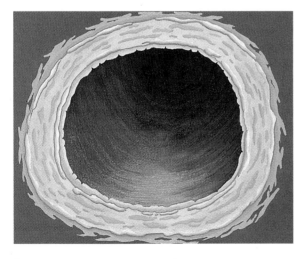
A

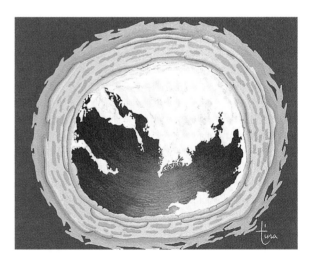
B

Figure 9–12 (*A*) Cross-section of normal coronary artery. (*B*) Coronary artery with atherosclerosis narrowing the lumen. (From Scanlon, VC, and Sanders, T: Essentials of Anatomy and Physiology, ed 3. FA Davis, Philadelphia, 1999, p 263, with permission.)

DIAGNOSTIC PROCEDURES X-rays, arteriograms, and blood pressure measurements may be done for diagnosis.

TREATMENT Vasodilators, exercise, and a diet low in saturated fats, cholesterol, and calories may be tried. Any infections, ulcers, or gangrene of the toes and foot need immediate attention. Surgery may be necessary in some cases and may involve arterial grafting, **thromboendarterectomy,** and **sympathectomy.**

PROGNOSIS The prognosis varies and depends on the site and amount of arterial occlusion and the person's overall physical condition. Complications include **gangrene,** infections, and coronary artery disease.

PREVENTION Prevention includes adequate rest and exercise, avoidance of stress, and a diet low in cholesterol, calories, and saturated fats.

▓ THROMBOPHLEBITIS

DESCRIPTION *Thrombophlebitis* is inflammation of a vein in conjunction with the formation of a clot from the streaming blood constituents. An abnormal mass of platelets is formed, then the mass deposits on the vascular surface. The affected vein may be either partially or completely obstructed. The condition usually occurs in an extremity, most frequently in a leg, and can affect both superficial and deep veins.

ETIOLOGY Thrombophlebitis may be caused by trauma, reduced or turbulent blood flow, infection, chemical irritation, or prolonged immobility, or it may be idiopathic.

SIGNS AND SYMPTOMS The person may be asymptomatic. Symptoms, however, will depend on the site of the affected vein and may include a dull aching and tight feeling at the site; **induration,** redness, and tenderness along a superficial vein; and anxiety. Fever, chills, and malaise also may develop.

DIAGNOSTIC PROCEDURES Physical examination may reveal the inflammation. Phlebography (which shows filling defects and diverted blood flow), Doppler ultrasonography, and a radioactive fibrinogen uptake test may be used to diagnose thrombophlebitis.

TREATMENT In superficial thrombophlebitis, the person may be advised to rest in bed, elevate the affected limb, and apply heat over the site of the affected vein. In deep-vein thrombophlebitis, the affected limb may be elevated and possibly wrapped with elastic bandages. **Lysis** may be injected for acute, deep-vein thrombophlebitis. Anticoagulant therapy may be prescribed. Surgical procedures such as vein ligation and femoral vein thrombectomy may be used in cases of deep-vein thrombophlebitis.

PROGNOSIS If only superficial veins are involved, the condition may be self-limiting, and the prog-

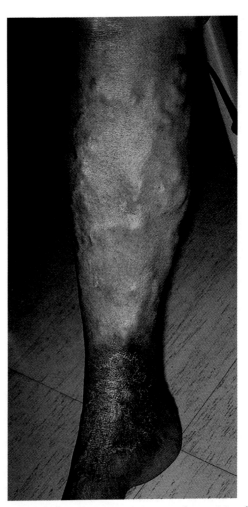

Figure 9–13 Varicose veins and stasis dermatitis of the ankle. (From Thomas, CL [ed]: Taber's Cyclopedic Medical Dictionary, ed 18. FA Davis, Philadelphia, 1997, p 2063, with permission.)

nosis is good. When deep veins are involved, the prognosis is guarded. A serious complication of thrombophlebitis is the formation of a pulmonary embolism, a life-threatening condition.

PREVENTION Individuals with a history of varicose veins or other conditions predisposing to thrombophlebitis should wear elastic hose. It may be advisable to allow for walking after long periods of sitting, such as when traveling or working.

▇ VARICOSE VEINS

DESCRIPTION *Varicose veins* are enlarged, twisted, superficial veins. They may occur in almost any part of the body, but most frequently they occur in the lower legs, involving the greater and lesser saphenous veins (Fig. 9–13).

ETIOLOGY Varicose veins may be due to an inherited defect or venous diseases. They also may be produced by conditions that cause venostasis, such as pregnancy or jobs requiring prolonged standing or heavy lifting.

SIGNS AND SYMPTOMS The person may be asymptomatic even though the varicose vein condition is severe. Quite frequently, however, the affected veins are visually evident. Characteristic symptoms with varicose veins of the legs include dull, aching heaviness or a feeling of fatigue after standing. Cramping may occur, followed by edema, and **stasis pigmentation.**

DIAGNOSTIC PROCEDURES In most cases, visual observation may be all that is necessary. Phlebography may be performed for diagnosis. Doppler ultrasonography detects possible backflow in deep or superficial veins.

TREATMENT The use of elastic stockings, a moderate exercise program, and avoidance of prolonged periods of standing or lifting may be recommended initially. Compression sclerotherapy may be done to collapse and produce permanent fibrosis of the affected veins. Severe varicose veins may require stripping and ligation.

PROGNOSIS The prognosis is good; however, further varicose veins may develop, requiring further treatment.

PREVENTION Prevention includes avoidance of prolonged standing or lifting, avoiding constrictive clothing, and elevating the legs when possible.

Anemias and Other Red Blood Cell Disorders

Anemia is a reduction in the number of circulating red blood cells, the amount of **hemoglobin,** or the volume of packed red blood cells (Fig. 9–14). It exists when the hemoglobin content of the blood is less than that required to satisfy the oxygen demands of the body. Anemias may be due to blood loss in the vascular system either externally or internally. Anemias may be hemolytic, in which case there is destruction of red blood cells within the body.

There are many types and classifications of anemias. Two of the less common, but still significant, anemias are *sideroblastic anemia* and *thalassemia* (also called *Cooley's anemia, Mediterranean disease,* and *erythroblastic anemia*).

Sideroblastic anemia is characterized by an inability to utilize the available iron in the blood. The iron deposits itself in the **mitochondria** of normoblasts (the precursors to blood cells in the bone marrow). These cells have the appearance of a ring around the cell nucleus and are called *ringed sideroblasts.* Sideroblastic anemia is a rare X-linked hereditary disorder; it also may be acquired, through the use of some drugs and toxins, as a result of some neoplastic diseases, or through the use of some chemotherapeutic agents.

Thalassemia is a Mendelian-dominant hereditary trait resulting in defective production of the globin portion of the hemoglobin. The result is a continual production of fetal hemoglobin, past the stage of infancy. Thalassemia is more common in persons of Mediterranean ancestry.

Iron deficiency anemia, folic acid deficiency anemia, pernicious anemia, aplastic anemia, and sickle cell anemia are covered in more detail in the following sections (Fig. 9–15).

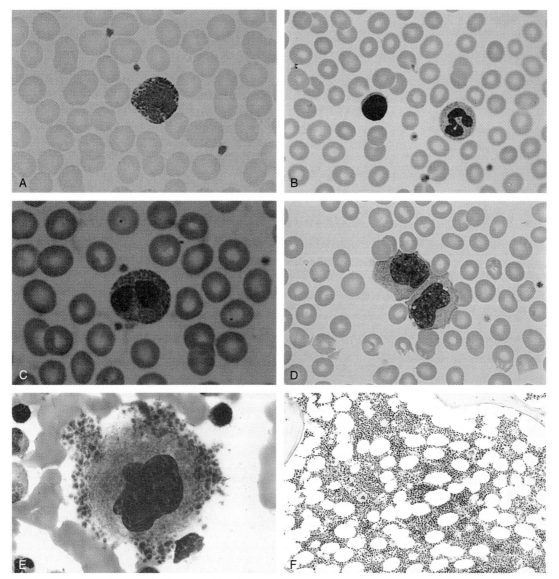

Figure 9–14 Blood cells. (*A*) Red blood cells, platelets, and a basophil (magnification ×600). (*B*) Lymphocytes (left) and neutrophil (right) (magnification ×600). (*C*) Eosinophil (magnification ×600). (*D*) Monocytes (magnification ×600). (*E*) Megacaryocyte with platelets (magnification ×600). (*F*) Normal bone marrow (magnification ×200). (From Harmening, DM: Clinical Hematology and Fundamentals of Hemostasis, ed 3. FA Davis, Philadelphia, 1997, with permission.)

▩ IRON DEFICIENCY ANEMIA

DESCRIPTION *Iron deficiency anemia* is characterized by inadequate reserves of iron in the body and the formation of unusually small, hemoglobin-poor red blood cells. These cells are smaller and paler than normal cells because red blood cells derive their color from hemoglobin. Iron deficiency anemia occurs more frequently in premenopausal women and in adolescents. It is the most common chronic disease in the United States.

ETIOLOGY Excessive blood loss from **menorrhagia,** gastrointestinal bleeding, or excessive blood donation may cause this deficiency. The condition

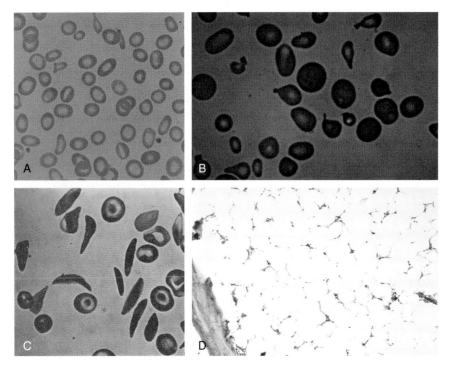

Figure 9–15 Anemia. (*A*) Iron-deficiency anemia; notice the pale, oval RBCs (magnification ×400). (*B*) Pernicious anemia, with large, misshapen RBCs (magnification ×400). (*C*) Sickle cell anemia (magnification ×400). (*D*) Aplastic anemia, bone marrow (magnification ×200). (*A, B,* and *C* from: Listen, Look, and Learn, Vol 3, Coagulation, Hematology. The American Society of Clinical Pathologists Press, Chicago, 1973, with permission; *D* from Harmening, DM: Clinical Hematology and Fundamentals of Hemostasis, ed 3. FA Davis, Philadelphia, 1997, with permission.)

also may result from low dietary intake during pregnancy; from breast feeding; in the menstrual years; from chronic intestinal diseases associated with malabsorption of iron; or merely from low dietary intake of iron-rich foods.

SIGNS AND SYMPTOMS Common symptoms include pallor, lassitude, headache, and irritability. If the anemia progresses, symptoms become more severe, such as dyspnea, tachycardia, and brittle hair and nails.

DIAGNOSTIC PROCEDURES Blood testing typically indicates low hemoglobin and hematocrit values. Levels of serum iron and serum ferritin may be low as well. The red blood count will typically reveal unusually high numbers of microcytic red cells. Bone marrow studies may be done to differentiate iron deficiency anemia from closely related blood disorders.

TREATMENT Iron deficiency anemia may be treated with oral or **parenteral** iron supplements. Dietary modifications, however, are often sufficient to restore lost bodily iron reserves.

PROGNOSIS The prognosis for iron deficiency anemia is good if the underlying cause, such as unusual bleeding, is detected and treated. The condition may be chronic in some cases, however.

PREVENTION Prevention includes a diet with adequate iron for daily needs and identification of high-risk individuals.

FOLIC ACID DEFICIENCY ANEMIA

DESCRIPTION *Folic acid deficiency anemia* is characterized by the appearance of large-sized, abnormal red blood cells (megaloblasts), which form when there are inadequate stores of folic acid within the body. Folic acid is one of the B complex of vitamins.

ETIOLOGY The cause of this anemia is often inadequate intake of folic acid. This may be due to poor diet or overcooking of vegetables, or it may be a consequence of alcoholism. The disease also may arise from increased utilization of folic acid, such as may occur during pregnancy, in infancy, or as a result of other blood disorders. Impaired absorption of folic acid by the body and drug-related folic imbalances also may produce the disease. The deficiency is more common in pregnant women, infants, children, and adolescents.

SIGNS AND SYMPTOMS Symptoms may include weakness, fatigue, **anorexia,** pallor, forgetfulness, and irritability.

DIAGNOSTIC PROCEDURES Serum folate levels will typically be decreased. Bone marrow studies may be done to determine if there is a secondary cause of the disease.

TREATMENT Folic acid supplements may be given orally, or they may be administered parenterally if the person's condition indicates that more immediate intervention is needed.

PROGNOSIS The prognosis depends on the underlying cause of the folic acid deficiency. For most, the prognosis is good.

PREVENTION Prevention includes a diet with adequate folic acid content, such as found in beef liver, cooked collards, red beans, and asparagus spears.

■ PERNICIOUS ANEMIA

DESCRIPTION *Pernicious (megaloblastic) anemia* is characterized by the appearance of large, abnormal red blood cells, which form when there are inadequate levels of vitamin B_{12} within the body. The disease is most common in persons of Scandinavian and Northern European descent and affects those between the ages of 50 and 60.

ETIOLOGY Pernicious anemia is caused by the failure of certain cells in the gastric mucosa to secrete adequate levels of a protein called *intrinsic factor* (IF). This protein is necessary for the absorption of dietary vitamin B_{12}, which is essential for red blood cell formation. Certain forms of the disease appear to be inherited, whereas other forms appear to be autoimmune disorders. Persons with other autoimmune diseases are more likely to develop pernicious anemia.

SIGNS AND SYMPTOMS The onset of symptoms is usually insidious but may eventually be manifested as fatigue, dyspnea, palpitations, sore tongue, and numbness and tingling of the extremities. Weakness, nausea, vomiting, **neuritis,** impaired coordination, altered vision, light-headedness, and tachycardia also may be present.

DIAGNOSTIC PROCEDURES A thorough medical history and physical examination are essential in the diagnosis of pernicious anemia. Laboratory studies

may reveal decreased levels of hemoglobin and serum levels of vitamin B_{12}. A Schilling test, specific for pernicious anemia, will confirm the diagnosis. Bone marrow aspiration and gastric analysis may be done.

TREATMENT Parenteral administration of vitamin B_{12}, initially in high doses, is typically the first course of treatment. Maintenance injections of vitamin B_{12} are necessary for life. Bed rest and transfusions may be necessary in extreme cases.

PROGNOSIS The damaged IF-secreting cells in the gastric mucosa will not regenerate, but if treatment is prompt and properly maintained, the person with pernicious anemia typically is able to lead a normal life.

PREVENTION There is no known prevention.

■ APLASTIC ANEMIA

DESCRIPTION *Aplastic anemia* is characterized by insufficient or totally absent red blood cell production as a result of injury or destruction of the blood-forming tissue in the bone marrow. In over half the cases, aplastic anemia is idiopathic. The bone marrow stops producing red and white blood cells and platelets. The result is that the person cannot fight infection and has a tendency to bleed.

ETIOLOGY Unknown causes include exposure to toxins, such as chloramphenicol, cytotoxic agents, radiation, and the hepatitis virus.

SIGNS AND SYMPTOMS Lassitude, pallor, **purpura,** bleeding, tachycardia, infections with high fever, dyspnea, headache, and congestive heart failure may all be symptomatic of aplastic anemia. Pancytopenia, a decrease in all cellular components of the blood, may occur if the bone marrow is damaged to the point that healthy blood-forming tissues are replaced by fatty abnormal tissue.

DIAGNOSTIC PROCEDURES The red blood count (RBC), WBC, and **reticulocyte** counts will be low in the majority of cases. Bone marrow studies may show evidence of fatty tissue with **megakaryocytes.** The medical history may provide evidence of recent exposure to a toxin.

TREATMENT Exposure to a known toxin must be discontinued. Bone marrow transplantation is the treatment of choice in young persons with severe aplastic anemia. Androgenic steroids or corticosteroids may be tried. Transfusions may be necessary.

PROGNOSIS The prognosis is poor for an individual with aplastic anemia. Death results in about 50 percent of cases. Those who live with the condition may go into partial or complete remission or need to be treated with transfusions for years. Complications include infections, hemorrhage, or transfusion-related problems.

PREVENTION Prevention includes avoidance of any chemical or physical agents that have the capacity to damage bone marrow.

◼ SICKLE CELL ANEMIA

DESCRIPTION *Sickle cell anemia* is a hereditary, chronic anemia in which abnormal sickle- or crescent-shaped red blood cells are present. These abnormally shaped red blood cells tend to clump together within capillaries, impairing circulation, damaging blood vessels, and producing chronic organ damage. The incidence of sickle cell anemia is highest among African-Americans and those of Mediterranean ancestry.

ETIOLOGY The condition is due to the presence of an abnormal form of hemoglobin, called *hemoglobin S,* within the red cells. The defective hemoglobin is synthesized by individuals inheriting homozygous hemoglobin S genes.

If the individual is heterozygous for the hemoglobin S gene, that individual is said to possess *sickle cell trait*. This is a comparatively benign condition that typically produces no symptoms; however, the red blood cells of such individuals may sickle as a consequence of any condition that produces **hypoxia.** If two individuals with the sickle cell trait marry, their offspring has a 25 percent chance of inheriting sickle cell anemia.

SIGNS AND SYMPTOMS Signs and symptoms characteristic of sickle cell anemia are episodic attacks of intense pain in the arms, legs, or abdomen. The sclera (the white of the eye) is jaundiced. Recurrent bouts of fever, chronic fatigue, dyspnea, tachycardia, and pallor may be additional manifestations of the disease. Infections, stress, and extremes in temperature may trigger the painful crises.

DIAGNOSTIC PROCEDURES If parents are known carriers of the sickle cell trait, the infant should be screened for the condition. A positive family history and a physical examination will confirm the diagnosis. Hemoglobin electrophoresis is the lab test of choice. It can be done on an umbilical at birth.

TREATMENT Treatment of sickle cell anemia is symptomatic and typically involves the prescription of analgesics and the maintenance of adequate hydration. Hospitalization may be required during attacks, and transfusions may be necessary. Experimental treatment using umbilical cord blood in transplant may be effective.

PROGNOSIS The prognosis is highly variable. Sickle cell anemia is a life-threatening disease. Many affected individuals die in childhood; however, because of improvements in the care of sickle cell patients, some live into the middle years. Complications include leg ulcers, **cholelithiasis,** orthopedic disorders, cerebral hemorrhage, and shock.

PREVENTION There is no prevention for sickle cell anemia other than genetic counseling for those at risk.

◼ POLYCYTHEMIA VERA

DESCRIPTION *Polycythemia vera* is a chronic blood disorder characterized by increased numbers of red blood cells, leukocytosis, thrombocytosis, and increased hemoglobin concentration. The disease is more common to men in late middle age than to others.

ETIOLOGY The cause of the uncontrolled and rapid cellular reproduction and maturation of all bone marrow cells is essentially unknown.

SIGNS AND SYMPTOMS The increased mass of red blood cells results in hyperviscosity of the blood and inhibits blood flow. This increase in red cells gives the skin a purplish appearance. The eyes appear bloodshot, and the mucous membranes are extremely red. An elevated hematocrit is evident. Altered circulation may cause headache, dizziness, and a feeling of fullness in the head. The spleen is enlarged. Hyperviscosity may lead to thrombosis of smaller vessels and ruddy cyanosis.

DIAGNOSTIC PROCEDURES The increased mass of red blood cells along with normal arterial oxygen saturation is the confirming diagnosis. Splenomegaly, thrombocytosis, and leukocytosis are also likely to be present.

TREATMENT Phlebotomy is the primary treatment to reduce hematocrit to the normal range. After repeated phlebotomies, iron deficiency develops and stabilizes red blood cell production. **Myelosuppression** may be necessary in clients with extreme thrombocytosis and splenomegaly.

PROGNOSIS Prognosis depends on the age at diagnosis, the treatment used, and complications. Mortality is high if polycythemia is untreated or is associated with leukemia.

PREVENTION There is no known prevention.

Leukemias

Leukemias are progressive, malignant diseases of the blood-forming organs and are marked by the unrestrained growth of abnormal leukocytes and their precursors in the blood and bone marrow (Fig. 9–16). The term *leukemia* refers to a neoplasm of **hematopoietic** tissue. The leukemia cells infiltrate the bone marrow and lymph tissue, then advance into the blood stream and the various organs of the body. There may or may not be a rise in circulating white blood cells, depending on whether the white cells are confined to the bone marrow.

Leukemia is classified according to the dominant abnormal cell type and the severity of the disease. Leukemia may be further classified as acute or chronic depending on the maturity of the cell. Although other variants occur, five of the more common leukemias are described here. They are acute myeloblastic (myelogenous) leukemia (AML), acute lymphoblastic (lymphocytic) leukemia (ALL), acute monoblastic (monocytic) leukemia, chronic myelocytic leukemia (CML), and chronic lymphocytic leukemia (CLL).

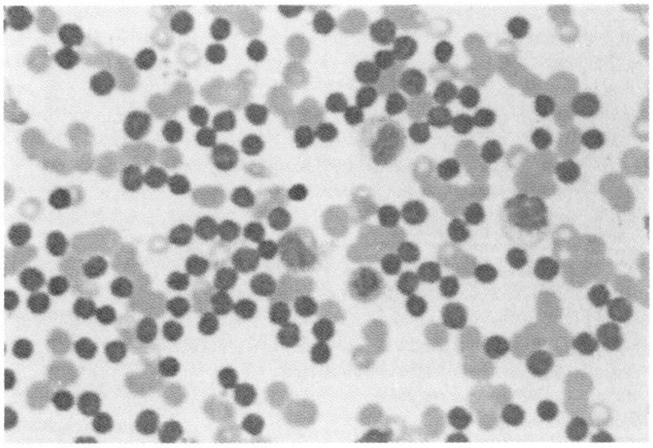

ACUTE MYELOBLASTIC (MYELOGENOUS) LEUKEMIA (AML)

DESCRIPTION *Acute myeloblastic leukemia* is a neoplasm characterized by the hyperproliferation of abnormal, immature white cell precursors called **blasts.** These abnormal cells accumulate in the blood, bone marrow, and body tissues. In AML, the white cells are immature, so that there is resultant rapid accumulation of myeloid precursors called myeloblasts. It is the most common type of nonlymphatic leukemia, occurring most frequently in men and in persons 30 to 60 years old.

ETIOLOGY The cause of acute leukemia is unknown. Predisposing factors may include infection by certain viruses, abnormal exposure to radiation, and hereditary tendencies.

SIGNS AND SYMPTOMS Symptoms may be sudden in onset. Initial symptoms include weakness, malaise, bone and joint pain, and anorexia. These may be followed by a pallor, fever, **petechiae,** and swollen lymph nodes. Unexplained bleeding and prolonged menses may also signal the onset of acute leukemia.

Figure 9–16 Leukemia. Notice the many darkly stained WBC (magnification ×800). (From Sacher, RA, and McPherson, RA: Widmann's Clinical Interpretation of Laboratory Tests, ed 10. FA Davis, 1991, color plate No. 44, with permission.)

DIAGNOSTIC PROCEDURES Bone marrow aspiration and biopsy are necessary for diagnosis. Laboratory findings may include **thrombocytopenia** and **neutropenia.**

TREATMENT A variety of chemotherapeutic agents are typically used in treating those with acute leukemias. Such treatments generally require hospitalization. Bone marrow transplants may be used for some acute leukemias, especially in young persons during a period of remission who have a tissue-compatible sibling. Supportive care may include transfusion of whole blood or blood products and the use of antibiotics to prevent secondary infection.

PROGNOSIS In AML, generally the survival time is only 1 year after diagnosis. One- to two-month remissions may occur in half of childhood cases.

PREVENTION There is no known prevention.

ACUTE LYMPHOBLASTIC (LYMPHOCYTIC) LEUKEMIA (ALL)

DESCRIPTION *Acute lymphoblastic leukemia* is similar to AML except that there is abnormal growth of lymphocyte precursors called lymphoblasts. The disease is more common in children aged 2 to 5 years old. Children account for about 80 percent of the ALL cases.

ETIOLOGY The cause of ALL, as in all acute leukemias, is unknown; however, radiation, certain chemicals, and genetic abnormalities may be contributing factors.

SIGNS AND SYMPTOMS The presenting symptoms may be high fever, abnormal bleeding, fatigue, and night sweats. There may be bruising after minor trauma, weakness, recurrent infections, and petechiae. The signs are similar to AML.

DIAGNOSTIC PROCEDURES As with AML, diagnostic procedures for ALL include bone marrow aspiration and biopsy, and blood tests to confirm the presence of thrombocytopenia and neutropenia.

TREATMENT Treatment includes chemotherapy to induce remission. Hospitalizations may be required to perform bone marrow transplants. Radiation therapy may be ordered. Supportive treatment is essential, including antibiotics for treatment and prevention of infection and transfusions for anemias.

PROGNOSIS In ALL, the treatment may induce remissions in the majority of cases; the remissions last on an average of 5 years. Children who undergo intensive treatment have the best survival rate.

PREVENTION There is no known prevention.

ACUTE MONOBLASTIC (MONOCYTIC) LEUKEMIA

DESCRIPTION *Acute monoblastic leukemia* is also called Schilling's leukemia, and is characterized by an increase in monoblasts, the monocytic precursors.

ETIOLOGY As in all forms of acute leukemia, the cause is unknown, but contributing factors include radiation exposure, chemotherapeutic agents, and genetic predisposition.

SIGNS AND SYMPTOMS All acute leukemias present with repeated infections, bruising from minor injury, fever and fatigue. The course of the disease is generally brief and hectic.

DIAGNOSTIC PROCEDURES Bone marrow aspiration and biopsy are used for diagnosis. A differential white blood count will be ordered.

TREATMENT Chemotherapeutic agents will be used in treatment, and a bone marrow transplantation may be performed. Antibiotics will be ordered for any infections, and supportive treatment is important.

PROGNOSIS The disease is fatal if untreated. With treatment the prognosis varies but is generally poor.

PREVENTION There is no known prevention.

CHRONIC MYELOCYTIC LEUKEMIA (CML)

DESCRIPTION *Chronic myelocytic (myelogenous) leukemia* is characterized by the proliferation of abnormal white cell precursors called *granulocytes* in the bone marrow. These abnormal granulocytes later enter the blood and invade other body tissues. CML usually affects adults 40 to 60 years of age.

ETIOLOGY Ninety percent of individuals with chronic myelocytic leukemia have what is termed the *Philadelphia chromosome,* an abnormality on chromosome 22. This abnormality is thought to be acquired rather than inherited. Factors that may cause this genetic abnormality include viruses, radiation, and carcinogenic chemicals.

SIGNS AND SYMPTOMS The symptoms occur in two phases. The first, an insidious chronic phase, lasts from 2 to 4 years and is followed by an acute phase, lasting 3 to 6 months. Symptoms include pallor, weakness, fever, purpura, skin nodules, sternal tenderness, headache, retinal hemorrhages, bleeding gums, nosebleeds, weight loss, and anorexia.

DIAGNOSTIC PROCEDURES Laboratory findings may reveal leukocytosis, neutropenia, and anemia. The Philadelphia chromosome can be detected through bone marrow or blood testing.

TREATMENT Chemotherapy may be used to treat both the chronic and acute phases. Secondary infections must be treated immediately.

PROGNOSIS The disease is rapidly fatal after the onset of the acute phase. The average survival time is 3 years.

PREVENTION There is no known prevention.

CHRONIC LYMPHOCYTIC LEUKEMIA (CLL)

DESCRIPTION *Chronic lymphocytic leukemia* is characterized by the accumulation of immature, immunologically ineffective B lymphocytes. These cells accumulate to an enormous extent in the lymphoid tissue, blood, and bone marrow. It is the most common form of leukemia in the United States, usually affecting people over the age of 50.

ETIOLOGY The cause is unknown, but the disease is suspected to be genetic or immunologic in origin.

SIGNS AND SYMPTOMS The onset is usually insidious. Symptoms eventually include pallor, weakness, lymph node enlargement, fatigue, fever, and weight loss. As the disease progresses, tachycardia, palpitations, and an increased incidence of infections are common.

DIAGNOSTIC PROCEDURES The disease often is found by accident during a routine physical examination. Laboratory findings indicating CLL include granulocytopenia, neutropenia, and anemia. The WBC often rises as the disease progresses. Bone marrow aspiration and biopsy confirm the diagnosis.

TREATMENT Treatment may be withheld until the person manifests symptoms. When the person exhibits signs or symptoms or has anemia or thrombocytopenia, treatment with chemotherapy is usually initiated. Radiation therapy or corticosteroids may be tried, too. Complications such as anemia, hemorrhage, or secondary infections must be treated promptly.

PROGNOSIS The progression of CLL is slow, but the prognosis is guarded and depends on a person's age, signs, and symptoms. If the person has anemia, death usually occurs in less than 2 years. Various immunologic disorders may accompany CLL, worsening the prognosis.

PREVENTION There is no known prevention.

Lymphatic Diseases

LYMPHEDEMA

DESCRIPTION *Lymphedema* is an abnormal accumulation of lymph, usually in the extremities.

ETIOLOGY Lymphedema results from the inflammatory or mechanical obstruction of the lymph vessels or nodes (Fig. 9–17). Such a condition may arise directly as a result of infections, neoplasms, allergic reactions, or thrombus formation. The condition also may arise secondary to surgery, trauma, burns, or radiation. Some forms of lymphedema are congenital. Young women seem more susceptible than others to developing lymphedema.

SIGNS AND SYMPTOMS The affected limb, in part or whole, will typically be swollen and hypertrophied, with thickened and fibrotic skin. Lymphedema is

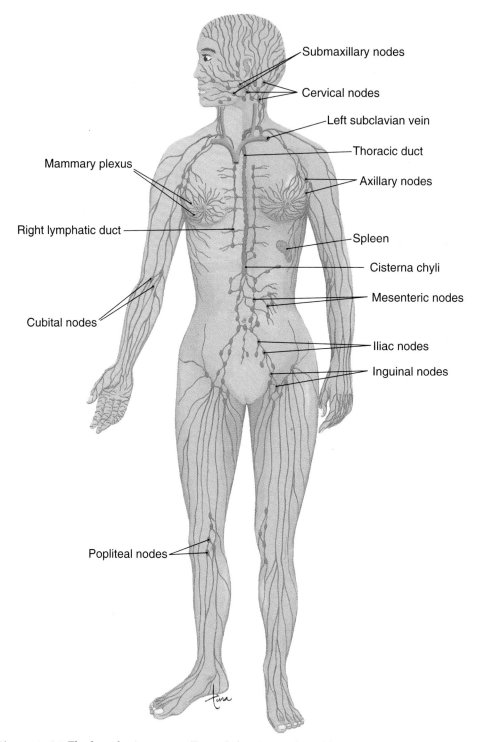

Figure 9–17 The lymphatic system. (From Gylys, BA, and Wedding, ME: Medical Terminology: A Systems Approach, ed 3. FA Davis, Philadelphia, 1995, p 182, with permission.)

usually painless, and it may be accompanied by episodes of **lymphangitis** and **cellulitis.** The edema may be either pitting or nonpitting.

DIAGNOSTIC PROCEDURES A thorough patient history and physical examination are necessary. Lymphangiography and radioactive isotope studies are helping in detecting the site of lymphatic obstruction.

TREATMENT Treatment is difficult. It usually includes elevation of the affected part, especially at night, the use of special fitted elastic stockings put on prior to getting up and worn all day, and massaging the limb toward the trunk to "milk" the edema out of the extremity. **Diuretics** may be prescribed in some instances. Surgery to correct lymphatic obstruction and promote drainage is a last resort.

PROGNOSIS The prognosis for lymphedema depends on the cause. Infections worsen the prognosis.

PREVENTION There is no known prevention.

HODGKIN'S DISEASE

DESCRIPTION *Hodgkin's disease* is a neoplastic malignancy of the lymphatic system characterized by painless enlargement of the lymph nodes, spleen, and other lymphatic tissues. It occurs more frequently between the ages of 25 and 55.

ETIOLOGY The exact cause of Hodgkin's disease is not known. There is even disagreement on whether the disease is a true malignancy or an inflammatory immunologic disorder. Certain viruses are strongly suspected as etiologic agents.

SIGNS AND SYMPTOMS The usual presenting symptom is enlarged, firm, nontender, painless regional lymph nodes, generally in the neck, chest, or abdomen. Fever, fatigue, weight loss, diaphoresis, and **pruritus** may follow. The disease is characterized by exacerbation and remission of symptoms.

DIAGNOSTIC PROCEDURES Laboratory findings may reveal **lymphocytopenia** and anemia. Definitive diagnosis is established by identifying the presence of Reed-Sternberg cells in lymphatic tissue. These are giant connective-tissue cells that usually possess two large nuclei. A lymph node biopsy, bone marrow biopsy, chest x-ray, lower extremity lym-

phangiogram, scintiscan of the liver and spleen, and liver function studies may be used to confirm the diagnosis. It is extremely important that the extent of the disease process be known and that it be staged prior to the initiation of therapy.

TREATMENT Treatment depends on the stage of the disease. It can range from some combination of chemotherapy, with or without irradiation, to massive combination chemotherapy and full-body irradiation.

PROGNOSIS The prognosis varies with the staging. When the disease is at stages I and II, the prognosis is good if there are no manifestations for the first 5 years.

PREVENTION There is no known prevention.

LYMPHOSARCOMA

DESCRIPTION *Lymphosarcomas, or non-Hodgkin's lymphomas,* are a group of malignant diseases of the lymphatic system. They are categorized as follows:

1. Well-differentiated lymphatic
2. Poorly differentiated lymphocytic
3. Histiocytic (formerly called *reticulum cell sarcoma*)
4. Mixed lymphocytic and histiocytic
5. Undifferentiated or stem-cell malignant lymphoma.

ETIOLOGY The cause is unknown, although viruses have been suggested as etiologic agents. Lymphosarcomas occur in all age groups; they are more common in men.

SIGNS AND SYMPTOMS Swollen lymph glands, especially enlarged tonsils and adenoids, are common presenting symptoms. Coughing, dyspnea, fatigue, sweating, fever, and weight loss may follow.

DIAGNOSTIC PROCEDURES Diagnosis is by lymph node biopsy and/or bone marrow biopsy. Non-Hodgkin's lymphomas need to be distinguished from Hodgkin's disease.

TREATMENT Treatment includes radiation therapy or chemotherapy. Staging is important prior to beginning any treatment. Refer to Chapter 3 for further information on staging.

PROGNOSIS The prognosis is good if the person is in remission; however, if a remission cannot be produced by treatment, the prognosis is poor.

PREVENTION There is no known prevention.

SPECIAL FOCUS BONE MARROW TRANSPLANTATION

Bone marrow is the soft organic material that fills the cavities of the bone. Bone marrow transplantation (BMT) is used in the treatment of aplastic anemia, thalassemia and sickle cell anemia, and immunodeficiency disorders. Other diseases in which BMT may be used include acute leukemia, chronic myelogenous leukemia, non-Hodgkin's lymphoma, Hodgkin's disease, and testicular cancer.

The BMT procedure involves the use of a special needle to aspirate 500 to 700 mL (500 mL is a bit more than half a quart) of marrow from the iliac crest of the pelvic bone, or from the upper portion of the sternum, of a human leukocyte antigen (HLA)–compatible donor (an allogenic transplantation) or of the recipient himself or herself during complete remission (an autologous transplantation). After aspiration, the marrow is filtered and infused into the recipient so that the recipient's marrow can then be repopulated.

SPECIAL FOCUS CIRCULATORY DISEASE OF CHILDHOOD

Reye's syndrome, because it affects more than one body system, could have been considered in several chapters of this text. The disease is discussed in this chapter because one common symptom of the disease is the accumulation of ammonia in the blood.

■ REYE'S SYNDROME

DESCRIPTION *Reye's syndrome* is an acute illness that disrupts the body's urea cycle, resulting in the accumulation of ammonia in the blood, **hypoglycemia,** severe brain edema, and dangerously high intracranial pressure. The disease almost exclusively affects those under 15 years of age.

ETIOLOGY The etiology is not known, but Reye's syndrome almost always follows an upper respiratory infection and is especially associated with type B influenza and varicella. The incidence of the disease also may be linked to the use of aspirin during influenza or varicella infections.

SIGNS AND SYMPTOMS The symptoms of Reye's syndrome develop in five stages:

- Stage I: Lethargy, vomiting, and hepatic dysfunction, which may be followed by a few days' recovery
- Stage II: Hyperventilation, delirium, and hyperactive reflexes
- Stage III: Coma, rigidity of organ cortices (*cortices* [singular *cortex*] are outer layers)
- Stage IV: Deepening coma, large and fixed pupils, and loss of cerebral functions
- Stage V: Seizures, loss of deep tendon reflexes, flaccidity, and respiratory arrest.

DIAGNOSTIC PROCEDURES A medical history of prior viral infection accompanied by any of the clinical features mentioned previously is strongly suggestive of Reye's syndrome. An increased level of ammonia in the blood confirms the diagnosis. Liver function studies, liver biopsy, and cerebral spinal fluid analysis may be necessary.

TREATMENT Reye's syndrome requires hospitalization and intensive treatment to restore blood sugar levels, control cerebral edema, and correct acid-base imbalances. Intracranial pressure must be decreased to prevent seizures. Endotracheal intubation and mechanical ventilation may be necessary.

PROGNOSIS The prognosis is largely dependent on the stage of progression of the disease. Monitoring intracranial pressure and early treatment measures have greatly reduced the mortality rate from 90 percent to 20 percent.

PREVENTION The risk of developing Reye's syndrome as a consequence of influenza or varicella infection is lessened by avoiding the use of aspirin during the course of those diseases. Parents should be advised to give nonsalicylate analgesics and antipyretics.

COMMON SYMPTOMS OF CIRCULATORY SYSTEM DISEASES

Individuals with circulatory diseases may present with the following common complaints, which deserve attention from health professionals:

- Fatigue
- Dyspnea
- Fever
- Weakness
- Tachycardia and palpitations
- Pallor
- Chest pain
- Unusual sweating, especially at night
- Edema
- Nausea, vomiting, or anorexia
- Anxiety
- Headache

 ## ALTERNATIVE MEDICINE

Marching along the route of traditional treatment for heart disease, alternative medicine identifies the following treatment modalities:

- Reduce stress.
- Exercise regularly.
- Eat organic foods and a diet high in fiber, with reduced fat. Avoid processed foods, reduce consumption of meat, sugar, and alcohol.
- Reach, and maintain, a reasonable weight.
- Increase levels of nutrients such as vitamin B_6, magnesium, and antioxidants that include vitamins E and C and selenium. However, note that high doses of any vitamin are not recommended unless under the supervision of a medical practitioner.

BIBLIOGRAPHY

The Burton Goldberg Group (ed): Alternative Medicine: The Definitive Guide. Future Medicine Publishing, Fife, Wash., 1995.

Burns, MV: Pathophysiology: A Self-Instructional Program. Appleton & Lange, Stamford, Conn., 1998.

Fauci, AS, et al: Harrison's Principles of Internal Medicine, ed 14. McGraw-Hill, New York, 1998.

Frazier, MS, Drzymkowski, JA, and Doty SJ: Essentials of Human Disease and Conditions. WB Saunders, Philadelphia, 1996.

Gordon, D: Too Big a Heart. Time (special issue) 150(19): 35–37, 1997.

Morrow, L: A Broken Heart. Time 152(21):93–96, 1998.

Mulvihill, ML: Human Diseases: A Systemic Approach. Appleton & Lange, Stamford, Conn., 1995.

Professional Guide to Diseases, ed 6. Springhouse Corporation, Springhouse, Pa., 1998.

CASE STUDIES

I A woman calls the medical office to make an appointment for her 80-year-old husband. He has been complaining of shortness of breath and fatigue. His wife has noticed prominent pulsations in the artery in his neck. She also reports that his ankles tend to swell.

1. How soon will you set the requested appointment?

2. Is age a factor in this patient's condition?

3. What dietary restrictions might the doctor recommend for this patient?

II A single woman, active both socially and professionally, complains to the doctor of light-headedness and palpitations. She is about 70 pounds overweight, smokes two packs of cigarettes a day, and enjoys fine dining.

1. What circulatory condition do the patient's circumstances and symptoms suggest? What are the contributing factors?

2. What diagnostic procedures might the physician call for in this situation? What procedures might be indicated?

3. What is the prognosis?

REVIEW QUESTIONS

MATCHING

Match the following infectious heart diseases with their definitions:

_____ 1. Inflammation of cardiac muscle

_____ 2. Inflammation of the sac surrounding the heart

_____ 3. Inflammation of the heart valves and chambers

a. Endocarditis
b. Pericarditis
c. Myocarditis

Match the following diseases with their correct definitions:

_____ 4. Heart suddenly ceases to pump

_____ 5. Local dilation of artery or chamber of heart

_____ 6. Inflammation of vein with thrombus formation

_____ 7. Dilated, tortuous veins

a. Thrombophlebitis
b. Cardiac arrest
c. Aneurysm
d. Varicose veins
e. Aplastic anemia
f. Lymphedema

TRUE/FALSE

T   F   1. In pulmonic insufficiency, backflow of blood into the right ventricle causes ventricular hypertrophy.

T   F   2. In aortic insufficiency, backflow of blood into the left ventricle causes ventricular hypertrophy.

T   F   3. In tricuspid stenosis, backflow of blood into the right atrium causes atrial hypertrophy.

T   F   4. In mitral stenosis, backflow of blood into the left atrium causes atrial hypertrophy.

T   F   5. Polycythemia is the result of a deficient supply of red blood cells.

MULTIPLE CHOICE

1. Select all the high-risk individuals for hypertension:
   a. Persons under a great deal of stress
   b. Persons who are of African-American descent
   c. Persons who are obese
   d. Persons who eat food high in salt
   e. Persons who lead sedentary lifestyles
   f. Persons on oral contraceptives

SHORT ANSWERS

1. Define the five types of anemias:

   a. Iron deficiency anemia:

   b. Folic acid deficiency anemia:

   c. Pernicious anemia:

   d. Aplastic anemia:

   e. Sickle cell anemia:

2. Define the five types of leukemia:

   a. Acute myeloblastic leukemia:

   b. Acute lymphoblastic leukemia:

   c. Acute monoblastic leukemia:

   d. Chronic myelocytic leukemia:

   e. Chronic lymphocytic leukemia:

3. Define:

   a. Atherosclerosis:

   b. Arteriosclerosis:

4. List the causes of heart murmurs:

   a.

   b.

   c.

   d.

5. Rheumatic fever, an inflammatory disease in children, generally follows

   _____ .

6. List and describe the five stages of Reye's syndrome:

   a.

   b.

   c.

   d.

   e.

7. The classic symptom of myocardial infarction is _____ .

8. The medication taken sublingually or topically for angina pectoris is

   _____ .

9. Are lymphosarcoma and Hodgkin's disease similar? _____ . Explain.

ANSWERS

MATCHING

1. c	3. a	5. c	7. d
2. b	4. b	6. a	

TRUE/FALSE

1. T	4. T
2. T	5. F
3. T	

MULTIPLE CHOICE

1. a, b, c, d, e, f

SHORT ANSWERS

1. a. Iron deficiency anemia: Inadequate supply of iron resulting in smaller blood cells.
   b. Folic acid deficiency anemia: Inadequate intake of folic acid, a nitrogenous acid found in some foods.
   c. Pernicious anemia: Failure of the gastric mucosa to secrete adequate intrinsic factor, resulting in malabsorption of vitamin B_{12}.
   d. Aplastic anemia: Absence of regeneration of red blood cells.
   e. Sickle cell anemia: Genetically determined defect of hemoglobin synthesis occurring almost exclusively in African-Americans.
2. a. Acute myeloblastic leukemia: A neoplasm of proliferating abnormal white cell blasts.
   b. Acute lymphoblastic leukemia: Proliferation of abnormal white cells called lymphoblasts.
   c. Acute monoblastic leukemia: Proliferation of abnormal white cells called monoblasts.

  d. Chronic myelocytic leukemia: Proliferation of abnormal white cells that invade the bone marrow, blood, and body tissue.

  e. Chronic lymphocytic leukemia: An abnormal accumulation of small lymphocytes that have lost the capacity to divide.

3. a. Atherosclerosis: A form of arteriosclerosis where the lumen of the coronary arteries is narrowed by fatty, fibrous plaques; it generally affects large and medium-sized arteries.

  b. Arteriosclerosis: Sclerosis and thickening of the walls of arterioles.

4. a. Blood leaking back through an incompetent or deformed valve

  b. Blood forcing its way through a stenosed valve

  c. Dilation of the heart

  d. A rapid diastolic flow

5. A streptococcal infection

6. a. Stage I: Lethargy, vomiting, and hepatic dysfunction.

  b. Stage II: Hyperventilation, delirium, hyperactive reflexes.

  c. Stage III: Coma, rigidity of organ cortices.

  d. Stage IV: Deepening coma, large and fixed pupils, loss of cerebral functions.

  e. Stage V: Seizures, loss of deep tendon reflexes, flaccidity, respiratory arrest.

7. Crushing chest pain that may radiate to the left arm, neck, and jaw.

8. Nitrates, usually nitroglycerin.

9. Yes and no. Lymphosarcoma is a non-Hodgkin's lymphoma. Both involve the lymph system, and signs and symptoms may be similar, as may the treatment; however, the prognoses differ.

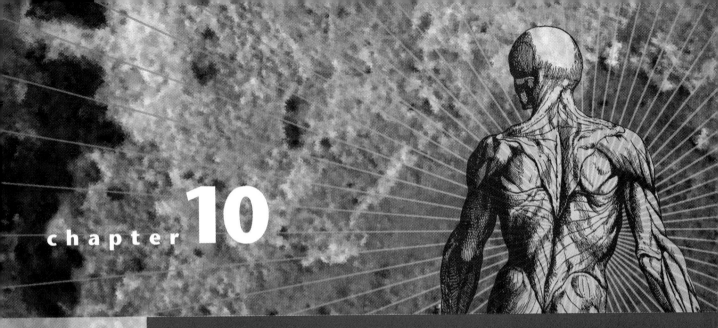

Nervous System Diseases

CHAPTER OUTLINE

Headaches
Acute and Chronic Headache
Migraine Headache
☐ ALTERNATIVE MEDICINE

Head Trauma
Epidural and Subdural Hematoma (Acute)
Cerebral Concussion
Cerebral Contusion

Paralysis
Hemiplegia
Spinal Cord Injuries: Paraplegia and
    Quadriplegia

Infections of the Central Nervous
    System
Acute Bacterial Meningitis
Encephalitis
Brain Abscess

Peripheral Nerve Diseases
Peripheral Neuritis

Bell's Palsy

Cerebral Diseases/Disorders
Cerebrovascular Accident (Stroke)
Transient Ischemic Attacks (TIAs)
Epilepsy

Degenerative Diseases
Alzheimer's Disease
Parkinson's Disease
Multiple Sclerosis
Amyotrophic Lateral Sclerosis (ALS)

Cancer
Tumors of the Brain

Common Symptoms of Nervous System
    Diseases

Bibliography

Case Studies

Review Questions

LEARNING OBJECTIVES

Upon successful completion of this chapter, you will:

- Identify the three main divisions of the nervous system.
- Describe the basic unit of the nervous system and how it functions.
- List the causes for headache.
- Compare the prognoses for migraine and chronic headaches.
- Compare epidural to subdural hematomas.
- Contrast concussion to contusion.
- Recall four courses of treatment for spinal cord injuries.
- Distinguish the signs and symptoms of paraplegia and quadriplegia.
- Restate the noninjury cause of hemiplegia.
- Discuss the signs and symptoms of meningitis and encephalitis.
- Recall the prognosis for brain abscess.
- Identify at least three classifications of epilepsy.
- Describe the disease process of peripheral neuritis.
- Explain the characteristic symptoms of Bell's palsy.
- Discuss cerebrovascular accident (CVA).
- Recognize the signs and symptoms of Parkinson's disease.
- Recall the etiology of multiple sclerosis.
- Discuss appropriate treatment protocol for amyotrophic lateral sclerosis.
- Describe the progression of brain tumors.
- List at least four signs and symptoms characteristic of nervous system diseases.

KEY WORDS

Adrenocorticotropic hormone (ACTH)
(ăd•rē•nō•cŏr•tĭ•cō•trō′pĭk hor′mōn)
Agnosia (ăg•nō′zē•ă)
Agraphia (ă•grăf′ē•ă)
Alexia (ă•lĕk′sē•ă)
Analgesics (ăn•ăl•jē′zĭks)
Antibiotics (ăn•tī•bī•ŏt′ĭks)
Anticholinergic (ăn•tī•kō•lĭn•ĕr′jĭk)
Aphasia (ă•fā′zē•ă)
Apraxia (ă•prăk′sē•ă)
Arrhythmia (ă•rĭth′mē•ă)
Bacteremia (băk•tĕr•ē′mē•ă)
Bradycardia (brăd•ē•kăr′dē•ă)
Brudzinski's sign
Cerebrospinal fluid (CSF)
(sĕr•ē•brō•spī′nal flū′ĭd)
Cheyne-Stokes respiration (chān′stōks
rĕs•pĭr•ā′shŭn)

Coma (kō′mă)
Contracture (kŏn•trăk′chūr)
Craniotomy (krā•nē•ŏt′ō•mē)
Decubitus ulcer (dē•kū′bĭ•tŭs ŭl′sĕr)
Diplopia (dĭp•lō′pē•ă)
Dysphasia (dĭs•fā′zē•ă)
Embolism (ĕm′bō•lĭzm)
Hematoma (hē•mă•tō′mă)
Hemiparesis (hēm•ē•păr′ē•sĭs)
Hypotension (hī•pō•tĕn′shun)
Idiopathic (ĭd•ē•ō•păth′ĭk)
Ischemia (ĭs•kē′mē•ă)
Kernig's sign
Meninges (mĕn•ĭn′jēz)
Nuchal rigidity (nū′kăl rĭ•jĭ′dĭ•tē)
Stupor (stū′pŏr)
Thrombosis (thrŏm•bō′sĭs)
Tinnitis (tĭn•ī′tŭs)

The body's nervous system is an elaborate, interlaced network of nerve cells of astonishing complexity and sophistication. This network includes the brain, spinal cord, and nerves. The entire system functions to regulate and coordinate body activities and bring about responses by which the body adjusts to changes in its internal and external environment.

The nervous system is divided into two divisions. The *central nervous system* (CNS) consists of the brain and spinal cord. The CNS processes and stores sensory information and includes the parts of the brain governing consciousness. The CNS interacts with the second division of the nervous system, the *peripheral nervous system* (PNS). The PNS is composed of all other nervous tissue outside the CNS and includes 12 pairs of cranial nerves, 31 pairs of spinal nerves, all sensory nerves, and the sympathetic and parasympathetic nerves. The sympathetic and parasympathetic nerves comprise the *autonomic nervous system* (ANS), which regulates involuntary muscle movements and the action of glands. Figure 10–1 illustrates the major subdivisions of the nervous system. Figure 10–2 illustrates the major sections of the brain.

The basic functional and structural unit of the nervous system is the *neuron,* a cell specialized to initiate or conduct electrochemical impulses. A neuron receives impulses through its rootlike system of dendrites. Impulses pass along one or more dendrites, through the cell body of the neuron, and out a long stalklike extension of the cell called an *axon.* Figure 10–3 illustrates the dendrites, cell body, and axon of sensory and motor neurons.

Headaches

■ ACUTE AND CHRONIC HEADACHE

DESCRIPTION A *headache* is any diffuse pain occurring in any portion of the head. The condition may be acute or chronic. Headache is one of the most common maladies afflicting humans. In most cases, headache signals nothing more serious than fatigue or tension. Less frequently, but more important, headache may be the manifestation of an underlying disorder. For this reason, an individual's

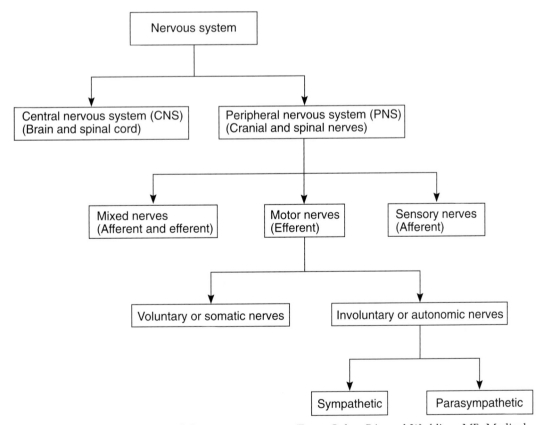

Figure 10–1 Subdivisions of the nervous system. (From Gylys, BA, and Wedding, ME: Medical Terminology: A Systems Approach, ed 4. FA Davis, Philadelphia, 1999, p 296, with permission.)

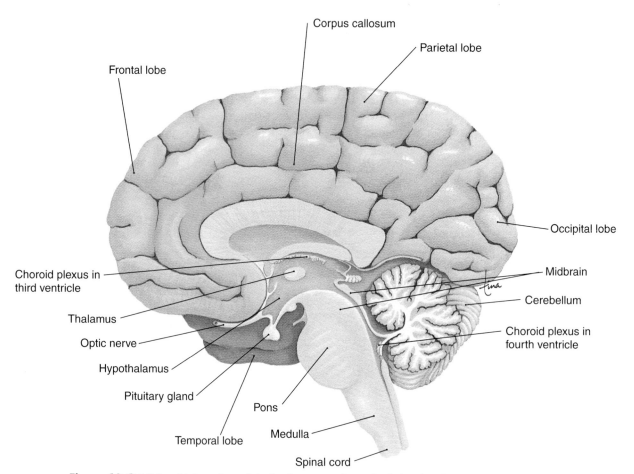

Figure 10–2 Midsagittal section of the brain as seen from the left side. The medical plane shows the internal anatomy as well as the lobes of the cerebrum. (From Scanlon, VC, and Sanders, T: Essentials of Anatomy and Physiology, ed 3. FA Davis, Philadelphia, 1999, p 165, with permission.)

complaint of headache should not be minimized or unthinkingly treated with **analgesics** before the underlying cause has been determined.

ETIOLOGY Headache is caused by irritation of one or more of the pain-sensitive structures or tissues in the head and neck. These structures include the cranial arteries and veins, the cranial and spinal nerves, the cranial and cervical muscles, and the **meninges.** (Curiously enough, most of the tissue of the brain itself is insensitive to pain.) Almost any disturbance of body function can lead to irritation of these structures and occasion a headache. Causes of headache can be grouped into organic, psychoneurological, and environmental categories. Table 10–1 summarizes possible causes of acute and chronic headaches for each of these categories.

SIGNS AND SYMPTOMS The character of headache pain varies markedly from individual to individual. It may be a dull, aching pain or an acute, almost unbearable pain. The pain may be intermittent and intense or throbbing. The pain may focus in the front, sides, or back of the head, or it may be confined to one side of the head or to a region over one or both eyes.

DIAGNOSTIC PROCEDURES If a medical history reveals a pattern of recurrent or unusually severe headaches, further medical testing is usually undertaken to try to detect an underlying cause. This may include a thorough physical examination and neurological testing. Diagnostic tests may include cranial computed tomography (CT) scans, an electroencephalogram (EEG), x-rays of the skull and

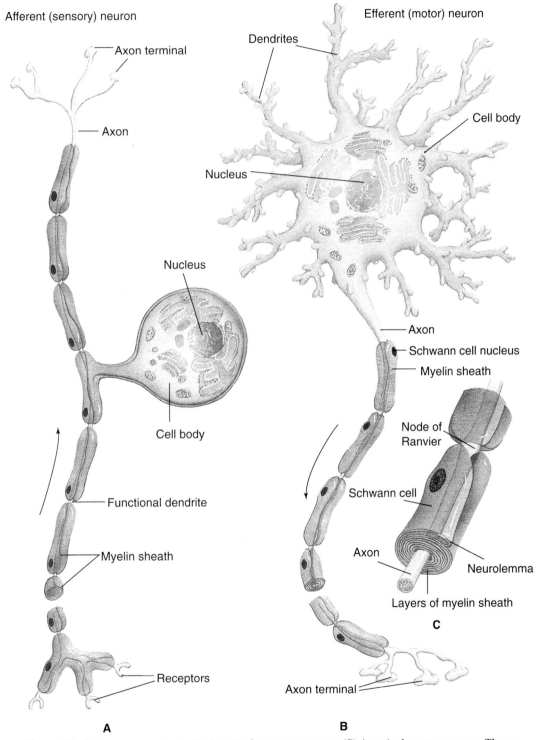

Figure 10–3 Neuron structure. (*A*) A typical sensory neuron. (*B*) A typical motor neuron. The arrows indicate the direction of impulse transmission. (*C*) Details of the myelin sheath and neurolemma formed by Schwann cells. (From Scanlon, VC, and Sanders, T: Essentials of Anatomy and Physiology, ed 3. FA Davis, Philadelphia, 1999, p 155, with permission.)

Table 10–1 Etiologies of Acute and Chronic Headaches

Organic	Toxins: Drugs, alcohol, tobacco, poisonous gases, nitrites in foods, toxins produced by local or systemic bacterial infections
	Systemic diseases: Nephritis, diabetes mellitus, arthritis, blood diseases
	Gastrointestinal disturbances: Gastric hyper- or hypoacidity, constipation
	Cardiovascular diseases: Congestive heart failure
	Endocrine diseases: Tumors of the adrenal, pituitary, thyroid glands; ovarian tumors
	Gynecologic disturbances: Menstruation, pregnancy, menopause, dysmenorrhea
	Respiratory disturbances: Infection or blockage in paranasal sinuses, adenoidal infection, deviated nasal septum
	Organic brain disease: Brain tumor, abscess, cyst, hydrocephalus, intracranial hemorrhage, embolus, thrombus, meningitis, encephalitis
	Sensory organ diseases: Glaucoma, conjunctivitis, iritis, otitis media
Psychoneurological	Nervous tension or exhaustion
	Fatigue
	Worry
	Excitement
	Psychoneuroses
Environmental insults	Head trauma
	Bright lights
	Noise
	Rapid altitude change
	Rapid temperature change
	Irritants: Smoke, dust, pollen
	Sunstroke
	Motion sickness

Source: Adapted from Thomas, CL (ed): Taber's Cyclopedic Medical Dictionary, ed 18. FA Davis, Philadelphia, 1997, p 844, with permission.

spine, and a lumbar puncture to detect abnormalities in the **cerebrospinal fluid** (CSF).

TREATMENT The course of treatment chosen is entirely determined by the cause of the headache. Analgesics are generally effective in providing temporary, symptomatic relief of headache pain. Ultimately, though, any underlying cause must be treated as well.

PROGNOSIS The prognosis for most acute headaches is good. The prognosis for chronic headaches is more variable and is usually determined by the nature and severity of the underlying cause.

PREVENTION Prevention of acute and chronic headaches is dependent on the cause.

MIGRAINE HEADACHE

DESCRIPTION A *migraine headache* is a recurrent, frequently incapacitating type of headache characterized by intense, throbbing pain often accompanied by nausea and vomiting. Migraine headaches usually begin in adolescence or early adulthood and diminish slowly in frequency and intensity with advancing age. Women are affected more than twice as frequently as men.

ETIOLOGY Migraine headaches are occasioned by changes in the cerebral blood flow, presumably due to vasoconstriction and subsequent vasodilation of cerebral-cranial arterioles. What initiates this process, however, is not known. Susceptibility to migraine headaches may be hereditary.

SIGNS AND SYMPTOMS Prior to the onset of pain, many migraine sufferers report symptoms such as flashing lights before their eyes, photophobia, or **tinnitus.** Other symptoms occurring before the migraine attack (called *premonitory symptoms*) may include unusual thirst, craving for sweet foods, and alterations in mood or mental clarity. Once the pain of the attack begins, it is typically accompanied by nausea, vomiting, and photophobia.

DIAGNOSTIC PROCEDURES The diagnosis depends on the medical history. A recurrent pattern of severe headaches preceded by any of the classic premonitory symptoms noted previously suggests the diagnosis of migraine headache.

TREATMENT Drug therapy may include the use of ergot preparations, which in some cases forestall an impending attack or lessen the severity of an ongoing attack. Simple analgesics, however, may be all that are necessary. In some cases, no treatment is chosen other than bed rest in a quiet, darkened room for the duration of the attack. More recently, biofeedback and relaxation exercises have been used successfully in some cases to lessen the number of attacks.

PROGNOSIS The prognosis varies. No form of therapy has proved successful in permanently disrupting the cycle of migraine attacks. As noted earlier, migraine headaches tend to become less frequent and less severe with age.

PREVENTION There is no specific prevention for migraine headaches.

 ALTERNATIVE MEDICINE

Alternative medicine suggests several methods for treating headaches:

- **Diet:** Food allergies can be a major source of headache pain. Common offenders include refined sugars, chocolate, sodas, alcohol, nuts, and dried fruit. These should be omitted from the diet if they are suspected of causing pain.
- **Herbs:** Ginkgo biloba, garlic, and onion may be effective in providing headache relief. Powdered ginger, cayenne pepper, chamomile, coriander, and bay leaves also can be useful.
- **Bodywork:** Massage and acupressure are beneficial in releasing muscle tension, thereby reducing headaches. Many bodywork therapies require a professional, but acupressure self-help techniques can be practiced by anyone. Acupressure involves placing pressure with the thumbs and the index fingers on various points on the back of the neck and near the bridge of the nose. Pressing fingertips into any area of the neck that is sore and tender can be helpful. Moving shoulders in a gentle rhythmic motion encourages relaxation and tension release.
- **Relaxation:** Techniques for relaxation include meditation, biofeedback, and yoga. Deep-breathing for five minutes is relaxing, and progressive muscle relaxation exercise can help prevent some headaches.
- **Hydrotherapy:** Another method of treating headaches without drugs is hydrotherapy. Hot baths, saunas, heat lamps, and steam baths reduce tension, increase circulation, and remove metabolic wastes from the body.

Head Trauma

Head trauma usually results from an accident, a blow to the head, or a serious fall. Recovery may be rapid or extended, depending on the severity of the trauma. It is important to watch an individual who has suffered head trauma for any signs of dizziness, nausea, severe headache, and loss of consciousness. The forms of head trauma considered here are hematomas, concussions, and contusions.

EPIDURAL AND SUBDURAL HEMATOMA (Acute)

DESCRIPTION An *epidural hematoma* is a mass of blood (usually clotted) formed between the skull and the outer membrane covering the brain, the *dura mater.* In a *subdural hematoma,* the blood collects between the dura mater and the second membrane covering the brain, the *arachnoid membrane* (Fig. 10–4). In both cases, pressure from the mass of blood can be sufficient to impair brain function.

ETIOLOGY Both epidural and subdural hematomas are caused by blood seeping from ruptured vessels above or below the dural membrane. The blood vessel damage occasioning an epidural hematoma is usually the result of a blow to the head, whereas a subdural hematoma is more often caused by the head striking an immovable object. Skull fractures are almost always accompanied by cerebral hematomas.

SIGNS AND SYMPTOMS The symptoms of epidural hematoma typically include an initial loss of consciousness followed by an intervening period of consciousness that may last from a few minutes to several hours. As the condition worsens, there may be **hemiparesis,** severe headache, and dilated pupils. These symptoms may appear within a short period of time or over a period of days, depending on the rate at which blood accumulates. Subdural hematomas generally exhibit similar symptoms but with a delayed onset because the blood typically accumulates more slowly. Loss of consciousness will occur, however, as well as weakness on one or both sides of the body. Nausea, vomiting, dizziness, and convulsions may also be found.

DIAGNOSTIC PROCEDURES The individual's clinical picture and a medical history revealing head trauma should suggest a potential diagnosis of epidural or subdural hematoma. Skull x-rays or CT scans and cerebral angiography may be ordered to pinpoint the position of the hematoma.

TREATMENT It may be necessary to perform a **craniotomy** to aspirate the accumulated blood and control further bleeding. Surgery may be performed on an emergency basis if rising intracranial pressure proves life-threatening.

PROGNOSIS The prognosis for both epidural and subdural hematomas is always guarded. Barring any complications, a person can recover with few,

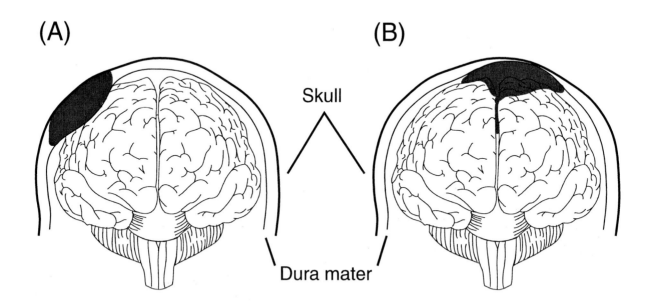

(A)

(B)

Skull

Dura mater

Epidural hematoma

Subdural hematoma

Figure 10–4 Intracranial hemorrhage. (*A*) Epidural hematoma—arterial bleeding between the skull and dura mater. (*B*) Subdural hematoma—venous bleeding between the dura mater and brain. Note that the meningeal spaces have been enlarged for clarity. (From Starkey, C, and Ryan, JL: Evaluation of Orthopedic and Athletic Injuries. FA Davis, Philadelphia, 1996, p 494, with permission.)

if any, residual effects. In serious cases, however, irreversible brain damage may result.

PREVENTION The best prevention is to minimize the risk of head trauma.

CEREBRAL CONCUSSION

DESCRIPTION A *cerebral concussion* is an immediate loss of consciousness, typically lasting from a few seconds to a few minutes, followed by a short period of amnesia. The reaction of a boxer who has just been "knocked out" is a classic example of cerebral concussion.

ETIOLOGY This condition is usually caused by a blunt impact to the head of sufficient force to cause the brain to strike and rebound from the skull. The loss of consciousness, subsequent amnesia, and other bodily symptoms of cerebral concussion are due to disruption of normal electrical activity in the brain. The brain tissue itself is usually not injured.

SIGNS AND SYMPTOMS Primary symptoms are temporary loss of consciousness with shallow respirations, depressed pulse rate, and flaccid muscle tone. After regaining consciousness, there is usually a variable period of amnesia that may be accompanied by **bradycardia,** faintness, pallor, **hypotension,** and photophobia. Delayed symptoms may include headache, nausea, vomiting, and blurred vision.

DIAGNOSTIC PROCEDURES A careful neurological assessment will typically be performed. Cranial CT scans will usually reveal no evidence of brain tissue damage (compare with Cerebral Contusion). Skull x-rays and magnetic resonance imaging (MRI) may prove helpful.

TREATMENT Treatment usually involves nothing more than quiet bed rest. The affected individual should be closely watched for any behavioral changes that may indicate progressive brain injury. If pain exists, a mild analgesic may be ordered.

PROGNOSIS If the individual remains alert with only one or two symptoms such as headache, nausea, a brief episode of vomiting, impaired concentration, or slightly blurred vision, the prognosis is usually good, with a low risk of subsequent complications.

Brain edema is a life-threatening complication most often seen in child and adolescent concussion victims.

PREVENTION Prevention of concussions includes following safety measures that minimize the risk of head injury, such as the use of approved head protection when playing sports and riding bikes, and the use of seat belts while driving.

CEREBRAL CONTUSION

DESCRIPTION A *cerebral contusion* is a serious injury in which the tissue along or just beneath the surface of the brain is bruised. Blood from broken vessels usually accumulates in the surrounding brain tissue.

ETIOLOGY Cerebral contusions are produced by a blow to the head or the impact of the head against a surface that causes the hemispheres of the brain to twist against or slide along the inner surface of the skull. The twisting or shearing force may be sufficient to damage deep structures in the brain as well.

SIGNS AND SYMPTOMS The signs and symptoms of cerebral contusions vary according to the location and extent of the tissue injury to the brain. Symptoms may range from transient loss of consciousness to coma. When conscious, an individual may exhibit hemiparesis, severe headache, and a variety of behavioral disturbances, ranging from lethargy, apathy, and drowsiness on the one hand, to hostility and combativeness on the other.

DIAGNOSTIC PROCEDURES A thorough neurological assessment is required. Skull x-rays may be necessary to rule out a fracture. Cranial CT scans will typically reveal the location and extent of tissue damage produced by a cerebral contusion.

TREATMENT The treatment required varies according to the location and severity of the contusion. Contusion victims need to be hospitalized so that their vital signs can be monitored and so that rapid medical intervention can take place should it be required.

PROGNOSIS The prognosis for cerebral contusion is always guarded, ultimately depending on the extent of the brain injury. Sudden, progressive edema of the brain with a consequent escalation of intracranial pressure is a serious, life-threatening complication of cerebral contusion. Other complications include cerebral hemorrhage and epidural or subdural **hematoma.** Permanent neurological deficits may result from contusions, including epilepsy caused by scar tissue formation at the site of the contusion.

PREVENTION See preventive measures for cerebral concussion.

Paralysis

HEMIPLEGIA

DESCRIPTION *Hemiplegia* is the loss of voluntary muscular control and sensation on one side of the body only.

ETIOLOGY Hemiplegia is most frequently caused by disease processes such as cerebrovascular accident (CVA) that disrupt the blood supply to the brain and brain stem. The condition also may result from cerebral contusion and epidural or subdural hematoma resulting from head trauma. Damage to the right side of the brain causes left-sided paralysis, and vice versa.

SIGNS AND SYMPTOMS Symptoms of hemiplegia include paralysis or weakness of the arm, leg, and (usually) face on one side of the body. The condition often is accompanied by communication disorders such as **aphasia, agnosia, apraxia, agraphia,** and **alexia.** The onset of these symptoms may be sudden, as in the case of CVA, or may occur more gradually, as in the case of a tumor.

DIAGNOSTIC PROCEDURES A thorough neurological assessment is necessary. Cranial CT scans, a complete blood analysis, and an electroencephalogram (EEG) may be performed as well.

TREATMENT Treatment is directed at the cause of the hemiplegia. Otherwise, treatment measures are largely supportive. Physical rehabilitation should begin as soon as possible.

PROGNOSIS The extent of neurological damage determines, in part, the prognosis. Physical rehabilitation, always an arduous process, is the best hope for recovering lost motor and sensory function.

PREVENTION There are no specific preventive measures for hemiplegia.

SPINAL CORD INJURIES: PARAPLEGIA AND QUADRIPLEGIA

DESCRIPTION Spinal cord injuries often are characterized by the degree of motor and sensory disability they occasion. *Paraplegia* is the loss of voluntary motion or sensation (paralysis) of the trunk and lower extremities. *Quadriplegia* is paralysis of all four extremities and, usually, the trunk.

ETIOLOGY In general, spinal cord injury resulting in paraplegia or quadriplegia is a consequence of fracture, dislocation, or both, of the vertebral column. The location of the spinal cord injury, the type of trauma inflicted on the cord, and the severity of that trauma determines whether paraplegia or quadriplegia may result. Refer to Figure 10–5 while reading the remaining discussion for a better understanding of the location of spinal cord injuries resulting in paraplegia or quadriplegia.

Spinal cord injury resulting in paraplegia is usually due to trauma to the thoracic and lumbar portions of the vertebral column (T1 or lower). Trauma that produces vertical compression and twisting (flexion) of this portion of the spinal cord is the usual mechanism of injury.

Spinal cord trauma at or above C5 in the cervical portion of the vertebral column may result in quadriplegia. Injuries between C5 and C7 may result in varying degrees of motor and sensory weakness in the arms and shoulders. Injuries above C3 usually result in death. Trauma that produces stretching (hyperextension) or flexion of this portion of the spinal cord is the usual mechanism of injury.

SIGNS AND SYMPTOMS Loss of motor and sensory functions in the legs and trunk are the symptoms of paraplegia. Bowel, bladder, and sexual function also may be lost.

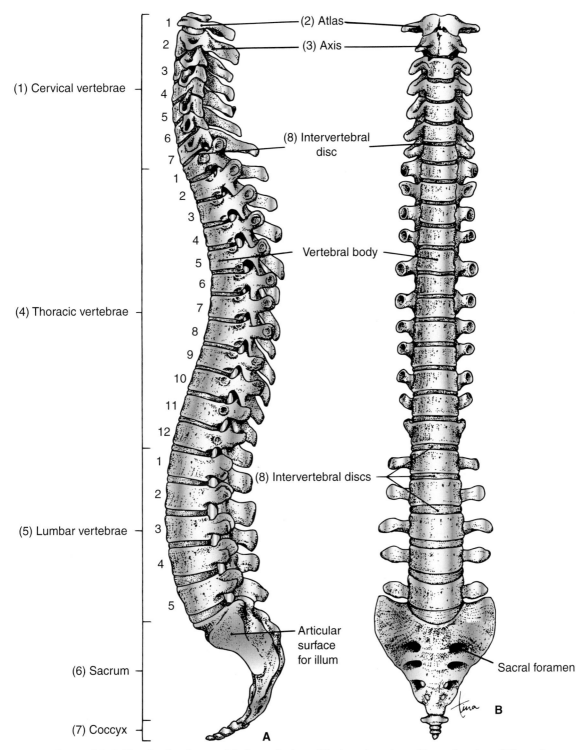

(1) Cervical vertebrae

(2) Atlas

(3) Axis

(8) Intervertebral disc

(4) Thoracic vertebrae

Vertebral body

(5) Lumbar vertebrae

(8) Intervertebral discs

Articular surface for illum

(6) Sacrum

Sacral foramen

(7) Coccyx

A

B

Figure 10–5 Vertebral column. (*A*) Lateral view. (*B*) Anterior view. (From Scanlon, VC, and Sanders, T: Understanding Human Structure and Function. FA Davis, Philadelphia, 1997, p 95, with permission.)

The symptoms of quadriplegia are those of paraplegia and total or partial loss of motor and sensory functions in the upper limbs and trunk. These symptoms also may be accompanied by falling blood pressure and body temperature, bradycardia, and respiratory difficulties. In some cases, unassisted respiration may cease.

DIAGNOSTIC PROCEDURES A thorough neurological assessment is necessary. Spinal x-rays, spinal CT scans, and magnetic resonance imaging (MRI) will typically be performed to gauge the nature of the spinal cord injury, as well as to detect possible spinal **ischemia**, edema, or blockage of the flow of cerebrospinal fluid.

TREATMENT The treatment goals for all spinal cord injuries include (1) restoration of spinal alignment, (2) stabilization of the injured spinal area, (3) decompression of compressed neurological structures, and (4) early rehabilitation to an active, productive life. Much of the early treatment effort is directed at preventing progressive spinal cord tissue damage that may occur following the initial trauma. This may involve surgery, the use of specialized drugs, or cooling the affected portion of the spine.

PROGNOSIS The prognosis for individuals with spinal cord injuries is always guarded. It may take several months to adequately assess the extent of the paralysis. If the damage to the spinal cord is complete, there is little hope of regaining lost motor and sensory functions. In general, though, the sooner treatment procedures are begun following an incident of spinal cord trauma, the better the prognosis.

PREVENTION Preventing paraplegia and quadriplegia involves following safety measures that minimize the risk of spinal cord injury. Such measures include wearing seat belts while driving, checking the water depth before diving into any body of water, and wearing protective gear when participating in contact sports.

Infections of the Central Nervous System

Infections of the CNS can be caused by almost any bacterial or viral agent. Certain symptoms of CNS infections are fairly common. These include headache, fever, sensory disturbances, neck and back stiffness, positive **Kernig's** and **Brudzinski's signs,** and CSF abnormalities. Such infections usually constitute a medical emergency, and immediate steps must be taken to diagnose and treat the condition.

■ ACUTE BACTERIAL MENINGITIS

DESCRIPTION *Acute bacterial meningitis* is inflammation of the three-layer membrane called the *meninges* that surrounds the brain and spinal cord (Fig. 10–6). This disease is considered a medical emergency.

ETIOLOGY The principal bacterial agents causing this disease are *Hemophilus influenzae* type B, *Neisseria meningitidis,* and *Streptococcus pneumoniae.* Many other bacteria also may cause the condition. The disease often arises as a complication of other bacterial infections elsewhere in the body, such as pneumonia, osteomyelitis, endocarditis, and otitis media. The disease also may follow in the wake of head trauma.

SIGNS AND SYMPTOMS In addition to the common signs noted above, acute bacterial meningitis is usually marked by the sudden onset of severe headache, vomiting, and seizures. **Nuchal rigidity,** particularly upon bending the neck forward, is a classic sign of acute bacterial meningitis. Initial drowsiness may progress to **stupor** or **coma.**

DIAGNOSTIC PROCEDURES A thorough medical history and physical examination are essential. The diagnosis is usually established by performing a lumbar puncture to confirm elevated cerebrospinal fluid pressure and to analyze the CSF for the presence of bacteria and elevated levels of proteins and leukocytes (Fig. 10–7). Blood, urine, and throat cultures also may be useful in isolating the infectious agent. Chest, skull, and sinus x-rays and an EEG may be ordered.

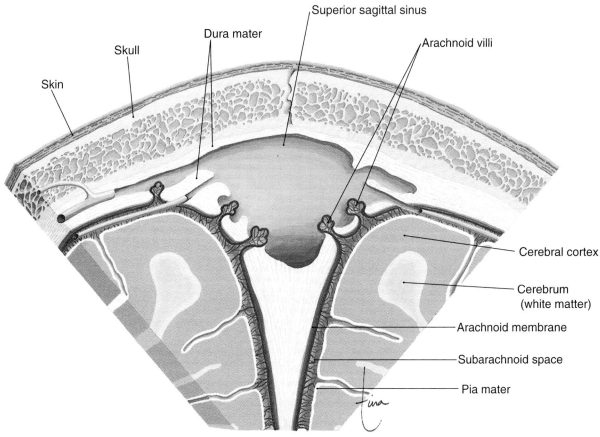

Skin

Skull

Dura mater

Superior sagittal sinus

Arachnoid villi

Cerebral cortex

Cerebrum
(white matter)

Arachnoid membrane

Subarachnoid space

Pia mater

Figure 10–6 The structure of the meninges. The frontal section through the top of the skull shows the double-layered dura mater and one of the cervical venous sinuses. (From Scanlon, VC, and Sanders, T: Essentials of Anatomy and Physiology, ed 3. FA Davis, Philadelphia, 1999, p 172, with permission.)

TREATMENT An aggressive, sustained course of antibiotic therapy is usually begun as soon as possible. Supportive therapy includes measures to lessen brain swelling and prevent blockage in the movement of cerebrospinal fluid. Isolation may be required. Good nutrition and adequate fluid intake are important.

PROGNOSIS Acute bacterial meningitis can prove fatal, especially among infants and elderly persons. The prognosis is good, however, in the event of prompt diagnosis and effective treatment. Meningitis can cause lasting neurological damage in children, particularly hearing loss, retardation, and epilepsy.

PREVENTION There is no known prevention, but careful handling of excretions and proper hand-

washing techniques help prevent the spread of the disease.

◼ ENCEPHALITIS

DESCRIPTION *Encephalitis* is inflammation of the brain, especially of the cerebral hemisphere, cerebellum, or brain stem. The disease sometimes occurs in epidemic outbreaks.

ETIOLOGY The disease can be caused by any one of a group of four arboviruses (arthropod-borne viruses). As their name implies, these viruses are often spread by insects, principally mosquitoes. Less frequently, encephalitis arises following measles, varicella, rubella, herpes virus infection, and as a consequence of vaccination.

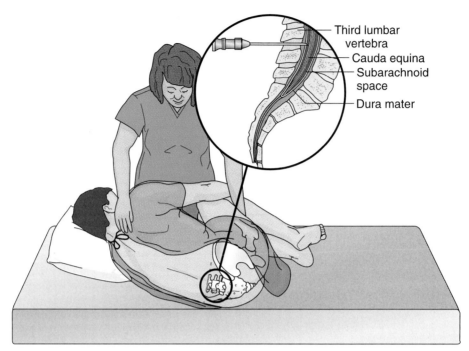

Third lumbar vertebra
Cauda equina
Subarachnoid space
Dura mater

Figure 10–7 Position for lumbar puncture. (From Williams, LS, and Hopper, PD [eds]: Understanding Medical-Surgical Nursing. FA Davis, Philadelphia, 1999, p 942, with permission.)

SIGNS AND SYMPTOMS Symptoms of encephalitis vary with age. The disease is frequently manifested in infants by the sudden onset of fever and convulsions. Children may experience headache, fever, and drowsiness followed by nausea, vomiting, muscular pain, and stiff neck. Adults typically experience an abrupt onset of fever, nausea, and vomiting, accompanied by a severe headache. Varying degrees of mental confusion and disorientation are a hallmark of encephalitis in adults. Other symptoms may include diffuse muscle aching and photophobia.

DIAGNOSTIC PROCEDURES A careful medical history is necessary. Lumbar puncture and analysis of the cerebrospinal fluid is the most important diagnostic tool. Detection of a virus or its antibody in the CSF or blood serum will confirm the diagnosis. The fluid also may show evidence of increased leukocyte counts and high protein levels. EEGs, cranial CT scans, or MRI may prove useful in isolating a focal point of the infection.

TREATMENT Treatment is mostly supportive. Drug therapy may be employed to control convulsions and reduce inflammation and edema. It is important for the patient to receive adequate rest, nutrition, and fluid intake.

PROGNOSIS The prognosis varies according to the infecting species of virus, but it is generally guarded. Certain forms of the disease have high mortality rates. Severe bouts of the disease can leave survivors with lasting neurological impairments.

PREVENTION Control of insects known to be arbovirus carriers is the major way of preventing encephalitis.

■ BRAIN ABSCESS

DESCRIPTION *Brain abscess* is a collection of pus, usually found in the cerebellum or the frontal or temporal lobes of the cerebrum (Fig. 10–8). The pus accumulation may be free or encapsulated, may vary in size, and may occur at single or multiple sites.

ETIOLOGY Generally, a brain abscess is secondary to some other infection, such as otitis media, sinusi-

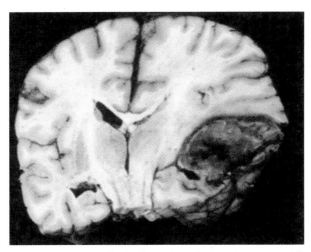

Figure 10–8 Cerebral abscesses. A young man with chronic otitis media developed an abscess in the temporal lobe, which then ruptured into the temporal horn of the lateral ventricle. (From Rubin, E, and Farber, JL [eds]: Pathology, ed 3. Lippincott-Raven, Philadelphia, 1999, p 1484, with permission.)

tis, or mastoiditis. Other causes include **bacteremia,** pulmonary infections, cranial trauma, or congenital heart disease.

SIGNS AND SYMPTOMS Signs and symptoms may include headache (which is usually worse in the morning), nausea, vomiting, disturbances in vision, hemiplegia, slowed pulse and respiration, fever, pallor, and drowsiness.

DIAGNOSTIC PROCEDURES A medical history revealing a recent or ongoing infection in the sinuses, ears, or respiratory tract and the clinical symptoms mentioned should suggest a diagnosis of brain abscess. Skull x-rays, an EEG, cranial CT scans, and cerebral angiography may help to localize the site of the infection. Lumbar puncture may confirm increased intracranial pressure.

TREATMENT Elimination of the abscess is the goal of treatment. **Antibiotics** are used in the treatment of the underlying infections. The pus needs to be drained, but surgery is not attempted unless the pus is encapsulated.

PROGNOSIS A brain abscess is usually fatal if untreated. With treatment, the prognosis is guarded owing to potential for damage to brain tissue.

PREVENTION The only known prevention is prompt treatment of any infections.

Peripheral Nerve Diseases

■ PERIPHERAL NEURITIS

DESCRIPTION *Peripheral neuritis* is a degeneration of the nerves supplying the distal muscles of the extremities. The syndrome is noninflammatory, most frequently affecting men between 30 and 50 years of age.

ETIOLOGY Causes include chronic alcohol intoxication or toxicity from poisons, drugs, or heavy metals. Infections such as meningitis, pneumonia, and tuberculosis may induce peripheral neuritis, as may metabolic disorders such as gout, diabetes mellitus, and lupus erythematosus. Additional causes include nutritional deficiencies and tumors.

SIGNS AND SYMPTOMS The onset is slow in most cases and may be marked by progressive muscular weakness, paresthesia, tenderness and pain, usually in the distal portions of the extremities. Physical wasting, loss of reflexes, and clumsiness may result.

DIAGNOSTIC PROCEDURES A thorough history and physical examination to determine motor and sensory deficits are necessary. Electromyography may be ordered.

TREATMENT The treatment depends on the cause. Toxins must be neutralized, infections and metabolic diseases treated, and nutritional deficiencies corrected. Analgesics and bed rest, especially of the affected limb, are essential. Physical therapy may be required to recover function of the affected limb or limbs.

PROGNOSIS The prognosis depends on how successfully the underlying cause can be treated and the extent of existing nerve damage.

PREVENTION Prevention includes prompt treatment of nutritional deficiencies, infections, and metabolic diseases. Avoidance of toxins is also essential for prevention.

BELL'S PALSY

DESCRIPTION *Bell's palsy* is a disorder of the facial nerve (the seventh cranial nerve) causing paralysis of the muscles on one side of the face. It is more common in persons between 20 and 60 years of age.

ETIOLOGY Bell's palsy is idiopathic, although possible causes may be tumors, vascular ischemia, autoimmune disease, or viral disease.

SIGNS AND SYMPTOMS Symptoms include facial weakness and characteristic drooping mouth. The sense of taste may be disrupted. Pain in the jaw or behind the ear may precede or accompany the paralysis. Another sign is *Bell's phenomenon,* where the eye cannot close completely. When the person attempts to close the eye, the eyeball rolls upward and the eye may tear excessively (Fig. 10–9).

DIAGNOSTIC PROCEDURES The clinical picture of the sudden, unexplained onset of facial paralysis suggests the diagnosis.

TREATMENT The affected portion of the face, particularly the eye, must be protected from trauma, wind, or temperature extremes. Electrical stimulation, massage, warm moist heat, and analgesia may be prescribed. Corticosteroid drugs may be prescribed in some instances.

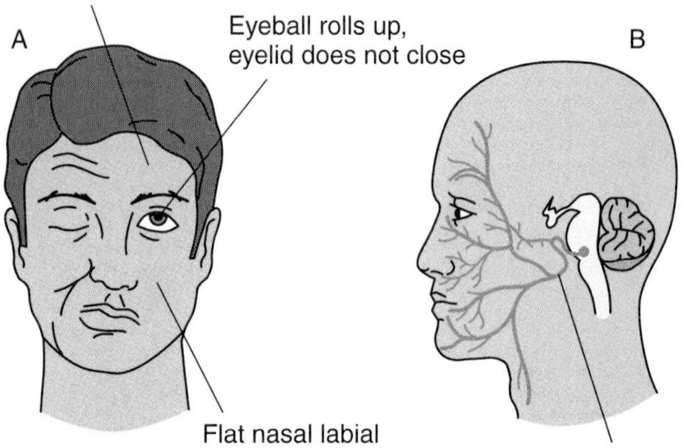

Forehead not wrinkled

Eyeball rolls up, eyelid does not close

Flat nasal labial fold, paralysis of lower face

Facial nerve

Figure 10–9 Bell's palsy. (*A*) Note the weakness of the affected side of the face. (*B*) The distribution of the facial nerve. (Modified from Lewis, SM, Collier, IC, and Heitkemper, MM: Medical-Surgical Nursing: Assessment and Management of Clinical Problems, ed 4. Mosby, St. Louis, p 1795, with permission.)

PROGNOSIS The prognosis is good in the majority of cases. The palsy usually disappears spontaneously within 1 to 8 weeks, but it can recur. If the palsy remains, facial **contractures** may develop.

PREVENTION There is no known prevention for Bell's palsy.

Cerebral Diseases/Disorders

CEREBROVASCULAR ACCIDENT
(Stroke)

DESCRIPTION *Cerebrovascular accident* (CVA) is a clinical syndrome marked by the sudden impairment of consciousness and subsequent paralysis. It is caused by occlusion or hemorrhaging of blood vessels supplying a portion of the brain. Deprived of adequate blood supply, the tissue in the affected portion of the brain becomes necrotic. The condition is commonly known as a *stroke*.

ETIOLOGY Three mechanisms may produce a stroke: cerebral hemorrhage, **thrombosis,** and **embolism** of cerebral arteries. These processes are chiefly a consequence of atherosclerotic disease. They also may result from a variety of blood disorders, hypertension, cardiac **arrhythmias,** systemic diseases such as diabetes mellitus or syphilis, head trauma, cerebral aneurysms, or rheumatic heart disease. Contributing factors include smoking, lack of exercise, a poor or high-fat diet, obesity, a family history of atherosclerotic disease, or the use of oral contraceptives.

SIGNS AND SYMPTOMS The signs and symptoms of CVA reflect the portion of the brain involved in the attack and whether the attack is caused by a thrombus, an embolus, or a hemorrhage. The symptoms of strokes caused by an embolus or a hemorrhage are often sudden in onset, whereas those caused by a thrombus may appear more gradually. Common symptoms include impaired consciousness ranging from stupor to coma, **Cheyne-Stokes respiration,** full and slow pulse, and hemiparesis. Other symptoms include **dysphasia,** numbness, sensory disturbances, **diplopia,** poor coordination, confusion, and dizziness.

DIAGNOSTIC PROCEDURES Cerebral angiography and EEGs are useful in confirming the diagnosis. Cranial CT scans and MRI often prove useful in pinpointing the affected portion of the brain and in determining the mechanism that produced the stroke.

TREATMENT Treatment of CVA depends on the severity of the event and whether it was hemorrhagic, thrombotic, or embolic in origin. General treatment protocols may include drug therapy (anticoagulant or antiplatelet agents) or surgery to improve cerebral circulation or to remove clots. Other therapeutic procedures may include measures to guard against or to control brain edema. Physical rehabilitation is necessary for most stroke clients; it needs to be started early and continued until they are able to do as much for themselves as possible.

PROGNOSIS The prognosis for an individual experiencing a CVA is determined by the extent of damage to the affected portion of the brain. In general, the greater the delay in recovery following the event, the poorer the ultimate prognosis. Some individuals may remain permanently disabled or have a recurrence.

PREVENTION Prevention includes prompt treatment of cardiac and circulatory problems and avoidance of predisposing factors such as smoking, lack of exercise, and a high-fat diet.

■ TRANSIENT ISCHEMIC ATTACKS (TIAs)

DESCRIPTION *Transient ischemic attacks* are temporary, often recurrent episodes of impaired neurological activity resulting from insufficient blood flow to a part of the brain. These "little strokes" may last for seconds or hours, after which the symptoms gradually subside. TIAs share a common pathophysiology with strokes and may serve as a warning of an impending CVA.

ETIOLOGY TIAs are caused by the temporary obstruction of cerebral arterioles by very small emboli or by ischemia of a small portion of brain tissue due to arterial narrowing in that region. These processes are usually the result of atherosclerotic disease. (See Cerebrovascular Accident [Stroke] for other potential causes and risk factors.)

SIGNS AND SYMPTOMS The particular combination of symptoms during a TIA, like those for a CVA, depend on which portion of the brain is affected. Symptoms may include the sudden onset of muscle weakness in the arm, leg, or foot on one side of the body. Other symptoms may include double vision, speech deficits, dizziness, and staggering or uncoordinated gait. TIAs generally do not result in unconsciousness.

DIAGNOSTIC PROCEDURES EEGs, cranial CT scans, and cranial MRIs are helpful in isolating the area of ischemia within the brain.

TREATMENT The course of treatment selected depends on the location of the area of ischemia and the underlying cause. Antiplatelet agents and aspirin or anticoagulant drugs are typically used to treat an ongoing attack and minimize the chance of another. Surgery to promote blood flow to the affected area may be attempted in certain cases.

PROGNOSIS The prognosis for an individual experiencing transient ischemic attacks is dependent upon the underlying cause. Although the symptoms subside, TIAs tend to be recurrent and may signal an impending cerebrovascular accident.

PREVENTION See preventive measures for cerebrovascular accident.

■ EPILEPSY

DESCRIPTION *Epilepsy* is a chronic brain disorder characterized by recurring attacks of abnormal sensory, motor, and psychological activity. During these attacks, the individual may or may not lose consciousness. Each attack of epileptic episode is called a seizure. Not all seizures are epilepsy, though. Epileptic seizures exhibit a chronic pattern, with similar characteristics at each recurrence. Epilepsy represents a disruption of the normal pattern of electrical activity within the brain. During an epileptic seizure, neurons within the brain discharge in a random, intense manner. This hyperactivity may be focused within a small section of the brain or involve several areas of the brain at once. Epilepsy can begin at any time of life.

Seizures generally are categorized as partial or generalized. *Partial* seizures are focal in origin: that is, they affect only one part of the brain and cause specific symptoms. *Generalized* seizures are nonfocal in origin and may affect the entire brain.

ETIOLOGY Most cases of epilepsy are **idiopathic.** Epilepsies may follow birth trauma, congenital malformations of the brain, head trauma, CVA, CNS infections such as meningitis and encephalitis, or neoplasms. Other causes may include brain tissue damage produced by chemicals, drugs, and toxins, or degenerative brain disorders and structural defects of the brain.

SIGNS AND SYMPTOMS Individuals may experience a warning or "aura" of the impending seizure or no warning at all. Symptoms of the seizure may be a simple uncontrollable twitch of the finger, hand, or mouth. The person may be dizzy and experience unusual or unpleasant sights, sounds, or odors, all without losing consciousness. Some individuals experience sudden loss of consciousness and intense rigidity of the body, with alternating relaxation and contraction of muscles. A characteristic cry may be uttered. Cyanosis, inhibited respiration, incontinence, and chewing of the tongue may occur. After the seizure has passed, amnesia, headache, and drowsiness are common occurrences. Some individuals may sleep for hours following a seizure; others may not return to normal for days.

DIAGNOSTIC PROCEDURES A thorough medical history is essential. Recurrent seizures or a family history of epilepsy should suggest the diagnosis. Epilepsy is also indicated in the presence of seizures following head trauma, CNS infections, or CVA. Because many individuals with epilepsy exhibit abnormalities in brain-wave patterns, even between seizures, EEGs are very helpful in diagnosis. Cranial CT scans also are useful in pinpointing brain lesions that may be triggering seizures. MRIs provide clear images of the brain, show structural changes resulting from disorders, and also help to diagnose epilepsy.

TREATMENT An array of anticonvulsant drugs exists that have proved effective in controlling epileptic seizures. Because certain drugs are more effective in controlling specific forms of seizures, the client and the physician may have to engage in a process of trial and error before settling on one drug that best controls the individual's seizures with the fewest side effects. Neurosurgery may be attempted in some cases when a severe case of epilepsy can be traced to the presence of a specific, accessible brain lesion. Educating and counseling the person with epilepsy about the nature of the disease are an essential part of the treatment process.

PROGNOSIS The prognosis varies from case to case. The prognosis is good if a course of drug therapy can be found that effectively suppresses the seizures. An individual in these circumstances can generally expect to live a normal life. The prognosis is not so favorable if seizures cannot be controlled. Such individuals may have to lead a comparatively restricted existence.

PREVENTION Only certain forms of epilepsy are preventable. Preventive measures involve avoiding head injuries, prompt treatment of brain infections, and avoiding the abuse of drugs and alcohol.

Degenerative Diseases

ALZHEIMER'S DISEASE

DESCRIPTION *Alzheimer's disease,* formerly called *presenile dementia,* is a type of chronic organic brain syndrome characterized by the death of neurons in the cerebral cortex and their replacement by microscopic "plaques." The result is progressive intellectual impairment. The disease affects mainly people between 60 and 70 years old.

ETIOLOGY The cause of Alzheimer's disease is unknown, but hereditary factors, autoimmune reactions, and cellular changes of viral origin have all been proposed.

SIGNS AND SYMPTOMS The disease progresses through three distinct stages. The first stage exhibits mild mental impairment. This includes loss of short-term memory, inability to learn new things, and subtle changes in personality. In the second stage, there is increased forgetfulness, agitation, irritability, and extreme restlessness. In the third and final stage, clients are unable to care for themselves, are incontinent, and are unable to communicate. The rate at which an individual progresses through each stage varies. Within 5 to 10 years there is profound deterioration of intellectual ability and physical capability. The person becomes emotionally detached and may show sleep disturbances, restlessness, and hostility.

DIAGNOSTIC PROCEDURES The goal of diagnosis is to rule out other degenerative brain diseases producing similar symptoms. An EEG and cranial CT and MRI scans may be performed.

TREATMENT Treatment is merely palliative and directed toward maintaining nutrition, hydration, and safety. Emotional support of family members is important.

PROGNOSIS The prognosis is poor, with the disease progressing over a period of 5 to 10 years. Death may occur from secondary causes such as septic **decubitus ulcers** or pneumonia.

PREVENTION There is no known prevention. Research currently underway points increasingly to a genetic marker abnormality, which if identified and corrected may enable prevention of Alzheimer's disease.

■ PARKINSON'S DISEASE

DESCRIPTION *Parkinson's disease* is a chronic disease characterized by progressive muscle rigidity and involuntary tremors. Parkinson's is a common crippling disease in the United States, affecting more men than women, usually in their fifties and sixties.

ETIOLOGY The cause is unknown, but the condition may be related to a deficiency within the brain of a neurotransmitter chemical called *dopamine.* Dopamine is necessary for brain cell functioning.

SIGNS AND SYMPTOMS The onset of Parkinson's is slow and insidious. Symptoms eventually may include muscle weakness, progressively rigid extremities, and "pill-rolling" tremors beginning in the fingers. The individual's facial expression may appear fixed. Stress, fatigue, and anxiety tend to aggravate the tremors, whereas purposeful movement and sleep decrease the tremors. The person's intellect typically remains unaffected.

DIAGNOSTIC PROCEDURES Diagnosis is made on the basis of the unique set of physical symptoms characteristic of Parkinson's. The tremors and rigidity must be differentiated from the symptoms of other diseases. A urinalysis may be done to check the level of dopamine.

TREATMENT Treatment of Parkinson's disease is strictly palliative. Medical measures are usually withheld until the person has trouble with the activities of daily living. Then **anticholinergic** drugs may be prescribed. Levodopa, a dopamine replacement, may be used. Physical therapy and psychological support and reassurance are also necessary. If drug therapy is unsuccessful, certain surgical techniques may be attempted that destroy part of the thalamus and limit involuntary movement.

PROGNOSIS Although the disease is slowly progressive and debilitating, because of effective treatment strategies, many individuals with Parkinson's can live comparatively normal lives for many years. Dementia may ultimately result in a third of all cases.

PREVENTION There is no known prevention.

■ MULTIPLE SCLEROSIS

DESCRIPTION *Multiple sclerosis* (MS) is a chronic, progressive disease characterized by the destruction of the lipid and protein layer, the *myelin sheath,* that insulates and protects the axons of certain nerve cells. The demyelination process occurs at scattered sites throughout the CNS and results in progressive physical disability. The onset of MS usually occurs during early adulthood and rarely after 60 years of age. It occurs only slightly more frequently in women than men. The disease is a common cause of chronic disability.

ETIOLOGY The cause of MS is unknown, although immunologic, viral, and genetic etiologies have been proposed.

SIGNS AND SYMPTOMS Symptoms may include sudden, transient motor and sensory disturbances, impaired vision, muscle weakness, paralysis, incontinence, and mood swings such as euphoria or depression. The initial onset of symptoms, and later relapses, may occur following acute infection, trauma, serum injections, pregnancy, or stress. The symptoms usually come and go with no pattern or warning. They may last hours or weeks.

DIAGNOSTIC PROCEDURES A neurological examination, CSF analysis, and cranial CT and MRI scans may be useful in the diagnosis of MS. The disease is difficult to diagnose, however, because the onset may be mild and symptoms may take years to progress. Periodic testing and observation are usually necessary.

TREATMENT There is no specific treatment for MS. Treatment is directed at relieving symptoms and forestalling future attacks. Medications such as **adrenocorticotropic hormone** (**ACTH**), corticosteroids, and mood-altering drugs may be prescribed. Avoidance of temperature extremes and stress is important. Psychological counseling and physical therapy are essential.

PROGNOSIS Because the course of the disease is varied and unpredictable, the prognosis may be guarded. Individuals with MS experience remissions and exacerbations of symptoms, but as the disease progresses, remissions usually are incomplete and shorter in duration.

PREVENTION There is no known prevention for MS.

■ AMYOTROPHIC LATERAL SCLEROSIS (ALS)

DESCRIPTION *Amyotrophic lateral sclerosis,* commonly known as *Lou Gehrig's disease,* is a disease of motor neurons that result in progressive muscular atrophy and weakness. The disease generally occurs between 50 and 60 years of age, slightly more often in men when in women.

ETIOLOGY The cause is unknown, although some cases may be due to autosomal inherited traits.

SIGNS AND SYMPTOMS Symptoms of ALS include involuntary muscle contractions and muscular atrophy, weakness, and twitching, especially in the muscles of the extremities. The individual may have problems with speech, chewing, swallowing, and even breathing if the brain stem is affected. There is no sensory nerve involvement.

DIAGNOSTIC PROCEDURES The disease may be diagnosed on the basis of the presenting signs and symptoms. Electromyography and muscle biopsy will help ascertain whether there is nerve rather than muscle disease. It is necessary to rule out several other disorders that may produce similar symptoms, such as multiple sclerosis, spinal cord neoplasm, and myasthenia gravis.

TREATMENT There is no effective treatment for ALS. Treatment is symptomatic and may include emotional as well as physical support. Persons afflicted with the disease are likely to become confined to a wheelchair or a bed, need to be taught to suction themselves to prevent choking, require assistance with personal hygiene, and need a great deal of emotional support.

PROGNOSIS The prognosis is dependent on the area involved and the speed at which the disease progresses. ALS is usually fatal within 3 to 10 years after onset. Death most often results from respiratory failure or aspiration pneumonia.

PREVENTION There is no known prevention.

Cancer

■ TUMORS OF THE BRAIN

DESCRIPTION *Primary brain tumors* are benign or malignant neoplasms originating within the brain. *Secondary brain tumors* are the result of metastasis of neoplasms from elsewhere in the body. This latter category of tumors accounts for the majority of cases. Tumors cause neurological deterioration by replacing healthy brain tissue, by compressing brain tissue, or by blocking the blood supply or the flow of cerebrospinal fluid to a portion of the brain.

ETIOLOGY The cause is unknown.

SIGNS AND SYMPTOMS Brain tumors may be difficult to diagnose because of vague symptoms and their slow onset. The location of the growth in the brain will partially dictate the symptoms. Headache, vomiting, defective memory, mood changes, seizures, visual disturbances, motor impairment, and personality changes may occur.

DIAGNOSTIC PROCEDURES A complete history and physical examination, including neurological assessment, are essential. Skull x-rays, lumbar puncture, EEG, cranial CT and MRI scans, or biopsy of the lesion will confirm the diagnosis. Further studies may be done to locate the primary site of a metastatic brain tumor.

TREATMENT Surgery, radiation therapy, or chemotherapy—individually or in combination—may be used to treat the tumor. Medications may be ordered for symptomatic treatment of seizures, edema, and headache.

PROGNOSIS The prognosis is dependent on the size, location, and type of tumor.

PREVENTION There is no known prevention.

COMMON SYMPTOMS OF NERVOUS SYSTEM DISEASES

Individuals may present with the following common symptoms, which deserve attention from health professionals:

- Headache
- Weakness
- Nausea and vomiting
- Motor disturbances such as stiff neck or back, rigid muscles, seizures, convulsions, or paralysis
- Sensory disturbances of any kind, especially vision or speech
- Drowsiness, stupor, or coma
- Mood swings
- Fever

BIBLIOGRAPHY

The Burton Goldberg Group (ed): Alternative Medicine: The Definitive Guide. Future Medicine Publishing, Fife, Wash., 1995.

Fauci, AS, et al: Harrison's Principles of Internal Medicine, ed 14. McGraw-Hill, New York, 1998.

Frazier, MS, Drzymkowski, JA, and Doty, SJ: Essentials of Human Disease and Conditions. WB Saunders, Philadelphia, 1996.

Mulvihill, ML: Human Diseases A Systemic Approach. Appleton & Lange, Stamford, Conn., 1995.

Professional Guide to Diseases, ed 6. Springhouse Corporation, Springhouse, Pa., 1998.

CASE STUDIES

I You answer the phone at the medical office in which you work as a medical assistant. The call is from a client who is concerned about his aging mother who lives alone. She is extremely forgetful, is easily agitated, and has a compulsion to be busy at all times. She had been out to dinner last night and could not remember how to get home, although she is able to recall moments from her son's childhood.

1. What diseases or disorders may the physician wish to discuss with this client?

2. Would the client want to consider an alternative living arrangement for his mother? Why? What kind of arrangements might be considered?

II The husband of a 45-year-old woman calls for an appointment for his wife. She is exhibiting progressive muscular atrophy and weakness in all her extremities. She has difficulty talking, chewing, and swallowing.

1. What diagnostic procedures might the physician order?

2. What disease or disorder might be causing such symptoms?

3. What support services will this woman need?

REVIEW QUESTIONS

MATCHING

_____ 1. Sensory loss in lower extremities

_____ 2. Sensory loss in all extremities

_____ 3. Unilateral sensory loss

a. Quadriplegia
b. Paraplegia
c. Hemiplegia

SHORT ANSWER

1. List at least four common signs and symptoms of CNS infections:

   a.

   b.

   c.

   d.

2. Name and define the two classifications of seizures:

   a.

   b.

3. Another term for *cerebrovascular accident* is _____ .

4. What are TIAs?

5. List the three stages of Alzheimer's disease.

6. Can a brain abscess exhibit signs and symptoms similar to a brain tumor? Explain.

7. Name the disease:

   a. _____ is progressive demyelination throughout the CNS.

   b. _____ is progressive muscle rigidity and involuntary tremors.

TRUE/FALSE

T   F   1. Peripheral neuritis is an inflammatory degeneration of peripheral nerves.

T   F   2. The onset of peripheral neuritis is rapid in most cases.

T   F   3. Bell's palsy is a disease of a facial nerve, the fifth cranial nerve.

T   F   4. The prognosis of Bell's palsy is good.

ANSWERS

MATCHING

1. b   2. a   3. c

SHORT ANSWER

1. Headache, fever, sensory disturbances, neck and back stiffness, positive Kernig's and Brudzinski's signs, and cerebrospinal fluid abnormalities.
2. a. Partial seizures—focal in origin; affect only part of the brain.
   b. Generalized seizures—nonspecific in origin; affect the entire brain.
3. Stroke.
4. TIAs are transient ischemic attacks, recurrent episodes of neurological deficit resulting from lack of blood flow to a part of the brain, "little strokes."
5. The three stages of Alzheimer's disease are (1) mild mental impairment; (2) forgetfulness, agitation, irritability, and extreme restlessness; and (3) incontinence, inability to communicate, and inability to care for self.
6. Yes, the signs and symptoms of a brain tumor and abscess may be similar, that is, headache, nausea, vomiting, decreased vision, hemiparesis, slowed pulse and respiration, fever, pallor, and drowsiness. Both apply pressure on the brain; both are abnormal.
7. a. Multiple sclerosis.
8. b. Parkinson's disease.

TRUE/FALSE

1. False   3. False
2. False   4. True

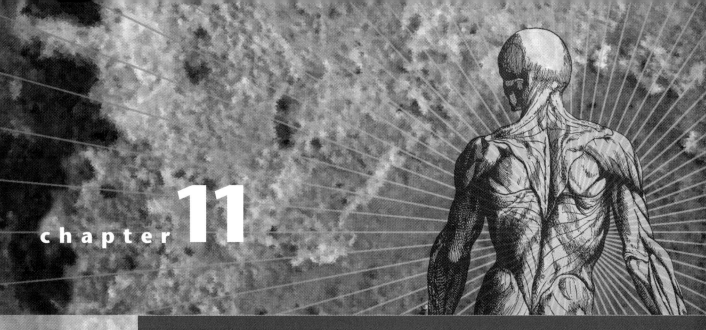

chapter 11

Endocrine System Diseases

CHAPTER OUTLINE

Pituitary Gland Diseases
Hyperpituitarism (Gigantism, Acromegaly)
Hypopituitarism
Diabetes Insipidus

Thyroid Gland Diseases
Simple Goiter
Hashimoto's Thyroiditis
Hyperthyroidism (Graves' Disease)
Hypothyroidism (Cretinism, Myxedema)

Parathyroid Gland Diseases
Hyperparathyroidism (Hypercalcemia)

Hypoparathyroidism (Hypocalcemia)

Adrenal Gland Disease
Cushing's Syndrome

Endocrine Dysfunction of the Pancreas
Diabetes Mellitus

**Common Symptoms of Endocrine
   System Diseases**

Bibliography

Case Studies

Review Questions

LEARNING OBJECTIVES
Upon successful completion of this chapter, you will:
- Describe the two forms of hyperpituitarism.
- Discuss the signs and symptoms of hypopituitarism.
- Identify the classic symptoms of diabetes insipidus.
- Recall the cause of simple goiter.
- Explain the treatment for Hashimoto's thyroiditis.
- Recognize the signs and symptoms of hyperthyroidism.
- Compare cretinism with myxedema.
- Relate hypercalcemia to hyperparathyroidism.
- Relate hypocalcemia to hypoparathyroidism.
- Review the classic symptoms of Cushing's syndrome.
- Recall the etiology of diabetes mellitus.
- Report the treatment of diabetes mellitus.
- Describe the complications of diabetes mellitus.
- List at least four common symptoms of endocrine diseases.

KEY WORDS
Adenoma (ăd•ĕ•nō′mă)
Amenorrhea (ă•mĕn•ō•rē′ă)
Cyanosis (sī•ă•nō′sĭs)
Dysphagia (dĭs•fā′jē•ă)
Exophthalmos (ĕks•ŏf•thăl′mōs)
Glycosuria (glī•kō•sū′rē•ă)
Goitrogens (goy′trō•jĕns)
Hyperplasia (hī•pĕr•plā′zē•ă)
Iatrogenic (ī•ăt•rō•jĕn′ĭk)
Idiopathic (ĭd•ē•ō•păth′ĭk)

Ketoacidosis (kē•tō•ă•sĭ•dō′sĭs)
Menorrhagia (mĕn•ō•rǎ′jē•ă)
Paresthesia (păr•ĕs•thē′zē•ă)
Polydipsia (pŏl•ē•dĭp′sē•ă)
Polyphagia (pŏl•ē•fā′jē•ă)
Polyuria (pŏl•ē•ū′rē•ă)
Pruritus (proo•rī′tŭs)
Retinopathy (rĕt•ĭn•ŏp′ă•thē)
Syncope (sĭn′kō•pē)
Tetany (tĕt′ă•nē)
Vasopressin (văs•ō•prĕs′ĭn)

The endocrine system consists of a group of ductless glands that act to regulate many of the body's physiological processes. Each type of endocrine gland produces one or more secretions that are discharged into the blood or lymph and circulated to all parts of the body. These secretions are called *hormones*. A hormone is a chemical substance that produces a specific effect on a particular type of tissue, on an organ, or on the body as a whole.

The principal organs of the endocrine system include the pituitary gland, the thyroid gland, the parathyroid glands, the adrenal glands, and the pineal body (the function of this gland is not known). In addition to their other roles, the pancreas and the testes or ovaries also have important endocrine functions. The hypothalamus releases hormones that offset the production of some other hormones. Figure 11–1 shows the location of the endocrine glands within the body. Table 11–1 lists the hormones produced by the principal endocrine glands and summarizes their major effects on the body.

The secretion of hormones by the endocrine system is governed by an amazingly intricate interrelationship between the glands themselves, the nervous system, and the levels of various substances in the blood. Dysfunction of an endocrine gland may result in either too little secretion of its hormone (*hyposecretion*) or too much (*hypersecretion*). Because of the effect this system has on the entire body, many disease conditions result from or are associated with endocrine dysfunction.

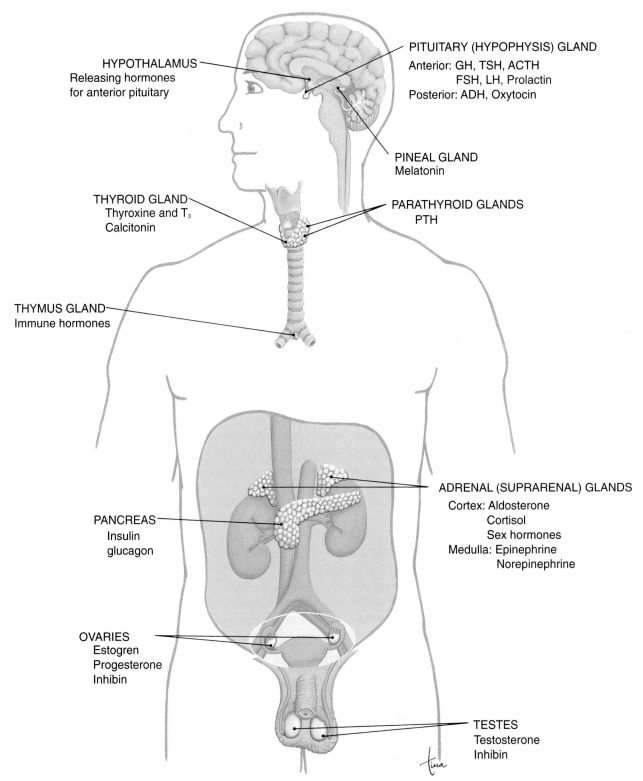

Figure 11–1 The endocrine system. The location of many endocrine glands. Both male and female gonads (testes and ovaries) are shown. (From Scanlon, VC, and Sanders, T: Essentials of Anatomy and Physiology, ed 3. FA Davis, Philadelphia, 1999, p 211, with permission.)

Table 11–1 **Principal Endocrine Glands**

Name	Position	Function	Endocrine Disorders
Adrenal cortex	Outer portion of gland on top of each kidney	Steroid hormones regulate carbohydrate and fat metabolism and salt and water balance	Hypofunction: Addison's disease Hyperfunction: Adrenogenital syndrome; Cushing's syndrome
Adrenal medulla	Inner portion of adrenal gland; surrounded by adrenal cortex	Effects mimic those of sympathetic nervous system; increases carbohydrate use of energy	Hypofunction: Almost unknown Hyperfunction: Pheochromocytoma
Pancreas (endocrine portion)	Abdominal cavity; head adjacent to duodenum; tail close to spleen and kidney	Secretes insulin and glucagon, which regulate carbohydrate metabolism	Hypofunction: Diabetes mellitus Hyperfunction: If a tumor produces excess insulin, hypoglycemia
Parathyroid	Four or more small glands on back of thyroid	Calcium and phosphorus metabolism; indirectly affects muscular irritability	Hypofunction: Tetany Hyperfunction: Resorption of bone; renal calculi
Pituitary, anterior	Front portion of small gland below hypothalamus	Influences growth, sexual development, skin pigmentation, thyroid function, adrenocortical function through effects on other endocrine glands (except for growth hormone, which acts directly on cells)	Hypofunction: Dwarfism in child; decrease in all other endocrine gland functions except parathyroids Hyperfunction: Acromegaly in adult; gigantism in child
Pituitary, posterior	Back portion of small gland below hypothalamus	Oxytocin increases uterine contraction Antidiuretic hormone increases absorption of water by kidney tubule	Unknown Hypofunction: Diabetes mellitus
Testes and ovaries	Testes—in the scrotum Ovaries—in the pelvic cavity	Development of secondary sex characteristics; some effects on growth	Hypofunction: Lack of sex development or regression in adult Hyperfunction; Abnormal sex development
Thyroid	Two lobes in anterior portion of neck	Increases metabolic rate; indirectly influences growth and nutrition	Hypofunction: Cretinism in young; myxedema in adult; goiter Hyperfunction: Goiter; thyrotoxicosis

Source: Thomas, CL (ed): Taber's Cyclopedic Medical Dictionary, ed 18. FA Davis, Philadelphia, 1997, p 637, with permission.

Pituitary Gland Diseases

■ HYPERPITUITARISM (Gigantism, Acromegaly)

DESCRIPTION *Hyperpituitarism* is the hypersecretion of growth hormone (GH) by a portion of the pituitary gland. Two distinct conditions may result from hyperpituitarism, depending on the time of life at which this dysfunction begins. *Gigantism* results from the hypersecretion of GH during an individual's growing years, especially prior to puberty (Figure 11–2). The person with gigantism grows abnormally tall, although the relative proportion of the body parts and sexual development remain unaffected. When GH hypersecretion occurs during adulthood, *acromegaly* results. Acromegaly is a chronic, disfiguring, life-shortening disease characterized by the overgrowth of bones and soft tissues (Fig. 11–3).

ETIOLOGY The hypersecretion of GH that produces gigantism and acromegaly is typically due to benign, slow-growing **adenomas** in the anterior pituitary. Not subject to normal control, these neoplastic cells release abnormally high levels of GH. A genetic cause has been suggested.

SIGNS AND SYMPTOMS The principal symptom of gigantism is excessive growth of the long bones of the body. This results in an abnormal increase in

Figure 11–2 Gigantism and dwarfism caused respectively by the overproduction or underproduction of the growth hormone (GH) during childhood and adolescence. (Photo by Michael Serino/ The Picture Cube.)

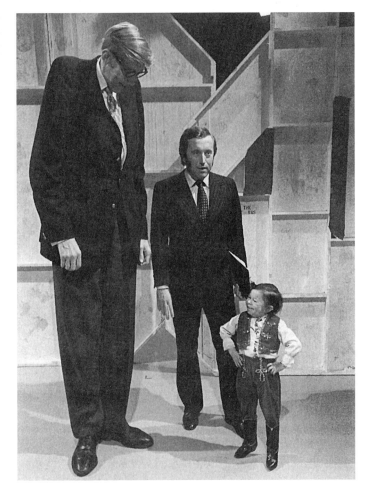

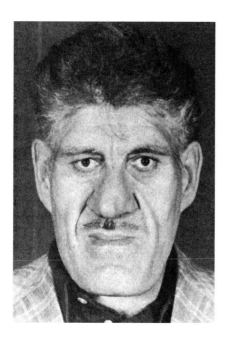
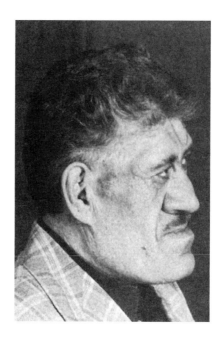

Figure 11–3 Acromegaly in a 56-year-old man. (From Martin, JB, Reichlin, S, and Brown, GM: Clinical Neuroendocrinology. FA Davis, Philadelphia, 1977, p 353, with permission.)

height. A child with the condition may grow as much as 6 inches a year.

The symptoms of acromegaly generally appear very gradually, causing the deformation and coarsening of facial features and enlargement of the hands, feet, head, and tongue. Serious physiological symptoms also may appear, such as increased sweating, oily skin, and chronic sinus congestion. The person with acromegaly will often complain of headaches, weakness, **paresthesia,** joint pain, and vision disorders.

DIAGNOSTIC PROCEDURES The clinical picture of symptoms will suggest the diagnosis. A glucose suppression test is the standard method for confirming elevated GH levels. Conventional skull x-rays or cranial computed tomography (CT) and magnetic resonance imaging (MRI) scans are useful in pinpointing the location and estimating the extent of the pituitary tumor. Bone x-rays may exhibit bone-thickening, especially of the cranium and long bones.

TREATMENT Treatment goals involve lowering GH levels to normal and stabilizing or removing the underlying tumor while minimizing damage to the pituitary gland itself. Surgery may be attempted depending on the size and location of the tumor.

Otherwise, radiation therapy or drug therapy may be used.

PROGNOSIS Hyperpituitarism is a chronic, progressive disease that generally reduces life expectancy. The prognosis for an individual with either gigantism or acromegaly depends on how far the condition has advanced before successful treatment. Gigantism is generally not life-threatening, and the prognosis is usually good. An individual with advanced acromegaly, however, may suffer serious complications such as congestive heart failure, diabetes mellitus, respiratory diseases, or cerebrovascular diseases. Even if successfully treated, the pituitary tumors may recur. Hypopituitarism may be an unintended consequence of treatment for either condition.

PREVENTION There is no specific prevention for hyperpituitarism.

■ HYPOPITUITARISM

DESCRIPTION *Hypopituitarism* is an endocrine deficiency in which any of the hormones produced by the anterior portion of the pituitary gland are secreted at insufficient levels or are absent. Growth hormone (GH) and gonadotropin are the most commonly deficient hormones in hypopituitarism. Less frequently, adrenocorticotropic hormone (ACTH) and thyroid-stimulating hormone (TSH) are deficient. When all the anterior pituitary hormones are affected, the condition is called *panhypopituitarism*. As Table 11–1 indicates, the major effect of some anterior pituitary hormones is the stimulation of hormone production by other endocrine glands. For this reason, hypopituitarism may have a cascading effect, resulting in hyposecretion of essential hormones by the "target" glands and producing symptoms that may mimic disorders of these glands.

ETIOLOGY Hypopituitarism is often caused by pituitary tumors or tumors of the hypothalamus. Less frequently, it is the result of infection and inflammation of these structures. Other significant causes include pituitary vascular diseases, especially postpartum hemorrhage of the pituitary gland, which occurs because the enlarged pituitary gland of pregnancy becomes vulnerable to ischemia. Head injuries and **iatrogenic** damage from surgery and radiation therapy also may result in hypopituitarism.

SIGNS AND SYMPTOMS The symptoms of hypopituitarism depend on the age and sex of the affected individual and on the specific hormones that are deficient. In children, GH deficiency will produce dwarfism, whereas gonadotropin deficiency may interfere with the emergence of secondary sexual characteristics. Gonadotropin deficiency in adult women may cause **amenorrhea** and infertility. In men, the deficiency can result in lowering of testosterone levels, decreased libido, and loss of body and facial hair. ACTH and TSH deficiencies may produce generalized symptoms such as fatigue, anorexia, weight loss, loss of skin pigmentation, low tolerance to cold, and a poor response to stress. Naturally enough, panhypopituitarism may result in all the preceding symptoms as well as mental and physiological abnormalities.

DIAGNOSTIC PROCEDURES The individual's clinical history of symptoms will suggest the diagnosis. A battery of laboratory tests to measure the levels of each of the principal pituitary hormones will typically be run to confirm the diagnosis. It is essential that laboratory tests also be run to measure the normal output of "target" glands (e.g., cortisol production by the adrenal glands), because deficiencies of these secretions may prove life-threatening. Cranial CT and MRI scans are useful in pinpointing pituitary tumors or lesions.

TREATMENT Hormone replacement therapy, both of pituitary hormones and of hormones secreted by the target glands, is the typical course of treatment. A bioengineered GH preparation is effective for treating GH-deficient growth abnormalities in children. Because hormonal balances normally change during growth and development, constant monitoring is necessary during hormone replacement therapy to make certain that appropriate hormonal levels are maintained. Surgical management of pituitary neoplasms may be required.

PROGNOSIS Despite the fact that lost pituitary function generally cannot be restored, the prognosis can be good with adequate hormone replacement therapy. Total loss of all hormonal secretions from the anterior pituitary may result in fatal complications.

PREVENTION There is no specific prevention for hypopituitarism.

■ DIABETES INSIPIDUS

DESCRIPTION *Diabetes insipidus* is characterized by **polyuria** and excessive thirst, which are the result of insufficient secretion of **vasopressin** by the posterior portion of the pituitary gland. Vasopressin, also known as *antidiuretic hormone* (ADH), helps regulate the amount of fluid the kidneys release as urine. Other things being equal, the higher the level of vasopressin, the greater the fluid reabsorption by the kidneys. In diabetes insipidus, the decreased vasopressin allows the filtered water to be excreted, which means that large quantities of diluted water must pass through the body. Diabetes insipidus usually starts in childhood or early adulthood and affects men more commonly than women.

ETIOLOGY Most cases of diabetes insipidus are **idiopathic,** especially those cases arising during childhood. Other causes include primary tumors of the pituitary gland and hypothalamus and damage to the posterior portion of the pituitary gland as a result of severe head injuries or from surgery.

SIGNS AND SYMPTOMS The classic symptom is polyuria. As much as 4 to 16 liters of dilute urine may be produced in 24 hours. This makes the person extremely thirsty because of the need to replace the fluids lost from the body. Consequently, there may be signs of dehydration such as weakness, fever, mental confusion, and prostration.

DIAGNOSTIC PROCEDURES Urinalysis will reveal a colorless urine with low osmolality (i.e., containing low levels of dissolved wastes). A "dehydration test" is often done to differentiate diabetes insipidus from other diseases causing polyuria. In this test, the person is denied fluids while hourly measurements are made of urine osmolality, body weight, and blood pressure. After a period of several hours, the individual is given a vasopressin medication. If the person has diabetes insipidus, the vasopressin will decrease the urine output and increase the urine's osmolality.

TREATMENT Hormone replacement therapy using various vasopressin medications is the most common treatment protocol for diabetes insipidus.

PROGNOSIS The prognosis of an individual with diabetes insipidus depends on the underlying cause of the condition. If the underlying cause is difficult to treat, such as cancer, the prognosis is guarded. In other cases, though, with effective vasopressin replacement therapy, the individual should be able to lead a normal life.

PREVENTION There is no specific prevention for diabetes insipidus.

Thyroid Gland Diseases

SIMPLE GOITER

DESCRIPTION A *goiter* is an enlargement (**hyperplasia**) of the thyroid gland. A *simple goiter* is any thyroid enlargement that is not caused by an infection or neoplasm and that does not result from another hypo- or hyperthyroid disorder. In certain parts of the world, simple goiter is an *endemic* condition (affecting many people in a given area). In the United States, however, simple goiter is now a *sporadic* condition (affecting only a few). Simple goiter is more common in women, especially during adolescence, pregnancy, and menopause. During these times, the body's demand for thyroid hormone is increased.

ETIOLOGY The thyroid gland hyperplasia that characterizes a goiter occurs when the thyroid gland cannot secrete sufficient levels of two iodine-rich hormones: tetraiodothyronine (T_4) and triiodothyronine (T_3). The thyroid gland tissue enlarges in order to compensate for the deficiency. In simple goiter, the inadequate secretion of these thyroid hormones may be caused by a dietary iodine deficiency, the ingestion of substances known to induce goiter (**goitrogens**), or some error in the hormone formation process within the thyroid gland. In many cases, though, the condition is idiopathic.

SIGNS AND SYMPTOMS The extent of thyroid enlargement will vary from case to case. A simple goiter may appear as a small nodule, or it can be quite massive, presenting a conspicuous swollen mass at the front of the neck, just above the sternum (Fig. 11–4). The goiter may compress the esophagus or trachea, producing **dysphagia,** dizziness, and **syncope.**

DIAGNOSTIC PROCEDURES Diagnosis of simple goiter is made on the basis of thyroid gland enlargement in the presence of normal levels of T_3 and T_4 hormones. A T_3 and T_4 radioimmunoassay test will accurately measure the levels of these two hormones.

TREATMENT The treatment goal is to reduce the size of the goiter. How this is accomplished will depend in part on the underlying cause of the condition. Treatment procedures may include dietary supplements of iodine, or T_3 and T_4 hormone replacement therapy. In the case of idiopathic simple goiter, treatment may involve thyroid suppression therapy (i.e., the use of certain drugs that slow thyroid gland activity). A large goiter that is unresponsive to therapy may require excision, resulting in lifelong thyroid replacement therapy.

PROGNOSIS The prognosis is generally good following effective treatment. Complications from severe

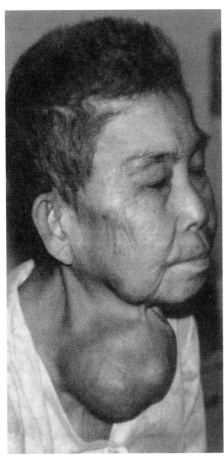

Figure 11–4 A middle-aged woman with nontoxic goiter. The thyroid has enlarged to produce a conspicuous neck mass. (From Rubin, E, and Farber, JL [eds]: Pathology, ed 3. Lippincott-Raven, Philadelphia, 1999, p 1164, with permission.)

cases of simple goiter include hemorrhage of thyroid gland blood vessels or hypo- or hyperthyroid conditions.

PREVENTION Prevention of simple goiter includes adequate dietary intake of iodine.

HASHIMOTO'S THYROIDITIS

DESCRIPTION *Hashimoto's thyroiditis* (lymphadenoid goiter) is an inflammatory autoimmune disease of the thyroid gland. It is a leading cause of nonsimple goiter and hypothyroidism. The disease is characterized by the infiltration of the thyroid gland with lymphocytes and by elevated blood serum levels of immunoglobulins and antibodies against thyroid tissue. Fibrous tissue slowly replaces healthy tissue within the thyroid gland as the disease progresses. This disease is more common in middle-aged women and in children. It sometimes accompanies other autoimmune diseases.

ETIOLOGY The cause of Hashimoto's thyroiditis is not known, but genetic factors are strongly suspected.

SIGNS AND SYMPTOMS Goiter is the principal symptom of Hashimoto's thyroiditis. As the disease advances, the individual typically begins to show symptoms of hypothyroidism such as cold, fatigue, and weight gain.

DIAGNOSTIC PROCEDURES Blood testing will typically reveal elevated immunoglobulin levels and the presence of antibodies that react with thyroid tissue. These findings in the presence of goiter suggest a diagnosis of Hashimoto's thyroiditis. A needle biopsy of thyroid tissue also may be performed to examine the tissue for changes that are characteristic of the disease. A radioactive iodine uptake (RAIU) test may be run to measure thyroid function.

TREATMENT Thyroid hormone replacement therapy is a standard form of treatment. The therapy usually must be continued for life.

PROGNOSIS The condition is chronic, but the prognosis is good if thyroid hormone replacement therapy is effective.

PREVENTION There is no known prevention for Hashimoto's thyroiditis.

HYPERTHYROIDISM (Graves' Disease)

DESCRIPTION *Hyperthyroidism* is a condition caused by the oversecretion of hormones by the thyroid gland. As Table 11–1 reveals, thyroid hormones such as T_4 and T_3 influence the metabolism of cells throughout the body. Consequently, when levels of these hormones are constantly elevated, as occurs in hyperthyroidism, profound changes can occur in the body's normal physiological processes. These changes frequently produce a cluster of symptoms called *thyrotoxicosis*.

A hyperthyroid state can result from a number of conditions and diseases. The most important and most common of these, though, is Graves' disease. Graves' disease may result from genetic and immunologic factors and is marked by an enlarged thyroid gland (goiter), characteristic changes in the structure of the eyes (ophthalmopathy), and characteristic skin lesions (dermopathy). This disease affects more women than men, and it typically appears between the ages of 30 and 50.

ETIOLOGY The cause of Graves' disease is not known, although a familial predisposition to the disease has led researchers to strongly suspect a genetic etiology.

SIGNS AND SYMPTOMS The classic manifestations of Graves' disease are goiter, symptoms of thyrotoxicosis, ophthalmopathy, and dermopathy. These symptoms may appear independently of one another and go through cycles of remission and exacerbation.

The symptoms of thyrotoxicosis include nervousness, loss of sleep, excessive perspiration, and heat intolerance. Wasting of muscle and decalcification of the skeleton may lead to persistent weight loss and fatigue. The symptoms of thyrotoxicosis also may include a host of cardiac manifestations such as tachycardia, arrhythmias, heart murmurs, and cardiomegaly.

The ophthalmopathy characteristic of Graves' disease includes **exophthalmos** (Fig. 11–5), protruding eyeballs that give the affected individual a "frightened" appearance. Inflammation of the muscles surrounding the eye may interfere with normal eye movements, including blinking. The dermopathy associated with Graves' disease is marked by the appearance of thickened patches of skin, usually on the feet or legs, having an "orange skin" texture and uneven pigmentation.

DIAGNOSTIC PROCEDURES Diagnosis is based largely on the characteristic physical manifestations of the disease. A radioimmunoassay will confirm increased serum levels of T_4 and T_3, and a thyroid radioactive iodine uptake (RAIU) test will confirm thyroid hyperactivity. Blood tests indicating elevated levels of certain antithyroid immunoglobulins also strongly suggest a diagnosis of Graves' disease.

TREATMENT The course of treatment chosen depends on the affected individual's age and sex, and on the severity of the case. One approach involves

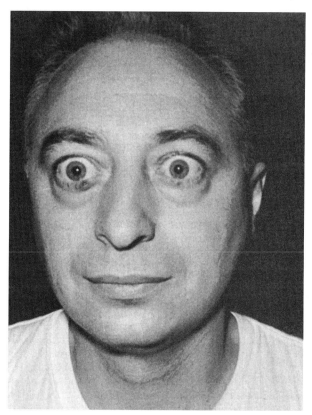

Figure 11–5 Exophthalmos caused by hyperthyroidism (Graves' disease). (Photo by Lester V. Bergman, NY)

the use of antithyroid agents (i.e., drugs that block hormone synthesis within the thyroid gland). Another approach involves altering the structure of the thyroid gland itself, through either surgery or radioactive iodine therapy. Short-term control of the hyperthyroidism of Graves' disease also may be obtained by administration of iodide compounds.

PROGNOSIS The prognosis of Graves' disease varies from case to case. If the course of treatment results in the remission of symptoms and the disappearance of immunoglobulins associated with the disease, then the prognosis for a complete recovery without recurrence is good. A potentially fatal complication of Graves' disease is *thyroid storm,* a severe episode of thyrotoxicosis. It is marked by the rapid onset of fever, sweating, tachycardia, pulmonary edema, and congestive heart failure. This condition requires emergency medical intervention.

PREVENTION There is no specific prevention for Graves' disease.

■ HYPOTHYROIDISM (Cretinism, Myxedema)

DESCRIPTION *Hypothyroidism* is undersecretion of hormones by the thyroid gland. Hypothyroidism is called *cretinism* when it appears as a congenital condition, and it is called *myxedema* when it is acquired later in childhood or during adulthood. Hypothyroidism is more common in women than men, and it is high in adults aged 40 to 50 in the United States.

ETIOLOGY Hypothyroidism may be caused by either an insufficient quantity of thyroid tissue or the loss of functional thyroid tissue. The former condition may be iatrogenic, resulting from thyroid surgery, radioactive iodine therapy performed to treat another thyroid disease, or a congenital thyroid abnormality. The progressive loss of functional thyroid tissue is generally idiopathic, but it shows strong evidence of being an autoimmune disorder.

Hashimoto's disease is a leading cause of hypothyroidism with goiter (see Hashimoto's Disease). Other forms of hypothyroidism accompanied by goiter may be caused by dietary or metabolic iodine deficiencies or be induced by certain drugs. Hypothyroidism also may arise secondarily from diseases of the anterior pituitary that result in hyposecretion of thyroid-stimulating hormone (TSH).

SIGNS AND SYMPTOMS Because the thyroid hormones T_4 and T_3 influence the metabolism of cells throughout the body, the persistently low levels of these hormones in hypothyroidism can result in a host of symptoms. The assortment of symptoms will vary with the age of the affected individual.

Newborns with hypothyroidism may exhibit constipation and feeding problems, may sleep too much, and may have a hoarse cry. Children with the condition (either congenital or acquired) will typically show retarded growth, a delayed emergence of secondary sexual characteristics, impaired intelligence, and one or more of the adult symptoms of hypothyroidism.

The onset of hypothyroidism during adulthood is often insidious. Initial symptoms may include fatigue, constipation, intolerance to cold, muscle cramps, and **menorrhagia.** Later symptoms may include mental clouding, diminished appetite, and weight gain. The skin may become dry, and the hair and nails may become brittle. In advanced forms of the disease, the affected individual may have an expressionless face and sparse hair. Other systemic conditions, such as cardiomegaly and megacolon, also may occur late in the disease.

DIAGNOSTIC PROCEDURES The composite picture of presenting signs and symptoms may suggest the diagnosis. Radioimmunoassay will typically show depressed levels of T_4 and T_3. A similar test will usually reveal elevated levels of TSH, except for hypothyroidism arising from pituitary gland dysfunction, in which case TSH levels may range from undetectable to near normal.

TREATMENT Treatment for hypothyroidism involves hormone replacement therapy with synthetic or animal-derived thyroid hormones. In the case of infants and children, therapy should begin as soon as possible to avoid or minimize intellectual impairment.

PROGNOSIS With effective thyroid hormone replacement therapy, the prognosis for an individual with hypothyroidism is great. A life-threatening complication of hypothyroidism is *myxedema coma.* This condition is marked by the onset of hypothermia and stupor, and it requires immediate medical attention.

PREVENTION Only hypothyroidism due to dietary iodine deficiency or drug-induced forms of the disease are preventable.

Parathyroid Gland Diseases

◼ HYPERPARATHYROIDISM
(Hypercalcemia)

DESCRIPTION *Hyperparathyroidism* is a general disorder of calcium and phosphate metabolism caused by excessive secretion of parathyroid hormone (PTH) by the parathyroid glands. The persistently high level of PTH typically depresses the concentration of phosphates in the extracellular fluid (*hypophosphatemia*) and elevates the concentration of calcium (*hypercalcemia*). It is hypercalcemia that creates most of the troubling effects associated with hyperparathyroidism. The disease is far more common than once suspected, and it affects women twice as frequently as men.

ETIOLOGY Hyperparathyroidism may have either a primary or a secondary etiology. The most common primary etiology is an adenoma on one of the parathyroid glands. Less commonly, the parathyroid glands may be affected by one of various forms of inherited endocrine system disorders.

Secondary etiologies of hyperparathyroidism are those which act to reduce levels of circulating calcium, causing the parathyroid glands to hypersecrete in an effort to counteract the shortage of serum calcium. Such etiologies include chronic renal failure, dietary insufficiency of calcium, or calcium malabsorption disorders.

SIGNS AND SYMPTOMS The onset of hyperparathyroidism is usually very gradual, with over half the affected individuals remaining asymptomatic for extended periods of time. Symptoms are usually related to hypercalcemia and may include weak, brittle bones; joint pain; or the presence of kidney stones. Polyuria is a common effect of hyperparathyroidism. Other hypercalcemic symptoms include CNS disturbances, such as personality disorders or intellectual impairment; or gastrointestinal disturbances, such as duodenal ulcers, nausea, and vomiting. Additional symptoms may include muscle weakness or atrophy, chronic fatigue, and cardiac disturbances.

DIAGNOSTIC PROCEDURES Radioimmunoassay will typically reveal elevated concentrations of serum PTH. Blood testing will usually reveal abnormally high serum calcium levels in primary forms of the disease and diminished or nearly normal levels in secondary forms. Serum phosphorus levels are decreased. Urinalysis may reveal elevated calcium. Conventional x-rays or CT scans of bone may reveal evidence of demineralization or increased bone turnover (i.e., newly formed bone mass balancing the reabsorption of older bone mass).

TREATMENT The treatment of hyperparathyroidism varies with the etiology. In primary forms of the disease, the goal is to reduce the level of circulating calcium. This may be accomplished surgically by removing the neoplastic or hypertrophic parathyroid glands. All but half of one parathyroid gland can be removed and the individual can still maintain normal PTH levels. Increased hydration and sodium intake also may be used to lower serum calcium levels. In some cases, drugs that increase the excretion of calcium by the kidneys or inhibit the reabsorption of calcium from bone may be employed. Secondary forms of hyperparathyroidism can only be corrected by treating the underlying cause.

PROGNOSIS The prognosis for an individual with hyperparathyroidism is generally good, given successful treatment. Complications may result from organ damage due to chronic hypercalcemia. Coma and cardiac arrest may result from severe hypercalcemia.

PREVENTION There is no known prevention.

◼ HYPOPARATHYROIDISM
(Hypocalcemia)

DESCRIPTION *Hypoparathyroidism* is undersecretion of parathyroid hormone (PTH) by the parathyroid glands. Consequently, circulating concentrations of calcium are reduced, resulting in hypocalcemia. There is excessive deposit of calcium into bone tissue.

ETIOLOGY Some cases of hypoparathyroidism are caused by hereditary disorders that result in underdevelopment of parathyroid tissue. Far more frequently, however, hyperparathyroidism is iatrogenic, usually resulting from the deliberate or inadvertent removal of parathyroid tissue during attempts to cure other endocrine disorders.

SIGNS AND SYMPTOMS The signs and symptoms of hypoparathyroidism are generally dependent on the degree of hypocalcemia. Symptoms may include numbness and tingling of the extremities, neuromuscular irritability, and muscle cramps. CNS symptoms may include general irritability and depression. **Tetany** also may occur, leading to laryngospasm, **cyanosis,** and grand mal seizures in severe cases. The affected individual may have brittle fingernails and hair loss.

DIAGNOSTIC PROCEDURES Radioimmunoassay revealing decreased PTH and serum calcium levels will suggest the diagnosis. Serum phosphorus will typically be increased. ECGs may indicate increased QT and ST cardiac waveform abnormalities due to hypocalcemia. X-rays may indicate increased bone density.

TREATMENT Treatment usually consists of lifelong vitamin D and calcium supplementation. Serum calcium levels should be tested regularly. A diet high in calcium and low in phosphorus is encouraged.

PROGNOSIS Although the condition is chronic, with successful treatment the individual with hypoparathyroidism can lead a relatively normal life.

PREVENTION There is no known prevention.

Adrenal Gland Disease

◼ CUSHING'S SYNDROME

DESCRIPTION *Cushing's syndrome* is hypersecretion of the adrenal cortex of the adrenal glands, resulting in the excess production of cortisol.

ETIOLOGY One cause of Cushing's syndrome is bilateral hyperplasia of the adrenal glands due to elevated serum levels of adrenocorticotropic hormone (ACTH). Elevated concentrations of ACTH may result from overproduction of this hormone by a malfunctioning pituitary gland or from ACTH-secreting neoplasms elsewhere in the body. In either case, the result is overstimulation of the cortices of the adrenal gland and hypersecretion of cortisol. Another cause of Cushing's syndrome is benign or malignant neoplasm of an adrenal cortex. Finally, the disease is frequently iatrogenic, produced as a side effect of the long-term administration of steroid drugs used to treat other diseases.

SIGNS AND SYMPTOMS The classic symptom of Cushing's syndrome is a round, "moon-shaped" face with acne. The head and trunk often are grossly exaggerated, with pencil-thin arms and legs. There may be impaired glucose tolerance, muscle weakness, stretch marks on the skin, a "buffalo" hump on the upper back, peptic ulcer, emotional changes, hypertension, and increased susceptibility to infection. The person also may have diabetes mellitus.

DIAGNOSTIC PROCEDURES The diagnostic procedures are chosen so as to establish a diagnosis of Cushing's syndrome and to pinpoint its etiology—frequently a difficult task. A 24-hour urine test will typically exhibit elevated free cortisol levels. It is important to determine steroid levels in both serum and urine. A low-dose dexamethasone suppression test confirms the diagnosis. Pituitary and abdominal CT scans may be helpful in locating tumors.

TREATMENT The treatment goal in each case is to restore the concentration of serum cortisol to normal levels. The approach chosen, however, will necessarily vary according to the etiology. In the case of adrenal hyperplasia due to elevated ACTH levels, surgery is usually performed to remove tumors on the pituitary gland or at ectopic sites. In some cases, drug therapy or radiation therapy may be attempted to suppress ACTH secretion. Occasionally, total adrenalectomy is the treatment of choice, but there is subsequently a requirement for lifelong cortisol replacement therapy. Surgery is again the treatment of choice when Cushing's syndrome is caused by tumors of the adrenal cortex. Chemotherapy also may be attempted in such cases.

PROGNOSIS The prognosis for Cushing's syndrome depends on the etiology of the case and on how far the disease has progressed before the institution of treatment. The prognosis is poor for an individual with Cushing's syndrome caused by a carcinoma of the adrenal cortex. The prognosis is generally good if the condition is caused by a localized adenoma of the pituitary gland.

PREVENTION Iatrogenic forms of Cushing's syndrome are preventable. Individuals receiving glucocorticoid steroids or ACTH preparations to treat other diseases should be carefully monitored for symptoms of Cushing's disease.

Endocrine Dysfunction of the Pancreas

■ DIABETES MELLITUS

DESCRIPTION *Diabetes mellitus* is a chronic disorder of carbohydrate metabolism resulting from insufficient production of insulin or from inadequate utilization of this hormone by the body's cells. Insulin is produced by the beta cells within structures called the *islets of Langerhans* scattered throughout the pancreas. Insulin acts to lower the levels of glucose in the blood by enabling glucose absorption by body cells. When the beta cells cannot produce sufficient levels of insulin, the glucose concentration in the blood rises to abnormally high levels, a condition called *hyperglycemia*. Deprived of glucose, their principal fuel, the body cells begin to metabolize fats and proteins, depositing unusually high levels of wastes called *ketones* in the blood and causing a condition called *ketosis*. These two conditions, hyperglycemia and ketosis, are responsible for the host of troubling and often life-threatening symptoms of diabetes mellitus. The diagnosis and classification of diabetes mellitus has changed. The new criteria are as follows:

- *Immune-mediated diabetes type 1* (formerly called *insulin-dependent diabetes mellitus* [IDDM]). This form of the disease has an abrupt onset, usually appearing before the age of 30. Type 1 diabetes mellitus is frequently marked by the complete absence of insulin secretion, making this form of the disease quite difficult to regulate.
- *Type 2 diabetes* (formerly called *non-insulin-dependent diabetes mellitus* [NIDDM]). The more common form of the disease typically has a gradual onset, usually appearing in adults older than 40. In type 2 diabetes mellitus, the pancreas generally retains some insulin-secreting ability, so that management of this disease is less problematic than that of type 1 diabetes mellitus. A few persons with type 2 diabetes are insulin-dependent.

- *Other specific types of diabetes.* This group refers to diabetes in persons with genetic defects of beta-cell function and persons with pancreatic dysfunction caused by drugs, chemicals, and infections.
- *Gestational diabetes mellitus (GDM).* This type of diabetes develops during pregnancy but most often resolves after delivery; however, this places women at increase risk of developing type 2 diabetes later in life.

ETIOLOGY The causes of type 1 and type 2 diabetes mellitus are still not known. The type 1 form of the disease, however, seems to be an autoimmune disorder. Individuals who develop this form of diabetes mellitus inherit a defective gene that renders them susceptible to the disease. At some point early in life, a triggering event occurs—perhaps a viral infection; this leads to the production of antibodies that destroy the beta cells. Type 2 diabetes mellitus also seems to be genetically linked, but little else is known about how this form of the disease arises. Other specific types of diabetes mellitus occur secondary to other diseases or conditions. Etiologies of this variety include chronic pancreatitis, pancreatic neoplasms, or drug-induced suppression of insulin production. Other endocrine disorders, such as Cushing's syndrome, also may induce diabetes mellitus. In addition, the disease may be caused by genetic abnormalities that render the body's cells insensitive to insulin.

Risk factors include obesity, sedentary lifestyle, family member with diabetes, having delivered a baby weighing 9 lb or more, and hypertension.

SIGNS AND SYMPTOMS The classic symptoms of most cases of diabetes mellitus are polyuria, **glycosuria,** and **polydipsia.** In addition to these symptoms, individuals with type 1 diabetes usually experience weight loss and **polyphagia,** and they are susceptible to **ketoacidosis.** Those with type 2 diabetes, on the other hand, are usually overweight and may experience symptoms such as repeated or hard-to-heal infections of the skin, gums, vagina, or bladder; blurred vision, and **pruritus.** Other generalized symptoms of both forms of the disease may include muscle weakness and fatigue. Because type 2 diabetes has such a gradual onset, individuals with this form of the disease often are still asymptomatic when the disease is discovered during routine screening.

DIAGNOSTIC PROCEDURES The individual's presenting symptoms may suggest a diagnosis of diabetes mellitus. A fasting plasma glucose test is the preferred way to diagnose diabetes.

TREATMENT A combination of diet, insulin, and exercise is used to treat most forms of diabetes mellitus. Individuals with type 1 diabetes typically need to follow a consistent dietary pattern that is closely linked to the injection of insulin. A consistent routine of exercise will lessen the need for insulin. Those with type 2 diabetes usually require a diet that restricts their caloric intake. Diet therapy alone may be all that is necessary to control their symptoms. If not, hypoglycemic drugs may be prescribed. These drugs act to stimulate insulin production or make body cells more sensitive to insulin. In some instances, those with type 2 diabetes also may require injected insulin. Self-management of the disease is the treatment goal for both forms of diabetes mellitus. Education and client compliance are essential for the control of diabetes. Diabetic individuals can test their blood glucose levels and urine glucose and acetone at home, so that they can make decisions about simple modifications of their diet, exercise, and insulin regimes. Regular medical supervision is required.

PROGNOSIS The prognosis for an individual with diabetes mellitus is uncertain. Even a well-motivated individual following a carefully balanced treatment regimen may eventually fall victim to one or more of the life-threatening late complications of the disease. In general, though, if diabetes mellitus is detected early and the affected individual's glucose levels can be stabilized near normal levels, persons with diabetes can reasonably expect to live for many years with few complications. Client motivation and knowledge of the disease process contribute significantly to effective management of the disease.

Complications affecting the prognosis may be classified as acute or late. The *acute* complications of diabetes mellitus are metabolic crises resulting from swings in the level of blood glucose of blood pH. One such complication is *diabetic coma*. This condition may be triggered by skipping or delaying an insulin injection or consuming too much food. It also may be occasioned by a period of emotional or physical stress. Whatever the precipitating event, the physiological process is the same. Severe hyperglycemia induces polyuria and subsequent dehydration, while severe ketosis raises blood acidity. The affected individual may experience intense thirst and abdominal pain with nausea or vomiting, and may become lethargic and drowsy. From that point, the individual may lapse into coma. A person in a diabetic coma will typically exhibit deep, slow breathing, have a "fruity" breath odor (from ketones in the blood transpiring through the lungs), and exhibit red, dry skin and a dry tongue. Individuals in a diabetic coma require emergency medical treatment consisting of a large dose of insulin and intravenous administration of fluids and salts.

Another acute complication is *insulin shock*. This situation may be occasioned by injecting too much insulin, inadequate food intake, or excessive exercise. As a result, blood glucose levels drop below normal (hypoglycemia). The affected person may begin feeling faint and shaky and begin to perspire. Speech disturbances, double vision, and clouded consciousness may follow. From this point, the individual may become comatose. Regrettably, coma produced by insulin shock is often difficult to distinguish from diabetic coma. A few distinguishing features of insulin-induced coma include short, shallow breathing with no characteristic breath odor and moist, clammy skin. Individuals experiencing insulin shock require emergency medical treatment consisting of intravenous administration of glucose.

The *late* complications of diabetes mellitus typically appear only after many years or even decades. Over time, the lipids that are released into the blood as a consequence of ketosis may cause arteriosclerotic disease. The subsequent impairment of blood flow in the extremities may produce intermittent claudication or even tissue necrosis and gangrene, especially in the feet and lower legs. Other arteriosclerotic complications may include coronary artery disease, cerebral vascular accident, and organic impotence in men.

The vascular system is not the only system subject to damage, however. Diabetes mellitus is a leading cause of kidney disease and renal failure, whereas diabetes-induced **retinopathy** is a leading cause of blindness. The nervous system also may be affected over time. CNS damage may produce numbness, paresthesias, and intermittent but severe bouts of pain. Autonomic nervous system damage may produce difficulties in swallowing, constipation or diarrhea, and neurogenic bladder problems. Diabetes mellitus also may hamper an individual's immune response, causing slow wound healing and leaving the person open to frequent infections.

PREVENTION There are currently no specific measures to prevent any form of diabetes mellitus. Some research has indicated, however, that insulin administration to people at risk for type 1 diabetes, such as relatives of insulin-dependent diabetics, may prevent the onset of the disease. The insulin may prevent the immune systems of these people from damaging insulin-producing beta cells. Studies in mice and some limited human tests have shown that doses of insulin cause the formation of smaller, more active cells that are not destroyed by the immune system.

COMMON SYMPTOMS OF ENDOCRINE SYSTEM DISEASES

Individuals may present with the following common symptoms, which deserve attention from health professionals:

- Mental abnormalities
- Unusual change in energy level
- Changes in skin
- Muscle atrophy

BIBLIOGRAPHY

The Burton Goldberg Group (ed): Alternative Medicine: The Definitive Guide. Future Medicine Publishing, Fife, Wash., 1995.

Burns, MV: Pathophysiology: A Self-Instructional Program. Appleton & Lange, Stamford, Conn., 1998.

Fauci, AS, et al: Harrison's Principles of Internal Medicine, ed 14. McGraw-Hill, New York, 1998.

Frazier, MS, Drzymkowski, JA, and Doty, SJ: Essentials of Human Disease and Conditions. WB Saunders, Philadelphia, 1996.

Professional Guide to Diseases, ed 6. Springhouse Corporation, Springhouse, Pa., 1998.

CASE STUDIES

I The client, a young woman who makes many of her own clothes, notices that she must increase the size of the neck in her dresses and blouses. A recent photograph suggests to her that her eyes are almost bulging. She complains that she "fidgets" a lot and constantly feels compelled to be doing something. During the general physical examination, she reports that she has recently gained weight.

1. What do these signs and symptoms suggest?

2. What diagnostic procedures might the physician perform or have performed?

3. What additional information about this patient would be helpful?

II A woman calls for an appointment for her 12-year-old son. He eats enormous amounts of food and seems to be thirsty all the time. His mother notes that he seems to be going to the bathroom more and more often, and his soccer coach has relayed to her his concern that the boy is tired all the time.

1. What endocrine dysfunction is suggested by these signs and symptoms?

2. If the boy does have the indicated dysfunction, what are the likely treatments?

3. What would the prognosis be for such a child?

REVIEW QUESTIONS

MATCHING

_____ 1. Gigantism

_____ 2. Acromegaly

_____ 3. Hypopituitarism

_____ 4. Diabetes insipidus

_____ 5. Simple goiter

_____ 6. Graves' disease

_____ 7. Myxedema

_____ 8. Hypoparathyroidism

_____ 9. Diabetes mellitus

a. Most common form of hyperthyroidism
b. Thyroid enlargement tumor of anterior pituitary
c. Thyroid enlargement
d. Hypothyroidism in adults
e. Hyperfunction of GH before puberty
f. Disorder caused by insulin lack or resistance
g. Hypocalcemia
h. Hyperfunction of GH after puberty
i. Classic symptom is polyuria
j. Caused by excessive glucocorticosteroid hormones
k. Hypothyroidism in children

SHORT ANSWER

Fill in the blanks:

1. A test that is likely to be ordered in a number of endocrine-related diseases to help determine hormone levels in blood serum is _____ .

2. An inadequate dietary intake of iodine may cause _____ .

3. Thyroid crisis or "storm" is a medical emergency; the symptoms include

   _____ , _____ , and _____ .

4. An infant who sleeps too much; shows signs of apathy, stupor, dry skin, constipation, has a large tongue and pot belly; and is slow in learning to talk may suffer from

   _____ .

5. The classic symptom of a round, moon-shaped face with acne are an indication of

   _____ .

DISCUSSION QUESTION

Discuss the interrelatedness of the endocrine diseases and why hyperfunction or hypofunction of one gland often affects the other endocrine glands.

ANSWERS

MATCHING

1. e	4. i	6. a	8. g
2. h	5. c	7. d	9. f
3. b			

SHORT ANSWER

1. Radioimmunoassay
2. Endemic goiter
3. High fever, tachycardia, delirium
4. Cretinism
5. Cushing's syndrome

DISCUSSION QUESTION

Answers will vary.

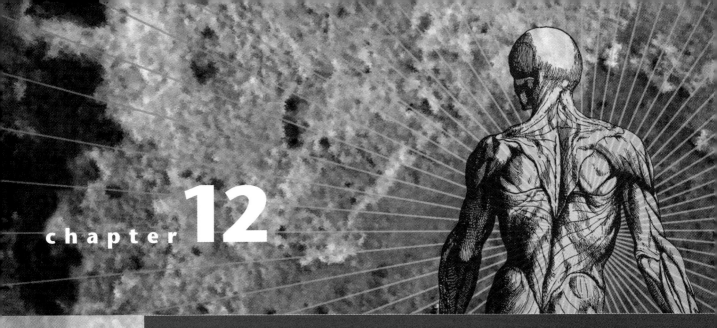

chapter 12

Musculoskeletal Diseases

CHAPTER OUTLINE

Bones
Deformities of the Spine: Lordosis, Kyphosis, Scoliosis
Herniated Intervertebral Disk
Osteoporosis
Osteomalacia
Osteomyelitis
Paget's Disease (Osteitis Deformans)
Fractures

Joints
Osteoarthritis
Rheumatoid Arthritis (RA)
Gout
□ ALTERNATIVE MEDICINE

Muscles and Connective Tissue
Sprains and Strains
Bursitis

Carpal Tunnel Syndrome
□ ALTERNATIVE MEDICINE
Tendonitis
Myasthenia Gravis
Polymyositis
Systemic Lupus Erythematosus (SLE)

Neoplasms

Special Focus: Childhood Disease of the Musculoskeletal System
Duchenne's Muscular Dystrophy

Common Symptoms of Musculoskeletal Diseases

Bibliography

Case Studies

Review Questions

LEARNING OBJECTIVES

Upon successful completion of this chapter, you will:

- Describe three spine deformities.
- Identify the common cause for intervertebral disk herniation.
- Compare osteoporosis to osteomalacia.
- Recall the description for osteomyelitis.
- List at least three diagnostic procedures used specifically for determining bone disorders.
- Illustrate at least four kinds of fractures with a simple drawing.
- Compare and contrast osteoarthritis and rheumatoid arthritis.
- Describe the treatment process for bursitis and tendonitis.
- Discuss signs and symptoms of Duchenne's muscular dystrophy.
- Identify the etiology of myasthenia gravis.
- Recall the signs and symptoms of polymyositis.
- Describe the prognosis for systemic lupus erythematosus.

KEY WORDS

Acetylcholine (ăs•ĕ•tĭl•kō′lēn)
Acidosis (ăs•ĭ•dō′sĭs)
Alopecia (ăl•ō•pē′shē•ă)
Analgesic (ăn•ăl•jē′sĭk)
Ankylosis (ăng•kĭ•lō′sĭs)
Ayurvedic (ă′yŭr•vă′dĭc)
Contracture (kŏn•trăk′chūr)
Crepitation (krĕp•ĭ•tā′shŭn)
Embolism (ĕm′bō•lĭzm)
Hypertrophy (hī•pĕr′trŏ•fē)

Idiopathic (ĭd•ē•ō•păth′ĭk)
Malaise (mă•lāz′)
Matrix (mā′trĭks)
Paresthesia (păr•ĕs•thē′zē•ă)
Ptosis (tō′sĭs)
Raynaud's phenomenon (rā•nōs′ fē•nŏm′ē•nōn)
Salicylate (săl•ĭs′ĭl•āt)
Tophus (pl. *tophi*) (tō′fŭs, tō′fī)
Virulence (vĭr′ū•lĕns)

The musculoskeletal system consists of bones, joints, bursae, muscles, tendons, and ligaments. It provides physical support and protection for the organs of the body. The action of muscles and bones allows physical movement, and the marrow within the bones produces blood cells. Figure 12–1 depicts the bones of the skeleton. Figures 12–2 and 12–3 illustrate the major muscles of the body. Any pathology of this system greatly affects activities of daily living.

Bones

■ DEFORMITIES OF THE SPINE: LORDOSIS, KYPHOSIS, SCOLIOSIS

DESCRIPTION *Lordosis* is an abnormal inward curvature of a portion of the spine, commonly called swayback. *Kyphosis* is an abnormal outward curvature of the spine, commonly known as *humpback or round back*. *Scoliosis* is an abnormal sideward curvature of the spine either to the left or right. Some rotation of a portion of the vertebral column also may occur. Scoliosis often occurs in combination with kyphosis and lordosis (Fig. 12–4). These three spinal deformities may affect children as well as adults.

ETIOLOGY Lordosis, kyphosis, and scoliosis may be caused by a variety of problems, including congenital spinal defects, poor posture, and disorders that cause overly rapid growth. These deformities also may result from tumors, trauma, osteoarthritis, tu-

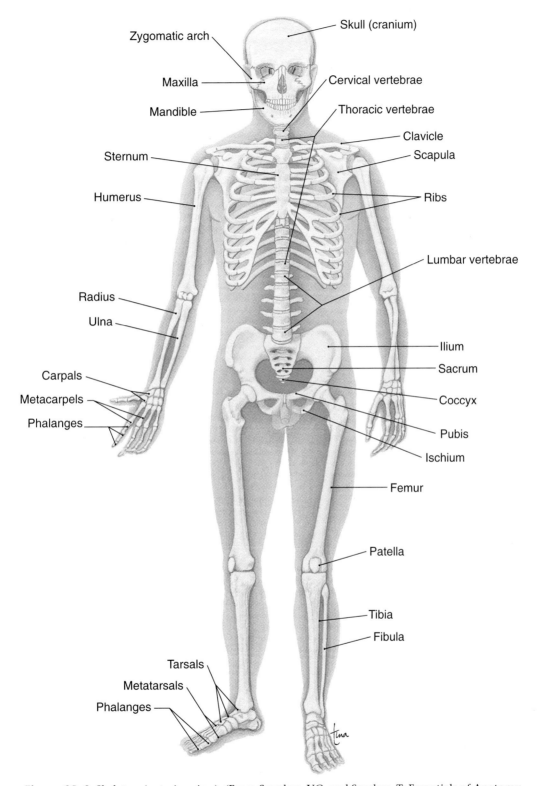

Figure 12–1 Skeleton (anterior view). (From Scanlon, VC, and Sanders, T: Essentials of Anatomy and Physiology, ed 3. FA Davis, Philadelphia, 1999, p 106, with permission.)

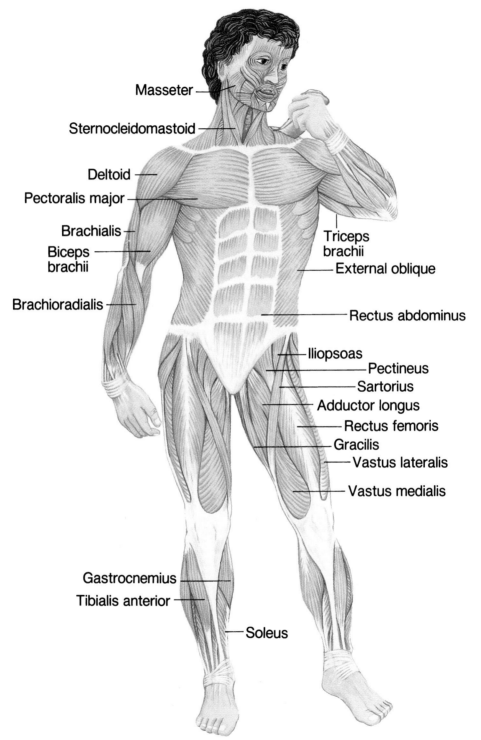

Masseter

Sternocleidomastoid

Deltoid

Pectoralis major

Brachialis

Biceps brachii

Brachioradialis

Triceps brachii

External oblique

Rectus abdominus

Iliopsoas

Pectineus

Sartorius

Adductor longus

Rectus femoris

Gracilis

Vastus lateralis

Vastus medialis

Gastrocnemius

Tibialis anterior

Soleus

Figure 12–2 Anterior view of muscles. (From Scanlon, VC, and Sanders, T: Essentials of Anatomy and Physiology, ed 3. FA Davis, Philadelphia, 1999, p 141, with permission.)

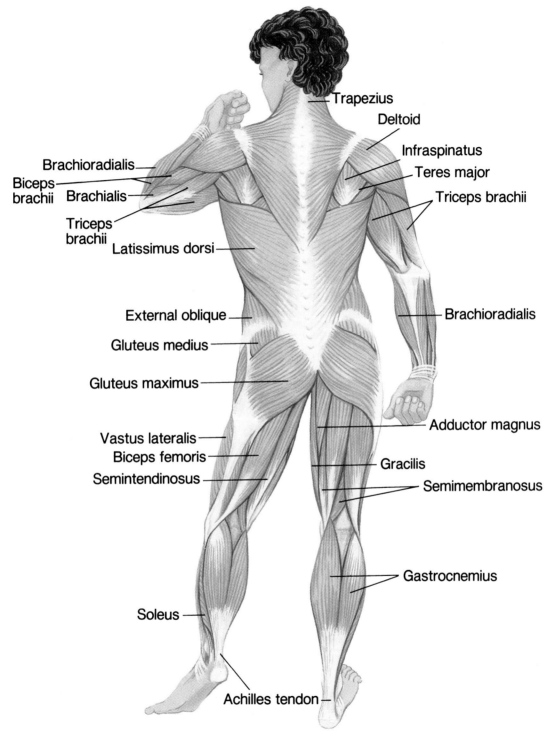

Figure 12–3 Posterior view of muscles. (From Scanlon, VC, and Sanders, T: Essentials of Anatomy and Physiology, ed 3. FA Davis, Philadelphia, 1999, p 140, with permission.)

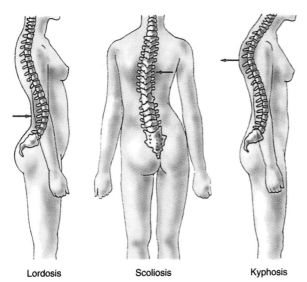

Lordosis   Scoliosis   Kyphosis

Figure 12–4 Common spinal cord deformities. (From Ignatavicius, DD, Workman, ML, and Mischler, MA [eds]: Medical-Surgical Nursing Across the Health Care Continuum, ed 3. WB Saunders, Philadelphia, 1999, p 1234, with permission.)

berculosis, muscle diseases, and degeneration of the spine associated with aging. Lordosis, kyphosis, and scoliosis also may be **idiopathic.**

SIGNS AND SYMPTOMS The onset of lordosis, kyphosis, and scoliosis frequently is insidious. Symptoms may eventually include chronic fatigue and backache. Scoliosis is often detected by individuals when they notice that their clothing seems longer on one side than the other. Or they may notice when looking in a mirror that the height of their hips and shoulders appears uneven.

DIAGNOSTIC PROCEDURES Physical examination and x-rays of the spine are the most commonly used procedures to detect these spinal deformities.

TREATMENT Treatment varies according to the nature and the severity of the spinal curvature, the age of onset, and the underlying cause of the disorder. Physical therapy, exercise, and back braces may all play a role in the treatment of these conditions. Surgery may be the treatment of choice in cases of adolescent scoliosis, if the curvature seriously interferes with mobility or breathing. In such cases, metal rods may be implanted to straighten the spine. **Analgesics** may be prescribed to alle-

viate the pain that frequently accompanies these disorders.

PROGNOSIS The prognosis of an individual with lordosis, kyphosis, or scoliosis depends on the underlying cause of the particular disease, how early it is detected, and whether it responds to treatment. In some cases, a spinal deformity may be arrested, but not corrected. Congestive heart failure and other cardiopulmonary difficulties may arise as complications of spinal deformities.

PREVENTION Prevention of lordosis, kyphosis, and scoliosis includes maintaining good posture. Scoliosis screening in public schools is mandated by law in some states.

◾ HERNIATED INTERVERTEBRAL DISK

DESCRIPTION An *intervertebral disk* is a saclike mass of cartilage. One is found between each of the 33 vertebrae. Within each intervertebral disk is the *nucleus pulposus,* a soft, gelatinous mass that helps each disk cushion the movements of the vertebrae. A *herniated intervertebral disk* occurs when the nucleus pulposus leaks through the wall of the disk and into the spinal canal, where it may press on spinal nerves and cause pain and disability (Fig. 12–5). The condition is commonly called a *slipped disk.* The most common sites for herniated disks are between the fourth and fifth lumbar vertebrae or between the fifth lumbar and the first sacral vertebrae. The condition is more common in men.

ETIOLOGY A herniated intervertebral disk usually is caused by spinal trauma from a fall, straining, or heavy lifting. The herniation may occur at the time of the trauma or sometime later. A herniated disk may be related to intervertebral joint degeneration. In this latter case, a minor trauma may result in a disk herniation.

SIGNS AND SYMPTOMS Symptoms depend on the particular site of herniation, but severe back pain that worsens with motion is common. **Paresthesia** and restricted mobility of the neck often occur. The sciatic nerve may be painful upon applying pressure. The sciatic pain may begin as a dull ache and progress to severe pain. Coughing, sneezing, or bending will intensify the pain and discomfort.

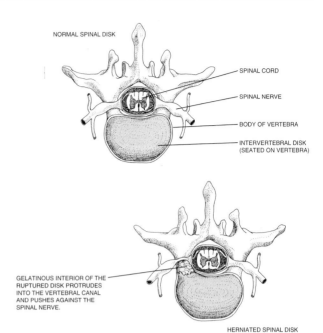

NORMAL SPINAL DISK

SPINAL CORD

SPINAL NERVE

BODY OF VERTEBRA

INTERVERTEBRAL DISK
(SEATED ON VERTEBRA)

GELATINOUS INTERIOR OF THE
RUPTURED DISK PROTRUDES
INTO THE VERTEBRAL CANAL
AND PUSHES AGAINST THE
SPINAL NERVE.

HERNIATED SPINAL DISK

Figure 12–5 Normal and herniated spinal disks. (From Thomas, CL [ed]: Taber's Cyclopedic Medical Dictionary, ed 18. FA Davis, Philadelphia, 1997, with permission.)

DIAGNOSTIC PROCEDURES Obtaining a thorough patient history is important to rule out other causes of back pain. The diagnosis is confirmed if the individual complains of sciatic pain when a straight-leg-raising test is performed. In addition spinal x-rays, computed tomography (CT) scans, and magnetic resonance imaging (MRI) may be ordered. Myelography may show the point of spinal compression caused by the herniated disk.

TREATMENT Bed rest, heat applied to the affected portion of the spine, and **salicylate** analgesics may be prescribed. Muscle relaxants may be helpful. Traction of the lower extremities and a back brace may be beneficial in the event of a herniated lumbosacral disk. A cervical halter or a cervical collar may be used to treat a slipped cervical disk. If conservative treatment is not successful, surgical removal of the herniated disk may be necessary. Spinal fusion may be necessary to stabilize the spine.

PROGNOSIS With surgery, the prognosis is improved.

PREVENTION Following proper lifting techniques may help prevent herniated intervertebral disks.

OSTEOPOROSIS

DESCRIPTION *Osteoporosis* is a metabolic bone disease affecting 5 to 10 million Americans. This disease especially affects women who are 50 years of age or older, postmenopausal, small-boned, or who come from a Northern European, especially Scandinavian, background. The total bone mass for someone affected by osteoporosis is less than expected for their age and sex. The proportion of bone mineral to bone **matrix** is normal, however, and there usually is no detectable abnormality of bone composition. Bones become brittle, porous, and vulnerable to fracture due to the decreased calcium and phosphate in bones (Fig. 12–6).

ETIOLOGY In most instances, osteoporosis is idiopathic, and it does not respond well to therapy. In some instances, osteoporosis is a manifestation of another disease, such as Cushing's disease. Possible contributing factors to osteoporosis include prolonged inadequate dietary intake of calcium, a sedentary lifestyle, poor or declining adrenal function, and faulty protein metabolism due to estrogen deficiency. Most commonly, osteoporosis occurs in postmenopausal women.

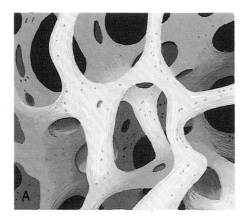 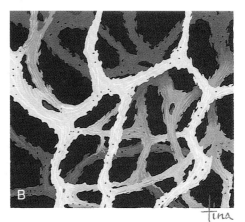

Figure 12–6 (*A*) Normal spongy bone, as in the body of a vertebra. (*B*) Spongy bone thinned by osteoporosis. (From Scanlon, VC, and Sanders, T: Essentials of Anatomy and Physiology, ed 3. FA Davis, Philadelphia, 1999, p 104, with permission.)

SIGNS AND SYMPTOMS Symptoms include bone pain, especially in the lower back and in the weight-bearing bones; spontaneous fractures, especially of vertebrae at the midthoracic level or thoracolumbar junction; and loss of height. Inspection may reveal a humpback.

DIAGNOSTIC PROCEDURES Blood tests are run to measure levels of phosphorus, alkaline phosphatase, total protein, albumin, and creatine. Excretion of calcium, phosphate, creatinine, and hydroxyproline also may be monitored through urinalysis. X-rays are helpful, but may be difficult to interpret in cases of osteoporosis because the density of skeletal parts may appear to be similar to that of soft tissue. A bone scintiscan, bone biopsy, or CT scan may be ordered if more specific diagnostic data are necessary.

TREATMENT The treatment depends on the cause. Increased dietary calcium, phosphate supplements, and multivitamins may be prescribed. In postmenopausal osteoporosis, estrogen therapy may be attempted to produce significant calcium retention, decrease the difference between the rates of bone formation and resorption, and to retard bone loss. Calcium and vitamin D may be supplemented to support bone metabolism. Calcitonin may be prescribed subcutaneously or via nasal spray to decrease bone resorption. Biophosphates (antiresorptive agents), parathyroid hormone (to stimulate bone resorption), or sodium fluoride (to increase

bone mass in the spine) may be tried. Exercise may help minimize osteoporosis by slowing loss of mineral calcium, but if the bones have become brittle, exercise of any kind may be prohibited. Analgesics and muscle relaxants may be needed if pain or muscle spasms are a problem. Frequent rest periods are advised if bone pain is severe.

PROGNOSIS The prognosis is mostly dictated by the cause. Osteoporosis can cause permanent disability if not arrested.

PREVENTION Prevention includes a calcium-rich diet. A person at risk may need to take more calcium and a multivitamin and to exercise daily. Table 12–1 lists the risk factors for osteoporosis.

■ OSTEOMALACIA

DESCRIPTION *Osteomalacia* is a disease in which there is a destructive mineralization of the bone-forming tissue. The disease is characterized by increasing softness of the bones, so that they become flexible and bend, causing deformities. When the disease occurs in children, it is called *rickets*, which is rarely seen in the United States.

ETIOLOGY Osteomalacia is caused by insufficient bodily stores or ineffective utilization of vitamin D, a substance that plays a central role in the physiological process of bone formation. Inadequate dietary intake of vitamin D may cause the disorder, as may inadequate exposure to sunlight, which the

Table 12–1 Risk Factors for Osteoporosis

Female
Advanced age
White or Asian
Thin, small-framed body
Positive family history
Low calcium intake
Early menopause (before age 45)
Sedentary lifestyle
Nulliparity
Smoking
Excessive alcohol or caffeine
High protein intake
High phosphate intake
Certain medications, when taken for a long time
   (high doses of glucocorticoid, phenytoin, thyroid
   medication more than 2 grains)
Endocrine diseases (hyperthyroidism, Cushing's
   disease, acromegaly, hypogonadism,
   hyperparathyroidism)

Source: Stanley, M, and Beare, PG: Gerontological Nursing,
   FA Davis, Philadelphia, 1995, p 167, with permission.

body needs to synthesize its own vitamin D. Other causes include intestinal malabsorption of vitamin D or defective metabolism of the substance. Conditions such as chronic **acidosis,** chronic renal failure, and other renal diseases or certain drugs and toxins also may cause osteomalacia.

SIGNS AND SYMPTOMS Symptoms may include mild, aching bone pain, loss of height, and muscular weakness. Bending, flattening, or deformation of bones is common in osteomalacia.

DIAGNOSTIC PROCEDURES Laboratory tests include blood analysis of phosphate, alkaline phosphatase, total protein, 25-hydroxyvitamin D_3, albumin, and creatinine. Urinalysis to determine levels of urine calcium, phosphorus, and creatinine may be performed. Skeletal x-rays will typically reveal zones of decalcification, called *pseudofractures,* appearing along the surface of certain bones, especially on the scapula, the rim of the pelvis, or the neck of the femur. Ultimately, a bone biopsy may be needed.

TREATMENT The treatment depends on the cause. Treatment may consist of vitamin D supplementation, possibly in conjunction with phosphorus supplementation, and a diet high in calcium. Analgesics may be prescribed to alleviate pain. Because the bones may be soft, the client may need to sit or

lie down more frequently. If the disease is caused by deficient absorption or metabolism of vitamin D, treatment of the underlying problem must accompany vitamin D supplementation.

PROGNOSIS Although osteomalacia is potentially curable, the underlying cause influences the prognosis.

PREVENTION Ensuring an adequate dietary vitamin D intake is necessary for prevention of osteomalacia.

■ OSTEOMYELITIS

DESCRIPTION *Osteomyelitis* is infection of the bone-forming tissue. Such infections are characterizes by inflammation, edema, and circulatory congestion of the bone marrow. As the infection progresses, pus may form and sustained inflammatory pressure may cause fracturing of small pieces of bone. Osteomyelitis usually begins as an acute infection, but it may evolve into a chronic condition. The disease is more common in children.

ETIOLOGY Osteomyelitis is most often caused by trauma that results in hematoma formation and an acute bacterial infection, particularly by *Staphylococcus aureus,* although other viruses and fungi also may cause the condition somewhere else in the body. The infectious microorganisms may reach the bone marrow through the blood or by spreading from infected adjacent tissue; they can also be introduced directly into the bone tissue following physical trauma or surgery. Diabetes mellitus may predispose an individual to osteomyelitis, as may the presence of prosthetic hardware (screws, plates, rods) within the bone.

SIGNS AND SYMPTOMS Specific symptoms depend on which bone or bones are affected and the **virulence** of the infecting microorganisms. Generalized symptoms may include the sudden onset of fever, chills, **malaise,** sweating, pain, and tenderness and swelling over the affected bone. Both the acute and chronic forms of osteomyelitis may exhibit the same clinical picture, although the chronic form may persist for years before it is detected following a flareup due to minor trauma.

DIAGNOSTIC PROCEDURES Blood cultures or aspiration and culture of fluid from the infection site are essential to isolate the causative microorganism. X-rays and bone scans may prove helpful in determining the site and extent of the infection.

TREATMENT Bed rest and parenterally administered antibiotics often suffice. If not, surgical drainage to remove pus and dead bone may be necessary. Immobilization of the affected part and analgesics may be required.

PROGNOSIS With today's therapeutic options, osteomyelitis frequently resolves favorably. If the acute form of the disease progresses to a chronic form, the prognosis is poor. Clients often suffer a fair amount of pain and require lengthy hospitalization.

PREVENTION Extreme care must be taken during surgery or following trauma to prevent contamination, so that the disease does not have a chance to develop.

■ PAGET'S DISEASE (Osteitis Deformans)

DESCRIPTION *Paget's disease* is a chronic metabolic skeletal disease. In the initial phase it is marked by a high rate of bone turnover. Bone is rapidly resorbed and replaced with bone of a coarse, irregular consistency. Consequently, the affected bone becomes thicker but softer. A later phase of the disease is characterized by the replacement of normal bone marrow with highly vascular fibrous tissue. The disease may occur in only one bone or at numerous sites throughout the skeletal system. The disease usually appears in individuals, primarily men, older than 40 years of age, and it becomes increasingly common with advancing age.

ETIOLOGY The cause of Paget's disease is not known.

SIGNS AND SYMPTOMS Many individuals with Paget's disease are asymptomatic. The nature of symptoms that do appear depends on the extent of the disease and which bone or bones are affected. Some individuals may first notice a swelling or other deformity in one of the long bones of the body or a need to increase their hat size if the bones of the skull are involved. The gradual onset of dull but persistent pain around the area of the affected bone may be the first symptom in some. The pain may become severe enough to be disabling, however. Gradual hearing loss may occur in the event of involvement of the ossicles or nearby skull bones.

DIAGNOSTIC PROCEDURES X-rays, bone scintiscans, and bone marrow biopsies may help diagnose the disease. Blood analysis and urinalysis are helpful. The high rate of bone turnover that is characteristic of the disease is indicated by high levels of alkaline phosphatase in the blood, together with high levels of hydroxyproline in the urine.

TREATMENT Treatment may include a high-protein, high-calcium diet and vitamin D supplementation. Aspirin may be prescribed for pain relief and to suppress the level of activity of the disease. Treatment with certain anti-inflammatory drugs and cytotoxic agents may be attempted. The use of calcitonins, hormone derivatives that prevent bone loss, also has been beneficial in many cases.

PROGNOSIS For severe forms of Paget's disease the prognosis is poor. Complications may include frequent fractures, hypercalcemia, kidney stones, deafness, blindness, and spinal cord injuries. An especially serious complication is bone sarcoma.

PREVENTION There are no preventive measures for Paget's disease.

■ FRACTURES

DESCRIPTION A *fracture* is a break or crack in a bone. Types of fractures are illustrated in Figure 12–7 and explained here:

- *Closed fracture.* A break in the bone with no external wound to the skin.
- *Open or compound fracture.* A break in the bone in which there is an open wound leading down to the site of the fracture or in which a piece of broken bone protrudes through the skin.
- *Greenstick fracture.* One in which the bone is partially bent and split, as a green stick or twig does when bent. This type of fracture occurs most frequently in children or among adults with soft bones.
- *Comminuted fracture.* One in which the bone is broken or splintered into pieces, often with fragments embedded in surrounding tissue.
- *Impacted fracture.* One in which the bone is broken with one end forced into the interior of the other.

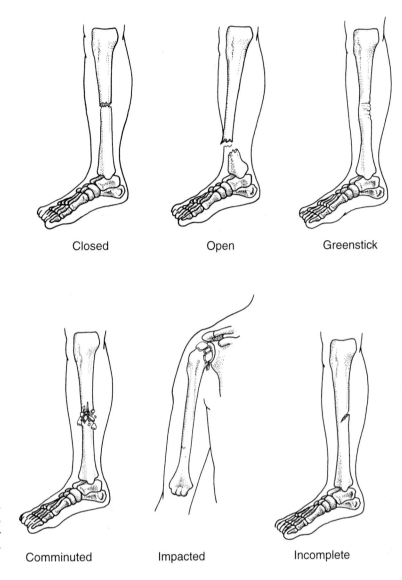

Figure 12–7 Common types of fractures. (Adapted from Gylys, BA, and Wedding, ME: Medical Terminology: A Systems Approach, ed 4. FA Davis, Philadelphia, 1999, p 203. With permission.)

Closed Open Greenstick

Comminuted Impacted Incomplete

- *Incomplete fracture.* One in which the fraction line does not include the whole bone (stress fracture).

ETIOLOGY Bone fractures are usually caused by physical trauma. A host of pathological processes, though, may occasion a bone fracture after only minimal trauma or following normal muscular contractions. Examples of diseases or conditions that may include fractures include bone neoplasms, osteoporosis, Paget's disease, osteomalacia, osteomyelitis, and nutritional and vitamin deficiency disorders.

SIGNS AND SYMPTOMS Common symptoms of fractures include acute pain at the affected site, muscle spasm, and perhaps hemorrhage and shock. Bone may protrude through the skin.

DIAGNOSTIC PROCEDURES X-rays are used to locate the fracture and determine its severity. A bone scintiscan may be ordered to detect hairline fractures.

TREATMENT Immobilization of the affected parts and control of any bleeding are paramount. Open or closed reduction may be needed to place the parts in their normal position for proper healing.

Open reduction is accomplished by surgery, followed by external fixation such as casting, or by internal fixation with the use of metal plates, screws, or rods. *Closed reduction* consists of manipulation and casting without a surgical incision. Traction may be used, especially for fractures of the leg bones, until healing takes place or until internal fixation can be performed. Rib fractures may require no treatment, or the chest may be bandaged or taped for support and pain control. Analgesics or muscle relaxants may be ordered to ease the pain accompanying many types of fractures.

PROGNOSIS The prognosis depends on the severity of the fracture and the age of the individual. The existence of an underlying pathological process worsens the prognosis by complicating the healing process. Complications can occur in any type of fracture and may include **embolism,** infection, delayed union or nonunion of the fracture, and complications resulting from immobilization.

PREVENTION The best prevention of fractures is conscientious adherence to safety rules at work and in play.

Joints

OSTEOARTHRITIS

DESCRIPTION *Osteoarthritis* is a chronic inflammatory process of the joints and bones resulting in degeneration of joint cartilage and subsequent **hypertrophy** of the surrounding bone. The disease may affect any joint in the body but especially weight-bearing ones such as the knee and hip. It is the most common form of arthritis, and it occurs with equal frequency in both sexes, especially among elderly persons. In fact, after age 60, most individuals will show evidence of osteoarthritis on x-ray, although they may be asymptomatic.

ETIOLOGY The cause of osteoarthritis is not known, but autoimmune factors may play a role. It seems to be related to aging. Secondary osteoarthritis generally occurs after trauma or a congenital abnormality such as dysplasia.

SIGNS AND SYMPTOMS The onset of osteoarthritis typically is insidious. The first symptom may include deep, aching joint pain that usually is relieved by rest. There may be stiffness, especially in the morning, and aching during weather changes. There usually is minimal inflammation. **Crepitation** may be heard on joint movement. Deformity may be minimal in some cases, but bony enlargement can occur.

DIAGNOSTIC PROCEDURES A thorough medical history will confirm symptoms. Skeletal x-rays from various angles may be necessary to diagnose the changes in the joint and bone. Synovial fluid analysis may be ordered to rule out inflammatory arthritis. Bone scans or MRI may be necessary for diagnosis.

TREATMENT Because osteoarthritis cannot be cured, the goal of treatment is to minimize pain and inflammation, to maintain joint function, and to minimize disability. Various analgesics and anti-inflammatory drugs may be prescribed. Physical activity restrictions, rest, and the use of crutches or a cane may be necessary. Local heat, such as a paraffin bath for the hands, and weight reduction may be helpful. If the condition is severe, various forms of orthopedic surgery may help to relieve pain and improve joint function. The replacement of hip and knee joints with prosthetic devices also may be attempted.

PROGNOSIS Prognosis depends on the site affected and the severity of the disease. Disability can range from minor to severe. The progression of osteoarthritis varies.

PREVENTION There is no known prevention.

RHEUMATOID ARTHRITIS (RA)

DESCRIPTION *Rheumatoid arthritis* is a chronic, systemic, inflammatory disease affecting the synovial membranes of multiple joints. The disease has the capacity to destroy cartilage, erode bone, and deform joints. The course of the disease is characterized by spontaneous remissions and unpredictable exacerbations. It occurs most frequently in women, with the prevalence of the disease increasing with advancing age.

As the disease develops, there is congestion and edema of the synovial membrane and joint. This causes formation of a thick layer of granulation tissue that invades the cartilage destroying the joint and bone (Fig. 12–8). Lastly, a fibrous **ankylosis** occurs, causing visible deformities and total immobility.

ETIOLOGY The cause of RA is not known. Research suggests that some individuals may be genetically predisposed to acquiring the disease. Infections and endocrine factors have also been named. Autoimmunity is considered a factor also.

SIGNS AND SYMPTOMS RA develops insidiously among most affected individuals. The earliest signs and symptoms may include malaise, persistent low-grade fever, fatigue, and weight loss. Joint pain and stiffness gradually emerge as the principal symptoms, usually affecting the joints of the fingers, wrists, knees, ankles, and toes in a symmetrical pattern. The pain is characteristically aggravated by movement of the affected joints. In advanced cases of RA affecting the hands, the inter-phalangeal joints are swollen and edematous and have a characteristic tapered appearance.

DIAGNOSTIC PROCEDURES A positive rheumatoid factor blood test is diagnostic in most cases. Other useful laboratory tests include antinuclear antibody, lupus erythematosus cell, serum protein electrophoresis, erythrocyte sedimentation rate (ESR), complete blood count (CBC), and synovial fluid analysis. X-rays are also useful.

TREATMENT The primary objectives of treatment are to reduce inflammation and pain, preserve joint function, and prevent joint deformity. Rest, salicylates (particularly aspirin), and physical therapy generally are prescribed. Advanced rheumatoid arthritis may require surgical repair of the hip, knee, or hand joints.

PROGNOSIS The course of the disease is generally unpredictable. Permanent spontaneous remission may occur with return to normal function or less disability than previously; however, the disease generally is progressive, with some degree of consequent deformity. Only a small percentage suffer total disability. RA usually requires lifelong treatment.

PREVENTION There is no known prevention.

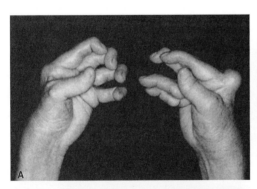
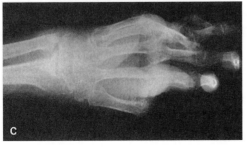
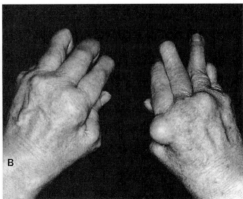

Figure 12–8 Severe rheumatoid arthritis can result in serious joint deformity (*A and B*) caused by the destruction of the joint tissues, as shown in the x-ray (*C*). (From Stanley, BG, and Tribuzi, SM: Concepts in Hand Rehabilitation. FA Davis, Philadelphia, 1992, p 405, with permission.)

GOUT

DESCRIPTION *Gout,* also called gouty arthritis, is a chronic disorder of uric acid metabolism. It is manifested as acute, episodic attacks of a form of arthritis in which crystals of uric acid compounds appear in the synovial fluid of joints. The disease also is marked by **tophi,** which are deposits of urate compounds in and around the joints of the extremities; these frequently lead to joint deformity and disability. Gout is also characterized by hyperuricemia, renal dysfunction, and kidney stones. The disease affects more men than women, usually appearing after the age of 30. Among women, gout usually appears after menopause.

ETIOLOGY The cause of gout may be metabolic, renal, or both. *Metabolic gout* is inherited, and several genetic factors have the potential to produce the condition. In this form of gout, the body produces more uric acid than can be cleared by the kidneys into the urine. *Renal gout* is caused by one of many possible renal dysfunctions. In this form of gout, the body may produce normal levels of uric acid, but the action of the kidneys is insufficient to clear the compound from the blood.

SIGNS AND SYMPTOMS The classic manifestation of gout is the sudden onset of excruciating joint pain, usually affecting the joints of the big toes. Other joints may be involved as well, especially those of the feet, ankles, and knees. The pain generally reaches a peak after several hours and then gradually subsides. An acute attack also may be accompanied by mild fever and chills. The individual is characteristically free of any symptoms between attacks. As the disease progresses, the interval between acute attacks diminishes, and tophi may appear around the affected joints or at other points of the body.

DIAGNOSTIC PROCEDURES Identification of urate crystals in joint fluid or the presence of tophi in and around joints is indicative of gout. Urinalysis will almost always reveal hyperuricemia. Other laboratory tests include ESR and white blood count (WBC). Skeletal x-rays may be used to assess the degree of damage to the affected joints.

TREATMENT Treatment of an acute attack may involve bed rest, immobilization of the affected part, local applications of heat or cold, and analgesics. Anti-inflammatory agents such as colchicine may be prescribed to alleviate the symptoms of an acute attack or to lessen the likelihood of a recurrence. Management of gout also may involve attempts to control the rate of uric acid formation by having the individual follow a low-purine diet. (Purines are end products of protein metabolism and are broken down to form uric acid.) Such a diet excludes sweetbreads, liver, kidney, poultry, fish, alcohol, rich pastries, and fried foods. In order to promote uric acid clearance by the kidneys, individuals with gout will usually be encouraged to drink fluids frequently and also may have to take various antihyperuricemic agents.

PROGNOSIS Because of modern treatment procedures, gout is seldom as permanently disabling as it once was. Treatment measures may need to be maintained indefinitely. Complications include hypertension, kidney stones, and renal damage.

PREVENTION There are no specific preventative measures for gout, but a low-purine diet and maintaining adequate hydration may lessen the chance of the disease occurring among those known to be at risk.

 ALTERNATIVE MEDICINE

Alternative treatment modalities for arthritis include proper diet and nutrition, detoxification, and stress reduction. Pain management and correction of postural or skeletal problems will also be addressed. The following recommendations are made:

- Lose excess weight to ease stress on weight-bearing joints.
- Choose a diet rich in vegetables, fruits, nuts, and whole grains.
- Eat cold water fish such as salmon, sardines, mackerel, and herring.
- Take a cod-liver oil supplement with the diet.
- Drink plenty of water.
- Consider acupuncture, chiropractic adjustments, deep massage, and proper body movement and alignment.

Nutritional supplements, herbal medicines, and **ayurvedic** medicine may be useful, but these treatments will need the direction of an alternative medicine specialist.

Muscles and Connective Tissue

■ SPRAINS AND STRAINS

DESCRIPTION A *sprain* is the tearing or stretching of a ligament surrounding a joint that usually follows a sharp twist. A *strain* is a tearing or stretching of a tendon or a muscle.

ETIOLOGY Sprains and strains may be caused by trauma or result from excessive use of a body part.

SIGNS AND SYMPTOMS Symptoms are localized pain and inflammation, black-and-blue discoloration at the site of the injury, and loss of mobility. Sprains and strains caused by chronic overuse of a ligament, muscle, or tendon will typically cause stiffness, soreness, and tenderness, whereas a sharp, transient pain may result when either condition is acute.

DIAGNOSTIC PROCEDURES A medical history revealing recent physical activities with the potential for causing sprains or strains may suggest the diagnosis. X-rays may be necessary to rule out the possibility of a fracture.

TREATMENT Sprains and strains usually require immediately elevating and resting the injured part. Cold compresses may be applied intermittently to the affected site for 12 to 48 hours to lessen swelling. Depending on the severity of the injury, immobilization of the affected part may be attempted by applying an elastic wrap or soft cast. Analgesics may be necessary to control pain or discomfort. Surgical repair may be indicated if the injury heals improperly or if a rupture results.

PROGNOSIS With proper treatment, healing of a strain or sprain generally occurs within 2 to 4 weeks.

PREVENTION Prevention of these injuries includes warming up when preparing for exercise or physical activity, following safety precautions, and recognizing personal physical limitations.

■ BURSITIS

DESCRIPTION *Bursitis* is inflammation of a bursa, a thin-walled sac lined with synovial tissue that facilitates movement of tendons and muscles over bony prominences. Common forms of bursitis include subacromial (shoulder); subdeltoid (arm); olecranon (elbow), which is commonly referred to as *miner's* or *tennis elbow;* prepatellar (knee), which is referred to as *housemaid's knee;* and ischial (pelvis), which is commonly referred to as *weaver's bottom.*

ETIOLOGY Bursitis may be caused by excessive frictional forces, trauma, and systemic diseases, such as gout or rheumatoid arthritis, or infection.

SIGNS AND SYMPTOMS The classic symptom is tenderness or pain, especially on movement of the affected part. Restricted movement, swelling, and edema at the site are common. Fluid accumulation in the bursae causes irritation, inflammation, and sudden or gradual pain.

DIAGNOSTIC PROCEDURES The client's clinical picture and a medical history may be all that are necessary for diagnosis. X-rays occasionally may show calcific deposits at the affected site.

TREATMENT Treatment may include application of cold or heat, immobilization of the affected part, analgesics, nonsteroidal anti-inflammatory agents, and local steroid injections. Active mobilization to prevent adhesions will prove helpful after the acute pain subsides.

PROGNOSIS The prognosis is good if the bursitis is treated as soon as possible. Bursitis may become chronic, in which case activity restrictions may be required or surgical intervention may be attempted to remove calcification. If infection results, surgical drainage or aspiration may be necessary, followed by antibiotic therapy.

PREVENTION Prevention of bursitis includes avoiding trauma and strenuous exercise that might stress or cause pressure on a joint.

■ CARPAL TUNNEL SYNDROME

DESCRIPTION *Carpal tunnel syndrome* is a most common syndrome that compresses the median nerve in the wrist, within the carpal tunnel. This compression causes sensory and motor changes in the hand. It is most commonly seen in individuals who use their hands and wrists for repetitive motion. These individuals include assembly-line workers, packers, data-entry clerks, dental hygienists, and any others who make strenuous use of their hands.

ETIOLOGY Overuse of the hands and fingers causes inflammation or fibrosis of the tendon sheaths that pass through the carpal tunnel. Edema and compression of the median nerve results.

SIGNS AND SYMPTOMS Pain, burning, weakness, numbness, or tingling in one or both hands are the classic symptoms. An individual will be unable to clench the fist or demonstrate a strong grip. Pain is usually worse at night and in the morning.

DIAGNOSTIC PROCEDURES The medical history usually indicates a tendency to the syndrome. There will be decreased sensation to light touch or pinpricks of the fingers and a positive Tinel's sign (tingling over the median nerve on light tapping). A blood pressure cuff inflated above systolic pressure on the forearm for 1 minute reproduces symptoms of the syndrome.

TREATMENT Rest of the wrist and support with a splint is the first treatment. If a client's occupation is the cause, ergonomic modifications of the work place may be implemented. Consideration may need to be given to another line of employment. Surgical decompression of the nerve by resecting the carpal tunnel ligament may be necessary.

PROGNOSIS The prognosis is good, especially if the client responds to wrist rest and a splint. Surgical techniques are quite effective, but a change of occupation may be necessary also.

PREVENTION Avoid repetitive movements of the wrist or hand. Use wrist rests at computer keyboards and mouse pads.

 ## ALTERNATIVE MEDICINE

Yoga-based stretching and postural alignment shows promise in the treatment of carpal tunnel syndrome. The yoga stretching may help relieve compression in the carpal tunnel. Better joint posture helps decrease intermittent compression and increases blood flow. A randomized trial study re-

ported in the November 11, 1998 *JAMA* showed that clients in the yoga-treated group demonstrated significant improvements for grip strength and pain reduction.

 ## TENDONITIS

DESCRIPTION *Tendonitis* is inflammation of a tendon or the tendon-muscle attachments to bone, usually in the shoulder rotator cuff, hip, Achilles tendon, or hamstring. The condition is characterized by inflammation, fibrosis, and tears in the tendon.

ETIOLOGY Tendonitis generally results from overuse, another musculoskeletal disease such as rheumatoid arthritis, postural misalignment, or hypermobility.

SIGNS AND SYMPTOMS Symptoms usually include dull aching in the affected tendon area and severe pain when the area is moved. At night, the pain often interferes with sleep.

DIAGNOSTIC PROCEDURES A medical history indicating physical strain or injury and the client's clinical picture generally are sufficient for diagnosis. X-rays may be normal or show bony fragments or calcium deposits. An arthrogram may establish the diagnosis.

TREATMENT Treatment of tendonitis may include rest or immobilization of the affected area, nonsteroidal anti-inflammatory drugs, application of cold or heat, local steroid injections, and physical therapy.

PROGNOSIS Tendonitis usually responds to medical treatment and a change in physical activities. If untreated, it can become disabling. Chronic tendonitis may require surgical intervention to remove calcium deposits.

PREVENTION Prevention of tendonitis includes avoidance of strenuous exercise or overuse that would stress or place pressure on a tendon.

 ## MYASTHENIA GRAVIS

DESCRIPTION *Myasthenia gravis* is a chronic, progressive neuromuscular disease that produces progressive, sporadic weakness and exhaustion of skeletal muscles. Curiously enough, neither the motor nerves nor the muscles themselves are directly affected by this disease. Rather, myasthenia gravis may be an autoimmune response resulting in the disappearance of receptors for the neurotransmitter **acetylcholine,** the substance that transfers a nerve impulse from the nerve ending across to the muscle fiber itself. The condition occurs more frequently in women than in men and has its highest incidence between the ages of 20 and 40. *Thymomas,* that is, tumors of the thymus gland, accompany myasthenia gravis in approximately 15 percent of cases.

ETIOLOGY The cause of this disease is not known, but it appears to be an acquired autoimmune disorder in which antibodies are produced that destroy the acetylcholine receptors.

SIGNS AND SYMPTOMS Skeletal muscle weakness and fatigability occur. Onset may be sudden, and most affected individuals will notice drooping eyelids and double vision as the first signs that something is wrong. Because the muscles most affected are usually those innervated by the cranial nerves (face, lips, tongue, neck, and throat), a blank expression, nasal regurgitation of fluids, difficulty swallowing, **ptosis,** and a bobbing head may result.

Muscle weakness typically occurs later in the day or after strenuous exercise. Although short rest periods characteristically restore muscle function, the muscle weakness is progressive in myasthenia gravis, and most muscles will be affected until paralysis occurs. Menses, emotional stress, prolonged exposure to sunlight or cold, and infections will heighten the symptoms. Respiratory muscle weakness or myasthenic crisis (the sudden inability to swallow and respiratory distress) may be severe enough to require mechanical ventilation.

DIAGNOSTIC PROCEDURES The improvement of muscle strength after resting or following injection of anticholinesterase drugs strongly suggests the diagnosis. Electromyography with repeated neural stimulation may be used to confirm the diagnosis. The confirming diagnosis of myasthenia gravis is improved muscle function after an injection (intravenous) of edrophonium or neostigmine.

TREATMENT Treatment is symptomatic and supportive. Anticholinesterase drugs are effective against fatigue and muscle weakness, but they become less effective as the disease progresses. Thymectomy is being used with some success. Corticosteroids may be beneficial. It is important to guard against myasthenic crisis and to treat it with emergency measures should it occur.

PROGNOSIS Unexplained, spontaneous remissions may occur, but usually the disease is a lifelong condition with periodic remissions, exacerbations, and day-to-day fluctuations. There is no known cure.

PREVENTION There is no known prevention.

■ POLYMYOSITIS

DESCRIPTION *Polymyositis* is a chronic, progressive disease of connective tissue characterized by edema, inflammation, and degeneration of skeletal muscles. When the disease occurs with skin involvement, it is called *dermatomyositis.* Polymyositis and dermatomyositis develop slowly and have frequent exacerbations and remissions.

ETIOLOGY Polymyositis is an idiopathic disease. Viral and autoimmune etiologies have been proposed but not confirmed. Nearly a third of cases are associated with other connective-tissue disorders such as rheumatoid arthritis and systemic lupus erythematosus. Other cases, particularly among elderly persons, are associated with malignancies.

SIGNS AND SYMPTOMS Polymyositis usually develops insidiously over a period of a few months to a few years. The most frequent initial manifestation of the disease is muscle weakness in the hips and thighs. Consequently, the affected individual will often report difficulty in ascending or descending stairs or difficulty in rising from a sitting or kneeling position. Occasionally, the disease will localize in specific muscle groups, weakening only the neck, shoulder, or quadricep muscles. Later symptoms include dysphagia and respiratory difficulties. In rare instances, the disease may appear as an acute condition, with the rapid onset and development of the symptoms noted.

When the disease develops as dermatomyositis, the previously mentioned symptoms may be preceded or accompanied by characteristic dermatologic changes. These include the appearance of a telltale lilac-colored rash on the eyelids, the bridge of the nose, and the cheeks, forehead, chest, elbows, and knees. The rash-covered portions of the body may itch severely. Dermatomyositis also may be accompanied by edema around the eye sockets.

DIAGNOSTIC PROCEDURES A muscle biopsy may reveal tissue changes characteristic of polymyositis, such as muscle fiber necrosis, infiltration of the muscle tissue with inflammatory cells (leukocytes), and patterns of tissue degeneration and regeneration. Blood testing will typically indicate increased serum levels of enzymes normally present in skeletal muscles. The ESR also will usually be elevated.

TREATMENT High doses of corticosteroid drugs are often administered to bring the disease under control, followed by lower, maintenance doses over a period of years. Cytotoxic drugs also may be used to lower the number of inflammatory cells affecting the muscles. Bed rest during an acute attack is beneficial. Physiotherapy and physical rehabilitation to regain muscle function are important components of the treatment process.

PROGNOSIS The prognosis is variable. Roughly half of those affected by polymyositis recover within 5 years and can discontinue therapy. Some individuals must remain on drug therapy indefinitely; others die from acute cardiac, pulmonary, or renal complications. Generally, the prognosis worsens with age.

PREVENTION There is no specific prevention for polymyositis.

■ SYSTEMIC LUPUS ERYTHEMATOSUS (SLE)

DESCRIPTION *Systemic lupus erythematosus* is a chronic, inflammatory connective-tissue disorder in which cells and tissues throughout the body are damaged by a variety of autoantibodies and immune complexes. The disease affects women eight times more often than men.

ETIOLOGY The cause of the autoimmune response that characterizes SLE is not known. Genetic factors, as well as environmental and hormonal factors, may predispose an individual to the disease. Stress, overexposure to ultraviolet light, immunization reactions, and pregnancy are events that may precipitate the condition. Certain drugs also have the capacity to induce an SLE-like syndrome.

SIGNS AND SYMPTOMS Because SLE can affect any part of the body, a host of symptoms are possible, including weight loss, fatigue, malaise, and fever. One manifestation of the disease is the "butterfly rash" (Fig. 12–9), which may be found on the face, neck, and scalp of about 50 percent of clients with SLE. Similar rashes may appear on other body surfaces, especially on exposed areas. There also may be photosensitivity of the skin, joint and muscle pain, joint deformities, malaise, fever, anorexia, and weight loss. Other signs and symptoms include oral or nasopharyngeal ulcerations, patchy **alopecia,** pleuritis or pericarditis, and **Reynaud's phenomenon.**

DIAGNOSTIC PROCEDURES CBC with differential, ESR, serum electrophoresis, antinuclear antibody, anti-DNA, and lupus erythematosus (LE) tests may be done. LE cells (polymorphonuclear leukocytes) often will be found in the bone marrow. The anti-DNA test, which detects a particular autoantibody,

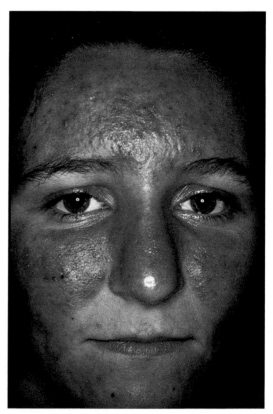

Figure 12–9 Butterfly rash of SLE. (From Lazarus, GS, and Goldsmith, LA: Diagnosis of Skin Disease. FA Davis, Philadelphia, 1997, p 230, with permission.)

is the most specific test for SLE, but it must be performed while the disease is in its active stage.

TREATMENT The mild stage of the disease requires only anti-inflammatory agents, including aspirin. Skin lesions will require topical treatment such as corticosteroid creams. Corticosteroid drugs remain the treatment of choice to control SLE, either for acute generalized exacerbations or for exacerbations of the disease localized to vital organ systems. Photosensitive patients should wear protective clothing when in the sun and use an effective sunscreen agent.

PROGNOSIS The prognosis improves with early detection and careful treatment, but it remains poor for those who develop cardiovascular, renal, or neurological complications or serious bacterial infections. There is a high death rate, usually within 5 years of onset.

PREVENTION There are no specific preventive measures for SLE.

NEOPLASMS

Primary neoplasms of the musculoskeletal system are uncommon, but when they do occur, the prognosis usually is poor. Primary malignancy may arise from osseous tissue. These tumors include the following:

1. Osteogenic sarcoma, which primarily affects the long bones of the body
2. Chondrosarcoma, which also affects the long bones but which tends to metastasize more slowly than osteogenic sarcoma
3. Malignant giant-cell tumor, which is common at the ends of long bones, especially near the knee and lower radius

Nonosseous tumors include fibrosarcoma, chondroma, and Ewing's sarcoma, which is a malignant tumor originating from bone marrow, usually in the long bones or pelvis.

Bone pain is the classic symptom. The pain is dull, localized, and may be more intense at night. A bone biopsy, bone x-ray, and bone scintiscan may be necessary for diagnosis. The treatments of choice are radiation and surgery, which usually involves amputation. With any amputation, rehabilitation is necessary.

SPECIAL FOCUS **CHILDHOOD DISEASE OF THE MUSCULOSKELETAL SYSTEM**

■ DUCHENNE'S MUSCULAR DYSTROPHY

DESCRIPTION *Duchenne's muscular dystrophy* is a congenital disorder characterized by progressive bilateral wasting of skeletal muscles; the symptoms of the disorder do not include neural or sensory defects. It generally strikes during early childhood and can cause death within 10 to 15 years of onset.

ETIOLOGY The disease is the result of an X-linked recessive disorder, which is usually inherited, but may also be due to mutation. The exact mechanism by which the genetic defect produces muscle wasting is not known.

SIGNS AND SYMPTOMS Manifestations of Duchenne's muscular dystrophy begin between the ages of 3 and 5 years. The disease first affects the leg and pelvic muscles, before spreading to involuntary muscles. The affected child may have a characteristic waddling gait, engage in toe-walking, and may suffer from lordosis or other spinal deformities. The child may have difficulty running and climbing stairs and may tend to fall easily. Muscle deterioration is progressive, and **contractures** typically develop.

DIAGNOSTIC PROCEDURES A family history of the disease together with the clinical picture of characteristic symptoms suggests the diagnosis. A muscle biopsy showing characteristic connective tissue and fat deposits will confirm the diagnosis. Electromyography can rule out muscle atrophy that is neurological in origin. Tests of urine creatinine, and serum levels of creatine phosphokinase (CPK) and transaminase, will usually be ordered.

TREATMENT No known treatment is successful in curing Duchenne's muscular dystrophy, but procedures to correct or preserve mobility are helpful. These include orthopedic appliances, exercise, physical therapy, and surgery.

PROGNOSIS The prognosis is poor for a child with Duchenne's muscular dystrophy. Children with this condition are usually confined to a wheelchair by the ages of 9 to 12. Within 10 to 15 years of the onset of the disease, death commonly results from cardiac or respiratory complications or infections.

PREVENTION Carriers of the genetic defect known to cause muscular dystrophy may want to receive genetic counseling regarding the risks of transmitting the disease.

COMMON SYMPTOMS OF MUSCULOSKELETAL DISEASES

Individuals may present with the following common symptoms, which deserve attention from health professionals:

- Pain
- Tenderness and swelling
- Malaise, weakness, and fatigue
- Fever
- Obvious bone deformation, including spontaneous fractures
- Inflammation
- Stiffness
- Weight loss

BIBLIOGRAPHY

The Burton Goldberg Group (ed): Alternative Medicine: The Definitive Guide. Future Medicine Publishing, Tiburon, Calif., 1995.

Diseases. Springhouse Corporation, Springhouse, Pa., 1993.

Fauci, AS, et al: Harrison's Principles of Internal Medicine, ed 14. McGraw-Hill, New York, 1998.

Frazier, MS, et al: Essentials of Human Disease and Conditions. WB Saunders Company, Philadelphia, 1996.

Garfinkel, MS, et al (eds): Yoga-based intervention for carpal tunnel syndrome. JAMA 280(18):1601–1603, 1998.

Professional Guide to Diseases, ed 6. Springhouse Corporation, Springhouse, Pa., 1998.

CASE STUDIES

I A postmenopausal woman slips while stepping off a curb, falls, and cracks her pelvic bone. During diagnosis, the physician begins to consider the possibility of osteoporosis.

1. What are the symptoms of osteoporosis?
2. What diagnostic procedures would the physician order to verify the diagnosis of osteoporosis?
3. If the diagnosis is verified, what treatment will the physician initiate?

II A mail carrier, in the middle of his daily 5-mile delivery route, suddenly experiences excruciating pain in his great left toe. As soon as his route is done, he calls his physician.

1. What are some possible diagnoses?
2. What additional information might the physician look for in making a diagnosis?
3. How might the mail carrier's profession be connected with his complaint?

REVIEW QUESTIONS

MATCHING

_____ 1. Posterior angulation of spine; roundback

a. Lordosis
b. Kyphosis

_____ 2. Lateral curvature of the spine

_____ 3. Spinal curvature with a forward convexity; swayback

_____ 4. Ruptured or slipped disk

c. Scoliosis

d. Herniated intervertebral disk

TRUE/FALSE

T   F   1. Osteomyelitis is a pyogenic infection.

T   F   2. Osteomyelitis involves both the bone marrow cavity and the bone itself.

T   F   3. Paget's disease is a metabolic bone disease.

T   F   4. Paget's disease is also called osteitis deformans.

T   F   5. Osteoarthritis is an acute degeneration and deterioration of joint cartilage.

T   F   6. Rheumatoid arthritis is a chronic, systemic inflammatory disease affecting joints.

T   F   7. Gouty arthritis is a metabolic disease affecting more men than women.

SHORT ANSWER

1. Name and define five types of fractures:

   a.

   b.

   c.

   d.

   e.

2. What is the difference between a sprain and a strain?

DISCUSSION QUESTION

Compare and contrast osteoporosis and osteomalacia.

MULTIPLE CHOICE

Circle all the correct responses:

1. Duchenne's muscular dystrophy is:

   a. Identified with a poor prognosis.

   b. Progressive bilateral wasting of skeletal muscles.

   c. A disease that first affects leg and pelvic muscles.

   d. Diagnosed by muscle biopsy.

2. Myasthenia gravis is:

   a. A failure in transmission of muscle impulses at the neuromuscular junction.

b. A condition in which there is too much acetylcholine released at the junction.

c. Diagnosed by muscle biopsy.

d. A disease that can be cured and prevented.

ANSWERS

MATCHING

1. b   2. c   3. a   4. d

TRUE/FALSE

1. True   5. False
2. True   6. True
3. False   7. True
4. True

SHORT ANSWER

1. a. Closed fracture: a break in the bone that does not break the skin.
   b. Compound or open fracture: more than one break in bone with a break in the skin.
   c. Greenstick fracture: an incomplete break in the bone where the bone bends and splits like green wood.
   d. Comminuted fracture: broken or crushed in small pieces; fragments may be embedded in surrounding tissue.
   e. Impacted fracture: one bone fragment is forced into another.
2. A sprain is a tear or stretching of a ligament, whereas a strain is a tear or stretching of a tendon or a muscle.

DISCUSSION QUESTION

Both are metabolic bone diseases; both have similar diagnostic tests including determination of serum calcium, phosphate, alkaline phosphatase, total protein, urine calcium, phosphorus, and creatinine. X-rays and bone scintiscans may be ordered. Osteoporosis: affects mostly women, 50 years or older, postmenopausal, small-boned; Northern European; total bone mass is less than expected; proportion of bone mineral to bone matrix is normal, with no detectable abnormality of bone composition; disease is idiopathic, senile, or juvenile; bone pain, especially low back; spontaneous fractures; loss of height. Osteomalacia: vitamin D deficiency; often familial; osteoid tissue increases; calcification does not occur; mild, aching bone pain; loss of height; muscular weakness; pseudofractures.

MULTIPLE CHOICE

1. All are correct.
2. All are incorrect.

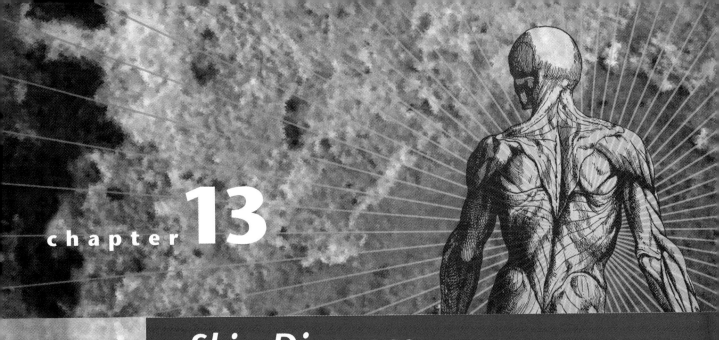

chapter 13

Skin Diseases

CHAPTER OUTLINE

Psoriasis

Urticaria (Hives)

Acne Vulgaris

Alopecia

Impetigo

Furuncles and Carbuncles

Pediculosis

Decubitus Ulcers

Dermatophytoses

Corns and Calluses

Warts

Discoid Lupus Erythematosus

Scleroderma

Dermatitis
Seborrheic Dermatitis

Contact Dermatitis
Atopic Dermatitis (Eczema)

Herpes-Related Skin Lesions
Cold Sores and Fever Blisters
Herpes Zoster (Shingles)

Cancer
Skin Carcinomas
Malignant Melanoma

Special Focus: Childhood Diseases of the Skin
Atopic Dermatitis
Diaper Rash
Pediculosis
Dermatophytosis

Common Symptoms of Skin Diseases

Bibliography

Case Studies

Review Questions

LEARNING OBJECTIVES

Upon successful completion of this chapter, you will:

- Compare and contrast seborrheic dermatitis and psoriasis.
- Identify the etiology of contact and atopic dermatitis.
- Compare the life of a normal skin cell to that of a psoriatic skin cell.
- Identify the signs and symptoms of urticaria.
- Discuss the progression that occurs when a comedo becomes an acne pustule or papule.
- List at least five causes of alopecia.
- Recall the sources of infection of herpes simplex.
- Describe the etiologic process of herpes zoster.
- Restate the prognosis and prevention for impetigo.
- Compare and contrast furuncle and carbuncle.
- List the three common locations for pediculosis.
- Discuss the prevention of decubitus ulcers.
- Recall the five areas where dermatophytosis is likely to occur.
- Recall the treatment for corns and calluses.
- Identify the etiology of warts.
- Describe the signs and symptoms of discoid lupus erythematosus.
- Restate the prognosis for scleroderma.
- Name the two most common types of skin cancers.
- Identify the four types of malignant melanomas.
- Explain the treatment of diaper rash.
- List at least four common symptoms of skin diseases.

KEY WORDS

Abrade (ă•brād′)
Antipruritic (ăn•tĭ•proo•rĭt′ĭk)
Bacteremia (băk•tĕr•ē′mē•ă)
Bulla (pl. *bullae*) (bŭl′lă), (bŭl′ē)
Comedo (kŏm′ē•dō)
Contracture (kŏn•trăk′chūr)
Cryosurgery (krī•ō•sĕr′jĕr•ē)
Débridement (dā•brēd•mŏn′)
Dysphagia (dĭs•fā′jē•ă)
Electrodesiccation
  (ē•lĕk•trō•dĕs•ĭ•kā′shŭn)
Erythema (ĕr•ĭ•thē′mă)
Induration (ĭn•dū•rā′shŭn)
Keratin (kĕr′ă•tĭn)

Keratolytic (kĕr•ă•tō•lĭt′ĭk)
Leukocytosis (loo•kō•sī•tō′sĭs)
Macule (măk′ūl)
Melanin (mĕl′ă•nĭn)
Nephritis (nĕf•rī′tĭs)
Papule (păp′ūl)
Plaque (plăk)
Pruritus (proo•rī′tŭs)
Pustule (pŭs′tūl)
Pyoderma (pī•o•dĕr′mă)
Raynaud's phenomenon (rā•nōs′
  fē•nŏm′ē•nŏn)
Stratum corneum (strā′tŭm kŏr•nē′ŭm)
Vesicle (vĕs′ĭ•kl)
Wheal (hwēl)

The integumentary system, comprising the skin and its accessory organs, provides protection for the body against infection, trauma, and toxic compounds. Skin contains the receptors for touch and other sensations that are important to our individual well-being from birth to death. The skin helps regulate body temperature and even synthesizes vitamin D when exposed to sunlight. Figure 13–1 illustrates the structure of the skin.

The three layers of the skin are the epidermis, the dermis, and the subcutaneous layer of tissue. The *epidermis,* or outer layer, produces **keratin**

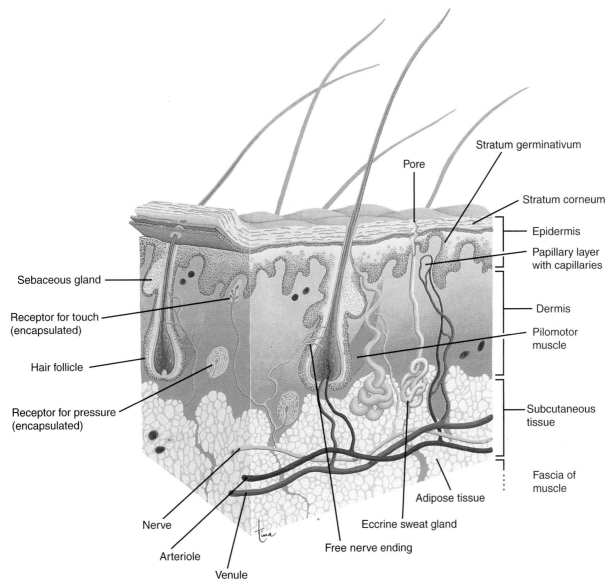

Figure 13–1 Skin. Structure of the skin and subcutaneous tissue. (From Scanlon, VC, and Sanders, T: Essentials of Anatomy and Physiology, ed 3. FA Davis, Philadelphia, 1999, p 85, with permission.)

and the pigment **melanin** that give the skin its color. The *dermis,* or middle layer, consists of fibrous proteins that give the skin strength and elasticity. The *subcutaneous layer* is mostly fat, providing insulation against heat loss. Nails, hair, sebaceous (oil) glands, and sudoriferous (sweat) glands are also part of the integumentary system.

Skin diseases are frequently manifested by alterations in the skin surface called *lesions.* Because most skin diseases produce a specific type of lesion or set of lesions, diagnoses are often made on the basis of the appearance of the lesions. Figure 13–2 illustrates nine basic types of skin lesions. Refer to this figure as you study the signs and symptoms of

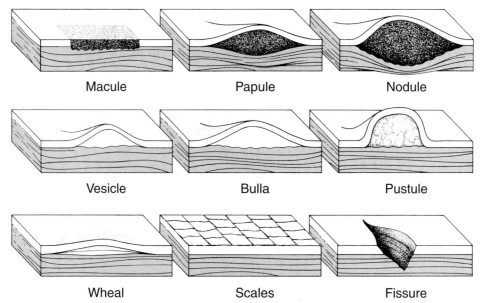

Figure 13–2 Skin lesions. (From Gylys, BA, and Wedding, ME: Medical Terminology: A Systems Approach, ed 3. FA Davis, Philadelphia, 1988, p 70, with permission.)

Table 13–1 Skin Lesions

Type	Characteristics	Examples
Flat Lesion		
Macule	Flat, discolored, circumscribed lesion of any size	Freckle, flat mole, hyperpigmentation
Elevated Lesion		
Papule	Solid elevated lesion, <1 cm in diameter	Nevus, warts, pimples
Nodule	Palpable circumscribed lesion, larger than a papule, 1–2 cm in diameter	Benign or malignant tumor
Wheal	Dome-shaped or flat-topped elevated lesion, slightly reddened and often changing in size and shape, usually accompanied by intense itching	Hives
Vesicle and bulla	Elevated lesion that contains fluid; a bulla is a vesicle >0.5 cm	Blister, herpes zoster, second-degree burn
Pustule	Elevated lesion containing pus that may be sterile or contaminated with bacteria; small abscess on the skin	Acne, pustular psoriasis
Scale	Excessive dry exfoliation shed from upper layers of the skin	Psoriasis, ichtryosis
Cyst	Elevated, encapsulated mass of dermis or subcutaneous layers, solid, or fluid-filled	Sebaceous cyst
Tumor	Swelling; well-demarcated, elevated lesion >2 cm in diameter	Fibroma, lipoma, steatoma, melanoma, hemangioma
Depressed Lesion		
Fissure	Small cracklike sore or break exposing the dermis; usually red	Athlete's foot, cheilosis
Ulcer	Loss of epidermis and dermis within a distinct border	Pressure sore, basal cell carcinoma

the various skin diseases discussed in this chapter. Table 13–1 identifies the characteristics of skin lesions and gives examples.

PSORIASIS

DESCRIPTION *Psoriasis* is a chronic skin disease marked by the appearance of discrete pink or red lesions surmounted by a characteristic silvery scaling (Fig. 13–3). The disease may begin at any age and is noninfectious.

ETIOLOGY The cause of psoriasis is not known, but it appears to be genetically determined. The disease may be an autoimmune disorder. Precipitating factors may include hormonal changes such as those occurring during pregnancy, emotional stress, or even changes in climate.

SIGNS AND SYMPTOMS A high rate of skin cell turnover produces the thick, flaky scaling that is characteristic of psoriasis. The affected areas of skin typically appear dry, cracked, and encrusted. These lesions may appear on the scalp, chest, buttocks, and extremities. **Pruritus** is a common complaint. In some individuals, psoriasis spreads to the nail beds, causing thickened, crumbling nails, which separate from the skin.

DIAGNOSTIC PROCEDURES Observation of the skin, a careful medical history, or a skin biopsy may suggest the diagnosis.

TREATMENT There is no cure for the disease, and the treatment is only palliative. The scales may be removed after they are softened with petroleum jelly or a preparation containing urea. Exposure to ultraviolet light may retard the cell reproduction, and coal tar preparations may be applied to affected areas. Steroid creams, low-dosage antihistamines, oatmeal baths, and open, wet dressings may be ordered. Careful skin hygiene is important.

PROGNOSIS Psoriasis is controllable, but remissions and exacerbations frequently occur. The unsightly lesions that characterize the disease may cause psychological distress.

PREVENTION There is no known prevention.

URTICARIA (Hives)

DESCRIPTION *Urticaria* (*hives*) is an episodic inflammatory reaction of the capillaries beneath a localized area of the skin.

ETIOLOGY Urticaria most frequently results following ingestion of certain foods such as shellfish or berries. The condition also may result from allergic reactions to insect stings or some inhalants, such as animal dander. Heat, cold, water, and sunlight may be predisposing factors of urticaria.

SIGNS AND SYMPTOMS The condition is characterized by the eruption of pale raised **wheals** on the skin, possibly surrounded by **erythema** (Fig. 13–4). The lesions usually form and then resolve quite rapidly, often moving from one portion of the body to another. This vascular reaction usually is accompanied by intense itching.

DIAGNOSTIC PROCEDURES The client's medical history should cover topics such as medications used, frequently ingested foods, environmental factors, and psychological status. The appearance of the in-

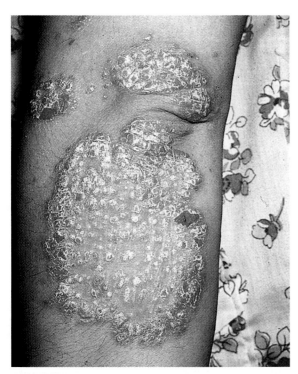

Figure 13–3 Psoriasis. This is a typical manifestation, occurring over a joint, with bright red scaly plaque and silvery scale. (From Reeves, JRT, and Maibach, H: Clinical Dermatology Illustrated: A Regional Approach, ed 3. FA Davis, Philadelphia, 1998, p 189, with permission.)

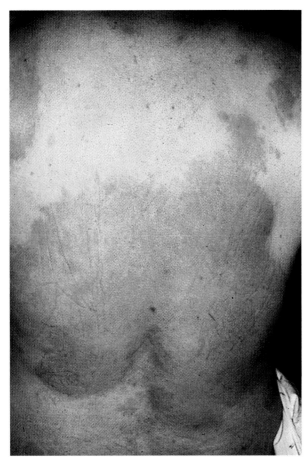

Figure 13–4 Urticaria (hives). These huge wheals occurred on a patient allergic to penicillin. (From Reeves, JRT, and Maibach, H: Clinical Dermatology Illustrated: A Regional Approach, ed 3. FA Davis, Philadelphia, 1998, p 212, with permission.)

flamed area and its history should help pinpoint a diagnosis of urticaria. Sensitization testing may help to identify the causative agent.

TREATMENT When the offending stimulus is removed, urticaria usually subsides. Antihistamines are often useful in controlling an ongoing attack. Epinephrine may be injected to control severe reactions. Hydrocortisone creams or lotions are helpful in providing symptomatic relief from itching.

PROGNOSIS The prognosis for an individual with this uncomfortable disorder is good.

PREVENTION Avoiding the causative agent is the best means of preventing urticaria.

ACNE VULGARIS

DESCRIPTION *Acne vulgaris* is an inflammatory disease of the sebaceous glands and hair follicles, and is characterized by the appearance of **comedos, papules,** and **pustules.** It is more common in adolescents, but the lesions can appear at an earlier or later age, too.

ETIOLOGY The cause of acne vulgaris is not known. The focus of research is on follicular occlusion and androgen-stimulated sebum production. Predisposing factors include hereditary tendencies and disturbances in hormonal balances affecting the activity of the sebaceous glands. Precipitating factors may include endocrine disorders, the use of steroid drugs, or psychogenic factors. The fact that bacteria are important in the disease process is indicated by successful results following antibiotic therapy.

SIGNS AND SYMPTOMS The acne plug often appears first as a comedo (whitehead) or a closed comedo (blackhead) (Fig. 13–5). The color in the blackhead is caused by the melanin produced by the hair follicle, not by dirt. Eventually, an enlarged plug may rupture or leak, spreading its contents to the dermis. This results in inflammation and acne pustules or papules. Scars can develop if chronic irritation continues over a period of time.

DIAGNOSTIC PROCEDURES A medical history and observation of the characteristic lesions confirm the diagnosis.

TREATMENT Therapy may include the use of a strong antibacterial solution applied to the skin, orally administered antibiotics, or both. Topically applied cleansing and peeling (**keratolytic**) agents may prove useful to some, but in general, the skin should be kept as clean and dry as possible.

PROGNOSIS Acne vulgaris is a persistent, often emotionally upsetting problem usually requiring prolonged treatment before it subsides. The ultimate prognosis for most acne sufferers is good. For a few, though, the disease can produce permanent scarring and disfigurement.

PREVENTION There is no known prevention.

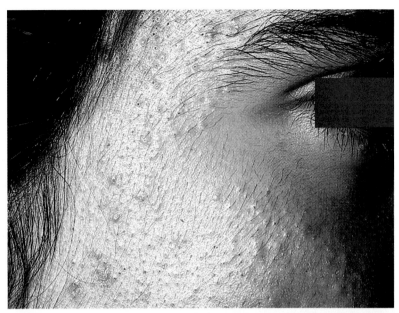

TOP

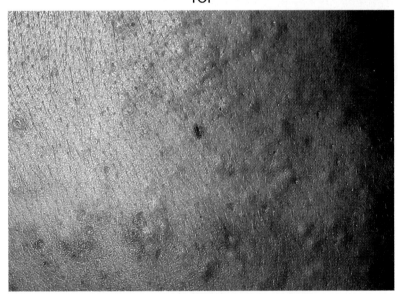

BOTTOM

Figure 13–5 Acne. (*Top*) Almost pure open-comedo (blackhead) acne with only a few inflamed papules. (*Bottom*) Close comedones or whiteheads. They are deep and tenacious. (From Reeves, JRT, and Maibach, H: Clinical Dermatology Illustrated: A Regional Approach, ed 3. FA Davis, Philadelphia, 1998, p 42, with permission.)

ALOPECIA

DESCRIPTION *Alopecia* is the absence or loss of hair, especially on the head.

ETIOLOGY Alopecia may result as a consequence of certain systemic illnesses, endocrine disorders, nutritional problems, and certain forms of dermatitis.

It may be caused by the use of certain drugs or occur as a consequence of chemotherapy or radiation therapy. More frequently, though, alopecia is not related to any specific pathological process. Among men, alopecia seems to be part of the aging process. This form of the condition, called *male pattern baldness*, seems to be related to levels of the hormone androgen and may be genetically determined. In

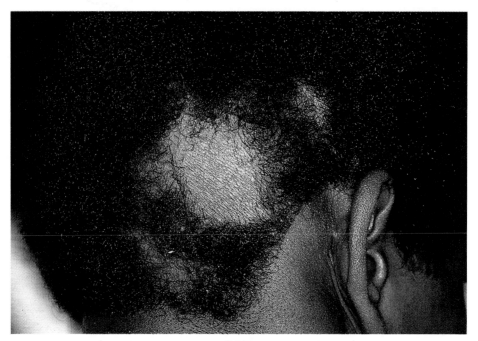

TOP

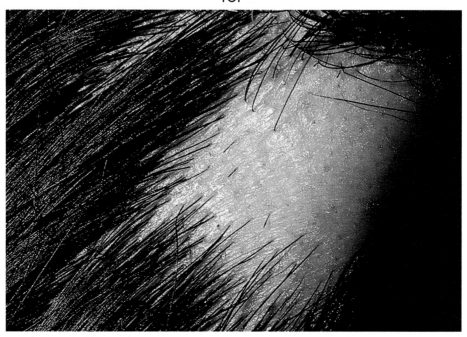

BOTTOM

Figure 13–6 Alopecia areata. (*Top*) Well-defined areas of complete hair loss. (*Bottom*) Short, blunt-ended "exclamation-point" hairs may be seen at the edge of the bald area. (From Reeves, JRT, and Maibach, H: Clinical Dermatology Illustrated: A Regional Approach, ed 3. FA Davis, Philadelphia, 1998, p 18, with permission.)

infants, alopecia is a common, temporary physiological condition.

SIGNS AND SYMPTOMS Alopecia may occur gradually with advancing age, or it may be more sudden, occurring all at once or in patchy spots (Fig. 13–6).

DIAGNOSTIC PROCEDURES The visual examination may be all that is necessary, but the cause must be determined, too.

TREATMENT Treatment varies with the cause of alopecia. For scarring alopecia, there is no treatment. In nonscarring alopecia, spontaneous regrowth may occur, requiring no treatment. If the cause is a change in androgen levels, medications may be ordered. Minoxidil preparations may be used to treat male pattern baldness. Another treatment is surgical redistribution of hair follicles by autografting.

PROGNOSIS The prognosis depends on the cause. Alopecia due to scarring is permanent.

PREVENTION There is no known prevention for some forms of alopecia. For others, early treatment of any disease known to cause alopecia is essential.

IMPETIGO

DESCRIPTION *Impetigo* is a contagious superficial skin infection marked by **vesicles** or **bullae** that become pustular, rupture, and form yellow crusts.

ETIOLOGY The disease is usually caused by *Streptococcus* or *Staphylococcus* bacteria. Predisposing factors include poor hygiene, malnutrition, and anemia. Impetigo occurs more frequently in warm weather.

SIGNS AND SYMPTOMS The lesions of impetigo begin as **macules,** vesicles, and pustules, usually accompanied by pruritus (Fig. 13–7). A thick, yellow crust eventually forms over the infected site. Impetigo can occur anywhere, but it is most common on the mouth, nose, or neck. Satellite lesions may appear as a result of autoinnoculation. Erythema with ulcerations and scarring may result.

DIAGNOSTIC PROCEDURES The characteristic lesions assist in the diagnosis. Viewing a Gram's stain of the vesicle fluid under the microscope usually confirms the infection.

TREATMENT Antibiotics are essential. Thorough cleansing of the lesions is necessary two to three times daily.

PROGNOSIS The prognosis is good.

PREVENTION Prevention includes good hygiene and avoidance of infected persons.

FURUNCLES AND CARBUNCLES

DESCRIPTION A *furuncle*, or boil, is an abscess involving the entire hair follicle and adjacent subcuta-

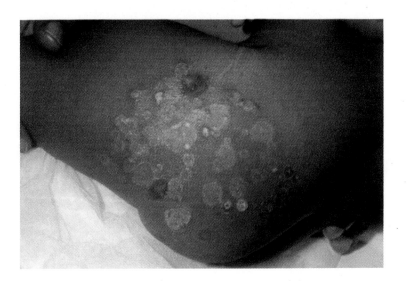

Figure 13–7 Early localized bullous impetigo in infant. Absence of inflammation in this infection is atypical. (Courtesy of John RT Reeves, MD.)

neous tissue. A *carbuncle* consists of several furuncles developing in adjoining hair follicles with multiple drainage sinuses (Fig. 13–8). The most common sites of these lesions are hairy parts of the body exposed to irritation, pressure, friction, or moisture.

ETIOLOGY Infection by *Staphylococcus* bacteria is the most common cause. Predisposing factors include diabetes mellitus, **nephritis,** debilitation, or an infected wound elsewhere in the body.

SIGNS AND SYMPTOMS The affected portion of skin may be extremely tender, painful, and swollen. The abscess may eventually enlarge, soften, and open, discharging pus and necrotic material. Erythema and edema may persist at the site for days or weeks. A mild fever may accompany this condition.

DIAGNOSTIC PROCEDURES Diagnosis is made on the basis of the appearance of the characteristic lesion. There may be slight **leukocytosis,** as evidenced through a complete blood count (CBC). Gram stains of the purulent content will reveal the causative organism.

TREATMENT The infected area must be cleansed with soap and water, and hot, wet compresses should be applied. Antibiotic agents are frequently prescribed. Surgical incision and drainage may be necessary after the lesion is mature.

PROGNOSIS The condition may recur for months or years. Complications from carbuncles may include **bacteremia.**

PREVENTION Prevention includes good personal hygiene and prevention of any infectious process.

PEDICULOSIS

DESCRIPTION *Pediculosis* is skin infestation with lice, a parasitic insect. The body (pediculosis corporis), the scalp (pediculosis capitis), or the pubic area (pediculosis pubis) are the most common sites for infestation to occur.

ETIOLOGY The lice feed on human blood and lay their eggs, or nits, in body hair or clothing, and the eggs hatch, feed, and mature in 2 to 3 weeks. The louse bite injects a toxin in the skin. Pediculosis is more common in people who live in overcrowded places with inadequate facilities and poor personal hygiene. Pediculosis can be transmitted from infected clothing, hats, combs, bed sheets, and towels. Pubic lice may be acquired through sexual intercourse with an infested person.

SIGNS AND SYMPTOMS Intense pruritus and evidence of nits (eggs) on hair shafts (Fig. 13–9) or lice on clothing or on skin are the most common signs and symptoms. There may be gross excoriation of

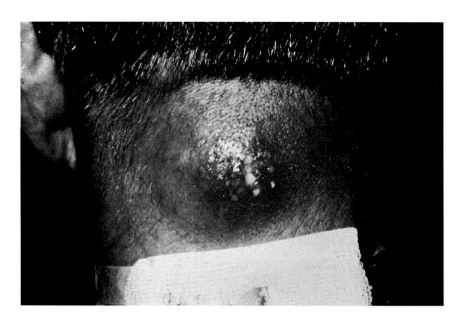

Figure 13–8 Carbuncle. (From Goldsmith, LA, Lazarus, GS, and Tharp, MD: Adult and Pediatric Dermatology: A Color Guide to Diagnosis and Treatment. FA Davis, 1977, p 364, with permission.)

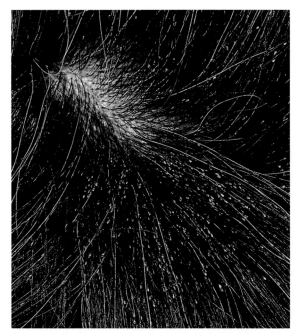

Figure 13–9 Nits attached to hairs of the head in a long-standing case of pediculosis capitis. (From Reeves, JRT, and Maibach, H: Clinical Dermatology Illustrated: A Regional Approach, ed 3. FA Davis, Philadelphia, 1998, p 14, with permission.)

patches of skin and **pyoderma.** Rashes or wheals may develop.

DIAGNOSTIC PROCEDURES Visual examination usually is all that is necessary. Nits can be found on the hair, body, or clothing.

TREATMENT For scalp lice, permethrin cream rinse is rubbed into the hair for 10 minutes. This is followed by the use of a fine-tooth comb to remove lice and nits. Body lice must be removed by washing with soap and water. All clothing and bedding must be washed or dry cleaned. Pubic lice may be treated with creams, lotions, or shampoos.

PROGNOSIS The prognosis is excellent with treatment.

PREVENTION Prevention includes good hygiene, avoiding contact with infested persons, and not sharing combs, brushes, or clothing.

■ DECUBITUS ULCERS

DESCRIPTION A *decubitus ulcer* is a localized area of dead skin and subcutaneous tissue.

ETIOLOGY These lesions are caused by impairment of the blood supply to the affected area as a result of persistent pressure against the skin surface. The condition is most frequently a consequence of prolonged immobilization and is often seen in the debilitated, the unconscious, or those who are paralyzed. Those with weak circulation, especially elderly persons, are at greatest risk of developing decubitus ulcers.

SIGNS AND SYMPTOMS Early signs of decubitus ulcer include shiny, reddened skin, usually appearing over a bony prominence (Fig. 13–10). Small blisters, erosions, necrosis, and ulceration eventually occur. If the ulcer becomes infected, it will be foul-smelling and purulent. Pain may or may not accompany the lesion.

DIAGNOSTIC PROCEDURES Visual examination of the lesion usually is enough to establish the diagnosis. Wound culture and sensitivity testing may be done to isolate the causative organism if infection is suspected.

TREATMENT Skin pressure must be alleviated and excellent skin hygiene provided. The affected area must be kept clean and dry. Topical antibiotic powders may be prescribed. Surgery may be necessary in severe cases.

PROGNOSIS The sooner the decubitus ulcer is diagnosed and treated, the better the prognosis. The healing process generally is slow and tedious.

PREVENTION Prevention includes frequent repositioning of patients who are immobilized and gentle massage of pressure areas to increase circulation.

■ DERMATOPHYTOSES

DESCRIPTION *Dermatophytosis* is a chronic, superficial fungal infection. Dermatophytoses can occur in the scalp (tinea capitis), body (tinea corporis), nails (tinea unguium), feet (tinea pedis), or groin (tinea cruris).

ETIOLOGY Dermatophytosis is caused by several species of fungi that have the ability to invade the keratinous structures of the body. The infection is transmitted by direct contact with the fungus or its spores. Infection is more likely if the skin is traumatized or **abraded** or in cases of poor hygiene.

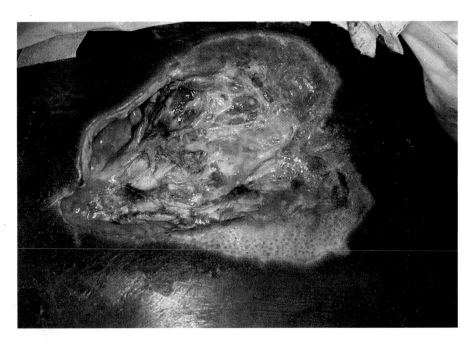

Figure 13–10 Deep decubitus ulcer over bony prominence. (From Goldsmith, LA, Lazarus, GS, and Tharp, MD: Adult and Pediatric Dermatology: A Color Guide to Diagnosis and Treatment. FA Davis, 1977, p 445, with permission.)

SIGNS AND SYMPTOMS

- *Tinea capitis* is a persistent, contagious, often epidemic infection occurring most frequently in children. The child may be asymptomatic or have slight itching of the scalp. The characteristic lesions are round, gray, and scaly (Fig. 13–11).
- *Tinea corporis,* or ringworm, occurs on exposed skin surfaces in persons with a history of exposure to infected domestic animals, especially cats. The lesions are ringed and scaled with small vesicles (Fig. 13–12).
- *Tinea unguium* is usually asymptomatic. The infection frequently starts at the tip of one or more toenails, with the affected nail appearing lusterless, brittle, and hypertrophic (Fig. 13–13).
- *Tinea pedis,* or athlete's foot, causes intense, persistent itching—this is its most common presenting symptom. Burning, stinging, and pain may result. The entire sole may become inflamed and dry with exfoliation and fissuring (Fig. 13–13).
- *Tinea cruris,* or jock itch, may be associated with tinea pedis and often occurs among male athletes. It is characterized by red, raised, sharply defined, itching lesions in the groin (Fig. 13–14).

DIAGNOSTIC PROCEDURES Diagnosis is dependent on the location and appearance of the skin lesion. The suspected lesions may be cultured to isolate the fungus. Skin tests or a Wood's light (a special ultra-

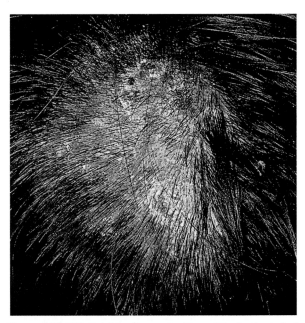

Figure 13–11 Patchy tinea capitis with broken hair stubs and spots of early inflammation, or kerion formation. (From Reeves, JRT, and Maibach, H: Clinical Dermatology Illustrated: A Regional Approach, ed 3. FA Davis, Philadelphia, 1998, p 9, with permission.)

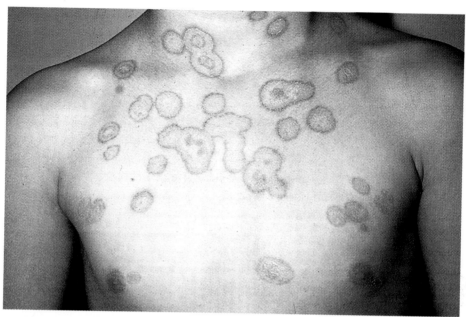

Figure 13–12 Dramatic widespread tinea corporis in a child. (From Reeves, JRT, and Maibach, H: Clinical Dermatology Illustrated: A Regional Approach, ed 3. FA Davis, Philadelphia, 1998, p 247, with permission.)

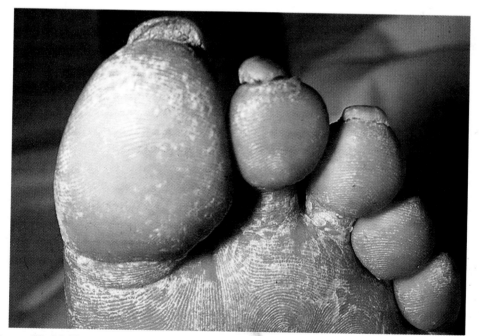

Figure 13–13 Tinea unguium and tinea pedis. Moderately severe tinea pedis with redness and scaling in "moccasin" distribution. (From Reeves, JRT, and Maibach, H: Clinical Dermatology Illustrated: A Regional Approach, ed 3. FA Davis, Philadelphia, 1998, p 126, with permission.)

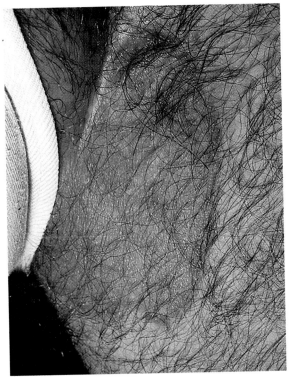

Figure 13–14 The inner thigh is the typical location of tinea cruris or "jock itch." The border is pronounced and scaly. (From Reeves, JRT, and Maibach, H: Clinical Dermatology Illustrated: A Regional Approach, ed 3. FA Davis, Philadelphia, 1998, p 99, with permission.)

violet light source) may be used to detect the lesions.

TREATMENT It may be necessary to treat the lesions by applying a topical fungicidal medication. Extreme caution is necessary when applying such preparations because they are strong irritants. Some medications may be prescribed orally, but these must be taken with caution, too, because of their side effects. The affected area of skin must be kept as dry and clean as possible. Loose-fitting clothing should be worn, and it should be changed frequently. Exercise and activity may need to be limited for a time to prevent excessive perspiration.

PROGNOSIS All forms of dermatophytoses tend to be chronic and persistent. Scrupulous management is required to resolve the condition. Even so, recurrences may be common.

PREVENTION Following proper hygiene practices is the best means of preventing dermatophytoses.

CORNS AND CALLUSES

DESCRIPTION *Corns* are horny **indurations** and thickenings of the **stratum corneum** of the skin. Corns have a central keratinous core. *Calluses* are localized hyperplasia of the stratum corneum. A callus will exhibit as a lesion with an indefinite border. Corns and calluses usually appear on areas of the body that receive repeated trauma (especially the feet).

ETIOLOGY Both conditions may be caused by pressure or friction from ill-fitting shoes, orthopedic deformities, or faulty weight-bearing. Persons who expose their skin to repeated trauma, such as manual laborers or string instrument players, are prone to calluses. Also, individuals with diabetes or impaired circulation are more apt to develop corns and calluses.

SIGNS AND SYMPTOMS Tenderness and pain are common symptoms. Corns have a glassy core, are smaller and more clearly defined, and are more painful than calluses.

DIAGNOSTIC PROCEDURES A physical examination of the affected area and medical history are usually sufficient for diagnosis.

TREATMENT Treatment consists of relieving pressure or friction points along the skin as soon as possible. Surgical **débridement** under local anesthetic may be necessary. Local injections of corticosteroids to relieve pain may be tried. Metatarsal and corn pads may be worn.

PROGNOSIS The prognosis is good with proper foot care and if the causative factor is removed.

PREVENTION Prevention includes wearing well-fitting shoes and avoiding any trauma to the feet or hands.

WARTS

DESCRIPTION *Warts* (verrucae) are circumscribed, elevated skin lesions resulting from hypertrophy of the epidermis (Fig. 13–15). Warts may be solitary or clustered, occurring most often on the exposed surfaces of the fingers and hands. Children are affected most frequently.

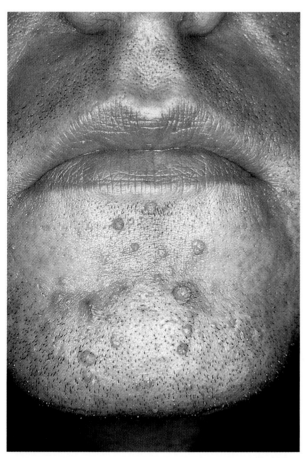

Figure 13–15 Large warts in beard area, spread by shaving. (From Reeves, JRT, and Maibach, H: Clinical Dermatology Illustrated: A Regional Approach, ed 3. FA Davis, Philadelphia, 1998, p 61, with permission.)

ETIOLOGY Warts are caused by infection from one of five possible papilloma viruses, each tending to infect different parts of the body. Generally, the mode of transmission is through direct contact or autoinnoculation.

SIGNS AND SYMPTOMS The size, shape, and appearance of warts will vary widely. Tenderness and itching may accompany the lesions.

DIAGNOSTIC PROCEDURES Visual examination of the wart usually is sufficient for diagnosis.

TREATMENT The wart may be removed by surgical excision, cryosurgery, or the use of keratolytic (peeling) agents. Immunotherapy may be tried for resistant warts. Treatment can be tedious and often is painful.

PROGNOSIS Spontaneous cures occur in about 50 percent of cases, but warts may resist any treatment, and recurrences are frequent. Secondary infection and scarring are possible.

PREVENTION Because warts can be transmitted by direct contact, avoidance of warts is important for prevention.

■ DISCOID LUPUS ERYTHEMATOSUS

DESCRIPTION *Discoid lupus erythematosus* (DLE) is a connective-tissue disorder characterized by a superficial, localized inflammation of the skin. It occurs most frequently on exposed skin surfaces. (The systemic form of the disease is discussed in Chapter 12.)

ETIOLOGY The cause of lupus is unknown; there is some evidence to suggest an autoimmune defect. It affects women more frequently than men.

SIGNS AND SYMPTOMS Macules, papules, **plaques,** plugged follicles, and atrophic areas are evident, usually on the face, neck, upper extremities, or any part of the body exposed to sunlight. The lesions are dusky red, well-localized, and covered by dry, horny, adherent scales.

DIAGNOSTIC PROCEDURES Generally, the patient's clinical picture and rash are enough to confirm the diagnosis. There is no specific test for discoid lupus erythematosus, but the disease may be differentiated from the systemic form by means of an antinuclear antibody test. Laboratory tests may include CBC, erythrocyte sedimentation rate (ESR), and urinalysis (UA).

TREATMENT The skin lesions may be treated with a topical corticosteroid cream or injected with the medication. Systemic drugs may be tried if topical forms do not work. The individual may be advised to avoid extreme fatigue and stress, as well as overexposure to sunlight, reflected sunlight, and fluorescent lighting.

PROGNOSIS DLE is a chronic condition, but it can be successfully controlled. The prognosis is good if the disease does not develop into its systemic form.

PREVENTION There is no known prevention.

■ SCLERODERMA

DESCRIPTION *Scleroderma,* also called systemic sclerosis, is a progressive, chronic, systemic disease characterized by diffuse fibrosis of the skin and internal organs. It may appear in two forms: morphea and systemic scleroderma. *Morphea* is purely a cutaneous disease, in which the skin becomes thickened and densely fibrous. In *systemic scleroderma* both skin and internal organs are involved. Parts of the gastrointestinal tract may become fibrotic and may exhibit impaired peristalsis.

ETIOLOGY The cause is unknown, but scleroderma appears to be an autoimmune disorder. Women are more frequently affected than men, especially those 30 to 50 years old.

SIGNS AND SYMPTOMS Raynaud's phenomenon generally is the first symptom, followed by pain, stiffness, and swelling of the fingers and joints. The skin becomes thick, shiny, and taut. **Contractures** eventually develop. Gastrointestinal symptoms include heartburn, reflux, diarrhea, constipation, weight loss, **dysphagia,** malabsorption, and mild anemia.

DIAGNOSTIC PROCEDURES The typical cutaneous clinical picture will help pinpoint the disease. Hand, chest, and gastrointestinal x-rays may show systemic changes. Urinalysis may indicate renal involvement. A skin biopsy may be done.

TREATMENT Treatment is palliative. Chemotherapy with immunosuppressive drugs may be tried. Raynaud's phenomenon may be treated with vasodilators and antihypertensive drugs. Any digital ulcerations require immediate treatment. Physical therapy may be prescribed to promote muscle function.

PROGNOSIS The disease course is quite variable. The systemic form is more serious and the prognosis is poor, with death usually resulting from renal, cardiac, or pulmonary failure.

PREVENTION There is no known prevention, except to prevent complications of the disease. The client is to avoid cold, stress, and trauma. About a third of individuals with scleroderma die within a year of onset.

Dermatitis

Dermatitis is inflammation of the skin manifested by itching, redness, and the appearance of various skin lesions. The disease may be acute, subacute, or chronic. This chapter considers the following forms of dermatitis: seborrheic dermatitis, contact dermatitis, and atopic dermatitis.

■ SEBORRHEIC DERMATITIS

DESCRIPTION *Seborrheic dermatitis* is a chronic functional disease of the sebaceous glands marked by an increase in the amount and often alteration in the quality of the sebaceous secretion. When the disease occurs in infancy, it is called *cradle cap.* Seborrheic dermatitis also is common in the diaper area.

ETIOLOGY Seborrheic dermatitis is an idiopathic disease. Heredity may predispose an individual to develop the condition; emotional stress may precipitate it.

SIGNS AND SYMPTOMS The disease is characterized by skin eruptions on areas of the scalp, eyelids, cheeks, beard, chest, axillae, groin, or trunk that produce dry, moist, or greasy scales (Fig. 13–16). The lesions are brown-yellow or red. Such scaling produced by the scalp is commonly called *dandruff.* The affected area of the skin frequently itches and may appear reddened.

DIAGNOSTIC PROCEDURES The diagnosis is usually made on the basis of the medical history and observation of the characteristic lesions. The disease must be differentiated from psoriasis (see the Psoriasis section in this chapter).

TREATMENT Shampoos containing selenium sulfide or zinc pyrithione are often helpful in controlling

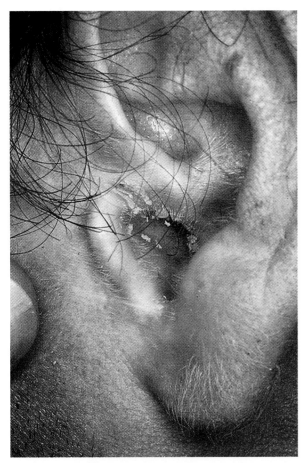

Figure 13–16 Seborrheic dermatitis in the ear canal. The ear is a common site of this inflammation. (From Reeves, JRT, and Maibach, H: Clinical Dermatology Illustrated: A Regional Approach, ed 3. FA Davis, Philadelphia, 1998, p 23, with permission.)

the scaling. Hydrocortisone creams may be prescribed to relieve redness and itching. Generalized seborrheic dermatitis requires careful attention, including scrupulous skin hygiene and keeping the skin as dry as possible.

PROGNOSIS Seborrheic dermatitis is a chronic condition, but the prognosis is good, given effective treatment. The presence of secondary infections may complicate treatment.

PREVENTION Adequate diet and sleep, regular exercise, sensible work habits, and a reduction of stress may help prevent the disease in those who are susceptible.

CONTACT DERMATITIS

DESCRIPTION *Contact dermatitis* is any acute skin inflammation caused by the direct action of various irritants on the surface of the skin or by contact with a substance to which an individual is allergic or sensitive.

ETIOLOGY A wide variety of animal, vegetable, or mineral substances may induce contact dermatitis. These may include drugs, acids, alkalies, or resins from plants such as poison ivy, poison oak, or poison sumac. The dyes used in colored toilet or facial tissue or in some soaps also may cause the condition. Some individuals are even sensitive to the composition of certain metals and may experience contact dermatitis as a consequence of wearing jewelry. Others may find that they develop dermatitis as a result of wearing latex gloves or wool fibers.

SIGNS AND SYMPTOMS The symptoms include erythema and the appearance of small skin vesicles that ooze, scale, itch, burn, or sting. The affected area may be hot and swollen (Fig. 13–17).

DIAGNOSTIC PROCEDURES Diagnosis is usually made on the basis of the appearance of the inflamed area of skin. A medical history revealing prior outbreaks of the condition and the location of the affected area of skin may help in isolating the specific irritant or allergen. A patch test with the offending agent may be done to determine the exact irritant.

TREATMENT The skin surface must be thoroughly cleansed of the suspected irritant. Lotions or creams may be the treatment of choice.

PROGNOSIS Contact dermatitis is generally self-limiting. The problem will tend to recur if the individual is reexposed to the particular irritant or allergen.

PREVENTION The best prevention is avoidance of known allergens or irritants.

ATOPIC DERMATITIS (Eczema)

DESCRIPTION *Atopic dermatitis* is an inflammation of the skin, of unknown etiology, in an individual with inherently irritable skin. The disease is common among infants, but it may occur at any time of life.

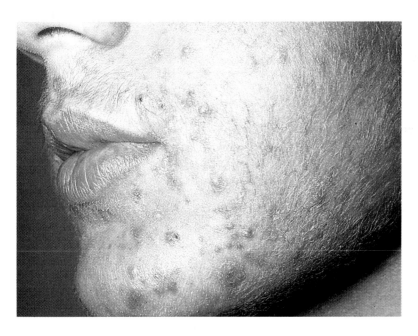

Figure 13–17 "Dishpan face" or irritant contact dermatitis. Dry, irritated skin from excessive washing with an acne soap. (From Reeves, JRT, and Maibach, H: Clinical Dermatology Illustrated: A Regional Approach, ed 3. FA Davis, Philadelphia, 1998, p 29, with permission.)

ETIOLOGY Although the condition is idiopathic, it appears to have allergic, hereditary, or psychological components. In about 70 percent of cases there is a family history of the disease. An allergic component is nearly always present, because the symptoms are frequently exacerbated by contact with wool, soaps, or oils and marked by an allergic sensitivity to certain foods.

SIGNS AND SYMPTOMS There will be pruritus and often severe characteristic lesions on the face, neck, upper trunk, and bends of the knees and elbows.

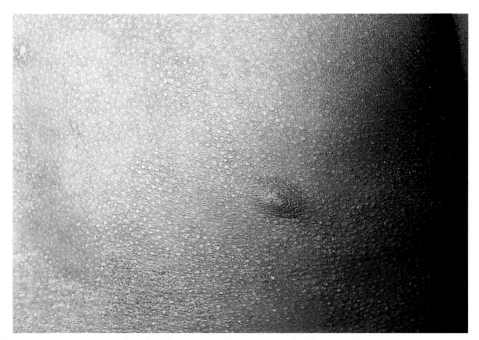

Figure 13–18 Mild papular eczema (atopic dermatitis) in a black child. (From Reeves, JRT, and Maibach, H: Clinical Dermatology Illustrated: A Regional Approach, ed 3. FA Davis, Philadelphia, 1998, p 167, with permission.)

Atopic dermatitis may cause vesicular and exudative eruptions in children (Fig. 13–18) and dry, leathery vesicles in adults.

DIAGNOSTIC PROCEDURES Observation of the skin and a medical history revealing a family tendency toward developing atopic dermatitis assist in diagnosing the condition. Serum immunoglobulin E (IgE) levels may be elevated.

TREATMENT Local and systemic agents may be prescribed to prevent itching. Careful daily skin care and total avoidance of known irritants are important. In addition, creams and ointments may be prescribed. Maintaining high humidity with a room humidifier may be helpful.

PROGNOSIS The prognosis is good, but the disorder is often frustrating to control and may have to be dealt with throughout most of the individual's life. Eczema frequently becomes infected with bacteria and less commonly with viruses.

PREVENTION The best prevention is avoidance of known irritants.

Herpes-Related Skin Lesions

■ COLD SORES AND FEVER BLISTERS

DESCRIPTION *Cold sores* and *fever blisters* are skin eruptions occurring about the perimeter of the mouth, lips, and nose, or on the mucous membranes within the mouth. Sometimes tingling and numbness may precede or follow these eruptions. The condition is common in children, but it affects people of any age.

ETIOLOGY These lesions are produced by the herpes simplex virus type 1 (HSV-1). This virus may lie dormant within the body for extended periods, reactivating during periods of lowered resistance or emotional and physical stress. Cold sores may erupt following a rise in body temperature, such as may occur during a common cold or even preceding menstruation. In some instances, however, they may occur prior to the onset of illness or for no apparent reason at all.

SIGNS AND SYMPTOMS The characteristic lesions are small pale vesicles appearing individually or in clusters, especially on the lips or about the mouth (Fig. 13–19). The affected area may burn and sting. The lesions may eventually break, forming ulcers or crusts.

Figure 13–19 Herpes simplex. Primary infection in adult, with typical widespread distribution around the mouth. (From Reeves, JRT, and Maibach, H: Clinical Dermatology Illustrated: A Regional Approach, ed 3. FA Davis, Philadelphia, 1998, p 64, with permission.)

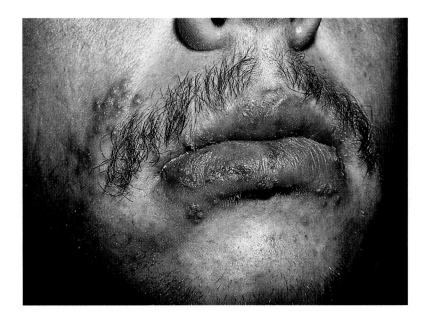

DIAGNOSTIC PROCEDURES The diagnosis is made on the basis of the individual's characteristic lesions. The virus may need to be isolated by histological examination of the scrapings.

TREATMENT Treatment is strictly symptomatic. The lesions should be kept as dry and clean as possible and protected from trauma. Topical analgesics or ointments may be applied to relieve burning and itching. Antibiotic ointments may be recommended to prevent secondary infection of open lesions.

PROGNOSIS Cold sores and fever blisters usually resolve within 1 to 3 weeks. The herpes simplex virus resumes dormancy, however, and may reappear again given favorable conditions. Sometimes another infection, or exposure to wind or sun can reactivate the virus.

PREVENTION There is no specific prevention other than avoiding contact with persons with visible cold sores.

■ HERPES ZOSTER (Shingles)

DESCRIPTION *Herpes zoster* (*shingles*) is an acute inflammatory eruption of highly painful vesicles on the trunk of the body or occasionally on the face. Adults past the age of 50 are primarily affected.

ETIOLOGY Shingles is caused by reactivation of the varicella-zoster virus (VZV), the same virus that causes chickenpox. What triggers this reactivation is not known. The lesions occur on a segment of skin lying above the course of a nerve that has been infected by the virus.

SIGNS AND SYMPTOMS The first symptom is pain along the course of the affected nerve, usually occurring 1 to 3 days prior to the appearance of the lesions. The skin eruption begins as an erythematous maculopapular rash that develops quite rapidly into vesicles. The site of these lesions is usually on one side of the trunk of the body, but if nerves supplying the face are involved, lesions also may appear on one side of the face, mouth, or tongue, or around one eye (Fig. 13–20). The region around the affected site is often intensely painful.

DIAGNOSTIC PROCEDURES The condition is diagnosed by its characteristic pattern of painful lesions. Confirmation of the diagnosis can be made by isolating the virus in cell cultures grown from scrapings of the lesions or by detecting varicella-zoster antibodies in the blood.

TREATMENT Sedatives, analgesics, and **antipruritics** may be prescribed. If the vesicles are infected, antibiotics may be given to prevent secondary infection.

PROGNOSIS The prognosis is usually good. Shingles runs its course within 7 to 10 days; however, recurrent bouts of severe pain may persist for weeks or months after the lesions have resolved. The disease may cause serious damage to the structure of the eye if nerves supplying the eye are involved. Unlike cold sores or fever blisters, shingles will not recur.

PREVENTION There is no specific prevention for shingles.

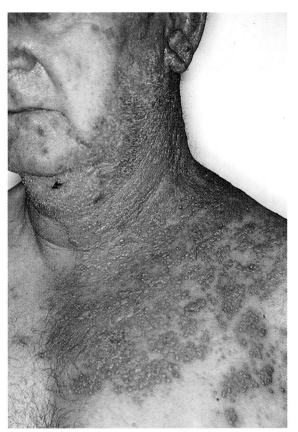

Figure 13–20 Herpes zoster (shingles). (From Reeves, JRT, and Maibach, H: Clinical Dermatology Illustrated: A Regional Approach, ed 3. FA Davis, Philadelphia, 1998, p 255, with permission.)

Cancer

SKIN CARCINOMAS

DESCRIPTION The most common skin cancers are basal cell carcinoma and squamous cell carcinoma. *Basal cell carcinomas* arise from the basal cell layer of the epidermis or hair follicles, are locally invasive, but very rarely metastasize. Basal cell carcinoma is the most common tumor affecting Caucasians. It occurs more frequently in blonde, fair-skinned men. *Squamous cell carcinomas* also arise from the epidermis and produce keratin. Squamous cell carcinoma is the more serious of the two because of its tendency to metastasize. This carcinoma occurs more frequently in fair-skinned white men over 60 years old.

ETIOLOGY Repeated overexposure to the sun's ultraviolet rays is the most important etiologic factor in skin carcinomas. Other causes include radiation exposure, chronic skin irritation and inflammation, and exposure to carcinogens.

SIGNS AND SYMPTOMS Cancerous skin lesions may appear any place on the body, but the common sites are sun-exposed areas of the body, such as the face, chest, back, ears, forearms, and the back of hands. Initially, both forms are painless. Basal cell carcinoma appears as a smooth, small, waxy nodule that appears translucent. Squamous cell carcinoma is characterized by a firm, red nodule with visible scales. Both carcinomas often ulcerate and form a crust.

DIAGNOSTIC PROCEDURES A medical history, careful observation of the skin noting characteristic lesions, and biopsy of the lesions are necessary for diagnosis.

TREATMENT The goal of treatment is to completely eradicate the lesions. The size, shape, location, and invasiveness of the carcinoma will determine treatment. Five methods of treatment include surgery (used in 90 percent of the cases), radiation therapy, **electrodesiccation, cryosurgery,** and laser therapy. Treatment of squamous cell carcinoma may involve local application of chemotherapeutic agents or cryosurgery.

PROGNOSIS The prognosis for carcinomas of the skin is good, with a 90 percent cure rate if they are detected and treated in the early stage. Although basal cell carcinomas rarely metastasize, untreated they may result in the loss of an ear, nose, or lip. Because squamous cell carcinomas may metastasize, individuals should be followed closely for a minimum of 5 years to detect new lesions or metastasis.

PREVENTION The best prevention is to avoid overexposure to the sun. Sun damage to the skin is cumulative, so sunscreens and protective measures should be used throughout life.

MALIGNANT MELANOMA

DESCRIPTION A *malignant melanoma* is a neoplasm composed of abnormal melanocytes appearing in both the epidermis and dermis. Malignant melanoma appears in one of four forms: *superficial spreading melanoma* occurs on any body site and is the most common form of melanoma; *lentigo maligna melanoma* occurs on exposed skin areas, especially the head and neck, and is a slowly evolving pigmented lesion; *nodular melanoma* occurs on any site and directly invades tissue below the dermis; *acral-lentiginous melanoma* occurs where hair follicles are absent (palms of hands, soles of feet, nail beds) and appears as irregular pigmented macules that develop into nodules and become invasive early. The incidence of malignant melanoma is increasing and has doubled in the past 10 years. It causes more deaths than all other skin diseases.

ETIOLOGY Although ultraviolet rays are suspect, the etiology is unknown. The persons at greatest risk have fair complexions, blue eyes, red or blonde hair, and freckles. There is a possible link between severe sunburn as a child and greatly increased risk of melanoma in later life.

SIGNS AND SYMPTOMS Malignant melanomas are characterized by lesions having irregular borders and a diversity of colors. The lesion of *superficial spreading* melanoma tends to be circular, flat, and visibly or palpably elevated. Color variations include tan, brown, black mixed with gray, bluish black, or white. There may be a whitish pink color in a small area within the lesion. The *lentigo ma-*

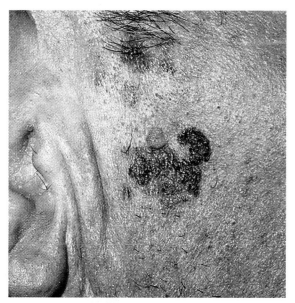

Figure 13–21 Dark lentigo maligna on cheek and in sideburn. Apparently clear area between the sites was probably involved in the past but resolved. Seborrheic keratosis is present at upper edge of lower lesion. (From Reeves, JRT, and Maibach, H: Clinical Dermatology Illustrated: A Regional Approach, ed 3. FA Davis, Philadelphia, 1998, p 338, with permission.)

ligna melanoma appears as a brown or black, flat lesion that undergoes changes in size and color with time (Fig. 13–21). The *nodular* melanoma is generally blue-black in color, resembling a "blood blister" that fails to resolve. The lesion is spherical with a relatively smooth surface. The *acral-lentiginous* melanoma appears as a dark brown, flat lesion or a blue-black or brown-black raised lesion.

DIAGNOSTIC PROCEDURES Suspicious skin lesions must be biopsied to determine the diagnosis.

TREATMENT The level of invasion and measure of the melanoma's thickness will determine the appropriate treatment. Surgical excision of the lesion is the most common treatment modality, and it may be necessary to remove nearby lymph nodes. Chemotherapy may be recommended.

PROGNOSIS The prognosis is related to the level of the dermal invasion and the thickness of the lesion. The prognosis is poorer if the melanoma grows vertically rather than horizontally. If metastasis occurs, it can affect every organ of the body. If the melanoma is detected and treated early, there is a 5-year relative survival rate of 88 percent.

PREVENTION Avoiding overexposure to the sun and ultraviolet rays and seeking prompt treatment for any suspected lesions are the best prevention. Figure 13–22 lists the warning signs for suspicious lesions.

SPECIAL FOCUS CHILDHOOD DISEASES OF THE SKIN

ATOPIC DERMATITIS

Atopic dermatitis is a common childhood skin disease that may be chronic and familial in nature. The condition is characterized by erythema and edema, with papules, vesicles, and crusts forming, usually on the cheeks and then spreading to the neck and creases of the arms and legs. Generally, there is itching associated with the rash. The most common allergens producing atopic dermatitis in infancy are foods, especially cow's milk and egg albumin. Later, environmental inhalants and pollen become stronger allergens. Although atopic dermatitis may be self-limiting in infancy, about half the affected infants develop asthma as children, and hay fever or other allergies as adults. It is important to stop the child from scratching so as to prevent secondary infection. The best prevention is the removal of known offending agents.

DIAPER RASH

DESCRIPTION *Diaper rash* is a maculopapular and occasionally excoriated eruption in the diaper area of infants (Fig. 13–23).

ETIOLOGY The condition is caused by irritation from heat, moisture, feces, or ammonia produced by the bacterial decomposition of urine.

SIGNS AND SYMPTOMS A rash in the diaper area will be evident. The infant may become irritable as a result of the discomfort of the rash.

DIAGNOSTIC PROCEDURES Observation of the characteristic rash is usually sufficient to establish the diagnosis.

TREATMENT Exposing the affected area to air and applying a heat lamp may be effective in many cases. Topical antimicrobial medication

A Asymmetry—one-half unlike the other half

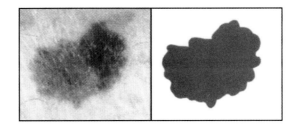

B Border irregularity—scalloped or poorly circumscribed border

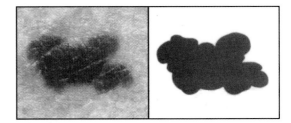

C Color varied from one area to another; shades of tan and brown; black; sometimes white, red, or blue

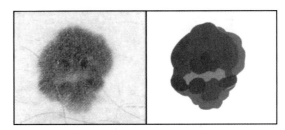

D Diameter larger than 6 mm as a rule (diameter of a pencil eraser)

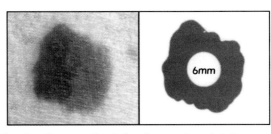

Figure 13–22 The ABCD rule for warning signals of melanoma. Look for danger signs in pigmented lesions of the skin. (Adapted from the American Academy of Dermatology, P.O. Box 4014, Schaumburg, Ill. 60168–4014, © Copyright 1993, with permission.)

may be necessary in the event of secondary infection.

PROGNOSIS The prognosis is good with treatment.

PREVENTION Prevention includes frequently changing diapers and keeping the perianal area dry and clean.

PEDICULOSIS

Pediculosis is skin infestation with lice, a parasitic insect. It is more common in children than in adults, especially in girls who share combs, brushes, and clothing. The prognosis is good with topical treatment.

DERMATOPHYTOSIS

Dermatophytoses is a general term referring to superficial fungal infections of the skin. *Tinea capitis*, a fungal infection of the scalp, is a persistent, contagious, often epidemic infection occurring most frequently in children. *Tinea corporis*, a fungal infection of the body, occurs on exposed skin surfaces in persons with a his-

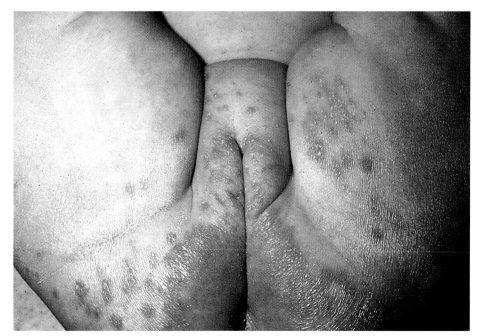

Figure 13–23 Typical yeast diaper eruption in older infant. (From Reeves, JRT, and Maibach, H: Clinical Dermatology Illustrated: A Regional Approach, ed 3. FA Davis, Philadelphia, 1998, p 109, with permission.)

tory of exposure to domestic animals, especially cats. Both conditions can be treated by topical fungicidal medication. The prognosis is good for these conditions. Both may clear spontaneously after puberty.

COMMON SYMPTOMS OF SKIN DISEASES

Individuals may present with the following common complaints, which deserve attention from health professionals:

- Skin eruptions
- Pruritus
- Erythema
- Pain
- Swelling
- Inflammation

BIBLIOGRAPHY

Goldsmith, LA: Adult and Pediatric Dermatology: A Color Guide to Diagnosis and Treatment. FA Davis, Philadelphia, 1997.

Professional Guide to Diseases, ed 6. Springhouse Corporation, Springhouse, Pa., 1998.

Reeves, JRT, and Maibach, HI: Clinical Dermatology Illustrated: A Regional Approach, ed 3. FA Davis, Philadelphia, 1998.

CASE STUDIES

I You have three preschool children. The mother of a neighborhood playmate calls to tell you that her child has impetigo.

1. What signs and symptoms should you look for?

2. What actions should you take with your children? What should you do in relation to the other neighborhood children?

3. What is the cause of impetigo?

II A client requests an appointment to have the physician examine a growth on her neck. She is 60 years old, blond, fair-skinned, and an avid tennis player. She did not call the physician when she first noticed the growth; it has grown since she first noticed it. The growth is raised, darkened, and irregular around the edges. The physician arranges for the growth to be removed. Biopsy indicates malignant melanoma.

1. What factors have contributed to this disease in this individual?

2. What treatment is indicated?

3. What do you think the prognosis is in this situation?

REVIEW QUESTIONS

MATCHING

_____ 1. Seborrheic dermatitis

_____ 2. Contact dermatitis

_____ 3. Atopic dermatitis

_____ 4. Psoriasis

_____ 5. Urticaria

_____ 6. Acne vulgaris

_____ 7. Alopecia

_____ 8. Herpes simplex virus type 1

_____ 9. Herpes zoster

_____ 10. Impetigo

a. Shingles
b. Hives
c. Inflammatory disease of sebaceous follicles
d. Appears to have allergic, hereditary, or psychological components
e. Produces dry, moist, or greasy scaling
f. Characterized by high rate of skin turnover
g. Cold or fever sores
h. Baldness
i. Contagious strep, or staph, skin infection
j. Causes erythema and small skin vesicles
k. Boil or abscess
l. Bedsore

SHORT ANSWER

Fill in the blanks:

1. A _____ or boil is an abscess involving the hair follicle and subcutaneous tissue. A _____ consists of several furuncles developing in adjoining hair follicles with multiple drainage sinuses.

2. Pediculosis is skin infestation with _____ .

3. Dermatophytosis is caused by _____ infections of the skin.

4. A skin disorder you might find on a person who is elderly, debilitated, or paralyzed is

   _____ .

5. Warts, or verrucae, are caused by the _____ .

6. Describe the classic symptom of discoid lupus erythematosus.

7. Name three skin cancers:

   a.

   b.

   c.

8. One important factor in skin cancers is _____ .

DISCUSSION QUESTIONS

1. Discuss the health problems that may occur from tanning booths.
2. Discuss the treatment for diaper rash.

ANSWERS

MATCHING

1. e	4. f	7. h	9. a
2. j	5. b	8. g	10. i
3. d	6. c		

SHORT ANSWER

1. Furuncle, carbuncle
2. Lice
3. Fungal
4. Decubitus ulcer
5. Papilloma viruses
6. Dusky red, butterfly-patterned lesion over the nose and cheeks
7. a. Basal cell carcinoma
   b. Squamous cell carcinoma
   c. Malignant melanoma
8. Excessive exposure to sunlight

DISCUSSION QUESTIONS

1. Answers will vary.
2. Expose the area to air; use a heat lamp; change diapers frequently; keep skin clean, dry, and cool.

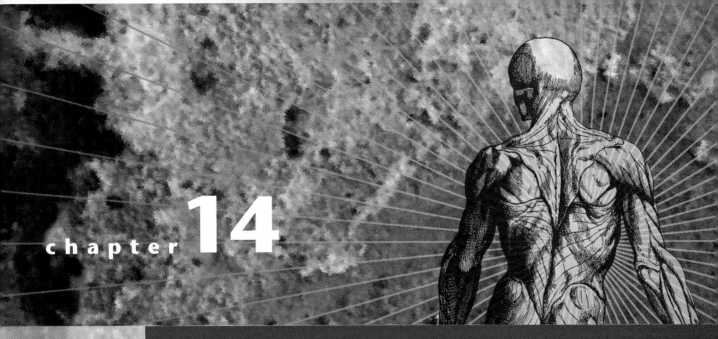

chapter 14

Eye and Ear Diseases

CHAPTER OUTLINE

Eye Diseases
Refractive Errors
Nystagmus
Stye (Hordeolum)
Corneal Abrasion
Cataract
Glaucoma
Retinal Detachment
Macular Degeneration

Eye Inflammations
Conjunctivitis
Uveitis
Blepharitis
Keratitis

Special Focus: Childhood Disease of the Eye
Strabismus

Common Symptoms of Eye Diseases

Ear Diseases
Impacted Cerumen
External Otitis (Swimmer's Ear)
Otitis Media
Otosclerosis
Motion Sickness
Ménière's Disease

Special Focus: Childhood Diseases of the Ear
Deafness
Otitis Media

Common Symptoms of Ear Diseases

Bibliography

Case Studies

Review Questions

LEARNING OBJECTIVES

Upon successful completion of this chapter, you will:

- Describe four common refractive errors.
- Identify the signs and symptoms of nystagmus.
- Recall the treatment for stye.
- Discuss the prognosis of corneal abrasions.
- List the various causes of cataracts.
- Restate the prognosis for and prevention of glaucoma.
- Describe the process that causes retinal detachment.
- List the prevention of macular degeneration.
- Identify the signs and symptoms of conjunctivitis.
- Describe uveitis.
- Recall the signs and symptoms of blepharitis.
- Restate the etiology of keratitis.
- Describe the treatment for impacted cerumen.
- Identify the etiology of external otitis or swimmer's ear.
- Compare and contrast serous otitis media to suppurative otitis media.
- Define otosclerosis.
- Discuss the treatment for motion sickness.
- Recall the etiology for hearing loss.
- Restate the treatment for Ménière's disease.
- Review the prognosis and prevention of strabismus.
- List at least three common symptoms of both eye and ear diseases.

KEY WORDS

Amblyopia (ăm•blē•ō′pē•ă)
Anticholinergic (ăn•tǐ•kō•lǐn•ěr′jǐk)
Atropine (ăt′rō•pēn)
Cellulitis (sěl•ū•lī′tǐs)
Conjunctiva (kŏn•jŭnk′tǐ•vă)
Cryotherapy (krī•ō•thěr′ă•pē)
Curet (kū•rět′)
Diaphoresis (dī•ă•fō•rē′sǐs)
Diplopia (dǐp•lō′pē•ă)
Macula (măk′ū•lă)
Myringotomy (mǐr•ǐn•gŏt′ō•mē)

Phacoemulsification
(făk″ō•ē•mŭl′sǐ•fī•kā″shŭn)
Photophobia (fō•tō•fō′bē•ă)
Pruritus (proo•rī′tǔs)
Radial keratotomy (rā′dē•ăl kěr•a•tŏt′ō•mē)
Seborrhea (sěb•ŏr•ē′ă)
Stapedectomy (stā•pě•děk′tō•mē)
Suppurative (sūp′ū•ră•tǐv)
Tinnitus (tǐn•ī′tǔs)
Tonometer (tŏn•ŏm′ě•těr)
Tympanoplasty (tǐm•păn•ō•plăs′tē)
Vertigo (věr′tǐ•gō)

Our most important sensory receptors are the eyes and the ears. The eye is the primary organ of sight, and the ear is the primary organ for sound and equilibrium. Obviously, any impairment of either of these sensory receptors can be a traumatic experience and can cause serious disability.

When studying the material in this chapter, it will be helpful to refer to Figures 14–1 and 14–5, which indicate the major parts of the eye and ear.

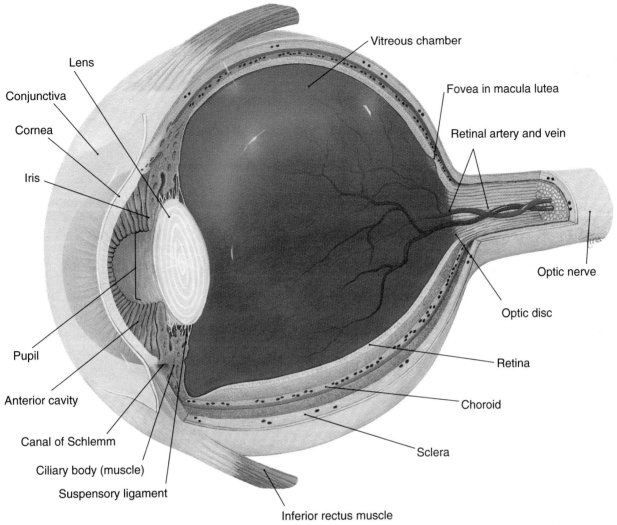

Figure 14–1 The internal anatomy of the eyeball. (From Scanlon, VC, and Sanders, T: Essentials of Anatomy and Physiology, ed 3. FA Davis, Philadelphia, 1999, p 192, with permission.)

Labels: Lens, Conjunctiva, Cornea, Iris, Pupil, Anterior cavity, Canal of Schlemm, Ciliary body (muscle), Suspensory ligament, Inferior rectus muscle, Vitreous chamber, Fovea in macula lutea, Retinal artery and vein, Optic nerve, Optic disc, Retina, Choroid, Sclera

Eye Diseases

■ REFRACTIVE ERRORS

DESCRIPTION *Refractive errors* are defects in visual acuity resulting from the inability of the eye to effectively focus light on the surface of the retina (refer to Fig. 14–2). Four common refractive errors are:

- *Hyperopia.* This condition occurs when light entering the eye comes to a focus behind the retina so that vision is better for distant objects. For this reason, the condition is commonly referred to as *farsightedness*. Hyperopia often results when the globe of the eye is abnormally short in length from front to back.

- *Presbyopia.* This refractive error is a form of farsightedness. Unlike hyperopia, however, presbyopia results from a loss of elasticity in the crystalline lens of the eye. When the eye fo-

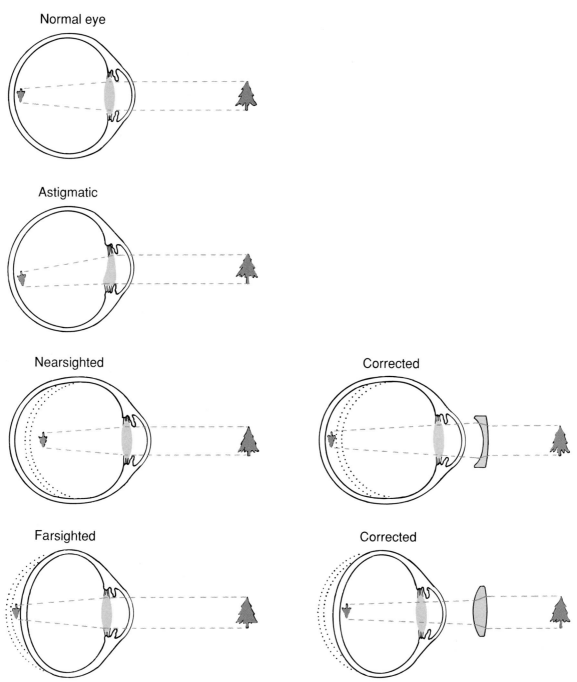

Figure 14–2 Errors of refraction compared with the normal eye. Corrective lenses are shown for nearsightedness and farsightedness. (From Scanlon, VC, and Sanders, T: Essentials of Anatomy and Physiology, ed 3. FA Davis, Philadelphia, 1999, p 195, with permission.)

cuses on a distant object, muscles encircling the lens contract, stretch, or flatten it. When the eye focuses on a nearby object, the muscles relax, allowing the lens to resume a more spherical shape. In presbyopia, however, the lens remains in a comparatively flattened position after the muscles have relaxed. This condition is a consequence of advancing age.

- *Myopia.* This condition occurs when light entering the eye comes to a focus in front of the retina so that vision is better for nearby objects. Consequently, the condition is commonly called *nearsightedness*. Myopia often results when the eyeball is abnormally long from front to back.

- *Astigmatism.* This refractive error occurs when light entering the eye is focused unevenly or diffusely across the retina so that some of the visual field appears properly focused while some does not. The condition is caused by variations in the curvature over certain portions of the lens or cornea of the eye.

ETIOLOGY It is not known what causes some individuals to develop these visual defects while others do not. Some types of refractive errors, however, show a strong familial pattern, suggesting a genetic predisposition to acquiring them.

SIGNS AND SYMPTOMS In addition to the characteristic visual deficits just described, general symptoms of refractive errors may include squinting, headaches, and frequent rubbing of the eyes.

DIAGNOSTIC PROCEDURES The diagnosis of refractive errors usually involves testing for visual acuity using the Snellen eye chart, ophthalmoscopic examination of the interior of the eye, and tests to detect eye muscle function.

TREATMENT Treatment of refractive errors involves the prescription and fitting of corrective lenses, either in the form of eyeglasses or contact lenses (Fig. 14–2). **Radial keratotomy** is a surgical procedure to correct myopia. About two-thirds of the clients who have this procedure are able to do without corrective lenses.

PROGNOSIS With corrective lenses the prognosis is good for persons with refractive errors.

PREVENTION There are no specific preventive measures for any of these refractive errors.

◼ NYSTAGMUS

DESCRIPTION *Nystagmus* is repetitive, involuntary movement of the eye. The condition is classified into various subcategories, according to the characteristic pattern of eye movements that occurs. One or both eyes may be affected.

ETIOLOGY Nystagmus may be either congenital or acquired. Acquired nystagmus results from disease processes that produce lesions in the portions of the brain, or the structures within the ears, that help govern eye movement. Diseases that may cause nystagmus include Ménière's disease and multiple sclerosis (see Ménière's Disease). Chronic visual impairment, certain drugs, or alcohol abuse also may produce this condition.

SIGNS AND SYMPTOMS The symptoms of nystagmus are continuous horizontal, vertical, or circular eye movements (or a combination of these). The individual also may report blurred vision.

DIAGNOSTIC PROCEDURES A number of tests to assess eye movement such as an opticokinetic drum test may be performed to help determine which structures within the ear or the central nervous system (CNS) may be causing the nystagmus.

TREATMENT Treatment must be directed at the underlying cause of the nystagmus if possible.

PROGNOSIS The prognosis depends on the underlying cause.

PREVENTION There is no specific prevention for nystagmus.

◼ STYE (Hordeolum)

DESCRIPTION A *stye* (*hordeolum*) is a localized, purulent, inflammatory infection of one or more of the sebaceous glands of the eyelid. Styes commonly occur on the skin surface at the edge of the lid or on the surface of the **conjunctiva.**

ETIOLOGY Styes usually result from infection by *Staphylococcus* bacteria. Often an eyelash is found in the center of the stye. It is often secondary to blepharitis (see Blepharitis).

SIGNS AND SYMPTOMS The chief symptom is pain and tenderness of an intensity directly related to the amount of swelling. There is redness at the site.

DIAGNOSTIC PROCEDURES Visual examination is all that is necessary in most cases; however, a culture may be taken to isolate *Staphylococcus.*

TREATMENT Warm compresses may be prescribed to hasten the pointing of the abscess. Antibiotic eye drops or ointment may be used. If the infection warrants it, oral antibiotics may be ordered. Removal of the eyelash may be followed by pus drainage. An incision of the abscess may be necessary.

PROGNOSIS The prognosis is good with treatment, but recurrences are common. A complication of a stye is **cellulitis** of the eyelid.

PREVENTION Prevention includes cleanliness and proper eye care.

CORNEAL ABRASION

DESCRIPTION A *corneal abrasion* is a scratch on the transparent anterior cellular layer of the eye.

ETIOLOGY Corneal abrasions may be produced by foreign bodies such as dirt, dust, or metal particles trapped between the cornea and the eyelid. A scratch also may result from fingernail contact with the cornea or from wearing poorly fitting or scratched contact lenses.

SIGNS AND SYMPTOMS Pain, redness, and tearing are common symptoms. The person may experience a sensation that something is constantly in the eye. Visual acuity may be impaired depending upon the size and location of the abrasion.

DIAGNOSTIC PROCEDURES A medical history and visual examination may be all that is necessary to suggest the diagnosis. Instilling the affected eye with a fluorescein stain may help highlight the presence of any corneal lesion. The injured area will appear green when examined with a flashlight. This technique may be used alone or in combination with a slit-lamp examination.

TREATMENT If a foreign body is indeed present in the eye, irrigation of the corneal surface may be attempted, or a topical anesthetic may be administered and the object removed. Once the eye surface is clear of debris, an antibiotic ophthalmic ointment will often be prescribed, followed by the application of an eye bandage to reduce movement of the eyelid across the cornea.

PROGNOSIS The prognosis is good with treatment. Complications of untreated corneal abrasion include ulceration of the cornea and permanent vision loss.

PREVENTION Prevention of corneal abrasions includes wearing protective eyewear when engaging in hazardous occupations or sports and following recommendations for cleaning and wearing contact lenses.

CATARACT

DESCRIPTION A *cataract* is an opacity or clouding of the crystalline lens of the eye or its surrounding membrane. The condition may be unilateral or bilateral. A cataract develops slowly, affecting visual acuity.

ETIOLOGY Cataracts are caused by a change in the chemical composition of the lens so that there is a loss of lens transparency. These changes can be caused by aging (senile cataracts), eye injuries (traumatic cataracts), certain diseases (secondary cataracts), and heredity or birth defects (congenital cataracts).

SIGNS AND SYMPTOMS A gradual loss or blurring of vision is the common symptom. Some people report seeing halos around lights, and some have problems driving at night because of glare from the lights of oncoming cars. As a cataract matures, the pupil of the eye may appear white to an observer. The condition is painless.

DIAGNOSTIC PROCEDURES Ophthalmoscopy, penlight examination, or slit-lamp examination will be used to confirm the diagnosis.

TREATMENT Treatment depends on the degree of visual impairment and on the age, general health, and occupation of the affected individual. Once the cloudy, natural lens of the eye is removed, the person needs a substitute lens to focus the eye. Surgical extraction of the defective lens is followed by refractive correction using eyeglasses, contact lenses, or surgically implanted artificial lenses called *intraocular lenses* (IOLs). The two most common surgical methods to remove cataracts are intracapsular and extracapsular extraction and **phacoemulsification.** Laser is used less frequently.

PROGNOSIS The prognosis is good with surgery, and visual acuity is improved in 95 percent of cases.

PREVENTION There is no known prevention for most cataracts.

GLAUCOMA

DESCRIPTION *Glaucoma* is a condition in which accumulating fluid pressure within the eye damages the retina and optic nerve, often causing blindness. The buildup of pressure occurs because more fluid, called *aqueous humor,* is produced than can be drained from the eye. The most common form of this condition, called *open-angle glaucoma,* results from obstruction of passages within the eye that form the *trabecular meshwork,* which drains the aqueous humor into the lymphatic system. In the United States, glaucoma affects 2 percent of the population older than age 40. The condition may be unilateral or bilateral.

ETIOLOGY Primary forms of the condition, such as open-angle glaucoma, are idiopathic; however, a strong familial tendency toward developing this condition suggests that unknown genetic factors may be involved. Glaucoma also may arise secondary to a wide variety of other diseases, or it may be induced by certain drugs or toxins.

SIGNS AND SYMPTOMS The most common forms of glaucoma develop asymptomatically and are often not detected until irreparable damage has already occurred to the retinas or optic nerves. When symptoms appear late in the course of the disease, they may include mild aching in the eyes and visual disturbances such as seeing halos around lights or a noticeable loss of peripheral vision.

DIAGNOSTIC PROCEDURES A positive family history for the disease should suggest a potential diagnosis of glaucoma. One of various types of **tonometers** will be used to detect elevated intraocular pressure. Ophthalmoscopic inspection of the retinal surface is essential to determine whether retinal damage has occurred. Vision field testing can help determine the extent of peripheral vision loss.

TREATMENT Drug therapy is the standard course of treatment for glaucoma and may take one of two forms. Certain types of drugs may be applied to the surface of the eye to decrease intraocular pressure. Other drugs may be prescribed that act to decrease the production of aqueous humor. Severe cases of glaucoma may be treated using a laser surgery that promotes drainage of aqueous humor through the trabecular meshwork.

PROGNOSIS The prognosis usually is good with early treatment. Drug therapy must be maintained for life.

PREVENTION It is important for all persons 20 years of age and older to have ophthalmoscopic examinations that include a test for glaucoma every 3 to 5 years.

RETINAL DETACHMENT

DESCRIPTION *Retinal detachment* is the complete or partial separation of the retina from the choroid layer of the eye (Fig. 14–3); it leads to the loss of

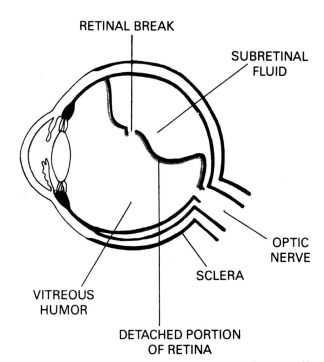

Figure 14–3 Retinal detachment. (From Thomas, CL [ed]: Taber's Cyclopedic Medical Dictionary, ed 15. FA Davis, Philadelphia, 1985, with permission.)

retinal function and blindness. The condition occurs as a result of a hole or break in the retina that allows fluid, the *vitreous humor,* to accumulate between the two layers.

ETIOLOGY Retinal detachment usually is caused by head trauma. Hemorrhages or tumors of the outer (choroid) layer also may cause the condition. Certain systemic diseases such as diabetes mellitus may predispose to the condition. Spontaneous retinal detachments also may occur among elderly persons.

SIGNS AND SYMPTOMS An individual with retinal detachment may report seeing floating spots or flashes of light. These worsen and are followed by a dark shadow extending from the periphery inwards. As more of the retina detaches from the choroid surface, there will be a progressive loss of vision. The condition is painless.

DIAGNOSTIC PROCEDURES Ophthalmoscopic examination while the pupils are fully dilated reveals the detached portion of the retina suspended in the vitreous humor of the eye.

TREATMENT Treatment depends on the location and extent of the detachment, but generally it involves restriction of eye movement through sedation, bed rest, or the use of an eye patch. Surgery, often using laser techniques, photocoagulation (a relatively simple procedure used to seal retinal tears), or **cryotherapy,** may be required to reattach the floating portion of the retina to the choroid surface.

PROGNOSIS The prognosis is good if surgical repair is successful. The prognosis is worse if the portion of the retina that produces the sharpest vision (the macula lutea) is detached. Without treatment, retinal detachment may become total in a few months.

PREVENTION There is no specific prevention for retinal detachment other than following safety measures that minimize the risk of head trauma.

■ MACULAR DEGENERATION

DESCRIPTION *Macular degeneration* is a slow progressive disease that produces changes in the pigmented cells of the retina and **macula.** These pigmented cells are more concentrated in the macula. The result is progressive loss of fine vision in one or both eyes. It is the leading cause of new blindness in the United States and it affects millions of elderly Americans.

ETIOLOGY Macular degeneration generally is a result of the aging process. Risk factors include increasing age (60 years or older), farsightedness, light iris color, positive family history, and cigarette smoking. Macular degeneration may be inherited or it may result from injury, inflammation, or infection.

SIGNS AND SYMPTOMS Macular degeneration usually starts with the appearance of spots on the retina called *drusen.* Drusen, similar to age spots, do not change vision very much; rather, the person will notice relatively mild visual loss with distortion. Early in macular degeneration, there may be no symptoms; however, as the degeneration continues, the person will experience painless visual loss and/or distortion and should have an immediate eye examination. This individual usually notices that sharp vision is affected and often is unable to read or do close work.

DIAGNOSTIC PROCEDURES Macular degeneration may be detected during a routine eye examination. A fluorescein angiography may be used. An Amsler's chart or grid is used to detect small changes in vision when they first appear. The Amsler's chart is a grid that looks similar to graph paper with horizontal and vertical lines. The person with macular degeneration may notice distortion of the grid pattern, such as bent lines and irregular box shapes or a gray shaded area.

TREATMENT Laser therapy may be used and may delay or prevent the onset of blindness. Some types of macular degeneration are untreatable. If scarring or atrophy has occurred, the condition cannot be reversed.

PROGNOSIS The disease slowly progresses, especially without treatment, and can lead eventually to blindness. Early diagnosis and treatment is helpful.

PREVENTION Zinc supplements may be helpful in preventing complications in individuals with some types of macular degeneration. Wearing sunglasses may help prevent ultraviolet light from entering the eye and help some people see better. Periodic vision testing is advisable for everyone, but especially for those who have a family history of retinal problems.

Eye Inflammations

CONJUNCTIVITIS

DESCRIPTION *Conjunctivitis* is inflammation of the conjunctiva, the mucous membrane structure that lines the inner surface of the eyelids and the anterior portion of the eyeball. The condition may be unilateral or bilateral.

ETIOLOGY Acute, sometimes epidemic, outbreaks of conjunctivitis are caused by infection from certain viruses or bacteria. These highly infectious forms of the disease commonly are referred to as *pinkeye.* Commonly the infection is transmitted by the person's own hand or by contaminated washcloths or towels. It usually lasts about 2 weeks. Conjunctivitis also may be caused by irritation from heat, cold, chemicals, allergies, or exposure to ultraviolet light.

SIGNS AND SYMPTOMS Conjunctivitis is marked by red, swollen conjunctivae, that may itch, burn, or cause pain, especially when blinking. The eyes may tear excessively and may be overly sensitive to light, although conjunctivitis rarely affects vision.

DIAGNOSTIC PROCEDURES Physical examination will reveal inflammation of the conjunctivae. Stained smears of conjunctival scrapings may reveal monocytes, polymorphonuclear leukocytes, and macrophages. Culture and sensitivity tests will identify the specific causative organism and indicate appropriate treatment.

TREATMENT Treatment varies depending on the causative agent, but antibiotic therapy may take the form of eyedrops or systemic medication. Often, warm compresses applied to the eye three to four times a day for 10 to 15 minutes are recommended.

PROGNOSIS The prognosis is good if degeneration of the conjunctiva or corneal damage does not occur. The disease normally is benign and self-limiting.

PREVENTION Prevention involves careful hygiene, proper handwashing, and the use of clean washcloths and towels to prevent infection.

UVEITIS

DESCRIPTION *Uveitis* is inflammation of the uveal tract, which is the principal vascular connective tissue component of the eye (iris, ciliary body, choroid). The condition is usually unilateral. The iris, ciliary body, or choroid may be affected separately or in combination. It may occur in the anterior or posterior portion of the tract.

ETIOLOGY Uveitis may be caused by microbial infections or debilitating diseases, such as tuberculosis, toxoplasmosis, and histoplasmosis, or it may result from improperly healed corneal abrasions. Uveitis may be associated with autoimmune disorders. It also may be idiopathic.

SIGNS AND SYMPTOMS Symptoms include pain, intense **photophobia,** blurred vision, redness, and constricted pupils. The physician may note severe ciliary congestion, tearing, and a pupil that is nonreactive when exposed to light.

DIAGNOSTIC PROCEDURES A slit-lamp examination is necessary for diagnosis. Skin tests for tuberculosis, toxoplasmosis, and histoplasmosis may be helpful in detecting granulomatous forms of the disease.

TREATMENT Treatment is specific to the particular type of uveitis and should be prompt and vigorous. **Atropine** is used so that the pupil remains dilated to reduce the likelihood of adhesions. Anti-infective chemotherapy and corticosteroid drugs may be necessary. Analgesics may be prescribed, and intraocular pressure must be monitored. Steroids may be required.

PROGNOSIS Most uveitis usually subsides in a few weeks with treatment. It may persist despite treatment. Adhesions may develop that can cause glaucoma, cataracts, or even retinal detachment.

PREVENTION There is no known prevention other than prompt treatment of infections and the debilitating diseases mentioned.

BLEPHARITIS

DESCRIPTION *Blepharitis* is ulcerative or nonulcerative inflammation of the edges of the eyelids, involving hair follicles and glands that open onto the surface. It is a condition commonly seen in children.

ETIOLOGY Ulcerative forms of blepharitis usually result from infection by *Staphylococcus* bacteria. Nonulcerative forms may be due to allergy or exposure to dust, smoke, or chemical irritants. The condition also may arise secondary to **seborrhea** of the sebaceous glands of the eyelids or pediculosis of the eyelashes or eyebrows.

SIGNS AND SYMPTOMS The affected individual may experience burning and itching or the feeling of a foreign body in the eye. The eyes usually appear red-rimmed. Both dry and oily scales may be present on the eyelid margins.

DIAGNOSTIC PROCEDURES The characteristic symptoms, a bacterial culture that reveals *Staphylococcus,* and examination of the eyelids for nits will suggest the diagnosis.

TREATMENT Seborrheic blepharitis requires daily shampooing to remove the scales. An antibiotic ointment will be prescribed for blepharitis caused by *Staphylococcus.* Pediculosis blepharitis requires the removal of nits and treatment with an ointment.

PROGNOSIS The prognosis is good with proper treatment and care, but some forms of the disease tend to recur and become chronic. Blepharitis may lead to keratitis.

PREVENTION The best preventive measures are cleanliness and proper eye care.

▇ KERATITIS

DESCRIPTION *Keratitis* is inflammation of the cornea. The condition usually is unilateral.

ETIOLOGY Keratitis is most frequently due to infection of the cornea by herpes virus type 1 or certain bacteria or fungi. The condition also may arise secondary to syphilis and, rarely, tuberculosis. Noninfectious keratitis may be caused by prolonged exposure to dry air or intense light, or it may result from corneal trauma.

SIGNS AND SYMPTOMS Symptoms of keratitis include irritation, tearing, and photophobia. When the cause is herpes simplex virus 1, an upper respiratory infection with facial cold sores may be the precursor. When prolonged exposure to dry air or in-

tense light is the cause of keratitis, the symptoms are exhibited about 12 hours later. The person experiences severe photophobia.

DIAGNOSTIC PROCEDURES Slit-lamp examination of the corneal surface confirms the diagnosis. Vision testing may indicate decreased visual acuity, and the medical history may reveal a recent upper respiratory infection.

TREATMENT Topical treatment with eyedrops and ointment is likely to be prescribed. A broad-spectrum antibiotic may prevent secondary infection. An eye patch may be recommended for a period of time.

PROGNOSIS The prognosis is good when the condition is properly treated, but untreated keratitis may lead to blindness.

PREVENTION The best prevention is proper eye care.

SPECIAL FOCUS ▇ CHILDHOOD DISEASE OF THE EYE

▇ STRABISMUS

DESCRIPTION *Strabismus* is a disorder in which the eyes cannot be directed to focus on the same object. The condition may affect one or both eyes. The eye may turn inward—convergent strabismus (esotropia), or crosseye; or it may turn outward—divergent strabismus (extraopia), or walleye (Fig. 14–4).

ETIOLOGY The most common cause of strabismus in children is lazy eye, or **amblyopia.** Other causes include unequal ocular muscle tone, farsightedness, central nervous system disturbances, or hereditary factors.

SIGNS AND SYMPTOMS There may be **diplopia** and blurred vision. The affected eye will appear to wander. If both eyes are involved, they may appear crossed, or give the child a "walleyed" appearance.

DIAGNOSTIC PROCEDURES A complete ophthalmologic examination is necessary. A neurological examination may be indicated as well.

TREATMENT Treatment depends on the cause. It often consists of covering the normal eye, forc-

Esotropia

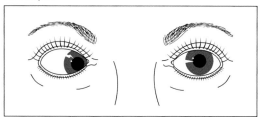

Exotropia

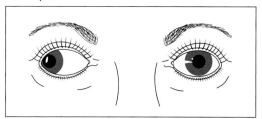

Figure 14–4 Strabismus: esotropia (left); exotropia (right). (From Gylys, BA, and Wedding, ME: Medical Terminology: A Systems Approach, ed 4. FA Davis, Philadelphia, 1999, p 324, with permission.)

ing the child to use the deviating one. Eye exercises and corrective lenses may be ordered. Surgical correction may be necessary.

PROGNOSIS Generally, the earlier treatment is begun, the more rapid is the improvement and the more effective the treatment. By the age of 6, the vision in the deviating eye usually has become so suppressed that treatment is not effective and visual loss is permanent.

PREVENTION There is no known prevention.

COMMON SYMPTOMS OF EYE DISEASES

Individuals may present with the following common symptoms, which deserve attention from health professionals:

- Any visual disturbance
- Pain or burning in the eye and any of its structures
- Eye redness

Ear Diseases

◼ IMPACTED CERUMEN

DESCRIPTION *Cerumen* is the soft, brown, waxlike secretion found in the external canal of the ear. The abnormal accumulation and eventual impaction of this substance within the ear canal can cause temporary hearing loss.

ETIOLOGY Abnormal cerumen accumulation may be due to dryness and scaling of the skin or excessive hair in the ear canal. Individuals with narrow or tortuous ear canals may be predisposed to the condition.

SIGNS AND SYMPTOMS There may be a gradual loss of hearing, and the person may notice a feeling of fullness in the ear or experience **tinnitus.**

DIAGNOSTIC PROCEDURES An otologic examination will reveal a soft or hard wax mass.

TREATMENT A dull ring **curet** put through a speculum may be all that is necessary to remove the wax. If the impaction adheres to the wall of the canal, it may be softened by repeated instillations of oil ear drops or hydrogen peroxide and then irrigated with water.

PROGNOSIS The prognosis is good with removal of the wax; however, the condition may recur.

PREVENTION There is no known prevention.

◼ EXTERNAL OTITIS (Swimmer's Ear)

DESCRIPTION *External otitis (swimmer's ear)* is inflammation of the external ear canal.

ETIOLOGY The inflammation may be caused by a bacterial or fungal infection or by a dermatologic condition such as seborrhea or psoriasis. Predisposing factors include swimming or bathing in con-

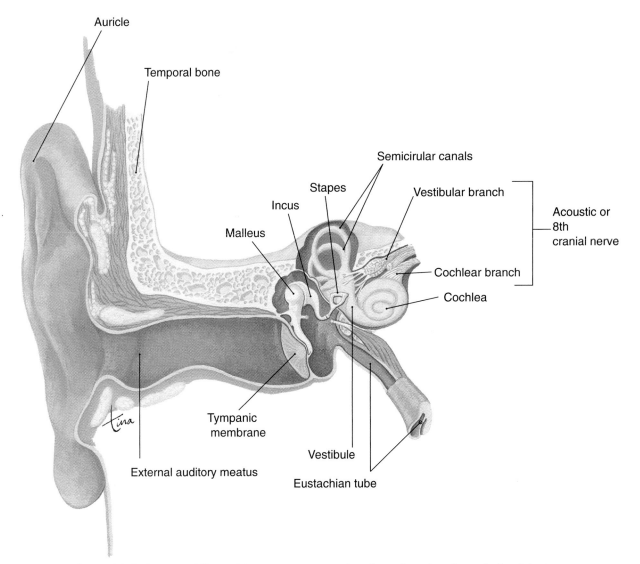

Figure 14–5 Outer, middle, and inner ear structures in a frontal section through the right temporal bone. (From Scanlon, VC, and Sanders, T: Essentials of Anatomy and Physiology, ed 3. FA Davis, Philadelphia, 1999, p 198, with permission.)

taminated water, or trauma to the ear canal from attempts to clean or scratch the ear. The frequent use of earphones, earplugs, or earmuffs may create a favorable environment within the ear canal in which bacteria and fungi may propagate.

SIGNS AND SYMPTOMS Severe pain, **pruritus,** and a red, swollen ear canal are common presenting symptoms. Drainage from the ear may be either purulent or watery. Fever and hearing loss may result.

DIAGNOSTIC PROCEDURES An otologic examination will confirm the diagnosis. WBC may be normal or elevated. A bacterial culture of ear canal scrapings, as well as sensitivity tests, may be carried out if an infection is suspected.

TREATMENT Antibiotics and analgesics may be prescribed. The ear must be kept dry and clean, and it should be protected from trauma. Ear drops or ointments may be instilled.

PROGNOSIS External otitis tends to recur and become chronic. When untreated, it can cause hearing loss.

PREVENTION Prevention includes wearing earplugs when swimming, bathing, or showering; also, cleaning the ear with any foreign objects should be avoided, to minimize the risk of trauma to the ear canal.

OTITIS MEDIA

DESCRIPTION *Otitis media* is an accumulation of fluid within the structure of the middle ear. The condition is subclassified into either serous or **suppurative** categories according to the composition of the accumulating fluid. In serous otitis media, the fluid is comparatively clear and sterile, secreted from the membranes lining the inner ear. In suppurative otitis media, the fluid is the product of pus-producing bacteria. The pressure from the accumulating fluid, in either form of the condition, may be enough to occasion temporary hearing loss. Both serous and suppurative forms of the disease may occur as acute or chronic conditions. Otitis media is most common among children.

ETIOLOGY Acute serous otitis media may occur spontaneously or following an upper respiratory tract infection. It also may be occasioned by rapid changes in atmospheric pressure, such as occur during flying, or by allergic reactions. The chronic form of serous otitis media may develop from the acute condition, or it may result from the overgrowth of adenoidal tissue or chronic sinus infections. Suppurative otitis media is caused by the introduction of pyogenic microorganisms into the middle ear, usually *Haemophilus influenzae, Streptococcus, Pneumococcus,* or *Staphylococcus.* The condition often follows the mumps, flu, or colds and may be induced by overly forceful nose blowing. Swimming in contaminated water also may result in a middle ear infection.

Irrespective of the particular form of the condition, or its ultimate cause, variations in the structure or function of the eustachian tube may strongly predispose an individual to developing otitis media. Narrowing or constriction of the eustachian tubes may interfere with the normal drainage of secretions from the middle ear. Conversely, those with eustachian tubes that are shorter, wider, or more horizontally placed than normal may be more prone to infectious forms of otitis media.

SIGNS AND SYMPTOMS A person with serous otitis media usually experiences only a sensation of fullness or pressure in the affected ear, along with varying degrees of hearing impairment. Suppurative otitis media, on the other hand, is usually manifested by pain in the affected ear and is often accompanied by general symptoms of infection such as fever and chills, nausea, and vomiting. Both conditions may occasion dizziness.

DIAGNOSTIC PROCEDURES Examination of the affected ear with an otoscope will reveal bulging of the eardrum. Often the eardrum will have a cherry-red discoloration. Fluid bubbles may be discernible behind the eardrum. The individual's WBC is usually elevated in cases of suppurative otitis media.

TREATMENT Antibiotics will be ordered to control suppurative otitis media, and analgesics may be prescribed to relieve pain and discomfort of either form. Decongestants may be ordered to promote drainage. In severe cases, drainage may be accomplished by **myringotomy** or needle aspiration. For chronic forms of otitis media, the acute attacks must be treated as previously described, but surgery, such as myringoplasty and **tympanoplasty,** may also be necessary. In some cases, tubes are inserted surgically into the tympanic membrane to equalize pressure between the atmosphere and the middle ear. In most cases, the tubes are removed after 6 to 12 months, or they may fall out on their own.

PROGNOSIS The prognosis for an individual with either form of acute otitis media usually is good, given prompt treatment. Chronic otitis media, however, may lead to scarring, adhesions, and severe ear damage with hearing loss. Complications are possible, ranging from either acute or chronic forms of suppurative otitis media to brain abscess, meningitis, or mastoiditis.

PREVENTION Prompt treatment of any upper respiratory tract infection and otitis media is necessary.

OTOSCLEROSIS

DESCRIPTION *Otosclerosis* is the formation of spongy bone, especially around the oval window, with resulting immobilization of the stapes. The condition is characterized by chronic, progressive deafness. The disease occurs primarily among women, usually appearing between the ages of 15 and 40 years.

ETIOLOGY Otosclerosis is an idiopathic condition, but because the disease shows a familial pattern, genetic factors are suspected. The condition is often aggravated by pregnancy.

SIGNS AND SYMPTOMS A gradual bilateral hearing loss of low tones or soft sounds is the first sign. Tinnitus may accompany the condition. Affected clients may turn their head to hear better or may notice they cannot use the phone on the affected ear.

DIAGNOSTIC PROCEDURES A Rinne's test is used to diagnose otosclerosis. An audiogram may reveal moderate to severe hearing loss, especially in the low range.

TREATMENT The ear that is most affected may undergo **stapedectomy** with a prosthesis inserted. The other ear will have the same surgery later. If surgery is not an option, a hearing aid may be tried.

PROGNOSIS The prognosis improves following surgery, although some degree of lasting hearing impairment is characteristic of the disease.

PREVENTION There is no known prevention.

MOTION SICKNESS

DESCRIPTION *Motion sickness* consists of nausea, vomiting, and **vertigo** induced by irregular or rhythmic movements, such as may occur during airplane, boat, or automobile travel.

ETIOLOGY This disorder is caused by any motion capable of disturbing the equilibrium of the organs of balance in the inner ear (the semicircular canals). Strong emotions such as fear and grief, digestive upset, or offensive odors may trigger or exacerbate the problem.

SIGNS AND SYMPTOMS An individual affected by motion sickness may experience loss of equilibrium, nausea, vomiting, dizziness, **diaphoresis,** headache, and anorexia. Symptoms may disappear almost immediately after the inciting motion has ceased, or they may persist for hours or days.

DIAGNOSTIC PROCEDURES Diagnosis is by history and complaints.

TREATMENT Ongoing attacks of motion sickness usually are successfully treated with antihistamines, antiemetics, or sedatives.

PROGNOSIS Although the condition may be severe enough to be debilitating for some, the symptoms of motion sickness usually disappear with the restoration of equilibrium.

PREVENTION Certain **anticholinergic** drug preparations taken prior to traveling are quite useful in preventing the onset of symptoms in susceptible individuals.

MÉNIÈRE'S DISEASE

DESCRIPTION *Ménière's disease* (pronounced mān•ē•ārz′) is a chronic inner ear syndrome marked by attacks of vertigo, progressive deafness, tinnitus, and a sensation of fullness in the ears. The condition usually appears in persons between the ages of 40 and 50 years.

ETIOLOGY The cause of Ménière's disease is not known, but the disease process appears to destroy the hair cells within the cochlea. There may be an overproduction or decreased absorption of the fluid within the cochlea and semicircular canals (endolymph). This change in fluid pressure disturbs or damages the sensory cells and thus transmission to the brain is affected. Head trauma, middle ear infection, autonomic nervous system dysfunction, and premenstrual edema may be predisposing factors.

SIGNS AND SYMPTOMS The classic symptoms are severe vertigo, tinnitus, and sensorineural hearing loss. An acute attack of vertigo may cause nausea, vomiting, sweating, and loss of balance. These attacks may occur several times a year. But remissions also can last several years.

DIAGNOSTIC PROCEDURES When all three symptoms are present, the diagnosis is not difficult. Further testing using audiometry and x-rays of the internal meatus of the ear may be necessary. The physician may request a magnetic resonance imaging (MRI) scan in order to rule out brain involvement.

TREATMENT A salt-free diet, diuretics, antihistamines, and mild sedatives are helpful in long-term care. Severe attacks may require epinephrine. If the disease persists and causes debilitating vertigo, surgical destruction of the affected labyrinth may be necessary. This relieves symptoms but causes irreversible hearing loss.

PROGNOSIS The prognosis varies, but usually recurrent attacks over several years lead to residual tinnitus and hearing loss.

PREVENTION There is no known prevention.

SPECIAL FOCUS CHILDHOOD DISEASES OF THE EAR

DEAFNESS

Deafness occurring during childhood may be congenital, and may be transmitted as a dominant, autosomal dominant, autosomal recessive, or sex-linked recessive trait. It may also be due to trauma, toxicity, or infection during pregnancy or delivery. The most common cause of sudden deafness in children is mumps. Other bacterial and viral infections, however, also can cause sudden deafness that may occasion permanent loss of hearing. Whatever the cause, deafness in children can contribute to difficulties in the development of language skills.

OTITIS MEDIA

Acute otitis media is common in children younger than 6 years of age. The most common organism causing the condition is *Hemophilus influenzae*. Predisposing factors in children include a eustachian tube that is shorter, wider, and more horizontal than normal, as well as abundant lymphoid tissue of the pharynx, which may cause obstruction of the nasopharynx. With prompt treatment, the prognosis is excellent.

COMMON SYMPTOMS OF EAR DISEASES

Individuals may present with the following common symptoms, which deserve attention from health professionals:

- Hearing loss
- Tinnitus
- Ear pressure
- Nausea and vomiting
- Pain
- Dizziness

BIBLIOGRAPHY

Burns, MV: Pathophysiology: A Self-Instructional Program. Appleton & Lange, Stamford, Conn., 1998.

Diseases. Springhouse Corporation. Springhouse, Pa., 1993.

Fauci, AS, et al: Harrison's Principles of Internal Medicine, ed 14. McGraw-Hill, New York, 1998.

Frazier, MS, et al: Essentials of Human Disease and Conditions. WB Saunders, Philadelphia, 1996.

Mulvihill, ML: Human Diseases: A Systemic Approach. Appleton & Lange, Stamford, Conn., 1995.

Professional Guide to Diseases, ed 6. Springhouse Corporation, Springhouse, Pa., 1998.

CASE STUDIES

I During a general physical examination, a 60-year-old woman complains of what appears to be a painless, gradual loss of sight. In response to questions, she reports that she perceives halos around most light sources, such as lamps and headlights. The physician notes that her eyes have a white cast to them.

1. What condition is indicated by these signs and symptoms?

2. What treatment options will the physician have to consider?

II A mother notices that her preschooler doesn't always respond when called. It also seems that the girl sits very close to the television and turns the volume up quite high. The mother suspects a hearing problem.

1. What ear diseases or disorders might cause hearing loss in a young child?

2. What treatments might be ordered for the various possible diseases?

3. Discuss the prognosis for each possible ear disease.

REVIEW QUESTIONS

TRUE/FALSE

T F 1. Hyperopia or farsightedness is a common refractive error.

T F 2. Myopia is nearsightedness.

T F 3. Presbyopia is an elliptical curvature of the cornea.

T F 4. Nystagmus is the medical term for stye.

T F 5. Complications of corneal abrasion are ulceration and permanent vision loss.

T F 6. In a mature cataract, the pupil of the eye becomes white.

T F 7. A common sign of a cataract is eye pain.

T F 8. Adults should be tested for glaucoma every 3 to 5 years.

T F 9. An uncommon eye disorder is conjunctivitis.

T F 10. Blepharitis may be caused by a *Staphylococcus* infection.

T F 11. *Photophobia* is the term to describe the eye's sensitivity to light.

T F 12. Keratitis may be caused by bacteria, virus, or fungus.

T F 13. Macular degeneration occurs more frequently in the young.

MATCHING

_____ 1. Cerumen

_____ 2. External otitis

_____ 3. Otitis media

_____ 4. Otosclerosis

a. Earache or inflammation of middle ear

b. Noise or ringing in ear

c. Causes severe vertigo

d. Swimmer's ear

e. Hearing loss due to aging

_____ 5. Tinnitus

_____ 6. Ménière's disease

_____ 7. Uveitis

f. Ear wax

g. Spongy bone in labyrinth's capsule

h. Inflammation of the uveal tract

i. Inflammation of the cornea

DISCUSSION QUESTIONS

1. Determine what a physician looks for in a physical examination of the eye and the ear.

2. Describe the prognosis for strabismus.

ANSWERS

TRUE/FALSE

1. T
2. T
3. F
4. F
5. T
6. T
7. F

8. T
9. F
10. T
11. T
12. T
13. F

MATCHING

1. f
2. d

3. a
4. g

5. b
6. c

7. h

DISCUSSION QUESTIONS

1. Answers will vary.
2. Answers will vary.

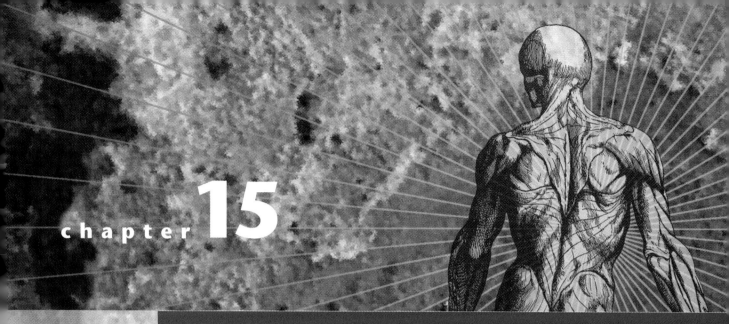

chapter 15

Pain and Its Management

CHAPTER OUTLINE

What Is Pain?
Definition of Pain
Purpose of Pain
Pathophysiology of Pain

Assessment of Pain

Acute, Chronic, and Terminal Pain

Treatment of Pain
Medications
Surgery
Biofeedback
Relaxation

Imagery
Autohypnosis
Transcutaneous Electrical Nerve Stimulation
   (TENS)
Massage
Humor, Laughter, and Play
Music
□ ALTERNATIVE MEDICINE

Conclusion

References

Bibliography

Review Questions

LEARNING OBJECTIVES

Upon successful completion of this chapter, you will:

- Define pain.
- List at least four factors that influence how we experience pain.
- Discuss the purpose of pain.
- Explain the gate control theory of pain.
- Describe the pain assessment tool.
- Compare and contrast acute pain, chronic pain, and terminal pain.
- List and describe at least six types of treatment for pain.

KEY WORDS

Acetylcholine (ăs•ĕ•tĭl•kō′lēn)
Cordotomy (kŏr•dŏt′ō•mē)
Endorphin (ĕn•dŏr′fĭn)
Histamine (hĭs′tă•mĭn)
Hypophysectomy (hī•pŏf•ĭ•sĕk′tō•mē)
Libido (lĭ•bī′dō)
Narcotic (năr•kŏt′ĭk)

Neuromodulator (nū•rō•mŏd′ū•lā•tŏr)
Neurotomy (nū•rŏt′ō•mē)
Neurotransmitter (nū•rō•trăns′mĭt•ĕr)
Patient-controlled analgesia (ăn•ăl•jē′zē•ă)
Substantia gelatinosa (sŭb•stăn′shē•ă
  jĕl•ă•tĭ•nō′să)
Synapse (sĭn′ăps)
Trigger point (trĭg′ĕr)

Pain affects each of us during our lifetime. In fact, pain is the most common reason why people seek medical advice.[1] Physiological pain accompanies many diseases and disorders of the body. Psychological pain often is expressed as sorrow over losses such as death or divorce. Psychological pain may become physiological pain, or the two may be concurrent. Although pain may be sensed as having a negative effect on the body, it may be positive, also. For instance, if pain could not be felt, you might not know you were burning your flesh on a hot stove.

Health professionals often are frustrated in their attempt to treat individuals who experience pain, especially when the cause of pain is not readily identifiable. Clients in pain may be frustrated and confused too, and may find the pain unbearable.

What is pain? What purpose, if any, does it serve? What happens in the body when a person feels pain? How does the health professional assess pain? What are the differences between acute and chronic pain? Can pain be treated? If so, how? These are some of the questions that are addressed in this chapter.

WHAT IS PAIN?

Definition of Pain

Dictionaries define *pain* as a sensation of hurting, or of strong discomfort, in some part of the body, caused by an injury, disease, or functional disorder and transmitted through the nervous system. *Pain* also may be defined as the distress or suffering (mental or physical) that is caused by great anxiety, anguish, grief, disappointment, or other psychological or emotional stimuli. A nurse who has worked for more than 20 years with clients in pain defines *pain* as "whatever the experiencing person says it is, existing when he says it does."[2] This definition is, perhaps, the most useful, for it acknowledges the client's complaint, recognizes the subjective nature of pain, and implicitly suggests that diverse measures may be undertaken to relieve pain.

How we experience pain is based, in part, on our early experiences of pain, our cultural backgrounds, our anxiety level, our attention level, and any suggestions we have or are given at the time we experience the pain. As health-care professionals, we too will be influenced by our past experience, our attitudes, and our beliefs regarding pain. Must there be an organic reason before pain is "real"? Who understands pain better—the person experiencing the pain or the health professional? Research suggests that health-care professionals may be overly concerned about the client's becoming addicted to pain medication or may feel that the person is merely malingering.

Purpose of Pain

Pain is a warning that something is wrong in normal body functioning. It is one of the most common complaints of a person seeking medical attention. It warns of inflammation, tissue damage, infection, bodily injury, or trauma—physical or emotional—somewhere in the body. Each disease produces characteristic patterns of tissue damage; hence, the quality, time, course, and location of a person's pain complaint and the location of tenderness provide important diagnostic clues.

Pathophysiology of Pain

What occurs at the cellular level when we experience pain? The gate control theory of pain offers a useful model of the physiologic process of pain (Fig. 15–1). According to gate control theory, "the experience of pain is the result of the summa-

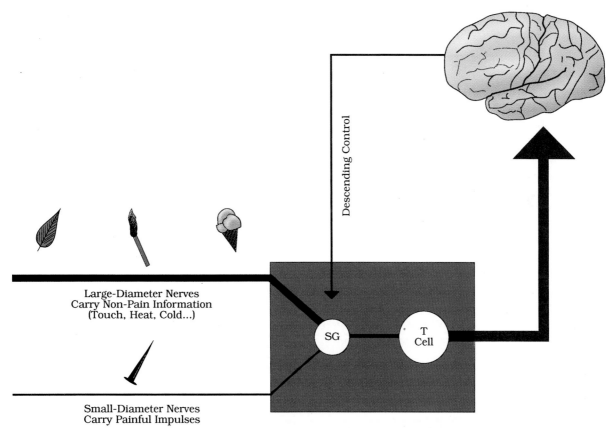

Figure 15–1 The gate control theory of pain transmission. The substantia gelatinosa (SG) accepts input both from large-diameter (nonpain) and small-diameter (pain) nerves. Based on the rate of input, the SG allows either the pain or nonpain stimulus to be passed on to the transmission cell (T cell) and up to the brain. Because nonpain impulses travel faster than pain impulses, stimulation of nonpain fibers can override the transmission of pain. In addition, the brain has an inhibiting influence both on the SG and the spinal cord that can work to limit the perception and reaction to pain. (From Starkey, C: Therapeutic Modalities for Athletic Trainers. FA Davis, Philadelphia, 1993, p 28, with permission.)

tion of the action of both **neurotransmitters** and **neuromodulators** at each neural receptor site from the site of injury to the cortex. At each neuron **synapse,** if the amount of neurotransmitter (**histamine, acetylcholine,** etc.) exceeds the amount of neuromodulators (**endorphin,** etc.), then the impulse continues to the next synapse where similar interactions are in operation."[3] In other words, we experience pain whenever the substances that tend to propagate a pain impulse across each "gate" in a nerve pathway overpower the substances that tend to block such an impulse. Amidst controversy and minor evolution, the gate control theory is presently recognized as a major basis of pain theory.

Studies of coping factors support a wider version of the gate control theory. These factors need to be considered before determining treatment for pain, and they raise a number of questions:

1. How well is the client coping with life?
2. Does the client have pain and if so, does he or she think that it is under control?
3. Does the client feel adequately informed about the painful condition?
4. Is the client occupied? How does the individual fill his or her time?
5. Does the client have other problems to cope with?
6. Does the client feel dissatisfied with his or her past life or does he or she have any substantial regrets?
7. Are there any reasons why the client may not be coping?[4]

These factors may help determine the best treatment for pain.

No current theory of pain is entirely satisfactory, and new theories will undoubtedly continue to be advanced and debated.

ASSESSMENT OF PAIN

Pain gives the body warning, and usually is accompanied by anxiety or the urge to relieve the pain. Pain is both sensation and emotion. Health care professionals may find the following mnemonic tool useful for assessing a client in pain:[5]

- *P = place* (client points with one finger to the pain's location).

- *A = amount* (client rates pain on a scale from 0, no pain, to 10, the worst pain possible).
- *I = interactions* (client describes what makes the pain worse).
- *N = neutralizers* (client describes what makes the pain less).

The scale of 1 to 10 as described above is the most useful method of assessing pain. Further pain assessment skills include observing the client's appearance and activity. Monitoring the client's vital signs may be of value in assessing acute pain, but not necessarily chronic pain.

ACUTE, CHRONIC, AND TERMINAL PAIN

Acute and chronic pain need to be differentiated prior to the beginning of treatment. *Acute pain* is recent in onset and has been experienced over a period lasting less than 6 months. Such pain may be manifested as an increase in heart rate, blood pressure, and muscle tension, and a decrease in salivary flow and gut motility. Acute pain frequently serves as a warning sign of a disturbance in some physiological process and usually is accompanied by anxiety.

Chronic pain may be either continuous or intermittent, occurring over a period longer than 6 months. Unlike the acute form, chronic pain may not serve as a warning of physiological disturbance. It is frequently debilitating, exhausting an individual's physical and emotional resources.

Chronic pain is often difficult to manage. Clients with chronic pain may have a disease with no cure that is characteristically painful. Other diseases have perpetuating factors such as sensory nerve damage that linger long after treatment is initiated. Also, the client may experience psychological effects that cause pain or exacerbate it. Often, the client is depressed and preoccupied with self. Chronic pain may be associated with a decrease in sleep, **libido,** and appetite. Because the parasympathetic nervous system tends to adapt to a state of chronic pain, however, there may be few, if any, outward physiological signs or behavioral changes noted in individuals experiencing such pain.

Terminal pain can be either acute or chronic but is the type of pain that occurs when the client is terminally ill. Although health-care professionals may be familiar with cancer or malignancy pain, clients who are terminally ill with diseases other than cancer may also experience pain. Like those suffering from chronic or acute pain, the terminally ill client should be offered analgesia for palliative treatment. The needs of the client's family and caregivers should be addressed, too. The assessment of the client with terminal pain is similar to that of any client experiencing pain, although the difference with the dying client is that he or she is dealing with emotions of anxiety, fear, anger, and depression, which are common to people whose condition is terminal. They are dealing with death in addition to pain.

TREATMENT OF PAIN

The objective of pain treatment is to remove the cause or lessen the pain's severity; however, there may be a lag in time between identifying the cause of the pain and providing relief. Treatment of pain is diverse and difficult. A multidisciplinary approach to pain management is being attempted by many pain clinics across the United States with success. This team approach involves both medical and nonmedical personnel. Pain therapy may include any of a number of approaches, as follows.

Medications

Medications tend to be the treatment of choice for many clients experiencing acute pain. Analgesics, anesthetics, and anti-inflammatory agents may be prescribed to decrease or eliminate pain, although they do not eliminate the cause of pain. Analgesics can be **narcotic** or nonnarcotic, prescription or over-the-counter, strong or weak.

A milestone in the treatment of some pain is the **patient-controlled analgesia** pump, or PCA (Fig. 15–2). The pump allows the patient to administer his or her own pain medication. In PCA, the amount of drug dispensed by the pump is determined by the physician. The device is designed not to release more than the prescribed amount within a set period of time, thus guarding against overmedication.

Research indicates that health-care professionals and family members tend to undermedicate for pain because of incorrect assumptions, prevailing attitudes, the complexity of pain assessment, and

unfounded fears, mainly those of addiction (psychological dependence). However, no medical research testifies to such an addiction. In fact, as the authors of one article on pain management state, what is "of greater clinical importance is that unrelieved pain adversely affects pulmonary, gastrointestinal and circulatory systems."[6] The same authors further describe the insomnia, depression, and irritability that result if the untreated pain becomes chronic.

Surgery

Surgery may be attempted to block the transmission of pain or to remove the cause of pain. Surgery for relief of pain may include such procedures as

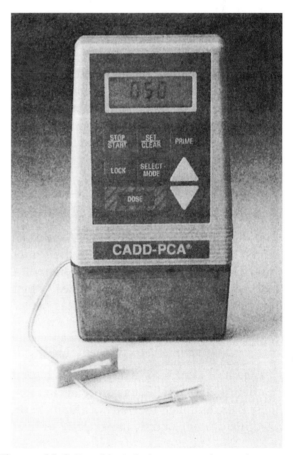

Figure 15–2 Portable infusion pump for patient-controlled analgesia (PCA). (Courtesy of Pharmacia Deltec, Inc., St. Paul, Minnesota; from Phillips, LD: Manual of IV Therapeutics, ed 2. FA Davis, Philadelphia, 1997, p 211, with permission.)

neurotomy, cordotomy, and **hypophysectomy,** as well as the removal of any causative factor. Surgery may be helpful to relieve the pain of pancreatic cancer, the severe intractable pain from other malignancies, or intractable abdominal pain.

Biofeedback

Biofeedback is aimed at helping an individual gain voluntary control over normally involuntary physiological functions. Various forms of electronic feedback produced by monitoring physiological events may promote blood flow and reduce muscle tension, which, in turn, may reduce the concentration of neurotransmitters at the site of pain. Currently, biofeedback of four different types is being used to control chronic pain.

1. Electroencephalogram (EEG) feedback
2. Skin temperature feedback
3. Cephalic blood volume-pulse feedback
4. Electromyographic feedback

The Biofeedback Society of America recommends the use of biofeedback for controlling pain in six major areas:

1. Vascular headache
2. Muscle contraction headache
3. Vasoconstrictive disorders
4. Psychophysiological disorders
5. Gastrointestinal disorders
6. Physical medicine and rehabilitation

Relaxation

Relaxation therapy can be utilized to modify muscle tension, which is believed to cause or exacerbate pain. The individual is taught a series of techniques for relaxation, which are used any time pain occurs. Audiotapes are used in beginning practice sessions; then the person learns to relax without any assistance. Relaxation therapy is especially successful when used in conjunction with biofeedback and imagery.

Imagery

Imagery is therapy used by a person experiencing pain to produce relaxation and increase the production of endorphins. The person imagines and concentrates on a pleasant scene or experience and is taught to relax. To be effective, imagery necessitates a positive relationship to the image scene; otherwise, the imagery may only exacerbate the pain.

Autohypnosis

Hypnosis is a state that resembles sleep but is induced by a hypnotist who makes readily accepted suggestions to the client. *Autohypnosis,* self-induced hypnosis, is most effective when a person is motivated—and pain is a strong motivating force. The period of pain relief from autohypnosis is from 4 to 6 hours, and the time of relief is extended with repeated hypnotic reinforcement. Autohypnosis can be learned in a few hours.

Transcutaneous Electrical Nerve Stimulation (TENS)

Transcutaneous electrical nerve stimulation is a therapeutic procedure in which an electrical impulse is induced in the large nerve fibers that carry non-pain information in order to block or reduce the transmission of painful impulses. The electrodes are connected by lead wires to a stimulator called a *TENS unit,* and the frequency and intensity of the electric current can be varied. Although still considered experimental by some, the use of TENS has proved effective for pain relief in some patients.

Massage

Massage is manipulation, methodical pressure, friction, and kneading of the body. A mentholated rub may be used to increase stimulation. Massage may be performed over or around an area of pain or at **trigger points.** This type of treatment stimulates blood flow, induces relaxation, and increases the production of endorphins.

Humor, Laughter, and Play

Norman Cousins, former editor of the *Saturday Review,* popularized the concept of making laughter and humor an antidote for pain. While quite ill in the hospital, he discovered he could go much longer without his pain medication when he had been doing a great deal of laughing. He watched comedy films and read humor books. Humor and laughter control pain in four ways: (1) by distracting attention, (2) by reducing tension, (3) by changing expectations, and (4) by increasing production of endorphins—the body's natural painkillers.[7]

Play is another activity that is helpful in reducing pain, even for the severely debilitated person. Play can be childlike or quite adult. Consider the following: Two toddlers, riding tricycles, approach the charge nurse on the floor of the burn unit in a major city hospital. The burns of both are obvious, but their "race" through the corridors has become part of their treatment. One child is quite concerned over the loss of his baseball hat—a gift to all the children from a major league team. The reason for the concern? All the children were leaving shortly to play ball with one of the therapists. Who can play ball without a cap? The tricycle race and the game afterwards focus the child's attention on play—not pain.

Music

Physicians and dentists have discovered that music will help alleviate pain. Dentists know that some patients are receptive enough to music to have their teeth extracted without anesthesia. Some hospitals allow music to be piped into their surgical rooms because it puts both patients and practitioners in a more relaxed state.

John Diamond, MD, practices preventive medicine and psychiatry in Valley Cottage, New York, and has spent more than 25 years researching music and its therapeutic value and life-enhancing quality. His books, *The Life Energy in Music,* volumes 1 and 2,[8] would be particularly interesting to any person seeking more knowledge about music therapy and its healing powers.

 ## ALTERNATIVE MEDICINE

Pain management is addressed in alternative medicine in the following ways:

Acupuncture: Acupuncture, which originated in China more than five thousand years ago, began to receive attention in Western culture in the 1970s. Acupuncture is a technique for treating certain painful conditions and for producing regional anesthesia by passing long, thin needles through the skin to specific points. The free ends of the needles are twirled or, in some cases, used to conduct a weak electric current. Most acupuncturists use only 10 to 12 needles per treatment, and the person feels only a slight pricking sensation when the sterile, disposable needles are inserted. The treatment is painless and can take anywhere from a few seconds to 45 minutes.

Acupuncture appears to stimulate the release of the body's natural painkillers, endorphins and enkephalins. It has been suggested that acupuncture influences the production and distribution of neurotransmitters and neuromodulators that, in turn, modify the person's perception of pain.

Aromatherapy: Aromatherapy is the use of essential oils found in plants and herbs to treat pain. This therapy is used extensively in Europe. Some believe the effects of the oils come from their pharmacological properties and their small molecular size, making them easier to penetrate the body tissues. Health-care professionals may use essential oils in massage to relieve pain and induce sleep. Oil baths, hot and cold compresses, or a simple topical application may also help alleviate pain.

Therapeutic Touch: In therapeutic touch generally there is no physical touching of the client. Sometimes, however, touching may be necessary, especially in pain associated with fractures or physical trauma. Proper use of therapeutic touch has been shown to reduce pain and ease problems associated with the autonomic nervous system.

The practitioner begins the therapeutic touch session with a client assessment wherein the practitioner places his or her hands 2 to 6 inches above the client's body, and makes rhythmic, slow hand motions so that the client's blockages in the energy field can be found. The practitioner's hand motions then replenish the client's energy field. The session lasts about 20 to 25 minutes. The technique has been taught to thousands of practitioners.

Yoga Therapy: Yoga, which means "union," is a system of beliefs and practices, the goal of which is to teach mind and body unity. In the Western world, yoga generally is associated with physical postures, relaxation, and regulation of breathing. These are yoga exercises, but not yoga in the spiritual sense. Yoga is often used in the treatment of pain to promote relaxation, aid circulation, reduce fatigue, stimulate particular body areas, strengthen muscles, and develop flexibility. For the best results, the regimen has to be practiced regularly.

CONCLUSION

Despite its multitude of forms and sometimes highly subjective qualities, pain is real. Pain needs to be understood and accepted in the terms of the person experiencing it. Each person experiences pain differently. Pain should be managed as aggressively as is its cause. The health professional and the person in pain should be willing to investigate many forms of pain management and seek the one or ones that best suit the individual's needs.

Finally, a useful attitude toward pain management is captured in the following statement by David Black in *The Laughter Prescription:* "Pain is an energy monster, we give it the power to hurt us. And we take that power away—depending on how we choose to view ourselves. All pain is real, but you can change your reality."[7]

REFERENCES

1. Cupples, SA: Pain as hurtful experience: A philosophical analysis and implications for holistic nursing care. Nursing Forum 27:5, 1992.
2. Zajac, J: Pediatric pain management. Critical Care Nursing Quarterly 15:35, 1992.
3. Donovan, M: Cancer pain: You can help! Nurs Clin North Am 17:713, 1982.
4. Walker, J: Elderly people in the community living with pain. Nursing Times 87:28–32, 1991.
5. McGuire, L: A short, simple tool for assessing your patient's pain. Nursing 81(11):48–49, 1981.
6. Slack, J, and Faut-Callahan, M: Pain management. Nurs Clin North Am 26:463, 1991.
7. Peter, LJ, and Dana, B: The Laughter Prescription. Ballantine Books, New York, 1982, p 8.
8. Diamond, J: The Life Energy in Music, Vols 1 and 2. Archaeus Press, Valley Cottage, NY, 1983.

BIBLIOGRAPHY

Cailliet, R: Pain: Mechanisms and Management. FA Davis, Philadelphia, 1993.
Ferrell, B, et al: Pain as a metaphor for illness. II. Family caregivers' management of pain. Oncol Nurs Forum 18: 1315–1321, 1991.
Friedman, DP: Pain patients just say "No" to drug addiction (letter to editor). J Pain Symptom Manage 6:351, 1991.
Greipp, ME: Undermedication for pain: An ethical model. Adv Nurs Sci 15:44–52, 1992.
Herr, K, and Mobily, PR: Interventions related to pain. Nurs Clin North Am 27:347–356, 1992.
Jacox, A, et al: A guide for the nation: Managing acute pain. Am J Nurs 92:5, 49–55, 1992.
McCaffrey, M, Ferrell, BR, and O'Neil-Page, E: Does life-style affect your pain-control decisions? Nursing 92(22):4, 58–61, 1992.
McCaggery, M: Addiction fear increasing among nurses (letter to editor). J Pain Symptom Manage 6:350, 1991.
Slack, J, and Faut-Callahan, M: Pain Management. Nurs Clin North Am 26:463–476, 1991.
Stephany, TM: When the family undermedicates. Home Healthcare Nurse 10:59, 1992.
Stevens, B: Assessment and management of pain in infants. The Canadian Nurse 88:31–34, 1992.
Wallace, KG: The pathophysiology of pain. Critical Care Nursing Quarterly 12:1–13, 1992.
White, J, and Strong, J: Measurement of activity levels in patients with chronic pain. The Occupational Therapy Journal of Research 12:5, 1992.

REVIEW QUESTIONS

1. Using the two definitions of pain given in the text, define pain in your own words, including *your* definition of pain.

2. Describe the purpose of pain.

3. Define the gate control theory of pain. What do you see as its limitations?

4. Give a short, simple tool for assessing pain.

5. Define acute, chronic, and terminal pain.

6. Of the 10 pain therapies outlined in the text, which have you tried? What works best for you? Which would you like to try the next time you have acute pain? Chronic pain? Which therapy would you *never* try and why?

ANSWERS

1. Answers will vary.
2. Pain can be a warning that something is wrong in normal body functioning. It warns of inflammation, tissue damage, infection, bodily injury, or trauma somewhere in the body.
3. The gate control theory of pain: Pain is the result of the summation of the action of both neurotransmitters and neuromodulators at each neural receptor site from the site of injury to the cortex. At each neuron synapse, if the amount of neurotransmitter exceeds the amount of neuromodulator, then the impulse continues to the next synapse where similar interactions are in operation.
4. McGuire describes a short, simple tool for assessing pain:
   P = *place* (client points with one finger to the pain's location).
   A = *amount* (client rates pain on scale from 0, no pain, to 10, the worst pain possible).
   I = *interaction* (client describes what makes the pain worse).
   N = *neutralizers* (client describes what makes the pain less).
5. Acute pain is recent in onset, usually lasting less than 6 months. There is an increase in heart rate, blood pressure, and muscle tension, but a decrease in salivary flow and gut motility. Chronic pain may be continuous or intermittent and lasts longer than 6 months. It generally serves no useful purpose and is associated with a decrease in sleep, libido, and appetite. Terminal pain may be acute or chronic and occurs when a client is terminally ill.
6. Answers will vary.

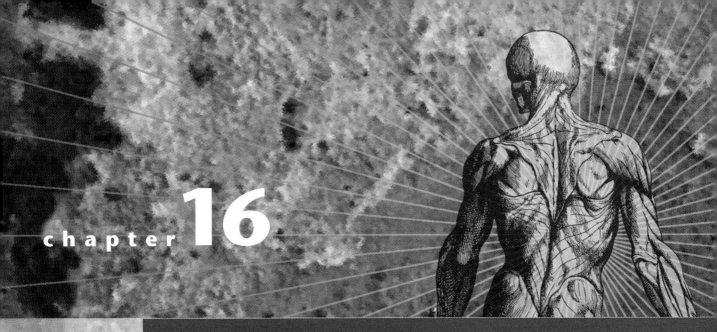

chapter 16

The Holistic Approach to Disease

CHAPTER OUTLINE

The Mind's Connection with Health and Disease

Holistic Health and Holistic Medicine Defined

Personal Responsibility

The Influence of Lifestyle
Environmental Influences—External and Internal

The Value of Good Nutrition
Stress and Distress

Managing Negative Emotions

Laughter and Play

Love, Friendship, and Faith

References

Bibliography

Review Questions

LEARNING OBJECTIVES

Upon successful completion of this chapter, you will:

- Describe the connection of mind and body in relation to the disease process.
- Define holistic health care.
- Discuss personal responsibility in relation to holistic health.
- Identify at least two external and two internal environmental factors that influence our health and well-being.
- List at least four influences of personal lifestyle on holistic health.
- Describe the effects of unexpressed negative emotions on our bodies.
- Identify at least seven constructive outlets for negative emotions.
- Define stress and distress.
- Identify at least three dietary goals for the United States.
- Discuss the importance of laughter and play in holistic health.
- List at least five "playful or fun" activities.
- Compare and contrast conditional and unconditional love.
- Discuss the effects of a personal faith on a holistic lifestyle.

One cannot think about any disease process without also thinking about health and healing. How is health defined? Do thoughts and feelings influence health? Can thoughts and feelings lead to ill health? What is the connection between the body and the mind? Is it important, perhaps even necessary, to identify the connection of body and mind in the treatment of an illness?

Technology has made extraordinary advances in modern medicine, yet most primary care providers will admit that the most sophisticated medical care may fail if the client, as well as the disease, is not part of the treatment protocol. This more holistic and complementary branch of medicine, aimed at treating and curing the client, requires looking at the mind-body connection and may include such modalities as reducing stress; encouraging laughter, play, relaxation, meditation, diet modification, guided imagery, and exercise; and helping the client take responsibility for managing his or her own life.

THE MIND'S CONNECTION WITH HEALTH AND DISEASE

It is difficult to identify or even define the mind. The mind has been described by Candace Pert, PhD, as "an enlivening energy in the information realm throughout the brain and body that enables the cells to talk to each other, and the outside to talk to the whole organism."[1] The mind has every-thing to do with our health. Moods and attitudes embodied in our emotions are part of the mind's physical expression. Our emotions affect all our organs and tissues. Negative emotions, especially over a long period of time, will have a negative effect on health; positive emotions have a positive effect on health.

It appears that sustained negative emotions over a long period of time can seriously hinder the body's immune system and keep it from functioning at an optimal level. Such linkages between our psychological state and the body's biological processes call upon the medical community and each of us to pay closer attention to our emotions and levels of stress. This approach to medical care is given several labels. Among them are holistic, complementary, and alternative health care. For the purposes of this chapter, the term "holistic" will be used.

HOLISTIC HEALTH AND HOLISTIC MEDICINE DEFINED

Holistic health is many things: It is a philosophy of life that relates to the whole rather than its parts; it is an attitude; it is an approach to life. Holistic health focuses on enabling good health to emerge in an individual. It encourages the individual to recognize the stresses of life and their impact on one's well-being.

Holistic medicine is a system of care that considers the needs of the whole person. Rather than focusing only on malfunctioning body parts, it also explores the broader dimensions of the individual's life—physical, nutritional, environmental, emotional, and spiritual. Holistic medicine encompasses all safe methods of diagnosis and treatment—including medication and surgery when appropriate. Holism in medicine can be traced, in part, to Hippocrates, who emphasized the environmental causes and treatment of illness, and the importance of emotional factors and nutrition. Both holistic health and holistic medicine emphasize personal responsibility and encourage cooperation and participation of client and practitioner to achieve and maintain good health.

PERSONAL RESPONSIBILITY

Because the body is not indestructible, we need to be taught self-care and responsibility from birth. Often, however, it is not until we see someone become disabled or die that we gain a proper appreciation for the body. From the moment of birth, the road to death begins. And during the period of life, we continually make choices about the body's well-being. Early in life, we are taught and learn by observation of those close to us either to respect or to ignore our bodies.

If we accept ourselves, feel self-worth, and have been taught well, we ought to listen to our body's signals and seek necessary attention. There is little or nothing even the most influential medical practitioner can do when the body breaks down if we do not want help or are unwilling to ask for it.

Andrew Weil, MD, a graduate of Harvard Medical School, and Director of the Program in Integrative Medicine at the University of Arizona, says that the most common correlation between mind and healing in people with chronic illness is total acceptance of the circumstances of one's life, including illness. This acceptance seems to allow and encourage a profound internal relaxation that enhances a person's spirit and immune system.[2]

THE INFLUENCE OF LIFESTYLE

Lifestyle is the consistent, integrated way of life of an individual, as typified by mannerisms, attitudes, and possessions. From the time one is born,

choices are made which influence lifestyle. These influences come from the following: (1) modeling of family members and peers, (2) education and knowledge, (3) personal attitudes, (4) degree of self-confidence, (5) individual responsibilities, (6) where we are in life, and (7) life's opportunities. From this list, we can see that an individual has a great deal of control over his or her own lifestyle. Such lifestyle choices have great influence, whether positive or negative, on one's own health and that of others. For example:

- Parents who provide a model of healthful living will influence their children toward a healthy lifestyle.
- Increased knowledge and awareness of blood cholesterol levels and their effect on health can encourage better diet.
- A person with self-confidence and a positive attitude is better equipped to cope with illness than a person racked by self-doubt or subject to a negative attitude. Acknowledgment of the internal healing system in the body leads to greater health.

Personal responsibility requires a person to act safely in a potentially dangerous situation. Conversely, being responsible for oneself requires that the individual avoid potentially harmful behaviors and attitudes, such as smoking, failing to exercise, driving without a seatbelt, or disregarding treatments prescribed by health-care providers. It requires that we listen to our bodies.

Environmental Influences—External and Internal

Personal health and well-being are greatly influenced by environment, both internal and external. Internal environmental factors include the genetic traits, familial tendencies, and physical and psychological characteristics inherent in each person. External environmental factors may be more easily defined. They include the air we breathe, the water we drink, the food we eat, and the surroundings in which we live and work.

Unfortunately, internal environmental factors are not easily controlled, changed, or altered. We are unable to change our genetic makeup; however, through genetic engineering, it is possible that we may influence the genetic makeup of our offspring. Familial tendencies are almost as difficult to influence as genetics, and we know that children will most often reflect the traits of their parents. Physical and psychological characteristics and attitudes can be altered; but deliberate, consistent, and continuous efforts must be instituted before change occurs. A choice may be made to alter the shape of the nose and a conscious effort can be made to modify a "type A" behavior; but even when such choices are deliberate, they may not greatly influence health.

Some, but not all, external environmental influences are more easily managed. A conscious effort may be made to refrain from smoking, but can one leave a job working in a coal mine? The air is cleaner in Seattle than in New York City, but can one move? Food may be purer with no preservatives or additives, but what about the risk of food poisoning? Should the government control the spraying of fruits and vegetables with pesticides, or should persons take their chances in the market? Is nuclear energy safe?

In the final analysis, one must recognize the influences that lifestyle and both internal and external environment have on health. It is important to understand that these factors also greatly affect the body's disorders and diseases.

The Value of Good Nutrition

How many times have you heard, "You are what you eat"? We understand the logic of advice such as "Beware of saturated fats," "Avoid refined sugar," and "Low salt, no salt, is the best salt." Why does eating often get out of control? Perhaps it comes from the philosophy that it is best to clean all the food from the plate. It may occur because food is used to relieve emotions and physical pain and as a reward for "being good."

Improper nutrition may result in body disorders or diseases. Bowel cancer is more common among groups of people who consume high amounts of animal fat and little fiber. There also is evidence that breast cancer may be linked to a high-fat and low-fiber dietary pattern and that where there is high meat consumption, cancer mortality rates are correspondingly high.

In *Dietary Goals for the United States* the following changes in food selection and preparation are suggested:[3]

- Increase consumption of fruits, vegetables, and whole grains.
- Decrease consumption of meat and increase consumption of poultry and fish.
- Decrease consumption of food high in fat and partially substitute polyunsaturated fat for saturated fat.
- Substitute nonfat milk for whole milk.
- Decrease consumption of butterfat, eggs, and other high-cholesterol sources.
- Decrease consumption of sugar and foods with high sugar content.
- Decrease consumption of salt and foods with high salt content.

Obviously, the list could go on and on. It is important, however, to realize that individuals have the power to improve their lifestyle by eating properly each and every day. Good nutrition can make a difference—if not in prolonging life, at least in enabling one to face life's stresses with greater ease.

Stress and Distress

It is generally believed that biological organisms require a certain amount of stress in order to maintain their well-being. Stress is always present. "Good" stress enables the body to meet the challenges of everyday activity. For example, stress keeps one alert when driving in heavy traffic or helps one respond to needs of family members in crises. Without a correct balance of stress, people would be unable to respond to any stimuli.

Distress, however, tends to be a negative influence. When stress occurs in quantities that the system cannot handle, it may produce pathological changes. These stressors can be either a person or a condition, for example, children, spouse, boss, the weather, traffic, noise, money, school, environment, retirement, divorce, death, disease—any change that occurs in one's life. The amount of distress experienced depends on how individuals respond to these stressors.

The recognition of stressors in life and their subsequent management constitute one of the keys to a healthy lifestyle. It has been shown that good nutrition, proper exercise, and a quality support system help alleviate distress.

MANAGING NEGATIVE EMOTIONS

Humans are emotional creatures. Feelings of joy, sorrow, anger, jealousy, love, resentment, fear, and hate are part of existence. How persons deal with their emotions has much to do with their physical health.

Emotions may be categorized as positive or negative. Fear is a negative emotion if, for instance, it keeps people from functioning as normal human beings; it is a positive emotion if it cautions people to be safe. A sense of joy may warm the body, cleanse the spirit, relax muscles, lighten air passages, and generally make people feel "good all over." Anger or resentment may cause the fist to clench, breathing to accelerate, the heart to pound, the head to ache, and muscles to tighten. Feelings of despair, panic, depression, fear, and frustration cause the healing resources of the human brain to be underutilized.

When we have a great will to live and expect the best in life, the brain has a greater ability to produce chemicals, such as encephalins and endorphins, that have a very positive effect on our bodies.

Some individuals may be sensitive to and recognize the physical signals given by the body. All too often, however, people have "buried" somewhere in their inner consciousness the negative impact emotions may have. Buried emotions later may exhibit themselves during an illness. Even then, illness may not be attributed to a negative emotion long since unexpressed. The kind of disease that results from unexpressed negative emotion is called *psychosomatic illness*. The symptoms of the disease are very real and are the result of one or more unexpressed negative emotions.

It is important to realize that negative emotions that are not dealt with in a wholesome manner probably will express themselves physically in the body. People must learn how to express negative feelings without destroying themselves or others if they wish to live a healthy life. Refer to Table 16–1 for suggestions on how to express negative feelings in a positive manner.

The next time anger or emotions have a negative effect, check the body to see which part is most affected. If you can feel a headache coming on, can feel the fire in your "gut," or feel your heart pounding, remember that you may be needing an emotional release.

LAUGHTER AND PLAY

Laughter has been described as "internal jogging." People cannot experience despair and joy at the same time. Therefore, it is important for individuals to allow, even plan for, laughter and play in their lives.

Table 16–1 Some Positive Ways of Working Out Negative Emotions

1. Chop wood.
2. Scrub and wax a floor.
3. Run a mile—or several.
4. Ride a bike.
5. Beat up a pillow.
6. Relax in a hot tub.
7. See a counselor.
8. Wash the car.
9. Knead bread.
10. Lift weights.
11. Cry, weep.
12. Accept yourself.
13. Read a funny book or go to a funny movie. Laugh!
14. Roll up the car windows, scream a little or a lot.
15. Make certain there is someone who loves you unconditionally.

There are several examples of the use of laughter and play in today's health care. Dr. O. Carl Simonton, noted radiation oncologist, tells of his work with teaching cancer patients how to juggle. On his first visit with patients, he gives them a set of juggling bags and one or two simple instructions. He juggles for them and tells them to practice every day and that they will do some juggling together each time they meet. Simonton reports that this activity (1) enables him and his patients to develop a relationship outside of "doctor-patient," (2) encourages a lot of laughing together, and (3) gives the patient something other than an illness to think about.

David Bresler, PhD, director of the Bresler Center for Allied Therapeutics in Los Angeles, uses long, slender balloons blown up and shaped into all kinds of animal forms to help children cope with chronic pain. This activity takes their minds off the pain and may stimulate the release of endorphins in the body.

A hospital chaplain whose avocation is that of a clown often visits hospital patients with clown paint on his face. Sometimes it is easier for patients to express their pain or grief in the "make-believe" vernacular. It also brings laughter and joy where there is pain and sorrow.

Norman Cousins reports in *Anatomy of an Illness* about the validity of laughter in healing his illness.[4] He watched old Marx Brothers movies several times a day, laughing to near tears. Following this time of laughter, he was always able to function without pain medication.

It seems obvious that play and laughter ought to be a more important and deliberate part of people's daily lives. All too frequently people forget to play as they become adults.

Some ways to interject laughter into life include:

- Become a collector of cartoons.
- Be a good jokester.
- Allow humor to get back at the "bad things" in life.
- Learn to smile, then chuckle, then laugh, then really roar with a deep belly laugh.
- Read humorous items.
- Watch a television program well known for its humor.
- Laugh at yourself—then share it!

Instituting play time in our lives may require more concentrated effort. Make a list of 40 playful or fun things that cost less than $5 each. Do something on this list every day. Your authors, who work hard at incorporating laughter and play, will share a few of their favorites:

- Find a beach, take off your shoes, and let the sand squiggle through your toes.
- Lay down in a snow drift and make an angel.
- Have a marshmallow or water-balloon fight.
- Finger paint.
- Throw a Frisbee to a dog—several times.
- Play in the water while everyone thinks you are watering the lawn.
- Be creative on April Fool's Day.
- Take a bubble bath and blow bubbles.
- Deliver May Day baskets and *run*.
- Plan a treasure hunt for the neighborhood.
- Dance.
- Go to the zoo.
- Sing crazy rhymes.
- Fly a kite or model airplane.
- Play volleyball, ping pong, and so on—for fun.
- Go to a playground—swing, slide, and go on the merry-go-round.
- If you see a road and wonder where it goes, take it.
- Feed ducks at a lake.
- Ride an elephant or camel.
- Play Hide and Seek.

Planned play every day may be hard work at first, but it is essential for a healthful lifestyle. The important principles of humor and play are practice, practice, practice, practice.

LOVE, FRIENDSHIP, AND FAITH

We learn in most psychology classes that we must love ourselves before we can love another. But what is love? Leo Buscaglia, in his book, *Love,* defines love as "a learned, emotional reaction. If one wishes to know love, one must live love, in action."[5] Love is spontaneous. If we love someone, we need to share that love now. Love must be given unconditionally. (Striking evidence of the positive effects of unconditional love comes from the successful use of pets in various kinds of therapy.) If we expect something in return for love, we are in error. We love because we feel it and want to share it. And we never "run out of" love.

Friendship is one part of love. Each of us needs at least one friend-mentor with whom we can share anything at any time. Our friend must love us as we are and not expect anything from us.

In both friendship and love, we must be willing to assume responsibility for ourselves and be able to take risks. Only then can personal growth occur. Read the following:

Risking

To laugh is to risk appearing unconcerned.
To weep is to risk appearing sentimental.
To express your independence is to risk losing your friends.
To trust others is to risk being taken advantage of.
To make a decision is to risk making a mistake.
To admit a mistake is to risk losing the respect of others.
To reach out to another is to risk involvement.
To show feeling is to risk exposing your true self.
To place your ideas, your dreams before the crowd is to risk their loss.
To love is to risk not being loved in return.
To live is to risk dying.
To hope is to risk despair.
To try at all is to risk failure.[6]

Not every person embraces religion or senses a strong spiritual influence in their lives, but at one time or another, all of us have witnessed its influence in the life of someone.

Some call it worship. Others refer to it as prayer. For your neighbor, it may be meditation. Yoga has been very helpful for many; for others, it is a mental discipline. The experience is a devotion, a setting aside, an adoration, a refreshing, or an enlightening. It may include service, witnessing, sharing, and a sense of community and belonging. Whatever it is, it is a very personal experience.

Practitioners of holistic health recognize the worth of such experiences in a person's life. A faith in something or someone greater and more powerful than ourselves can make the most desolate of times a little less frustrating.

REFERENCES

1. Quoted in Moyers, B. (ed): Healing and the Mind. Doubleday, New York, 1993, p 189.
2. Weil, A: Spontaneous Healing. Alfred A Knopf, New York, 1995.
3. Select Committee on Nutrition and Human Needs: Dietary Goals for the United States. U.S. Government Printing Office, Washington, DC, 1977, p 3.
4. Cousins, N: Anatomy of an Illness. WW Norton, New York, 1979.
5. Buscaglia, L: Love. Ballantine Books, New York, 1982, p 91.
6. Allen, C: Victory in the Valleys of Life. FH Revell, Old Tappan, N.J., 1981, p 114.

BIBLIOGRAPHY

Chopra, D: Perfect Health, The Complete Mind/Body Guide. Harmony Books, New York, 1991.
Kabat-Zinn, J: Full Catastrophe Living. Dell Publishing, New York, 1990.

REVIEW QUESTIONS

SHORT ANSWER

1. Internal environmental factors that influence health and well-being include:

   a.

   b.

   c.

   d.

2. External environmental factors that influence health and well-being include:

   a.

   b.

   c.

   d.

3. Personal lifestyle may be influenced by:

   a.

   b.

   c.

   d.

   e.

   f.

4. Emotions may be categorized as _____ or _____ .

5. The kind of disease that results from unexpressed negative emotion is called

   _____ .

6. List at least four constructive outlets for expression of negative feelings beneficial to you.

7. Describe situations that cause stress to have a positive or a negative impact on our lives.

8. Create a day's eating plan to allow for four servings of fruits and vegetables.

DISCUSSION QUESTIONS/PERSONAL REFLECTION

1. Identify a negative emotion you have difficulty expressing. Discuss with a friend what the consequences of such activity may be.

2. Share a cartoon, joke, or funny story with a classmate.

ANSWERS

SHORT ANSWER

1. a. Genetic traits
   b. Familial tendencies
   c. Inherent physical characteristics
   d. Inherent psychological characteristics
2. a. Air
   b. Water
   c. Food
   d. Surroundings
3. a. Education and knowledge
   b. Attitudes
   c. Individual responsibilities
   d. Modeling of family/peers

    e. Self-confidence

    f. Position in life

    g. Life's opportunities

4. Negative; positive
5. Psychosomatic illness
6. Chop wood, ride a bike, knead bread, run a mile, and so on.
7. Positive—stress keeps us alert in traffic
   Negative—insufficient money to pay heat bill
8. Varies: 6 oz orange juice in morning; 1 apple at noon; mixed vegetables for dinner; fresh strawberries for dessert

DISCUSSION QUESTIONS/PERSONAL REFLECTION

Answers will vary.

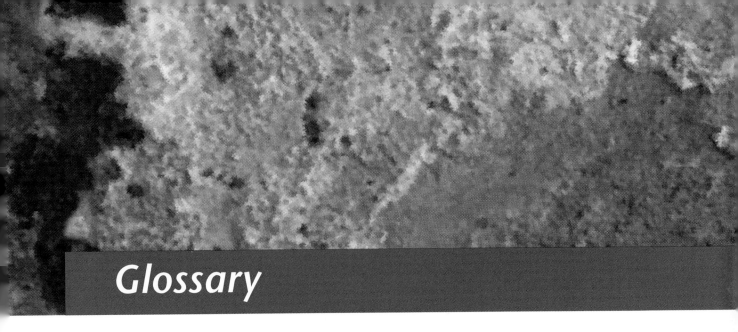

Glossary

A

ABRADE To chafe; to roughen or remove by friction.

ACETABULUM The rounded cavity on the outer surface of the hip bone that receives the head of the femur.

ACETYLCHOLINE A neurotransmitter substance that transfers nerve impulses across neuromuscular junctions, stimulating contraction of muscle fibers.

ACIDOSIS Higher than normal acidity in body fluids; due to the accumulation of acids or the excessive loss of bicarbonate.

ACUTE Designating a disease having rapid onset, severe symptoms, and a short course. (Compare with *Chronic*.)

ADENOMA Tumor of a gland or cancerous growth in glandular epithelial tissue.

ADRENOCORTICOTROPIC HORMONE (ACTH) Normally produced by the pituitary gland, it stimulates hormone production by the cortex of the adrenal gland. Sometimes administered as a therapeutic agent due to its anti-inflammatory properties.

AGNOSIA Loss of ability to understand or interpret auditory, visual, or other forms of sensory information even though the respective sensory organs are functioning properly.

AGRAPHIA Loss of ability to convert thought into writing.

ALEXIA Loss of ability to understand the written language.

ALKALOSIS Excessive alkalinity of body fluids due to accumulation of alkalines or reduction of acids.

ALLERGEN Any substance that, when introduced into the body, is capable of inducing an allergic reaction.

ALOPECIA Absence or loss of hair, especially on the head.

ALVEOLI (PULMONARY) The microscopic air sacs in the lungs through whose walls the exchange of carbon dioxide and oxygen occurs.

AMBLYOPIA Unilateral reduction in visual acuity, in which there is no apparent pathological condition of the eye.

AMENORRHEA Absence of menstruation.

AMINO ACID Any one of a large group of organic compounds constituting the primary building blocks of proteins.

AMNIOTIC FLUID The fluid inside the amniotic sac, the membranous enclosure within the uterus in which the fetus is suspended.

ANALGESIC A drug or other agent used to relieve pain.

ANAPHYLAXIS An allergic reaction of the body to a foreign or other substance. Sometimes used to refer exclusively to a sudden, unusually severe, and possibly life-threatening allergic reaction.

ANAPLASIA Loss of structural differentiation, as seen in malignant neoplasms.

ANASTOMOSIS Surgical, traumatic, or pathological formation of a connection between two normally separate tubular structures or organs in the body.

ANEURYSM An abnormal, saclike bulge in the wall of an artery, a vein, or the heart.

ANGIOGRAPHY Use of x-rays to show an image, on developed film or video monitor, of the blood vessels.

ANKYLOSIS Immobility of a joint.

ANOREXIA Loss of appetite for foods.

ANOXIA Absence of oxygen.

ANTIBIOTICS Any of a variety of natural or synthetic substances that inhibit the growth of or destroy microorganisms. Used in the treatment of infectious diseases.

ANTIBODY A protein substance produced by the body's immune system in response to and interacting with a specific antigen.

ANTICHOLINERGIC (DRUG) Drug or agent that inhibits the action of the neurotransmitter chemical acetylcholine, blocking parasympathetic nerve impulses, with consequent reduction of smooth-muscle contractions and various bodily secretions.

ANTIDIARRHEAL Drug or other agent used to prevent or treat diarrhea.

ANTIEMETIC Drug or other agent used to prevent or stop vomiting.

ANTIGEN Any substance that, when introduced into the body, causes the production of a specific antibody by the immune system.

ANTIPRURITIC An agent that prevents or relieves itching.

ANTIPYRETIC A drug or agent that reduces fever.

APHASIA Loss or impairment of the ability to communicate through speech, writing, or signs due to dysfunction of brain centers.

APNEA Temporary cessation in breathing.

APRAXIA Loss or impairment of ability to perform coordinated movements, especially impairment of the ability to use common objects for their intended purposes.

ARRHYTHMIA (CARDIAC) Irregularities in the force or rhythm of heart action caused by disturbances in the discharge of cardiac impulses from the heart's sinoatrial node or their transmission through the heart's conductile tissue.

ARTHRALGIA Pain in a joint.

ASCITES Abnormal accumulation of fluid in the peritoneal cavity.

ATELECTASIS In a neonate, the failure of the lung to completely expand at birth; generally, a collapsed lung. The collapse may be complete or partial.

ATROPINE Anticholinergic agent that counteracts effects of parasympathetic stimulation.

AUSCULTATION Listening to sounds produced by the internal organs or other body parts for diagnostic purposes.

AUTOINOCULATION Inoculation with organisms from one's own body.

AUTOSOMAL DOMINANT DEFECT A defect that will be expressed in the offspring even though it is carried on only one of the pair of homologous chromosomes.

AUTOSOMAL RECESSIVE DEFECT OR TRAIT A defect or trait carried in a chromosome other than the sex chromosomes (X and Y) that expresses itself only when a dominant gene is not present.

AYURVEDIC MEDICINE Practiced in India for 5000 years; combines natural therapies with a person's overall health profile; a metabolic body type is determined and a specific treatment plan is designed to bring the individual back into harmony with the environment. Modalities may include dietary changes, exercise, yoga, meditation, massage, herbal tonics and sweat baths, medicated enemas and inhalations.

AZOOSPERMIA Absence of spermatozoa in the semen.

B

BACTEREMIA Bacteria in the blood.

BILE A thick, brownish-yellow to greenish-yellow alkaline fluid produced by the liver, stored and concentrated in the gallbladder, and discharged into the duodenum. It is important as a digestive juice, facilitating the digestion of fats by the intestine.

BILIRUBIN An orange- to yellow-colored compound in the blood plasma, produced by the breakdown of hemoglobin following the normal or pathological destruction of red blood cells. It is collected by the liver to produce bile.

BILIRUBINURIA The presence of bilirubin in the urine. May be indicative of a liver or blood disorder.

BIOPSY Excision of a small piece of living tissue for microscopic examination. Usually performed to establish a diagnosis.

BIOTIN A component of the vitamin B complex essential for the metabolism of fat and carbohydrates.

BLAST A precursor of the final, mature form of a cell.

BLEB An irregularly shaped elevation of the epidermis. A blister.

BRADYCARDIA Abnormally slow heartbeat, generally characterized by a pulse rate below 60 beats per minute.

BRONCHIOLE One of the many smaller passages conveying air with the lung.

BRONCHODILATOR A drug or other agent that relaxes and expands the air passages of the lungs.

BRUDZINSKI'S SIGN A diagnostic indicator of meningitis, characterized by the involuntary flexion of the hips and knees in response to the forward flexion of the neck.

BRUIT An abnormal noise of venous or arterial origin heard during auscultation.

BULLA (PL., BULLAE) A large (generally greater than 0.5 cm) fluid-filled blister.

C

CACHEXIA A marked wasting away of the body, usually as a consequence of chronic disease.

CALYX (PL., CALYCES) One of the branches or recesses of the pelvis of the kidney into which the malpighian renal pyramids open.

CARCINOGEN Any substance or agent that can produce cancer.

CARDIOGENIC SHOCK Condition of acute circulatory failure caused by interruption of the heart's pumping action. Considered a medical emergency.

CARDIOMEGALY Increase in the volume of the heart or the size of the heart muscle tissue.

CARPAL TUNNEL SYNDROME A condition characterized by soreness, tenderness, and weakness of the muscles of the thumb; caused by pressure on the median nerve at the point where it goes through the carpal tunnel of the wrist.

CASTS (URINARY) An abnormal component of urine formed from proteins that have precipitated in the renal tubules.

CELLULITIS An inflammation of cellular or connective tissue.

CEREBROSPINAL FLUID (CSF) The clear fluid that bathes the ventricles of the brain and the central cavity of the spinal cord.

CERVICITIS An inflammation of the cervix.

CHANCRE A firm, red, ulcerated sore. A chancre is the primary indication of syphilis; it occurs at the point of entry of the infection.

CHEYNE-STOKES RESPIRATION A breathing pattern disturbance characterized by a period of deep, rapid respirations followed by a period of shallow respirations or no respirations at all. The cycle rhythmically repeats every 45 seconds to 3 minutes.

CHOLELITHIASIS The formation or presence of gallstones in the gallbladder or bile duct.

CHOLESTASIS A halt in production and secretion of bile by the liver.

CHOREA A nervous condition marked by involuntary muscular twitching of the limbs or facial muscles.

CHORIOCARCINOMA A highly malignant neoplasm of the uterus or fallopian tube.

CHROMOSOME In human cells, a linear structure in the nucleus composed of DNA and proteins and bearing part of the genetic information of the cell. Each human cell (except for egg or sperm cells) has 46 chromosomes, occurring in 23 pairs.

CHRONIC Designating a disease showing little change or of slow progression. (Compare with *Acute*.)

CHYME The nearly liquid mixture, composed of partially digested food and gastric secretions, that is found in the stomach and duodenum during digestion of a meal.

CILIA (BRONCHIAL) Microscopic, hairlike extensions of cells lining the interior of the bronchi, whose rhythmic beating moves fluids, mucus, and particulates out of the lungs.

CLAUDICATION Lameness; limping.

CLUBBING A condition characterized by bulbous swelling of the tips of the fingers and toes.

COITUS Sexual intercourse.

COLECTOMY Surgical removal of all or a portion of the colon.

COLOSTOMY A surgically created opening in a portion of the large intestine (colon), which is brought to the abdominal surface for the purpose of evacuating feces. May be temporary or permanent. (Compare with *Ileostomy*.)

COMA A state of profound unconsciousness occurring as a result of illness or injury. The affected individual cannot be aroused by external stimuli.

COMEDO A plug of dried, discolored fatty matter clogging a pore of the skin; commonly called a *blackhead*.

CONCEPTUS The products of conception from fertilization to birth.

CONIZATION The surgical removal of a cone of tissue, such as excision of cervical tissue for microscopic examination.

CONJUNCTIVA The mucous membrane structure that lines the inner surface of the eyelids and that is reflected onto the anterior portion of the eyeball.

CONTRACTURE Permanent shortening or contraction of a muscle, often producing physical distortion or deformity.

CORDOTOMY Surgical division of one or more of the lateral nerve pathways emerging from the spinal cord in order to relieve pain.

CORYZA Common cold. An acute inflammation of the nasal mucous membrane accompanied by profuse nasal discharge.

CORPUS LUTEUM A small yellow structure on the ovary formed from the mass of follicle cells left behind after an ovum is released. It secretes hormones necessary for the maintenance of pregnancy.

CRANIOTOMY Surgical incision through the cranium.

CREATININE A nitrogen-based compound formed in muscle tissue, passed into the bloodstream, and excreted in the urine. Elevated levels of creatinine in the blood may indicate a kidney disorder.

CREPITATION A crackling sound, such as that produced by the grating of ends of a broken bone.

CRYOSURGERY A technique used to destroy tissue by application of extreme cold. The cold is typically produced by use of a probe through which liquid nitrogen circulates.

CRYOTHERAPY The use of cold to treat disease or disorder.

CRYPTORCHIDISM Condition in which the testicles of an adult male have not descended into the scrotum.

CURET Surgical instrument shaped like a spoon or scoop for scraping and removing material from a cavity.

CYANOSIS A bluish discoloration of the skin and mucous membranes due to an increased proportion of unoxygenated hemoglobin in the blood.

CYSTECTOMY Removal of a cyst. Excision of the cystic duct and the gallbladder. Excision of the urinary bladder or a part of it.

DÉBRIDEMENT The removal of dead or damaged tissue or other matter, especially from a wound.

DECUBITUS ULCER An open sore or skin lesion resulting from impaired circulation to a portion of the body surface as a result of prolonged pressure from a bed or chair. Commonly called a *bedsore*.

DEMENTIA An irreversibly deteriorating mental state; characterized by impaired memory, judgment, and ability to think, and caused by cerebral damage due to an organic brain disease.

DIAPHORESIS Sweating, especially when profuse or medically induced.

DIASTOLIC PRESSURE The lowest arterial pressure reached during any ventricular cycle.

DIFFERENTIATION The process whereby cells take on functions and forms different from those of the cells from which they originated.

DILATATION The expansion or enlargement of an organ or vessel.

DIPLOPIA Double vision.

DISSEMINATED INTRAVASCULAR COAGULATION (DIC) A pathological form of coagulation of the blood that is diffuse rather than localized. The process damages rather than protects the area involved, and several clotting factors are consumed to such an extent that generalized bleeding may occur.

DIURETIC A drug or agent that promotes the secretion of urine.

DOWN SYNDROME Mild to severe mental retardation due to a birth defect; the physical manifestations of the defect include a sloping forehead, low-set ears, and a tendency to dwarfishness.

DUCTUS ARTERIOSUS A connection between the aorta and the pulmonary artery in the fetus; it allows most of the blood pumped by the left ventricle to bypass the lungs (which do not function in the fetus) and enter the systemic circulation. In some infants, the connection persists after birth; the condition is known as *patent ductus arteriosus.*

DYSPHAGIA Difficulty in swallowing or inability to swallow.

DYSPHASIA Impairment of speech resulting from a brain lesion.

DYSPLASIA Alteration in size, shape, and organization of mature cells.

DYSPNEA Labored or difficult breathing, generally indicating an insufficient amount of oxygen in the blood.

DYSTONIA Impaired or disordered muscle tone.

DYSURIA Difficult or painful urination, symptomatic of numerous conditions.

E

ECHOCARDIOGRAM The image produced by ultrasound examination of cardiac structures.

ECTOPIC Arising or occurring at an unusual location or in a tissue structure where it is not normally found.

EDEMA Excessive accumulation of fluid in bodily tissues. May be localized or general.

EFFACEMENT The dilation of the cervix.

EFFUSION The seeping of fluid into a body cavity or part.

ELECTROCAUTERY A technique used to destroy tissue by means of an instrument containing an electrode heated to red hot temperatures by an electric current.

ELECTRODESICCATION A method of electrosurgery in which tissue is destroyed by dehydration with a probe generating a series of short, high-frequency electric sparks.

ELECTROLYTES The ionized salts present in blood, tissue fluids, and within cells. They are involved in all metabolic processes and are essential to the normal functioning of all cells.

EMBOLISM Obstruction of a blood vessel by foreign substances or a blood clot.

EMBOLUS A clot or undissolved mass carried through the circulatory vessels by the blood or lymph flow. An embolus may be a blood clot, piece of tissue, fat globule, or air bubble. (Compare with *Thrombus.*)

EN BLOC (in surgery) To remove as one piece.

ENCAPSULATION Enclosure in a layer of tissue not normal to the part.

ENDEMIC (of a disease) Widespread throughout a population but not with a high mortality rate.

ENDOMETRIUM The mucous membrane lining the inner surface of the uterus.

ENDORPHIN One of a group of naturally occurring substances, produced by the central nervous system, that reduce the perception of pain.

ENTEROPATHY Any disease of the intestine.

EPIDIDYMO-ORCHITIS Inflammation of epididymis and testis.

EPIGASTRIC Pertaining to the epigastrium, the region of the abdomen over the pit of the stomach.

EPIGASTRIUM Region of the abdomen over the pit of the stomach.

EPISTAXIS Hemorrhage from the nose; a nosebleed.

EPITHELIAL Pertaining to the layer of cells forming the outer surface of the body, the lining of the body cavities, and principal tubes and passageways.

ERYTHEMA (ERYTHEMATOUS) Diffused redness of the skin due to dilation of the superficial capillaries.

EXCHANGE TRANSFUSION The repeated removal of small amounts of blood from an individual and its replacement with like amounts of donor blood. Usually performed until the volume of the exchange equals one or two total blood volumes.

EXCORIATION Abrasion of the skin or of the surface of any organ by trauma, chemical agents, burns, or other causes.

EXCRETION The process of eliminating or getting rid of waste products of the body.

EXFOLIATIVE CYTOLOGY The microscopic examination of cells that have been shed from or scaled off the surface epithelium. Performed for diagnostic purposes.

EXOCRINE Pertaining to glands that release their secretions into the digestive tract or to the outer surface of the body.

EXOPHTHALMOS Abnormal protrusion of the eyeball.

EXUDATE Fluid discharged through vessel walls and collecting in adjacent tissue. It has a high content of protein and cellular debris. (Compare with *Transudate.*)

FECALITH A hard, solid, intestinal mass formed around a core of fecal material.

FEMORAL HEAD The top or head of the femur, commonly called the *thigh* or *leg bone*.

FIBRILLATION (VENTRICULAR) A cardiac arrhythmia characterized by the rapid, incomplete, and uncoordinated contractions of the muscle fibers of ventricles of the heart. Can lead to cardiac arrest. (See *Arrhythmia*.)

FIBRIN A whitish protein that is the basis for the clotting of blood.

FISTULA An abnormal tubelike passage from a normal cavity or tube to a free surface or to another cavity.

FOLLICLE-STIMULATING HORMONE (FSH) A secretion of the pituitary gland that stimulates the growth and maturation of the graafian follicles in the ovary or the production of sperm in the testes.

FONTANELLES Incompletely ossified spaces or soft spots between the cranial bones of the skull of a fetus or infant.

GAMMA GLOBULIN A class of proteins formed in the blood that function as antibodies. Ability to resist infection is related to the concentration of these proteins.

GANGLION A mass of nervelike cell bodies lying outside the brain and spinal cord.

GANGRENE The death of masses of body tissue, followed by bacterial invasion and subsequent decay; usually, but not exclusively, associated with the loss or interruption of blood supply to a tissue area.

GENE One of the units of heredity, located at a definite position on a particular chromosome.

GENOTYPE A description of the combination of genes of an individual, either with respect to a single trait or with respect to a larger set of traits. (Contrast with *Phenotype*.)

GLYCOSURIA The presence of sugar, particularly glucose, in the urine.

GOITROGENS Substances that cause goiters. These occur in nature in certain foods, including turnips, rutabagas, and cabbage.

GONORRHEAL OPHTHALMIA NEONATORUM In the newborn, the severe, hyperacute inflammation of the membrane lining the inner surface of the eyelids and covering the white of the eye. Caused by infection with gonococci, and usually contracted during vaginal birth from an infected mother.

GRANULOMA One of a variety of growths of inflamed, granular-appearing tissue.

HALITOSIS Foul-smelling breath.

HEMATEMESIS Vomiting blood.

HEMATOMA Swelling and discoloration in an organ or tissue due to the accumulation of blood (usually coagulated) from a tear, leak, or break in a blood vessel.

HEMATOPOIETIC Related to the formation of red blood cells.

HEMATURIA Blood in the urine.

HEMIPARESIS Paralysis affecting only one side of the body.

HEMOGLOBIN The oxygen-carrying pigment in red blood cells.

HEMOLYSIS The rupturing of red blood cells with the resulting release of hemoglobin into the plasma.

HEMOPTYSIS The coughing and spitting up of blood due to bleeding in any portion of the respiratory tract.

HEPATOMEGALY Enlargement of the liver.

HETEROZYGOUS Possessing different genes from each parent for a particular trait.

HISTAMINE A substance present in all body tissues and released by injured cells as part of the body's inflammation process. It functions to dilate capillaries, lower blood pressure, increase gastric secretions, and constrict bronchial smooth muscle.

HOMEOSTASIS The tendency of the body systems to maintain stability even though they are exposed to continually changing outside forces.

HOMOZYGOUS Possessing identical genes from each parent for a particular trait.

HYDROCELE As used here, the painless swelling of the scrotum caused by the accumulation of fluid in the membrane surrounding a testicle.

HYDRONEPHROSIS Swelling of the renal pelvis of the kidney with urine due to obstructed outflow.

HYDROURETER: The swelling of the ureter with urine due to obstructed outflow.

HYPERGLYCEMIA Abnormally high levels of sugar in the blood.

HYPERLIPEMIA Excess levels of fatlike substances called lipids in the blood.

HYPERPARATHYROIDISM As used here, oversecretion of parathyroid hormone by the parathyroid glands as a consequence of chronic renal disease.

HYPERPLASIA The overproliferation of normal cells within a normal tissue structure.

HYPERTENSION Persistently high arterial blood pressure.

HYPERTROPHY An increase in size or volume of an organ or other body structure that is produced entirely by an increase in the size of existing cells, not by an increase in the number of cells.

HYPOALBUMINEMIA Abnormally low levels of a protein called albumin in the blood plasma.

HYPOGLYCEMIA Abnormally low levels of sugar in the blood.

HYPOKALEMIA Extreme potassium depletion in the circulating blood, commonly manifested by episodes of muscular weakness or paralysis and tetany.

HYPOPHYSECTOMY Removal of a pituitary gland.

HYPOTENSION Persistently low systolic and diastolic blood pressure.

HYPOTHYROIDISM Underactivity of the thyroid gland, marked by underproduction of the hormone thyroxine.

HYPOVENTILATION Reduced rate and depth of breathing.

HYPOVOLEMIC SHOCK A condition of severe physiological distress caused by a decrease in the circulating blood volume so large that the body's metabolic needs cannot be met.

HYPOXEMIA Insufficient oxygenation of the arterial blood.

HYPOXIA Insufficient oxygenation of the blood or tissue.

HYSTEROSALPINGOGRAPHY Use of x-rays to visualize the uterus and fallopian tubes.

I

IATROGENIC (of a disease or disorder) Caused by treatment; for instance, an infection caused by a failure of surgical antiseptic precautions.

IDIOPATHIC (of a disease) Of unknown cause.

ILEOSTOMY A surgically created opening in the lower small intestine (ileum), brought to the abdominal surface for the purpose of evacuating feces. May be temporary or permanent.

IMMUNOGLOBULIN One of a family of closely related though not identical proteins that are capable of acting as antibodies.

INCONTINENCE Inability to control the passage of urine, semen, or feces due to one or more physiological or psychological conditions.

INDURATION An area of hardened tissue; the process of hardening.

INSIDIOUS Of a disease, occurring or progressing with few or unnoticeable symptoms, so that the individual is unaware of the onset of the disease.

INTROMISSION The insertion of the penis into the vagina.

ISCHEMIA A temporary deficiency of blood in a body part due to a constriction or obstruction of a blood vessel.

ISOIMMUNIZATION Immunization of an individual against the blood group antigens (e.g., Rh antigens) of another individual.

J

JAUNDICE A condition characterized by a yellowish discoloration of the skin, whites of the eyes, and bodily fluids resulting from the accumulation of bilirubin in the blood. Caused by any of several disease processes in which the normal production and secretion of bile are disrupted.

K

KERATIN A hard, fibrous protein that is the primary constituent of hair and nails.

KERATOLYTIC An agent used to loosen and remove the outer layer of the epidermis.

KERNIG'S SIGN A diagnostic indicator of meningitis, characterized by the inability to straighten the knee while the hip is flexed.

KETOACIDOSIS Abnormally high concentrations in the blood or tissues of organic compounds called *ketone bodies:* beta-hydroxybutyric acid, acetoacidic acid, and acetone. The condition is frequently associated with diabetes mellitus.

KOPLIK'S SPOTS Small red spots with bluish white centers on the oral mucosa, particularly in the region opposite the molars. A diagnostic sign in measles.

KYPHOSCOLIOSIS Abnormal backward and lateral curvature of the spine.

LASSITUDE A state of exhaustion or profound listlessness.

LEIOMYOMA Tumor of smooth-muscle tissue.

LESION Any discontinuity or disruption of tissue caused by disease or trauma.

LEUKOCYTE Any of the white cellular components of blood or lymph.

LEUKOCYTOSIS A temporary increase in the number of white cells in the blood, typically, but not exclusively, caused by the presence of infection.

LEUKOPENIA An abnormal decrease in the number of circulating white blood cells.

LEUKORRHEA Whitish or yellowish mucous discharge from the vagina. Although generally considered a normal secretion of the vagina, leukorrhea may indicate an underlying disorder if the flow markedly increases; changes color, thickness, or odor; or is accompanied by a burning sensation or the presence of blood.

LIBIDO Conscious or unconscious sexual desire.

LIGATION Process of tying off blood vessels or constricting other body tissues for therapeutic purposes.

LIPID Any one of a group of fats or fatlike substances.

LIPIDURIA Lipids in the urine.

LUMBAR Pertaining to the part of the back between the thorax and pelvis.

LUMEN The space within an artery, vein, intestine, or other tubular structure.

LUTEINIZING HORMONE (LH) A secretion of the hypothalamus that stimulates development of the corpus luteum. (See *Corpus luteum.*)

LYMPHADENOPATHY Disease of the lymph nodes, usually manifested as swelling of the nodes.

LYMPHANGITIS Inflammation of lymph vessels.

LYMPHOCYTOPENIA The presence of abnormally small numbers of lymphocytes in the circulating blood.

LYSIS Destruction of red blood cells, bacteria, and other structures by a specific lysin.

MACROCEPHALY Larger than normal head.

MACROPHAGE Any of the class of cells within the body tissues having the ability to engulf particulate substances and microorganisms.

MACULA A small colored spot or thickening.

MACULAR Relating to or containing macules.

MACULE A discolored spot of skin that is neither elevated above nor depressed below the surrounding skin surface.

MACULOPAPULAR Containing both macules and papules.

MALAISE A generalized feeling of illness, discomfort, or depression indicative of some underlying disease or disorder.

MAMMOGRAM A low-dosage diagnostic x-ray of the breast.

MATRIX A mold in which something is cast; originating substance or network; the basic material from which a structure or tissue develops.

McBURNEY'S POINT A point of special abdominal tenderness indicating acute appendicitis. It lies over and corresponds with the normal position of the appendix.

MEGAKARYOCYTE A large bone marrow cell with large or multiple nuclei. It gives rise to blood platelets.

MELANIN A dark pigment that gives color to skin and hair.

MENARCHE The initial menstrual cycle, marking the onset of fertility.

MENINGES The three membranes covering the brain and spinal cord.

MENORRHAGIA Excessive menstrual flow, either in duration or quantity, or both.

METASTASIS (METASTASIZE) Movement of bacteria or body cells, especially cancer cells, from one part of the body to the other, typically by way of the circulatory system.

METRORRHAGIA Uterine bleeding, especially at a time other than the menstrual period.

MICTURITION Urination.

MITOCHONDRIA Cell organelles that are the chief energy conversion source of cells and contain many enzymes.

MITRAL REGURGITATION Backward flow of blood through the mitral valve of the heart.

MUTATION A permanent change in a gene that is potentially capable of being transmitted to offspring.

MYALGIA Muscle pain or tenderness.

MYELOSUPPRESSION Concerning inhibition of bone marrow function.

MYOCARDIUM The middle layer of the walls of the heart, composed of cardiac muscle.

MYOTONIA Any disorder involving sustained, involuntary contractions of muscle.

MYRINGOTOMY Surgical incision of the tympanic membrane (eardrum).

NARCOTIC A drug that in moderate doses depresses the central nervous system, relieving pain and producing sleep, but that in excessive doses produces unconsciousness, stupor, coma, and possibly death.

NEOPLASM Tumor or abnormal growth of new tissue. Neoplasm is undesirable because it has no function and detracts from the health of the organism.

NEPHRECTOMY Removal of a kidney.

NEPHRITIS Any form of inflammation of the kidney, acute or chronic.

NEPHROSCLEROSIS Hardening of structures within the kidney; generally associated with hypertension and disease of the renal arterioles.

NEURITIS Inflammation of a nerve or nerves.

NEUROBLASTOMA A malignant, highly invasive tumor composed of embryonic cells of the central nervous system, primarily affecting infants and children.

NEUROMODULATOR The alteration in function or status in response to a stimulus of the nerve.

NEUROTOMY Division or dissection of a nerve.

NEUROTRANSMITTER A substance produced and released by one neuron that travels across a synapse, exciting or inhibiting the next neuron in the neural pathway.

NEUTROPENIA The presence of abnormally small numbers of neutrophils in the circulating blood.

NEVUS (PL., NEVI) Birthmark or mole; congenital discoloration of the skin due to abnormal pigmentation or vascular tumor.

NOCTURIA Excessive urination at night.

NONVIRULENT Nonpathogenic.

NORMOBLAST A red blood cell with a nucleus, as opposed to an erythrocyte, which is nonnucleated.

NUCHAL RIGIDITY Stiff neck.

NYSTAGMUS Rhythmic, involuntary movement of the eyeball.

OCCULT BLOOD Minute quantities of blood in feces, urine, and gastric fluid, detectable only by microscopic examination or chemical test.

OLIGOMENORRHEA Abnormally infrequent and scanty menstrual flow.

OLIGOSPERMIA Deficient quantity of spermatozoa in the seminal fluid.

OLIGURIA Reduced urine secretion.

OPPORTUNISTIC INFECTIONS Infections with any organism, but especially fungi and bacteria, that occur due to the opportunity afforded by the altered physiological state of the host.

ORCHIDECTOMY Surgical removal of a testicle.

ORTHOPNEA Respiratory condition in which there is discomfort in breathing in any but erect standing or sitting positions.

ORTOLANI'S SIGN The click felt when an examiner abducts and lifts the femurs of a prone infant during physical assessment. The click indicates subluxation or displacement of the hip.

OSTEOLYTIC Causing osteolysis, which is the destruction of bone due to the loss of mineral because of metabolic disturbance, the abnormal presence of a certain enzyme, or some other disorder.

P

PALLIATIVE Treatment provided to relieve the symptoms of a disease rather than to effect a cure.

PALLOR Lack of color; paleness, as of the skin.

PANHYSTEROSALPINGO-OOPHORECTOMY Surgical removal of the entire uterus, including the cervix, ovaries, and fallopian tubes.

PAPANICOLAOU TEST (SMEAR) A diagnostic test for the early detection of cancer cells. Commonly called *Pap test, Pap smear.*

PAPILLOMA Wart or polyp; a benign growth in the epithelium.

PAPILLOMATOSIS The widespread formation of warts.

PAPILLOMAVIRUSES A family of viruses that cause warts or benign epithelial tumors in humans and animals.

PAPULAR Resembling or pertaining to a papule.

PAPULE A red, raised area of the skin, generally small and solid.

PARASYMPATHETIC Referring to a portion of the automatic (involuntary) nervous system. Activity of the parasympathetic nerves produces affects such as constriction of the pupil of the eye and slowed heart rate.

PARENTERAL Taken into the body or administered by some route other than the digestive system, for example, intravenous, subcutaneous, intramuscular, or mucosal.

PARESTHESIA Sensation of numbness, prickling, or tingling.

PARITY The condition of having borne viable offspring.

PARTURITION The act of giving birth.

PATENT (OF A VESSEL OR VEIN) Open, free-flowing.

PATHOGENIC Capable of causing disease.

PATIENT-CONTROLLED ANALGESIA (PCA) Pump allowing patients to administer their prescribed pain medications.

PERCUSSION Diagnostic technique in which various body surfaces are tapped; the resulting sounds indicate the size, position, and general condition of underlying organs or structures.

PERCUTANEOUS TRANSLUMINAL CORONARY ANGIOPLASTY (PTCA) A method of treating localized arterial narrowing due to atherosclerosis. A balloon-tipped catheter is guided to the site of the narrowing and briefly inflated, resulting in dilation of the vessel.

PERICARDIOCENTESIS Surgical puncture of the membranous sac surrounding the heart to draw out fluid.

PERISTALSIS The involuntary wavelike contraction occurring along the walls of the hollow tubes of the body, especially the esophagus, stomach, and intestines.

PETECHIA (PL., PETECHIAE) A small, reddish or purplish pinpoint spot on a body surface, such as the skin or mucous membranes, caused by a minute hemorrhage.

PH The degree of acidity or alkalinity of a solution, expressed in numbers from 0 to 14. Maximum acidity is pH 0 and maximum alkalinity is pH 14. A pH of 7 is neutral.

PHACOEMULSIFICATION An ultrasonic device that disintegrates cataracts so they can be aspirated and removed.

PHAGOCYTOSIS Ingestion and digestion of bacteria, other cells, and particles by a class of cells called phagocytes.

PHENOTYPE The observable physical characteristics of an individual, determined by the combined influences of the individual's genetic makeup and the effects of environmental factors. (Contrast with *Genotype*.)

PHOTOPHOBIA Unusual intolerance of light.

PHOTOTHERAPY Treatment of disease by exposure of the skin to natural or artificial light.

PITTING EDEMA A form of tissue swelling beneath the skin that, when pressed firmly with a finger, will maintain the indentation produced by the finger for a few minutes.

PLAQUE A solid, elevated patch of skin. Often formed from the combination of numerous, closely spaced papules. (See *Papule*.)

PLASMA The liquid part of the lymph and of the blood.

PLEURA The saclike membrane enveloping each lung and lining the adjacent portion of the thoracic cavity. The two layers form a potential space, the pleural cavity.

PLEURECTOMY Surgical excision of a portion of the pleura.

PLICATION Surgical procedure in which folds in the wall of an organ are stitched together to reduce its size.

PNEUMOCEPHALOGRAPHY Visualization of the brain using x-rays, after injecting air into the ventricles.

POLYCYTHEMIA VERA A chronic, life-shortening disorder of the bone marrow, involving the tissue producing blood cells. It is primarily characterized by abnormally high numbers of circulating red blood cells.

POLYDIPSIA Excessive thirst.

POLYLMORPHONUCLEAR LEUKOCYTE A white blood cell that possesses a nucleus composed of 200 or more lobes or parts.

POLYPHAGIA Eating abnormally large amounts of food at a meal.

POLYPOSIS The formation of numerous small growths or masses on a mucous membrane surface.

POLYURIA Excessive formation and discharge of urine.

POSTNATAL After birth.

POSTURAL DRAINAGE A therapeutic technique in which a patient is directed to assume a variety of positions that facilitate the drainage of secretions in the lobes of the lungs or the bronchial passages.

PRENATAL Before birth.

PRIMAGRAVIDA A woman during her first pregnancy.

PROJECTILE VOMITING Vomiting in which the stomach contents are ejected with great force.

PROLAPSE A falling or dropping down of an organ or internal part.

PROSTAGLANDINS A class of chemically related fatty acids present in many body tissues and having the ability to stimulate smooth-muscle contractions, lower blood pressure, and regulate or influence many other body functions.

PROSTHESIS Artificial organ or body part.

PROTEINURIA Excessive levels of serum protein in the urine.

PRURITUS Severe itching.

PTOSIS Draping or drooping of an organ or part, such as the upper eyelid from paralysis, or the visceral organs from weakness of the abdominal muscles.

PULMONARY INFARCTION The death of a localized area of lung tissue resulting from an interruption of blood flow to that area. Generally caused by a pulmonary embolism.

PURPURA A bleeding disorder with various manifestations and causes; characterized by hemorrhages into the skin, mucous membranes, internal organs, and other tissues.

PURULENT (DISCHARGE) Containing pus.

PUSTULE Small, raised area of the skin filled with pus or lymph.

PYLORUS (PYLORIC SPHINCTER) The lower opening of the stomach leading into the duodenum. The pylorus is closed most of the time by the pyloric sphincter, a ring of muscles that opens at intervals to allow the flow of chyme into the duodenum.

PYODERMA Any acute, pus-causing, inflammatory skin disease.

PYURIA Pus in the urine.

R

RADIAL KERATOTOMY A surgical procedure in which a series of spokelike incisions are made in the surface of the cornea. Intraocular pressure stretches the incisions, slightly flattening the curvature of the cornea. The procedure is used to correct certain refractive errors.

RADIOISOTOPE Radioactive form of an element. Some are commonly used for diagnostic or therapeutic purposes.

RALES An abnormal respiratory sound heard on auscultation of the lungs and produced by the movement of air through secretion-filled or constricted bronchial passages.

RAUWOLFIA (SERPENTINA) A plant whose roots are used to derive a number of hypotensive agents.

RAYNAUD'S PHENOMENON Intermittent interruptions of blood supply to the fingers, toes, and sometimes the ears, marked by severe pallor of these parts and accompanied by numbness, tingling, or severe pain.

REED-STERNBERG CELLS Giant connective tissue cells with one or two large nuclei that are characteristic of Hodgkin's disease.

REFLUX A flowing back or return flow of fluid or other matter.

RENAL CALCULI Small crystalline masses formed by the pathological accumulation of mineral salts in the kidney; kidney stones.

RESECTION Excision.

RETICULOCYTE An immature form of red blood cell, normally comprising about 1 percent of circulating red blood cells.

RETINOPATHY Any disease of the retina of the eye.

RETROVIRUS One of a family of viruses that contain RNA and reverse transcriptase.

RHINITIS Inflammation of the nasal mucous membranes.

RHONCHUS (PL., RHONCHI) A rale or rattling in the throat, especially when it resembles snoring.

RUBELLA German measles.

S

SALICYLATE Any of the salts of salicylic acid used for their pain-relieving, fever-reducing, and anti-inflammatory properties. The most widely used salicylate is aspirin (acetylsalicylic acid).

SEBORRHEA Functional disease of the sebaceous glands marked by an increase in the amount, and often an alteration of the quality, of the sebaceous secretion.

SEPTIC Pertaining to disease-causing organisms or their toxins.

SEPTICEMIA A condition associated with the presence or proliferation of disease-causing microorganisms or the accumulation of their toxins in the blood. Commonly called *blood poisoning.*

SEPTUM Any wall between two cavities, for example, the atrial septum divides the right and left atria of the heart.

SEROCONVERSION The development of detectable specific antibodies to a disease-causing organism or vaccine.

SHUNT Abnormal or artificial passage between two vessels, for instance, between the cavities of the heart.

SPIROCHETE Member of an order of microorganisms that have a slender, spiral shape.

SPLENOMEGALY Enlargement of the spleen.

SPUTUM Substance expelled by coughing or clearing the throat.

STAPEDECTOMY Excision of the stapes in the ear in order to improve hearing, especially in cases of otosclerosis. The stapes is replaced by a prosthesis.

STASIS PIGMENTATION A tan discoloration of the skin, a common result of venous insufficiency of the legs.

STENOSIS Abnormal constriction or narrowing in an opening or passageway of an organ or body part.

STRATUM CORNEUM The outermost or horny layer of the epidermis.

STRIDOR A harsh, high-pitched sound during respiration due to obstruction of air passages.

STUPOR A condition of unconsciousness or lethargy.

SUBSTANTIA GELATINOSA Gray matter of the spinal cord that surrounds the central canal and forms the apical part of the posterior horn of the spinal cord.

SUPPURATIVE Producing or generating pus.

SYMPATHECTOMY Surgical excision of a portion of a sympathetic nerve. The procedure causes dilation of the blood vessels affected by the interrupted nerve, resulting in improved blood supply to tissue supplied by those vessels.

SYNAPSE The narrow gap between two neurons in a neural pathway where the termination (axon) of one neuron comes in close proximity with the beginning (dendrite) or cell body of another neuron.

SYNCOPE A transient loss of consciousness due to inadequate blood flow to the brain.

SYSTEMIC Pertaining to or affecting the body as a whole.

SYSTOLIC PRESSURE The period of maximum arterial blood pressure. (Compare with *Diastolic Pressure.*)

TACHYCARDIA Abnormally rapid heart beat, generally defined as exceeding 100 beats per minute.

TACHYPNEA Abnormal, very rapid breathing.

TERATOGEN Anything that adversely affects normal cellular development in the embryo or fetus. It may be certain chemicals, some therapeutic and illicit drugs, radiation, and intrauterine viral infections.

TERATOMA A tumor composed of a number of different tissue types, none of which is normally found in the area of occurrence. Teratomas usually occur in the testes or ovaries.

TETANY A nervous condition characterized by sharp, painful, periodic muscle contractions, particularly those of the extremities.

THORACENTESIS Surgical puncture of the chest wall to remove fluid from either of the pleural cavities.

THORACOTOMY Surgical incision in the wall of the chest.

THREADY PULSE A fine, barely perceptible pulse.

THRILL An abnormal tremor accompanying a vascular or cardiac murmur; felt on palpation.

THROMBOCYTOPENIA A condition in which there is an abnormally small number of platelets in circulating blood.

THROMBOCYTOSIS An increase in the number of blood platelets.

THROMBOENDARTERECTOMY Surgical removal of a thrombus together with a portion of the inner lining from an artery.

THROMBOSIS The formation or presence of a blood clot within a blood vessel.

THROMBUS A blood clot formed along the wall of a blood vessel or in a cavity of the heart. It may be of sufficient size to obstruct blood flow; or all, or a portion, of it may break off to become an embolus. (See *Embolus.*)

TINNITUS A subjective, continuous ringing or buzzing sound in one or both ears.

TONOMETER Instrument for measuring pressure; for instance, the pressure of the aqueous humor of the eye.

TOPHUS (PL., TOPHI) A calculus (stone) or mineral deposit in bone or tissue.

TOXEMIA A condition in which poisonous products of body cells at a local source of infection or derived from the growth of microorganisms are spread throughout the body in the blood.

TRANSIENT VISUAL SCOTOMATA Temporary, islandlike, blind gaps in the visual field.

TRANSILLUMINATION Visual inspection of a body structure or organ by passing a light through its walls.

TRANSUDATE A fluid discharged through a membrane or vessel wall. In contrast to an exudate, a transudate has a low content of protein or cellular debris.

TRANSURETHRAL RESECTION Surgical procedure in which a portion of the prostate is removed using an instrument passed through the urethra.

TRIGGER POINT Any place on the body that when stimulated causes a sudden pain in a specific area.

TYMPANOPLASTY Surgery to correct the eardrum.

UNIVERSAL PRECAUTIONS Precautions for preventing the transmission of blood-borne viruses to be taken by all health-care professionals when facing exposure or possible exposure to blood, certain other body fluids, or body fluids visibly contaminated with blood. Universal precautions are listed as "Guidelines for Prevention of Transmission of Human Immunodeficiency Virus (HIV) and Hepatitis B Virus (HBV) to Health-Care and Public-Safety Workers," issued by the Centers for Disease Control of the National Institutes of Health. The guiding principle of universal precautions is that *all patients should be assumed to be infectious for HIV and other blood-borne pathogens.*

UREA The chief nitrogenous constituent of urine.

UREMIA Toxic condition associated with chronic renal failure and produced by excess levels of urea, creatinine, and other nitrogen-based compounds in the blood.

UROLITH A concretion, or stone, within the urinary tract.

URTICARIA A vascular reaction of the skin characterized by the temporary eruption of wheals; hives.

VALVOTOMY Surgical incision into a valve.

VARICES Abnormally dilated and twisted veins, arteries, or lymph nodes.

VARICOCELE Dilation of the complex network of veins that comprise part of the spermatic cord to form a palpable swelling within the scrotum.

VASOCONSTRICTION Decrease in the diameter of blood vessels.

VASODILATOR A drug or agent causing relaxation and expansion of the blood vessels.

VASOPRESSIN A hormone secreted by the hypothalamus that raises blood pressure, increases peristalsis, and promotes resorption of water by the kidney. Synthetic or prepared extracts are administered as antidiuretics. Also known as *antidiuretic hormone (ADH)*.

VENTRICLE A cavity in an organ, for instance the brain or the heart.

VENTRICULOGRAPHY The use of x-rays to visualize the ventricles of the heart, after injecting a contrast material, or the brain, after injecting air.

VENTRICULAR SEPTAL RUPTURE A breakage or tear in the septum between the left and right ventricles of the heart.

VERTIGO A sensation of spinning around in space or of having objects spin around oneself.

VESICLE A small (generally less than 0.5 cm) fluid-filled blister.

VILLI (INTESTINAL) The tiny finger-like projections lining the interior of the small intestine that absorb fluid and nutrients.

VIRULENCE The strength of a disease, its capacity to overcome the resistance of the organism.

WHEAL A generally round, transient elevation of the skin, which is white in the center, with pale red edges; often accompanied by itching.

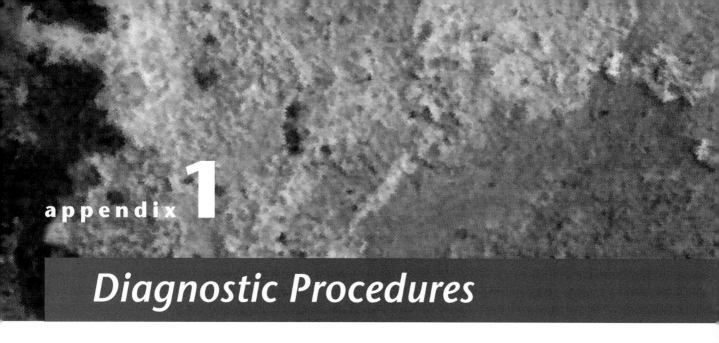

appendix 1

Diagnostic Procedures

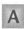 **A**

ALANINE AMINOTRANSFERASE A venipuncture is performed to measure this hepatic enzyme. Alanine aminotransferase is an enzyme necessary for tissue energy production. The presence of this enzyme in the blood may indicate acute hepatic disease such as hepatitis and distinguish myocardial from hepatic tissue damage.

ALKALINE PHOSPHATASE A venipuncture is performed to measure serum levels of alkaline phosphatase, an enzyme that influences bone calcification and lipid and metabolite transportation. The test is used in assessing bone and liver function.

AMNIOCENTESIS Surgical puncture of the amniotic sac, which surrounds the fetus in utero, to remove amniotic fluid; can detect over 100 genetic disorders and evaluate an adverse uterine environment.

ANGIOGRAPHY Often called *arteriography*. It consists of x-ray visualization of blood vessels, with or without the injection of a radiopaque material. Common types include cerebral, coronary, renal, pulmonary, and abdominal angiography.

ANTIBODIES TO EPSTEIN-BARR (EB) VIRUS The EB virus is found in patients with mononucleosis. The blood cells are cultured and the EB virus antibodies are diagnostic.

ANTI-DNA ANTIBODIES Measures antinative DNA antibody levels in a serum sample obtained by venipuncture.

ANTINUCLEAR ANTIBODY (ANA) A test diagnostic of systemic lupus erythematosus (SLE) where peripheral blood smears are taken and a fluorescein-tagged antihuman gamma globulin is used. If the LE factor is present, the specimen will fluoresce.

AORTOGRAPHY X-ray of the aorta after injection of an opaque medium into a vessel to assess possible aneurysm, arteriosclerosis, or congenital anomalies.

ARTERIAL BLOOD GASES (ABGs) A percutaneous arterial puncture is made to assess the gas exchanges of oxygen and carbon dioxide in the lungs by measuring the partial pressures of oxygen and carbon dioxide.

ARTERIOGRAM See *Angiography*. X-rays of arteries after the injection of a radiopaque material into the bloodstream.

ARTHROGRAM Visualization of a joint by radiographic study after injection of a contrast medium into the joint space.

ASPARTATE AMINOTRANSFERASE A venipuncture is performed to measure this cardiac enzyme. Aspartate aminotransferase is essential to energy production; used to detect recent myocardial infarction, to differentiate acute hepatic disease, and to monitor clients with cardiac and hepatic disease.

ASSAY The analysis of a substance to determine its constituents and the proportion of each.

361

AUDIOGRAM A record made by a delicate instrument, the audiometer, of the threshold of hearing.

AUSCULTATION AND PERCUSSION (A & P) *Auscultation* is listening to the sounds within the body, usually using a stethoscope. *Percussion* is using the fingertips to tap the body lightly to determine size, position, and consistency of body structures and fluids.

B

BCG VACCINE Bacille Calmette-Guérin, a form of tuberculosis vaccine that offers some protection to tuberculin-negative persons. Its use is recommended only where exposure to tuberculosis is great and the usual tuberculosis control measures are not possible.

BARIUM ENEMA X-ray of the lower gastrointestinal tract where barium, given as an enema, is the contrast medium.

BARIUM SWALLOW X-ray of the upper gastrointestinal tract where barium, given by mouth, is the contrast medium.

BILIRUBIN LEVELS Blood test to determine the level of bilirubin in the circulating blood.

BLOOD SERUM FOR HORMONES Radioimmunoassay (see *Radioimmunoassay*) and competitive protein binding are two testing methods commonly used to measure serum hormone levels; blood samples will be carefully drawn so as to correspond with or avoid times of peak secretions for the particular hormones being tested.

BONE MARROW BIOPSY Bone marrow fluid and cells can be removed through aspiration or needle biopsy of bone tissue; examination will give important data about blood disorders.

BRONCHOGRAPHY X-ray of the lung after instillation of an opaque iodine medium through a catheter into the trachea and bronchi. Bronchoscopy is more frequently used.

BRONCHOSCOPY Visualization of the larynx, trachea, and bronchi through a metal or fiberoptic scope with a light; also used for removal of foreign bodies and biopsy.

BRUDZINSKI'S SIGN When the neck of the client is bent, involuntary flexure movements of the ankle, knee, and hip are produced; seen in meningitis.

CARCINOEMBRYONIC ANTIGEN (CEA) Blood tests used to monitor the effectiveness of cancer therapy; serum CEA levels will fall within about 1 month if treatment is successful.

CARDIAC CATHETERIZATION A catheter is passed into the right (veins to inferior vena cava) or left (arteries to the aorta) side of the heart; can determine blood pressure and blood flow in the heart and permits collection of blood samples.

CARDIAC ENZYMES See *Creatinine phosphokinase (CPK), Lactate dehydrogenase (LDH),* and *Aspartate aminotransferase.*

CATHETERIZATION, URINE Introduction of a catheter through the urethra into the bladder for withdrawal of urine.

CATHETERIZATION OF EJACULATORY DUCTS A catheter is passed into the ejaculatory ducts to determine blockage or disease.

CEREBRAL ANGIOGRAPHY See *Angiography.* X-ray visualization of blood vessels of the brain after injection of radiopaque material into the arterial bloodstream. CT scan is a less hazardous procedure and is more commonly used.

CEREBROSPINAL FLUID (CSF) ANALYSIS Lumbar puncture between the third and fifth lumbar vertebrae is commonly used to measure CSF pressure and to obtain CSF to diagnose viral or bacterial meningitis, brain tumor and hemorrhages, and chronic central nervous system infections.

CHEMISTRY SCREENS Tests performed on blood to determine values of any number of factors, such as calcium, phosphorus, creatinine, uric acid, cholesterol, total protein, alkaline phosphatase, glucose, blood urea nitrogen, sodium, etc.

CHOLECYSTOGRAM Used to detect biliary tract disease. A series of x-rays of the gallbladder is taken after the ingestion of contrast medium.

COCCIDIODIN SKIN TEST A delayed hypersensitivity skin test used to detect an acute self-limiting disease of the respiratory organs—coccidioidomycosis.

COLONOSCOPY Visual examination of the lower bowel with a colonoscope. Biopsy and surgical excision can be accomplished through the scope.

COMPLETE BLOOD COUNT (CBC) A venipuncture usually is performed to give a complete picture of all the blood's formed elements. A CBC usually includes hemoglobin, hematocrit, red and white blood counts, and a differential white cell count.

COMPLETE NEUROLOGICAL EXAMINATION A series of tests and procedures to assess functioning of cranial nerves, motor and sensory systems, and superficial and deep tendon reflexes.

COMPUTERIZED TOMOGRAPHY (CT) SCAN Noninvasive x-ray technique more sensitive than conventional x-ray; a scanner and detector circle the patient sending an array of focused x-rays through the body; allows a specialist to distinguish tumors, abscesses, hemorrhages, and white and gray brain tissue.

CONVERGENCE TESTING Part of an eye examination to determine the movement of the eyes toward fixation of the same near point.

COOMBS' TEST, DIRECT A venipuncture is done to detect the presence of protein antibodies on the surface of red blood cells; helpful in diagnosing erythroblastosis fetalis.

CREATININE PHOSPHOKINASE (CPK) A venipuncture is performed to measure CPK, an enzyme that speeds up the creatine to creatinine transformation in muscle cells and brain tissue. Its purpose is to detect acute myocardial infarction or reinfarction and evaluate chest pain and skeletal muscle disorders.

CULTURE AND SENSITIVITY Withdrawing of tissue or fluid, placing it on a suitable culture media, and determining whether or not bacteria grow. If bacteria do grow, they are identified by bacteriologic methods. Tests are then done to determine the susceptibility of the client's bacterial infection to antibiotics.

CYSTOMETRY The study of urinary bladder efficiency using an instrument that measures the bladder's pressure and capacity. A catheter is passed into the bladder; then while saline, water, or air is instilled, the client reports any sensations or the need to void. Pressure and volume are recorded.

CYSTOSCOPY The urinary bladder is distended with water or air while the patient is sedated. Examination of the bladder with a fiberoptic scope is done to obtain biopsies and to remove polyps.

CYSTOURETHROGRAPHY X-ray examination of the bladder and urethra by use of contrast media cytology.

CYTOLOGY The science and study of cells; their structure and formation.

DILATION AND CURETTAGE (D & C) Involves widening of the cervical opening and scraping with a curet to remove the uterine lining.

DOPPLER ULTRASONOGRAPHY Noninvasive test evaluating blood flow in the major veins and arteries of arms, legs, and extracranial cerebrovascular system. A handheld transducer directs high-frequency sound waves to the area being tested.

ECHOCARDIOGRAPHY Noninvasive diagnostic test using ultrasound to visualize internal cardiac structures. A special transducer is placed on the client's chest, and it directs ultra high-frequency sound waves toward cardiac structures, which reflect these waves. The echoes are converted to electrical impulses and displayed on an oscilloscope.

ECHOENCEPHALOGRAPHY Involves the reflection of ultrasound waves from structures within the skull; less commonly used since CT scanning became so prevalent.

EJACULATORY OR SEMEN ANALYSIS Uses semen specimen to evaluate the volume of seminal fluid, sperm count, and sperm motility; also used to detect semen on a rape victim, identifying the blood group of an alleged rapist, or to prove sterility in a paternity suit.

ELECTROCARDIOGRAPHY (ECG) The recording of electric currents emanating from the heart muscle. Electrodes are placed on the client to obtain the reading.

ELECTROENCEPHALOGRAPHY (EEG) The process of recording the electric currents developed in the brain by placing electrodes on the skull.

ELECTROLYTE ANALYSIS See *Serum calcium, Phosphorus, Total protein,* or *Serum electrolytes* and *Chemistry screens.*

ELECTROMYOGRAPHY (EMG) Recording the changes in electrical potential of muscle using surface needle electrodes, insertion of needle electrodes into muscle, or stimulation of the muscle nerve.

ENDOSCOPIC RETROGRADE CHOLANGIOPANCREATOGRAPHY (ERCP) A radiographic examination of the pancreatic ducts and hepatobiliary tree after injection of a contrast medium into the duodenal papilla. It is used to diagnose pancreatic disease.

ENDOSCOPY Visual inspection of any cavity of the body by means of an endoscope.

ERYTHROCYTE SEDIMENTATION RATE (ESR) A blood specimen is obtained by venipuncture to measure the time required for erythrocytes in whole blood to settle to the bottom of a vertical tube; may be one of the earliest disease indicators.

EXFOLIATIVE CYTOLOGY Microscopic examination of desquamated cells or cells that have shredded or scaled off the surface epithelium. The cells are obtained from sputum, lesions, secretions, urine, aspirations, smears, or washings.

FLUORESCEIN STAIN A dye used to reveal corneal lesions and to test circulation in the retinas and extremities. A sterile fluorescin strip is moistened and touched to the eyelid, and the dye film spreads to the entire eye. A special slit-lamp (see *Slit-lamp examination*) is used to detect areas of concentrated dye.

FLUOROSCOPY Examination of deep structures using x-rays. Immediate projection of x-ray images can be visualized.

GASTRIC ANALYSIS Requires aspiration of gastric contents for culture to detect gastric pathogens; a nasogastric tube will be used to collect the washings.

GASTROSCOPY Inspection of the stomach interior using a gastroscope.

GRAM'S STAIN A staining procedure in which microorganisms are stained with crystal violet, followed by iodine solution; decolorized with alcohol; and counterstained with safranin. The retention of either the violet or pink color serves as a means to identify and classify bacteria. Gram-positive bacteria retain the violet color; gram-negative bacteria lose the violet color and are counterstained red.

HEMATOCRIT Used to measure the percentage of packed red cells in a whole blood sample obtained by finger stick or venipuncture.

HEMOGLOBIN A venipuncture or finger stick is done to measure the amount of hemoglobin found in whole blood; used to measure the severity of anemia or polycythemia.

HISTOPLASMIN SKIN TEST A form of delayed hypersensitivity skin testing to detect a systemic fungal respiratory disease due to *Histoplasma capsulatum.*

HYDROXY-25 See *Hydroxyproline.*

HYDROXYPROLINE A 24-hour urine catch is required to test for hydroxyproline; circulating hydroxyproline can also be checked by a blood sample.

HYSTEROSALPINGOGRAPHY X-ray of the uterus and uterine tubes after the introduction of an opaque material through the cervix.

INTRAVENOUS PYELOGRAM Contrast medium is injected intravenously, and x-rays are taken as the medium is cleared from the blood by glomerular filtration. The renal calyces, renal pelves, ureters, and urinary bladder are all visible on film.

KERNIG'S SIGN In a sitting position or when lying with the thigh flexed on the abdomen, the leg cannot be completely extended; a sign of meningitis.

KIDNEYS, URETERS, BLADDER (KUB) X-rays taken of the kidneys, ureters, and bladder.

LACTATE DEHYDROGENASE (LDH) A venipuncture is done to test for the LDH enzyme; helps to differentiate myocardial infarction, pulmonary infarction, anemias, and hepatic disease; supports CPK test results; monitors client response to some forms of chemotherapy.

LAPAROSCOPY A small incision is made in the abdominal wall to visualize the interior of the abdomen using a laparoscope. It is used to examine the ovaries or fallopian tubes and as a gynecologic sterilization technique.

LARYNGOSCOPY Visual examination of the interior of the larynx using a laryngoscope.

LOW-DOSE DEXAMETHASONE SUPPRESSION TEST This test may be performed whenever there is unexplained excessive glucocorticoid secretion. Dexamethasone is given orally every 6 hours for 2 days and adrenocorticotropic hormone (ACTH) stimulation is monitored to determine pathology.

LUMBAR PUNCTURE See *Cerebrospinal fluid (CSF) analysis.*

LUPUS ERYTHEMATOSUS (LE) TEST A blood sample is mixed with laboratory-treated antigens. If the sample contains antinuclear antibody, the LE factor will react with the antigen causing swelling and rupture of the nuclear material. Phagocytes from the serum engulf the foreign particles and form LE cells, which are then detected by microscopic examination.

LYMPHANGIOGRAPHY X-ray of the lymphatic vessels following injection of oil-based contrast medium into a lymphatic vessel in each foot.

MAGNETIC RESONANCE IMAGING (MRI) An imaging procedure that relies on irradiation in a magnetic field and the use of computers to produce images of different areas of the body. An individual is surrounded by a magnetic field, which causes hydrogen atoms to line up in a certain fashion. A signal is released when the atoms move back to their original places and is processed by the computer. Ionizing radiation is not required.

MAMMOGRAM X-ray of the mammary gland or breast.

MICROSCOPIC URINE A urine sample is centrifuged; then the cells, casts, and crystals are viewed to detect infection, obstruction, inflammation, trauma, or tumors.

MYELOGRAPHY X-ray of the spinal cord after the injection of a contrast medium; used to identify and study spinal lesions caused by trauma and disease. It has been largely replaced by CT scan or MRI.

OPHTHALMOSCOPY Allows magnified examination of inner structures of the eye; the ophthalmoscope used has a light source and a special viewing device.

OPTICOKINETIC DRUM TEST Used to determine and measure eye movements; patient looks at a rapidly rotating, vertically striped drum.

ORTOLANI'S SIGN A procedure to evaluate the stability of the hip joints in newborns and infants. With the infant on his or her back, the joints are manipulated, and if a clicking or popping sensation (Ortolani's sign) is felt or heard, the joint is unstable.

OTOLOGIC EXAMINATION An ear examination; may include the use of an otoscope, a tuning fork, and an audiometer.

OTOSCOPY Direct visualization of the external auditory canal and the tympanic membrane through an otoscope.

P

PAPANICOLAOU (PAP) TEST Diagnostic test for early detection of cancer cells by a simple smear method. The sample is usually taken from the cervix through a vaginal speculum.

PATCH TEST A skin test for identifying allergens to confirm allergic contact sensitization. The suspected substance is applied to an adhesive patch that is placed on the client's skin. Another patch with nothing on it acts as a control.

PELVIC EXAMINATION Includes both an inspection of the vulva, vagina, and cervix for abnormalities and a bimanual palpation of the uterus, fallopian tubes, and ovaries. A Pap smear often is done at the same time.

PENLIGHT EXAMINATION Performed with a lighted instrument to check pupil reactivity.

PERICARDIOCENTESIS Surgical puncture of the pericardium to remove purulent pericardial effusion.

pH STUDIES Determines the acidity or alkalinity level of gastrointestinal secretions. The pH electrode to be used is swallowed by the client. Studies also can be done on blood and urine.

PHENYLKETONURIA (PKU) TEST A heel stick on an infant is done to collect three drops of blood for screening to check for elevation of serum phenylalanine; performed about 4 days after milk feeding has begun. Also called the *Gutherie screening test.*

PHLEBOGRAPHY X-ray of the veins after the injection of a radiopaque contrast medium.

PPD TUBERCULIN TEST Intradermal injection of a purified protein derivative (PPD) tuberculin antigen. A delayed reaction occurs in clients infected with tubercle bacillus, whether or not there are clinical manifestations of disease.

PROCTOSCOPY Visual examination of the rectum using a proctoscope.

PROSTATE-SPECIFIC ANTIGEN (PSA) Serology test to detect, classify, and stage prostatic cancer.

PULMONARY ARTERY CATHETERIZATION (PAC) Permits evaluation of ventilation function through spirometer measurements; performed on clients with pulmonary dysfunction.

PULMONARY FUNCTION STUDIES A number of different tests to determine the ability of the lungs to exchange oxygen and carbon dioxide.

R

RADIOIMMUNOASSAY A technique in radiology used to determine the concentration of an antigen, antibody, or other protein in the serum. See *Blood serum for hormones.*

RADIOISOTOPE STUDIES Small quantities of radioisotopes, used as tracers or indicators, are added to the stable compound being studied so that the location of the latter in the body can be detected.

RECTAL EXAMINATION A digital examination to detect polyps, early cancer, lesions, inflammatory conditions, and hemorrhoids. It also can show how far the uterus is displaced in the female, and reveals the texture and size of the male prostate.

RECTAL MANOMETRY Measures rectal sphincter function and peristaltic contractions.

REFRACTION TEST Defines any vision or refractive error and determines any correction required with glasses or contact lenses.

RENAL FUNCTION TEST See *Urine concentration and Dilution tests.*

RETICULOCYTE COUNT A venipuncture is performed and the number of immature erythrocytes in the blood is determined; important in diagnosing certain blood disorders, especially anemia.

RETROGRADE PYELOGRAM Contrast medium is introduced through a urinary catheter into the ureters and calyces of the kidney while being observed on x-ray.

RHEUMATOID FACTORS Diagnostic blood test for immune-related diseases, for example, rheumatoid arthritis.

RINNE TEST Hearing test to evaluate air and bone conduction. A tuning fork is placed on the mastoid process.

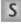

S

SCHILLING TEST Vitamin B_{12} is tagged with radioactive cobalt and administered orally. Gastrointestinal absorption is measured by determining the radioactivity of urine samples collected for the next 24 hours. Measures deficiencies of the vitamin; aids in diagnosis of megaloblastic anemia and central nervous system disorders of peripheral and spinal myelinated nerves.

SCINTISCAN Produces a map of scintillations observed when a radioactive substance is introduced into the body. The intensity of the record indicates the differential accumulation of the substance in the various body parts.

SEROLOGICAL STUDIES Samples of serum are taken and tests performed.

SERUM B$_{12}$ A venipuncture is done for a quantitative analysis of serum vitamin B$_{12}$ levels. Usually done concurrently with a serum folic acid, because deficiencies of the two are common causes of megaloblastic anemia. Also see *Schilling test.*

SERUM BILIRUBIN Measures serum levels of bilirubin; helps evaluate liver function, jaundice, biliary obstruction, and hemolytic anemia.

SERUM CALCIUM, PHOSPHORUS, TOTAL PROTEIN, OR SERUM ELECTROLYTES This series of tests performed on a blood sample will determine levels of calcium, phosphorus, and protein in the blood. See *Chemistry screens.*

SERUM CREATININE Creatinine in blood serum provides a sensitive measure of renal damage. Creatinine levels are directly related to the glomerular filtration rate. See *Chemistry screens.*

SERUM FERRITIN Serum ferritin levels are related to the amount of available iron stored in the body. This test screens for iron deficiency and overload, measures iron storage, and can distinguish between iron deficiency and chronic inflammation.

SERUM FOLATE See *Serum folic acid.*

SERUM FOLIC ACID This test on a blood sample measures the levels of folic acid; helps to diagnose megaloblastic anemia and to determine folate stores in pregnancy.

SERUM GONADOTROPIN See *Serum human chorionic gonadotropin.*

SERUM HUMAN CHORIONIC GONADOTROPIN (HCG) The production of HCG begins very quickly after the fertilized ovum is implanted into the uterine wall; the blood test reveals the presence of HCG if pregnancy has occurred.

SERUM IRON A blood sample will estimate iron storage in the blood and help distinguish between iron deficiency anemia and anemia of chronic disease.

SERUM PREGNANCY TEST See *Serum human chorionic gonadotropin.*

SERUM PROTEIN ELECTROPHORESIS Measures serum albumin and globulins in an electric field by separating the proteins on the basis of size, shape, and electric charge at pH 8.6; helps to diagnose hepatic disease, protein deficiency, blood and renal disorders, and gastrointestinal and neoplastic diseases.

SGOT (SERUM GLUTAMIC-OXALOACETIC TRANSAMINASE) See *Aspartate aminotransferase.*

SGPT (SERUM GLUTAMIC-PYRUVIC TRANSAMINASE) See *Alanine aminotransferase.*

SIGMOIDOSCOPY Visual inspection of the sigmoid flexure of the large intestine using a sigmoidoscope.

SKIN (INTRADERMAL OR SCRATCH) TEST A small quantity of solution containing a suspected allergen is put on a lightly scratched area of the skin, or an intradermal injection may be used. If a wheal forms within 15 minutes, allergy is indicated.

SLIT-LAMP EXAMINATION Allows an ophthalmologist to visualize the anterior portion of the eye. The slit lamp is an instrument with a special lighting system and a binocular microscope.

SNELLEN'S CHART A visual screening using a standardized chart with block letters arranged in rows of decreasing size. A large E chart or one with animals and familiar objects may be used for children.

SPUTUM CULTURE An examination of the material raised from the lungs and bronchi during deep coughing; important in the management of lung disease.

STOOL CULTURE The feces will be examined to determine pathogens that cause gastrointestinal disease; a chemical test may also be done on the stool specimen to detect occult blood.

STOOL OCCULT BLOOD A chemical test performed on a stool specimen to detect occult or hidden blood.

SYNOVIAL FLUID ANALYSIS A sterile needle is inserted into a joint space to obtain a fluid specimen; aids in arthritis diagnosis, relieving pain and distension, and administering local drug therapy.

THERMOGRAPHY A test that detects and records heat present in a body part; used to study blood flow to limbs and detect cancer of the breast.

THORACENTESIS Surgical puncture of the pleural space to remove fluid for analysis or treatment.

THYROID FUNCTION TESTS Tests of thyroid function, including physical examination; some tests include determination of thyroid hormone levels.

TONOMETRY Measurement of tension or pressure, especially of the eye for detection of glaucoma.

TRANSAMINASE See *SGOT* and *SGPT*.

TRENDELENBURG'S TEST The leg is raised above the heart level until veins are drained and then it is lowered quickly. If vein distention occurs immediately, valve incompetence is indicated.

ULTRASONOGRAPHY Use of ultrasound to produce an image or photograph of an organ or tissue. Ultrasound echoes are recorded as the sound waves strike tissues of different densities.

UPPER GASTROINTESTINAL ENDOSCOPY Allows visualization of the upper gastrointestinal tract to diagnose inflammatory, ulcerative, and infectious disease, neoplasms, and other lesions.

URATE CRYSTALS IN JOINT FLUID, OR TOPHI Synovial joint fluid is examined under the microscope. If urate crystals are found, the joints are acutely inflamed.

URINALYSIS A voided specimen in a clean container is obtained to test for color, appearance, formed elements, casts, odor, transparency, and specific gravity.

URINE CALCIUM AND PHOSPHATES Measures the urine levels of calcium and phosphates, which are essential for formation and resorption of bone; requires a 24-hour urine specimen.

URINE CATCH, 24-HOUR Urine is collected over a 24-hour period to measure quantity, and physical and chemical characteristics.

URINE CONCENTRATION AND DILUTION TEST Measures the levels of creatinine in urine; used to help assess glomerular filtration and to check the accuracy of 24-hour urine collection, based on relative contrast levels of creatinine excretion.

URINE CULTURE A clean-voided midstream sample is collected for evaluation of urinary tract infections; the specimen will be studied under a microscope and a colony count made to determine the presence of infection.

VAGINAL SMEARS With a cotton-tipped applicator or wooden spatula, vaginal secretions are collected for microscopic examination.

VENEREAL DISEASE RESEARCH LABORATORY TEST (VDRL) This test is widely used to screen for primary and secondary syphilis. A serum sample usually is used, but a specimen of cerebrospinal fluid may be used, also.

VISUAL ACUITY TEST Part of an eye examination; evaluates the patient's ability to distinguish the form and detail of an object.

WHITE BLOOD COUNT (WBC) Test made on whole blood to report the number of leukocytes in a cubic millimeter. The WBC may rise or fall in disease and is diagnostically useful only when interpreted in light of the patient's clinical status.

WOOD'S LIGHT An ultraviolet light used to diagnose certain scalp and skin diseases. The light causes hairs infected with a fungus to become brilliantly fluorescent.

X-RAY OF KIDNEYS, URETERS, AND BLADDER (KUB) Provides x-rays of the kidneys, ureters, and bladder, to evaluate the urinary tract, and kidney structure, size, and position.

Organ Function Tests*

Organ function tests are groupings of diagnostic and laboratory tests used to comprehensively evaluate how well an organ is working. Using several tests eliminates the risk of misdiagnosis because of inaccurate test results, and it presents a more complete picture of both the anatomic and physiologic alterations.

CARDIOVASCULAR SYSTEM

- *Cardiac enzymes:* Aspartate aminotransferase (AST, SGOT); creatine phosphokinase (CPK); creatine kinase (CK) and isoenzyme (CK-MB); lactate dehydrogenase (LH, LDH) and isoenzyme (LD_1, LD_2); hydroxybutyrate dehydrogenase (HBDH)
- *Lipids:* Total lipids, lipoprotein electrophoresis (HDL, LDL, VLDL); cholesterol; triglycerides; phospholipids
- *Electrolytes:* Potassium (K); sodium (Na)
- *Coagulation:* Prothrombin time (PT); activated partial thromboplastin time (APPT); coagulation time (CT); clotting time; Lee-White (LWCT)
- *Pericardial fluid:* Cytologic examination; other tests to measure red blood cell (RBC) count, white blood cell count (WBC), differential, and glucose; microbiologic examination if endocarditis is suspected (Gram stain, culture)

- *Drug levels:* Digoxin; digitoxin; diltiazem; nifedipine; propranolol; verapamil; others included in therapeutic regimen
- *Miscellaneous:* Erythrocyte sedimentation rate (ESR); WBC; glucose; blood gases (pH, Pco_2, Po_2)
- *Procedures:* Cardiac nuclear scanning; cardiac radiography; echocardiography; electrocardiography (ECG); phonocardiography; exercise electrocardiography; cardiac catheterization and angiography; heart and chest magnetic resonance imaging; non-nuclear computerized tomography (CT) of the chest

PULMONARY SYSTEM

- *Arterial blood gases (ABGs):* pH, Pco_2; Po_2; HCO_3; BE
- *Sputum:* Microbiologic examination (Gram and other stains, acid-fast bacillus [AFB] smear and culture); culture and sensitivity (C&S); cytologic examination
- *Pleural fluid:* Microbiologic examination (C&S, Gram stain); cytologic examination; other tests to measure LDH, RBC, WBC, differential, eosinophils, pH, and immunoglobulins
- *Drug levels:* Theophylline therapeutic regimen
- *Miscellaneous:* Alpha$_1$-antitrypsin; WBC
- *Procedures:* Bronchoscopy; mediastinoscopy, thoracoscopy, chest radiography and tomography; bronchography; pulmonary angiography; thoracic ultrasonography; lung nuclear

*From Watson, J, and Jaffe, MS: Nurse's Manual of Laboratory and Diagnostic Tests, ed 2. FA Davis, Philadelphia, 1995, pp 997–1002, with permission.

scanning; non-nuclear thoracic computerized tomography (CT); chest magnetic resonance imaging; pulmonary function studies; exercise pulmonary function; body plethysmography; sweat test; lung biopsy; thoracentesis; oximetry; skin tests for allergens and bacterial and fungal pulmonary diseases

NEUROLOGIC SYSTEM

- *Cerebrospinal fluid:* Routine analysis (cell count and differential, protein, glucose); other tests such as enzymes, electrolytes, urea, lactic acid, and glutamine; microbiologic examination (C&S, Gram, and AFS stains); cytologic examination; serologic examination (neurosyphilis tests)
- *Drug levels:* Anticonvulsants (phenobarbital, phenytoin, primidone), and others included in therapeutic regimen or considered for overdose in the comatose client (prescribed and otherwise)
- *Miscellaneous:* Electrolytes (K, Na, Cl, CO_2); glucose; alcohol; blood gases (ABGs); blood urea nitrogen (BUN); creatinine; toxicology screen (blood and urine)
- *Procedures:* Skull and spinal radiography; cerebral angiography; brain and cerebrospinal fluid flow nuclear scanning; echoencephalography; non-nuclear head, intracranial, neck, and spinal computerized tomography (CT) scanning; head and intracranial magnetic resonance imaging; electroneurography; evoked brain potentials; spinal nerve root thermography; oculoplethysmography; visual-auditory and optic-acoustic nerve tests

HEMATOLOGIC SYSTEM

- *Blood cell counts:* Complete blood count, including RBC, Hgb, Hct, RBC indices (MCV, MCH, MCHC), WBC, WBC differential, platelet, and reticulocyte
- *Blood cell types:* Hgb-electrophoresis; blood typing and cross-matching; sickle-cell screening
- *Coagulation:* Bleeding time; platelet aggregation; platelet survival; clot retraction time; capillary fragility; prothrombin time (PT); partial thromboplastin time (PTT); activated partial thromboplastin time (APTT); whole blood clotting time (CT); thrombin clotting time (TCT); prothrombin consumption time (PCT); factor assays; plasma fibrinogen; fibrin split products (FSP); euglobulin lysis
- *Iron deficiency:* Iron; total iron-binding capacity (TIBC); folic acid; ferritin
- *Hemolysis:* Red blood cell enzymes (glucose-6-phosphate dehydrogenase); haptoglobin, indirect Coombs; bilirubin
- *Miscellaneous:* Erythrocyte osmotic fragility; ESR; WBC enzymes; T and B lymphocyte assay; immunoglobulin assay
- *Procedures:* Schilling test; bone marrow aspiration; bone marrow nuclear scanning; red blood cell survival time study; platelet survival time study; lymph node biopsy

ENDOCRINE SYSTEM

- *Thyroid tests:* Calcitonin; thyroid-stimulating immunoglobulins (TSI); thyroxine-binding globulin (TBG); triiodothyronine (T_3); T_3 uptake; thyroxine (T_4); free T_4 index; thyroid antibodies; thyroid-stimulating hormone (TSH)
- *Thyroid procedures:* Thyroid nuclear scanning, radioactive iodine uptake study; thyroid-stimulating hormone study (TSH); thyroid cytomel and perchlorate suppression studies; ultrasonography, iodine-131 scanning
- *Parathyroid tests:* Parathyroid hormone (PTH); calcium; phosphorus; prednisone-cortisone suppression
- *Parathyroid procedures:* Ultrasonography; nuclear scanning
- *Pituitary tests:* Growth hormone (GH); growth hormone stimulation; growth suppression; prolactin (LTH); adrenocorticotropic hormone (ACTH); thyroid-stimulating hormone (TSH) and stimulation test; follicle-stimulating hormone (FSH); luteinizing hormone (LH), FSH-LH challenge; antidiuretic hormone (ADH)
- *Pituitary procedures:* Skull radiography; cerebral angiography; nuclear brain scanning; intracranial magnetic resonance imaging
- *Adrenal tests:* Cortisol; adrenocorticotropic hormone (ACTH); cortisol-ACTH challenge; aldosterone; aldosterone challenge; catecholamines; urinary hormones (cortisol, aldosterone, 17-hydroxycorticosteroids [17-OHCS], 17-ketosteroids [17-KS], 17-ketogenic steroids

[17-KGS], pregnanetriol, vanillylmandelic acid [VMA])

- *Adrenal procedures:* Non-nuclear computerized tomography (CT) scanning; adrenal nuclear scanning, ultrasonography; angiography; skull radiography
- *Pancreas tests:* Glucose; glucose tolerance; 2-hour postprandial glucose; ketones; glycosylated hemoglobin; BUN, creatinine; tolbutamide tolerance; insulin; amylase; lipase; aldolase; potassium (K); sodium (Na); glucagon; C-peptide
- *Pancreas procedures:* Endoscopic retrograde cholangiopancreatography (ERCP); ultrasonography; abdominal magnetic resonance imaging; pancreas nuclear scanning; non-nuclear computerized tomography (CT) scanning

RENAL-UROLOGIC SYSTEMS

- *Blood tests:* BUN, creatinine, electrolyte panel; osmolality; proteins; ammonia; uric acid; renin; aldosterone; gamma glutamyl transpeptidase (GGT)
- *Urine tests:* Routine analysis; creatinine clearance; insulin clearance; protein, complement C_3 and C_4; tubular function (phenosulfonphthalein [PSP]); concentration (osmolality, specific gravity); electrolytes; C&S
- *Procedures:* Kidney and renography nuclear scanning; nonnuclear abdominal computerized tomography (CT); ultrasonography; angiography; kidney, ureter, bladder radiography (KUB); antegrade pyelography; retrograde urethrography, cystography, and ureteropyelography; excretory urography (IVP); voiding cystourethrography; pelvic floor sphincter electromyography; cystometry; uroflowmetry and urethral pressure profile; cystoscopy; renal biopsy

MUSCULOSKELETAL SYSTEM

- *Muscle/bone enzymes:* Adolase; alkaline phosphatase (ALP); creatine phosphokinase (CPK); AST, SGOT
- *Electrolytes:* Calcium (Ca)
- *Joint tests:* Rheumatoid factor (RF); ESR; antistreptolysin O (ASO); immunoglobulins (IgG,

IgM); C-reactive protein (CRP); complement C_3 and C_4

- *Synovial fluid:* Routine analysis (RBC, WBC, neutrophils, protein, glucose, crystals); other tests such as rheumatoid factor (RA); complements
- *Procedures:* Bone and joint radiography; arthrocentesis; arthroscopy; arthrography; myelography; musculoskeletal magnetic resonance imaging; bone and joint nuclear scanning; electromyography; muscle biopsy

HEPATOBILIARY-GASTROINTESTINAL SYSTEMS

- *Liver enzymes:* Alkaline phosphatase (ALP) and isoenzymes (ALP$_1$); alanine aminotransferase (ALT, SGPT); 5′-nucleotidase (5′-N); lactic dehydrogenase (LDH) and isoenzymes (LDH$_5$); leucine aminopeptidase (LAP); gamma glutamyl transpeptidase (GTT); creatine phosphokinase (CPK) and isoenzymes (CPK$_3$)
- *Liver blood tests:* Bilirubin; protein (albumin, globulin) and protein electrophoresis; prothrombin time (PT); cholesterol; ammonia; hepatitis B–associated antigen and antibody tests
- *Liver procedures:* Abdominal radiography; liver nuclear scanning; non-nuclear computerized tomography (CT) scanning; abdominal magnetic resonance imaging; ultrasonography; hepatic and portal angiography; liver biopsy
- *Gallbladder procedures:* Abdominal radiography; oral cholecystography (OCG); intravenous cholangiography (IVC); percutaneous transhepatic cholangiography (PTC); operative cholangiography; T-tube cholangiography; biliary ultrasonography; non-nuclear computerized tomography (CT) scanning; gallbladder and biliary system nuclear scanning; endoscopic retrograde cholangiopancreatography (ERCP)
- *Esophageal and stomach tests:* Electrolyte panel; gastrin
- *Esophageal and stomach procedures:* Gastric analysis (macroscopic and microscopic); gastric acidity and acid stimulation; esophagogastroduodenoscopy (EGD); gastric emptying and gastrointestinal bleeding nuclear scanning; gastroesophageal reflux nuclear scanning; bar-

ium swallow; upper gastrointestinal series (UGI); fluoroscopy; esophageal manometry and associated tests; mesenteric angiography; esophageal or stomach biopsy

- *Small and large intestine tests:* Electrolyte panel, carotene, carcinoembryonic antigen (CEA); D-xylose absorption; lactose intolerance; fecal analysis (occult blood, fat, culture)
- *Small and large intestine procedures:* Duodenal contents analysis (macroscopic and microscopic); duodenal stimulation for cholecystokinin-pancreozymin and secretin; abdominal radiography; colonoscopy; proctosigmoidoscopy; barium enema; Meckel's diverticulum nuclear scanning; paracentesis; peritoneal fluid analysis; non-nuclear computerized tomography (CT) scanning; colon biopsy

REPRODUCTIVE SYSTEM

- *Female blood tests:* Prolactin; estrogen; follicle-stimulating hormone (FSH); luteinizing hormone (LH); progesterone
- *Female urine tests:* Pregnanediol; follicle-stimulating hormone (FSH); estrogen
- *Female procedures:* Colposcopy; culdoscopy; laparoscopy; hysterosalpingography; pelvic and breast ultrasonography; mammography; breast thermography; breast biopsy; cervical biopsy; Papanicolaou (PAP) smear; cytologic analysis (Barr chromatin body, chromosome analysis); non-nuclear computerized tomography (CT) pelvic scanning
- *Male blood tests:* Testosterone; semen analysis for fertility; cytology analysis for chromosomal and genetic abnormalities
- *Male urine tests:* 17-ketosteroids (17-KS)
- *Male procedures:* Scrotal nuclear scanning; scrotal-prostate ultrasonography; prostate biopsy
- *Pregnant female tests:* Complete blood count (CBC); ABO and Rh typing; albumin; syphilis serology (RPR, VDRL); renin; TORCH screen (cytomegalovirus, rubella, herpes virus, plasmal antibodies); human placental lactogen (HPL); creatine phosphokinase (CPK); human chorionic gonadotropin (HCG); progesterone and urinary pregnanediol; enzymes (heat-stable alkaline phosphatase [HSAP], diamine oxidase [DAO], oxytocinase); estriol (E_3) in blood and urine; endocrine panel for hormones; hematology panel for blood cells; coagulation; iron; folate; erythrocyte sedimentation rate (ESR); routine urinalysis; cytology analysis for sex chromatin and chromosome anomalies; amniotic fluid analysis for lecithin/sphingomyelin (L/S) ratio; genetic defects; creatinine; phosphatidylglycerol; uric acid

- *Pregnant female procedures:* Amnioscopy, amniocentesis, pelvimetry; contraction stress tests; pelvic ultrasonography; fetal monitoring (internal and external); fetoscopy
- *Newborn tests:* TORCH, type and Rh; bilirubin; glucose; calcium; albumin; phenylketonuria (PKU)

IMMUNE AND AUTOIMMUNE CONDITIONS

- *Immune and autoimmune tests:* T and B lymphocyte assay; immunoblast transformation; immunoglobulin assay (IgG, IgA, IgM, IgD, and IgE); antinuclear antibodies (ANA); antibody tests; uric acid; rheumatoid factor (RF); antistreptolysin O titer (ASO); C-reactive protein (CRP); protein electrophoresis for cryoglobulins; lupus erythematosus (LE); anti-DNA, complement C_3 and C_4 assay; ESR; human immunodeficiency virus antibody tests (HIV or AIDS)

TUMORS

- *Tumor marker tests:* Prostate (prostatic acid phosphatase [PAP], prostate-specific antigen [PSA]); thyroid (calcitonin); colon, lung, breast (carcinoembryonic antigen [CEA]); liver, testes (alpha-fetoprotein [AFP]); testes, trophoblastic (human chorionic gonadotropin [HCG]); ovary (CA 125); breast (CA 15-3); pancreas; colon (CA 19-9, CA 50); lymphoma, leukemia (lymphocyte B and T)
- *Other tumor tests:* Oncogenes (DNA sequences by polymerase chain reaction [PCR]); cytology examination for B- and T-cell gene rearrangement and DNA content of tumor cells; vasoactive intestinal peptide (VIP); squamous cell carcinoma antigen (SCC); tissue polypeptide antigen (TPA); neuron-specific enolase (NSE);

glycoprotein antigen (DU-PAN-2); metabolic tests (uric acid, albumin, cholesterol, triglycerides); hematologic tests (leukocytes, platelets); endocrine tests (antidiuretic hormone, cortisol, ACTH); isoenzymes (alkaline phosphatase [ALP], creatine kinase [CK-BB], galactosyl transferase [GT II], lactate dehydrogenase [LD_1]); electrolyte panel; and other tests based on suspected tumor location

- *Tumor procedures:* Radiography of suspected area; lymph node and retroperitoneal ultrasonography; mammography; bone marrow aspiration; nuclear body scanning (gallium-67); non-nuclear computerized tomography (CT) scanning of body and head; body and head/intracranial magnetic resonance imaging; endoscopy of area; lymphangiography; biopsy of affected organ

Profile or Panel Groupings and Laboratory Tests*

PROFILE OR PANEL GROUPINGS OF DIAGNOSTIC PROCEDURES

A profile or panel grouping refers to a measurement of multiple laboratory tests that reflects the function of several organ systems (health profile) or to a group of selected diagnostic tests and procedures that reflects the function or status of a specific organ or disease. In general, profiles or panels help to determine the client's state of health, support or rule out the presence of physiological abnormalities, determine the effectiveness of therapy, and provide preventive measures or teaching to reduce the progression of a disease. They are also used as screening tests for asymptomatic clients as a preventive measure, although it is generally felt that routine individual screening tests are all that are needed for those who are healthy.

The panel or profile consists of a battery or group of 4 to 12 biochemical tests performed on a few milliliters of serum with an instrument called the sequential multiple analyzer (SMA). The tests are ordered as a unit designated as SMA-4, SMA-6, or SMA-12. SMA-4 includes red blood cell (RBC) count, white blood cell (WBC) count, hemoglobin (Hgb), and hematocrit (Hct). SMA-6 includes sodium (Na), potassium (K), chloride (Cl), bicarbonate (HCO_3), glucose, and blood urea nitrogen (BUN). SMA-12 includes total protein, albumin, calcium (Ca), BUN, inorganic phosphorus, cholesterol, glucose, uric acid, creatinine, total bilirubin, alkaline phosphatase (ALP), and aspartate aminotransferase (SGOT [AST]). The electrolytes included in the SMA-6 can replace uric acid, creatinine, cholesterol, and phosphorus (P) to provide another variety of SMA-12. Another type of analyzer, known as SMAC, can accommodate a large profile of roughly 20 tests (CHEM 20), provide several tests from each of the panels, and analyze components of the blood singly or in combination to note organ or body system associations in a single procedure. Patterns of abnormalities can be recognized by the physician, and more conclusive diagnostic procedures can be ordered based on these profile results (Table A–3).

LABORATORY TESTS FOR DISEASES, ORGANS, OR ORGAN SYSTEMS

Cardiovascular System

- *Cardiac enzymes:* Aspartate aminotransferase (AST, SGOT), creatine phosphokinase (CPK), creatine kinase (CK) and isoenzyme (CK-MB), lactate dehydrogenase (LH, LDH) and isoenzyme (LD_1, LD_2), hydroxybutyrate dehydrogenase (HBDH)

*From Cavanaugh, BM: Nurse's Manual of Laboratory and Diagnostic Tests, ed 3. FA Davis, Philadelphia, 1999, pp 991–998, with permission.

Table A–3 Chem-20 Health Profile with Some Organ Associations of Each Analyte

Glucose *F, R*	Bilirubin, direct *L*
BUN *K, L, F*	Bilirubin, total *L*
Creatinine *K, F*	LDH *L, M*
Uric acid *K*	SGOT (AST) *L, M*
Sodium *K, F*	SGPT (ALT) *L*
Potassium *K, F*	Alkaline phosphatase *L, B*
Chloride *K, F*	Albumin *N, L, K*
Bicarbonate *K, F*	Total protein *N, L*
Calcium *B, F*	Cholesterol *N, R*
Phosphorus *K, B*	Triglycerides *N, R*

K = kidneys, *L* = liver, *B* = bone, *N* = nutrition, *M* = muscle, *R* = cardiac risk assessment, *F* = fluid and electrolyte balance.
Source: Sacher, RA, and McPherson, FA: Widmann's Clinical Interpretation of Laboratory Tests, ed 10. FA Davis, Philadelphia, 1991, p 14. Used with permission.

- *Lipids:* Total lipids, lipoprotein electrophoresis (HDL, LDL, VLDL), cholesterol, triglycerides, phospholipids
- *Electrolytes:* Potassium (K), sodium (Na)
- *Coagulation:* Prothrombin time (PT), activated partial thromboplastin time (aPTT), coagulation time (CT), clotting time, Lee-White coagulation time (LWCT)
- *Pericardial fluid:* Cytologic examination; other tests to measure RBC count, WBC count, differential, and glucose; microbiologic examination if endocarditis is suspected (Gram stain, culture)
- *Drug levels:* Digoxin, digitoxin, diltiazem, nifedipine, propranolol, verapamil, others included in therapeutic regimen
- *Miscellaneous:* Erythrocyte sedimentation rate (ESR), WBC, glucose, blood gases (pH, pCO_2, pO_2)
- *Procedures:* Cardiac nuclear scanning, cardiac radiography, echocardiography, electrocardiography (ECG), phonocardiography, exercise ECG, cardiac catheterization and angiography, heart and chest magnetic resonance imaging (MRI), non-nuclear computed tomography (CT) of the chest

Pulmonary System

- *Arterial blood gases* (ABGs): pH, pCO_2, pO_2, HCO_3, BE
- *Sputum:* Microbiologic examination (Gram and other stains, acid-fast bacillus [AFB] smear and culture), culture and sensitivity (C&S), cytologic examination
- *Pleural fluid:* Microbiologic examination (C&S, Gram stain); cytologic examination; other tests to measure LDH, RBC, WBC, differential, eosinophils, pH, and immunoglobulins
- *Drug levels:* Theophylline therapeutic regimen
- *Miscellaneous:* Alpha$_1$-antitrypsin, WBC
- *Procedures:* Bronchoscopy, mediastinoscopy, thoracoscopy, chest radiography and tomography; bronchography; pulmonary angiography; thoracic ultrasonography; lung nuclear scanning; non-nuclear thoracic CT; chest MRI; pulmonary function studies; exercise pulmonary function; body plethysmography; sweat test; lung biopsy; thoracentesis; oximetry; skin tests for allergens and bacterial and fungal pulmonary diseases

Neurological System

- *Cerebrospinal fluid:* Routine analysis (cell count and differential, protein, glucose); other tests such as enzymes, electrolytes, urea, lactic acid, and glutamine; microbiologic examination (C&S, Gram and AFB stains); cytologic examination; serologic examination (neurosyphilis tests)
- *Drug levels:* Anticonvulsants (phenobarbital, phenytoin, primidone) and others included in therapeutic regimen or considered for overdose in the comatose client (prescribed and otherwise)
- *Miscellaneous:* Electrolytes (K, Na, Cl, CO_2), glucose, alcohol, ABGs, BUN, creatinine, toxicology screen (blood and urine)
- *Procedures:* Skull and spinal radiography; cerebral angiography; brain and cerebrospinal fluid (CSF) flow nuclear scanning; echoencephalography; non-nuclear head, intracranial, neck, and spinal CT scanning; head and intracranial MRI; electroneurography; evoked brain potentials; spinal nerve root thermography; oculoplethysmography; visual-auditory and optic-acoustic nerve tests

Hematologic System

- *Blood cell counts:* Complete blood count (CBC), including RBC, Hgb, Hct, RBC indices (MCV,

MCH, MCHC), WBC, WBC differential, platelet, and reticulocyte
- *Blood cell types:* Hgb electrophoresis, blood typing and cross-matching, sickle cell screening
- *Coagulation:* Bleeding time, platelet aggregation, platelet survival, clot retraction time, capillary fragility, PT, PTT, aPTT, whole blood clotting time (CT), thrombin clotting time (TCT), prothrombin consumption time (PCT), factor assays, plasma fibrinogen, fibrin split products (FSP), euglobulin lysis
- *Iron deficiency:* Iron, total iron-binding capacity (TIBC), folic acid, ferritin
- *Hemolysis:* RBC enzymes (glucose-6-phosphate dehydrogenase [G-6-PD]), haptoglobin, indirect Coombs', bilirubin
- *Miscellaneous:* Erythrocyte osmotic fragility, ESR, WBC enzymes, T- and B-lymphocyte assay, immunoglobulin assay
- *Procedures:* Schilling test, bone marrow aspiration, bone marrow nuclear scanning, RBC survival time study, platelet survival time study, lymph node biopsy

Endocrine System

- *Thyroid tests:* Calcitonin, thyroid-stimulating immunoglobulins (TSI), thyroxine-binding globulin (TBG), triiodothyronine (T_3), T_3 uptake, thyroxine (T_4), free T_4 index, thyroid antibodies, thyroid-stimulating hormone (TSH)
- *Thyroid procedures:* Thyroid nuclear scanning, radioactive iodine uptake study, thyroid-stimulating hormone (TSH) study, thyroid Cytomel and perchlorate suppression studies, ultrasonography, iodine 131 (^{131}I) scanning
- *Parathyroid tests:* Parathyroid hormone (PTH), calcium, phosphorus, prednisone-cortisone suppression
- *Parathyroid procedures:* Ultrasonography, nuclear scanning
- *Pituitary tests:* Growth hormone (GH), GH stimulation, growth suppression, prolactin (LTH), adrenocorticotropic hormone (ACTH), TSH and stimulation test, follicle-stimulating hormone (FSH), luteinizing hormone (LH), FSH-LH challenge, antidiuretic hormone (ADH)
- *Pituitary procedures:* Skull radiography, cerebral angiography, nuclear brain scanning, intracranial MRI scanning

- *Adrenal tests:* Cortisol, ACTH, cortisol-ACTH challenge, aldosterone, aldosterone challenge, catecholamines, urinary hormones (cortisol, aldosterone, 17-hydroxycorticosteroids [17-OHCS], 17-ketosteroids [17-KS], 17-ketogenic steroids [17-KGS], pregnanetriol vanillylmandelic acid [VMA])
- *Adrenal procedures:* Non-nuclear CT scanning, adrenal nuclear scanning, ultrasonography, angiography, skull radiography
- *Pancreas tests:* Glucose, glucose tolerance (GT), 2-hour postprandial glucose, ketones, glycosylated hemoglobin, BUN, creatinine, tolbutamide tolerance, insulin, amylase, lipase, aldolase, potassium (K), sodium (Na), glucagon, C-peptide
- *Pancreas procedures:* Endoscopic retrograde cholangiopancreatography (ERCP), ultrasonography, abdominal MRI scanning, pancreas nuclear scanning, non-nuclear CT scanning

Renal-Urologic Systems

- *Blood tests:* BUN, creatinine, electrolyte panel, osmolality, proteins, ammonia, uric acid, renin, aldosterone, γ-glutamyl transpeptidase (GGT)
- *Urine tests:* Routine analysis, creatinine clearance, insulin clearance, protein, complement C_3 and C_4, tubular function (phenolsulfonphthalein [PSP]), concentration (osmolality, specific gravity), electrolytes, C&S
- *Procedures:* Kidney and renography nuclear scanning; non-nuclear abdominal CT; ultrasonography; angiography; kidney, ureter, bladder (KUB) radiography; antegrade pyelography; retrograde urethrography, cystography, and ureteropyelography; excretory urography (IVP); voiding cystourethrography; pelvic floor sphincter electromyography (EMG); cystometry; uroflowmetry and urethral pressure profile; cystoscopy; renal biopsy

Musculoskeletal System

- *Muscle/bone enzymes:* Adolase; alkaline phosphatase (ALP); creatine phosphokinase (CPK); AST, SGOT
- *Electrolytes:* Calcium (Ca)

- *Joint tests:* Rheumatoid factor (RF), ESR, anti-streptolysin O (ASO), immunoglobulins (IgG, IgM), C-reactive protein (CRP), complement C_3 and C_4
- *Synovial fluid:* Routine analysis (RBC, WBC, neutrophils, protein, glucose, crystals); other tests such as rheumatoid factor (RA), complements
- *Procedures:* Bone and joint radiography, arthrocentesis, arthroscopy, arthrography, myelography, musculoskeletal MRI scanning, bone and joint nuclear scanning, EMG, muscle biopsy

Hepatobiliary-Gastrointestinal Systems

- *Liver enzymes:* Alkaline phosphatase (ALP) and isoenzymes (ALP_1), alanine aminotransferase (ALT, SGPT), 5'-nucleotidase (5'-N), lactic dehydrogenase (LDH) and isoenzymes (LDH_5), leucine aminopeptidase (LAP), γ-glutamyl transpeptidase (GTT), creatine phosphokinase (CPK) and isoenzymes (CPK_3)
- *Liver blood tests:* Bilirubin, protein (albumin, globulin) and protein electrophoresis, PT, cholesterol, ammonia, hepatitis B–associated antigen and antibody tests
- *Liver procedures:* Abdominal radiography, liver nuclear scanning, non-nuclear CT scanning; abdominal MRI scanning, ultrasonography, hepatic and portal angiography, liver biopsy
- *Gallbladder procedures:* Abdominal radiography, oral cholecystography (OCG), intravenous cholangiography (IVC), percutaneous transhepatic cholangiography (PTC), operative cholangiography, T-tube cholangiography, biliary ultrasonography, non-nuclear CT scanning, gallbladder and biliary system nuclear scanning, endoscopic retrograde cholangiopancreatography (ERCP)
- *Esophageal and stomach tests:* Electrolyte panel, gastrin
- *Esophageal and stomach procedures:* Gastric analysis (macroscopic and microscopic), gastric acidity and acid stimulation, esophagogastroduodenoscopy (EGD), gastric emptying and gastrointestinal bleeding nuclear scanning, gastroesophageal reflux nuclear scanning, barium swallow, upper gastrointestinal (UGI) series, fluoroscopy, esophageal manometry and associated tests, mesenteric angiography, esophageal or stomach biopsy

- *Small and large intestine tests:* Electrolyte panel, carotene, carcinoembryonic antigen (CEA); D-xylose absorption; lactose intolerance; fecal analysis (occult blood, fat, culture)
- *Small and large intestine procedures:* Duodenal contents analysis (macroscopic and microscopic), duodenal stimulation for cholecystokinin-pancreozymin (CCK-PZ) and secretin, abdominal radiography, colonoscopy, proctosigmoidoscopy, barium enema, Meckel's diverticulum nuclear scanning, paracentesis, peritoneal fluid analysis, non-nuclear CT scanning, colon biopsy

Reproductive System

- *Female blood tests:* Prolactin, estrogen, follicle-stimulating hormone (FSH), luteinizing hormone (LH), progesterone
- *Female urine tests:* Pregnanediol, FSH, estrogen
- *Female procedures:* Colposcopy, culdoscopy, laparoscopy, hysterosalpingography, pelvic and breast ultrasonography, mammography, breast thermography, breast biopsy, cervical biopsy, Papanicolaou (Pap) smear, cytologic analysis (Barr chromatin body, chromosome analysis), non-nuclear CT pelvic scanning
- *Male blood tests:* Testosterone, semen analysis for fertility, cytology analysis for chromosomal and genetic abnormalities
- *Male urine tests:* 17-ketosteroids (17-KS)
- *Male procedures:* Scrotal nuclear scanning, scrotal-prostate ultrasonography, prostate biopsy
- *Pregnant female tests:* Complete blood count (CBC), ABO and Rh typing, albumin, syphilis serology (rapid plasmin reagin [RPR], Venereal Disease Research Laboratory [VDRL]), renin, TORCH screen (toxoplasmosis, other infections, rubella, cytomegalovirus, and herpes simplex), human placental lactogen (hPL), creatine phosphokinase (CPK), human chorionic gonadotropin (hCG), progesterone and urinary pregnanediol, enzymes (heat-stable alkaline phosphatase [HSAP], diamine oxidase [DOA], oxytocinase), estriol (E_3) in blood and urine, endocrine panel for hormones, hematology panel for blood cells, coagulation, iron, folate, ESR, routine urinalysis (UA), cytology analysis for sex chromatin and chromosomal anomalies, amniotic fluid analysis for

lecithin:sphingomyelin (L:S) ratio, genetic defects, creatinine, phosphatidylglycerol (PG), uric acid

- *Pregnant female procedures:* Amnioscopy, amniocentesis, pelvimetry, contraction stress tests, pelvic ultrasonography, fetal monitoring (internal and external), fetoscopy
- *Newborn tests:* TORCH, type and Rh, bilirubin, glucose, calcium, albumin, phenylketonuria (PKU)

Immune and Autoimmune Conditions

- *Immune and autoimmune tests:* T- and B-lymphocyte assay; immunoblast transformation; immunoglobulin assay (IgG, IgA, IgM, IgD, and IgE); antinuclear antibodies (ANA); antibody tests; uric acid; rheumatoid factor (RF); antistreptolysin O (ASO) titer; C-reactive protein (CRP); protein electrophoresis for cryoglobulins; lupus erythematosus (LE); anti-DNA, complement C_3 and C_4 assay; ESR; human immunodeficiency virus (HIV or AIDS) antibody tests

Infectious and Febrile Conditions

- *Infectious and febrile tests:* Heterophil, febrile agglutinins; blood culture analysis; culture of other body fluids; fungal antibody tests; antistreptococcal antibody tests; viral antibody tests; other antibody tests; differential WBC count, ESR
- *Infectious and febrile procedures:* Abscess-inflammatory nuclear scanning, gallium 67 (^{67}Ga) nuclear scanning, skin tests, chest x-ray

Tumors

- *Tumor marker tests:* Prostate (prostatic acid phosphatase [PAP], prostate-specific antigen [PSA]); thyroid (calcitonin); colon, lung, breast (carcinoembryonic antigen [CEA]); liver, testes (α-fetoprotein [AFP]); testes, trophoblastic (human chorionic gonadotropin [hCG]); ovary (CA 125); breast (CA 15-3); pancreas; colon (CA 19-9, CA 50); lymphoma, leukemia (lymphocyte B and T)
- *Other tumor tests:* Oncogenes (DNA sequences by polymerase chain reaction [PCR]), cytology

examination for B- and T-cell gene rearrangement and DNA content of tumor cells, vasoactive intestinal peptide (VIP), squamous cell carcinoma (SCC) antigen, tissue polypeptide antigen (TPA), neuron-specific enolase (NSE), glycoprotein antigen (DU-PAN-2), metabolic tests (uric acid, albumin, cholesterol, triglycerides), hematologic tests (leukocytes, platelets), endocrine tests (ADH, cortisol, ACTH), isoenzymes (alkaline phosphatase [ALP], creatine kinase [CK-BB], galactosyltransferase [GT II], lactate dehydrogenase [LD_1]), electrolyte panel, and other tests based on suspected tumor location

- *Tumor procedures:* Radiography of suspected area, lymph node and retroperitoneal ultrasonography, mammography, bone marrow aspiration, nuclear body scanning (^{67}Ga), non-nuclear CT scanning of body and head, body and head/intracranial MRI scanning, endoscopy of area, lymphangiography, biopsy of affected organ

Chronic Disorders

- *Hypertension:* Lipid panel (total lipids, HDL, LDL, cholesterol, triglycerides, phospholipids), glucose, ABGs, electrolyte panel, BUN, creatinine, creatinine clearance, uric acid, lactate dehydrogenase (LDH), aldosterone (blood and urine), catecholamines, CBC, renin, angiotensin-converting enzyme, urinalysis
- *Diabetes:* Blood and urine glucose and ketones: 2-hour postprandial, glucose tolerance (GT), triglycerides, glucagon, CBC, glycosylated hemoglobin, urinalysis, insulin assay
- *Arthritis:* Antinuclear antibodies (ANA), rheumatoid factor (RF), antistreptolysin O (ASO) titer, C-reactive protein (CRP), protein electrophoresis, uric acid, C_4 and total complement, immune complex assay, synovial fluid analysis
- *Chronic obstructive pulmonary disease (COPD):* Spirometry, theophylline level, ABGs, electrolyte panel, sputum culture, chest x-ray, pulmonary function
- *Coronary artery disease (CAD):* Glucose, lipid panel (see Hypertension above), electrolyte panel

- *Chronic heart failure (CHF):* Digoxin and other cardiac drug levels, coagulation profile (bleeding and clotting time, PT, PTT, and thrombin time; factor analysis; platelets), cardiac enzymes and isoenzymes (CK, GGTP, SGOT, SGPT, LD), CBC, electrolyte panel, ESR, ECG, cardiac radiography, angiography, echocardiography

- *Anemia:* Schilling test, iron, total iron-binding capacity (TIBC), ferritin, folate, CBC, bone marrow analysis
- *Drug abuse:* Opiates (meperidine [Demerol], codeine), heroin, cocaine, amphetamines, barbiturates, methaqualone, cannabinoids (marijuana, hashish), phencyclidine ("angel dust"), phenothiazines, tricyclic antidepressants

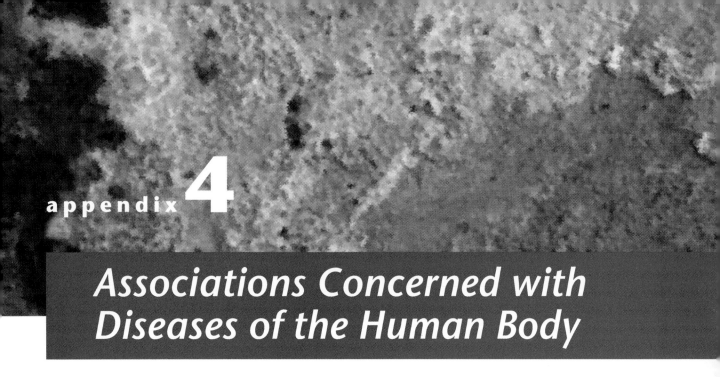

Associations Concerned with Diseases of the Human Body

APPENDIX 4–1 RESOURCE ORGANIZATIONS IN THE UNITED STATES*

AIDS

AMERICAN RED CROSS
National Headquarters
AIDS Education Program
Jefferson Park
8111 Gatehouse Road
Falls Church, VA 22042
(703) 206-7130

CDC NATIONAL AIDS CLEARINGHOUSE
P.O. Box 6003
Rockville, MD 20840-6003
(800) 458-5231
(800) 243-7012 (Deaf access)

CDC NATIONAL AIDS HOT LINE
P.O. Box 13827
Research Triangle Park, NC 27709
(800) 342-AIDS
(800) 344-7432 (Spanish)
(800) 243-7889 (Deaf access)

---

*Margolis, S, and Moses, H (eds): The Johns Hopkins Medical Handbook, Random House, New York, 1992; and Schwartz, CA, and Turner, RL: Encyclopedia of Associations: National Organizations of the U.S., ed 29, Gale Research, Detroit, 1995.

NATIONAL ASSOCIATION OF PEOPLE WITH AIDS
1413 K Street NW
Washington, DC 20005
(202) 898-0414

NATIONAL HOSPICE ORGANIZATION
1901 N. Moore Street, Suite 901
Arlington, VA 22209
(800) 658-8898

Alcoholism

SEE: *Substance Abuse*

Alzheimer's Disease

ALZHEIMER'S ASSOCIATION
919 N. Michigan Avenue, Ste. 1000
Chicago, IL 60611
(312) 335-8700
(800) 272-3900

Asthma

SEE: *Respiratory Disorders*

Blindness

SEE: *Visual Impairment*

Burns

AMERICAN BURN ASSOCIATION
c/o Secretary of Jeffrey R. Saffle, M.D.
University of Utah Medical Center
Department of Surgery
50 N. Medical Drive
Salt Lake City, UT 84132
(800) 548-2876

NATIONAL BURN VICTIM FOUNDATION
32–34 Scotland Road
Orange, NJ 07050
(201) 676-7700

Cancer

AMERICAN CANCER SOCIETY
1599 Clifton Road NE
Atlanta, GA 30329-4251
(800) ACS-2345

LEUKEMIA SOCIETY OF AMERICA
600 3rd Avenue
New York, NY 10016
(212) 573-8484
(800) 955-4LSA

NATIONAL CANCER INSTITUTE
Cancer Information Service
9000 Rockville Pike
Bethesda, MD 20892
(800) 4-CANCER

R.A. BLOCH CANCER FOUNDATION
4400 Main
Kansas City, MO 64111
(816) 932-8453

Cerebral Palsy

UNITED CEREBRAL PALSY ASSOCIATIONS
1660 L Street NW, Ste. 700
Washington, DC 20036
(800) USA-5UCP

Deafness

SEE: *Hearing Impairment*

Depression

SEE: *Mental Health*

Diabetes

AMERICAN DIABETES ASSOCIATION
1660 Duke Street
Alexandria, VA 22314
(800) ADA-DISC

JUVENILE DIABETES FOUNDATION INTERNATIONAL
120 Wall Street
New York, NY 10005
(800) JDF-CURE

Disability

JOB ACCOMMODATION NETWORK
918 Chestnut Ridge Road, Ste. 1
P.O. Box 6080
Morgantown, WV 26506
(800) 526-7234

NATIONAL REHABILITATION INFORMATION CENTER
8455 Colesville Road, Ste. 935
Silver Spring, MD 20919-3319
(301) 588-9824
(800) 346-2742

Diving Accidents

DIVERS ALERT NETWORK
3100 Tower Blvd., Ste. 1300
Durham, NC 27707
(919) 684-8111

Down Syndrome

NATIONAL DOWN SYNDROME SOCIETY
666 Broadway
New York, NY 10012
(800) 221-4602

Drug Abuse

SEE: *Substance Abuse*

Dyslexia

ORTON DYSLEXIA SOCIETY
Chester Bldg., Ste. 382
860 LaSalle Road
Baltimore, MD 21286-2044
(800) ABCD-123

Eating Disorders

NATIONAL ASSOCIATION OF ANOREXIA NERVOSA AND ASSOCIATED DISORDERS
Box 7
Highland Park, IL 60035
(708) 831-3438

Elderly

AMERICAN ASSOCIATION OF RETIRED PERSONS
801 E Street NW
Washington, DC 20049
(202) 434-2277

AMERICAN GERIATRIC SOCIETY
770 Lexington Avenue, Ste. 300
New York, NY 10015
(212) 308-1414

GERONTOLOGICAL SOCIETY OF AMERICA
1275 K Street NW, Ste. 350
Washington, DC 20005
(202) 842-1275

Emergency Response System

LIFELINE SYSTEMS, INC.
640 Memorial Drive
Cambridge, MA 01239
(800) 321-2042

Epilepsy

EPILEPSY FOUNDATION OF AMERICA
4351 Garden City Drive
Landover, MD 20785
(800) EFA-1000

Gastrointestinal

CROHN'S AND COLITIS FOUNDATION OF AMERICA
386 Park Avenue S.
New York, NY 10016-8804
(800) 932-2423

Hearing Impairment

ALEXANDER GRAHAM BELL ASSOCIATION FOR THE DEAF
3417 Volta Place NW
Washington, DC 20007
(202) 337-5220

BETTER HEARING INSTITUTE
P.O. Box 1840
Washington, DC 20013
(800) EAR WELL
(703) 642-6050

INTERNATIONAL HEARING SOCIETY
20361 Middlebelt Road
Livonia, MI 48512
(800) 521-5247

NATIONAL ASSOCIATION OF THE DEAF
814 Thayer Avenue
Silver Spring, MD 20910
(301) 587-1788

Heart Disease

AMERICAN HEART ASSOCIATION
7272 Greenville Avenue
Dallas, TX 75231-4596
(800) 242-8721

MENDED HEARTS
7272 Greenville Avenue
Dallas, TX 75231-4596
(214) 706-1442

NATIONAL HEART SAVERS ASSOCIATION
9140 W. Dodge Road
Omaha, NE 68114
(402) 398-1993

Hemophilia

NATIONAL HEMOPHILIA FOUNDATION
110 Greene Street, Ste. 303
New York, NY 10012
(800) 424-2634

Kidney Disease

AMERICAN KIDNEY FUND
6110 Executive Blvd., Ste. 1010
Rockville, MD 20852
(800) 638-8299

NATIONAL KIDNEY FOUNDATION
30 E. 33 Street, Suite 1100
New York, NY 10016
(800) 622-9010

Liver Disease

AMERICAN LIVER FOUNDATION
1425 Pompton Avenue
Cedar Grove, NJ 07009
(800) 223-0179

Lung Diseases

SEE: *Respiratory Disorders*

Lupus Erythematosus

LUPUS FOUNDATION OF AMERICA
4 Research Place, Ste. 180
Rockville, MD 20850-3226
(301) 670-9292
(800) 558-0121

Mental Health

ANXIETY DISORDERS ASSOCIATION OF AMERICA
6000 Executive Blvd., Ste. 513
Rockville, MD 20852
(301) 231-9350

DEPRESSION AND RELATED AFFECTIVE DISORDERS
600 N. Wolfe Street
Baltimore, MD 21287-7381
(410) 955-4647

NATIONAL DEPRESSIVE AND MANIC-DEPRESSIVE ASSOCIATION
730 N. Franklin Street, Ste. 501
Chicago, IL 60610
(312) 642-0049

NATIONAL MENTAL HEALTH ASSOCIATION
1015 Prince Street
Alexandria, VA 22314-2971
(703) 684-7722
(800) 969-NMHA

Neurological Disorders

AMYOTROPHIC LATERAL SCLEROSIS ASSOCIATION
21021 Ventura Blvd., Ste. 321
Woodland Hills, CA 91364
(800) 782-4747

MULTIPLE SCLEROSIS FOUNDATION
6350 N. Andrews Avenue
Fort Lauderdale, FL 33309
(800) 441-7055

MUSCULAR DYSTROPHY ASSOCIATION
3300 E. Sunrise Drive
Tucson, AZ 85718
(602) 529-2000

NATIONAL MULTIPLE SCLEROSIS SOCIETY
733 3rd Avenue, 6th Fl.
New York, NY 10017
(212) 986-3240
(800) FIGHT-MS

NORRIS MDA/ALS CENTER
California Pacific Medical Center
P.O. Box 7999
San Francisco, CA 94120
(415) 923-3604

Organ Donation

LIVING BANK
4545 Post Oak Place, Ste. 315
Houston, TX 77027
(800) 528-2971

UNITED NETWORK FOR ORGAN SHARING
P.O. Box 13770
Richmond, VA 23225
(800) 24-DONOR

Pain

AMERICAN CHRONIC PAIN ASSOCIATION
P.O. Box 850
Rocklin, CA 95677
(916) 632-0922

INTERNATIONAL ASSOCIATION FOR THE STUDY OF PAIN
909 NE 43rd Street, Ste. 306
Seattle, WA 98105-6020
(206) 547-6409

Parkinson's Disease

NATIONAL PARKINSON FOUNDATION
1501 N.W. 9th Avenue
Bob Hope Road
Miami, FL 33136
(800) 433-7022

PARKINSON'S DISEASE FOUNDATION, INC.
710 W. 168th Street
New York, NY 10032
(212) 923-4700
(800) 457-6676

Pesticides

NATIONAL PESTICIDE TELECOMMUNICATION NETWORK
Ag Chem Extension, Oregon State University
333 Weniger
Corvallis, OR 97331-6502
(800) 858-7378

Rare Disorders

NATIONAL ORGANIZATION FOR RARE DISORDERS
P.O. Box 9823
New Fairfield, CT 16812
(800) 999-6673

Respiratory Disorders

AMERICAN LUNG ASSOCIATION
1740 Broadway
New York, NY 10019
(212) 315-8700
(800) LUNG-USA

ASTHMA AND ALLERGY FOUNDATION OF AMERICA
11225 15th Street, NW, Ste. 502
Washington, DC 20005
(202) 466-7643
(800) 7ASTHMA

CYSTIC FIBROSIS FOUNDATION
6931 Arlington Road, No. 200
Bethesda, MD 20814
(800) 344-4823

Reye's Syndrome

NATIONAL REYE'S SYNDROME FOUNDATION
426 N. Lewis Street
Bryan, OH 43506
(800) 233-7393

Sickle Cell Anemia

SICKLE CELL DISEASE ASSOCIATION OF AMERICA, INC.
200 Corporate Pointe, Ste. 495
Culver City, CA 90230-7633
(800) 421-8453

Spina Bifida

SPINA BIFIDA ASSOCIATION OF AMERICA
4590 MacArthur Blvd. NW, Ste. 250
Washington, DC 20007
(202) 944-3285
(800) 621-3141

Spinal Cord Injury

NATIONAL SPINAL CORD INJURY ASSOCIATION
545 Concord Avenue, Ste. 29
Cambridge, MA 02138
(800) 962-9629

Substance Abuse

COTTAGE PROGRAM INTERNATIONAL
57 W. South Temple, Ste. 420
Salt Lake City, UT 84101-1511
(800) 752-6100

NATIONAL FAMILIES IN ACTION
2296 Henderson Mill Road, Ste. 300
Atlanta, GA 30345
(404) 934-6364

Tay-Sachs Disease

NATIONAL FOUNDATION FOR JEWISH GENETIC DISEASES
250 Park Avenue, Ste. 1000
New York, NY 10177
(212) 371-1030

Visual Impairment

AMERICAN FOUNDATION FOR THE BLIND
11 Penn Plaza, Ste. 300
New York, NY 10001
(212) 502-7600

LIGHTHOUSE NATIONAL CENTER FOR EDUCATION
111 E. 59th Street
New York, NY 10022
(800) 334-5497

NATIONAL ASSOCIATION FOR VISUALLY HANDICAPPED
22 W. 21st Street
New York, NY 10010
(212) 889-3141

RECORDING FOR THE BLIND AND DYSLEXIC
20 Roszel Road
Princeton, NJ 08540
(800) 221-4792

APPENDIX 4–2 RESOURCE ORGANIZATIONS IN CANADA†

AIDS

AIDS COMMITTEE OF OTTAWA
207 Queens Street, 4th Fl.
Ottawa, Ontario K1P 6E5
(613) 238-5014

---

†Thurn, L (ed): Encyclopedia of Associations: International Organizations, ed 30. Gale Research, New York, 1996.

CANADIAN PUBLIC HEALTH ASSOCIATION
National AIDS Information Clearing House
1565 Carling Avenue, Ste. 400
Ottawa, Ontario K1Z 8R1
(613) 725-3769

Alzheimer's Disease

ALZHEIMER SOCIETY OF CANADA
1320 Yonge Street, Ste. 201
Toronto, Ontario M4T 1X2
(416) 925-3552

Arthritis

ARTHRITIS SOCIETY
250 Bloor Street E, Ste. 901
Toronto, Ontario M4W 3P2
(416) 967-1414

Birth Defects

ABOUTFACE
99 Crowns Lane, 4th Fl.
Toronto, Ontario M5R 3P4
(800) 665-3223

Cancer

CANADIAN CANCER SOCIETY
National Office
10 Alcorn Avenue, Ste. 200
Toronto, Ontario M4V 3B1
(416) 961-7223

Diabetes

CANADIAN DIABETES ASSOCIATION
15 Toronto Street, Ste. 800
Toronto, Ontario M5C 2E3
(416) 363-3373

Eating Disorders

NATIONAL EATING DISORDERS INFORMATION CENTRE
College Wing, 1-211
200 Elizabeth Street
Toronto, Ontario M5G-2C4
(416) 340-4156
(416) 340-3440

Hearing Impairment

CANADIAN ASSOCIATION OF THE DEAF
205-2435 Holly Lane
Ottawa, Ontario K1V 7P2
(613) 526-4785
(613) VOICE/TTY

Heart Disease

CANADIAN ADULT CONGENITAL HEART NETWORK
The Toronto Hospital
200 Elizabeth Street, Rm. 12NU-119
Toronto, Ontario M5G 2C4
(416) 340-3872
(416) 340-5014

CANADIAN CARDIOVASCULAR SOCIETY
360 Victoria Avenue, Rm 401
Westmont, Quebec H3Z 2N4
(514) 482-3407
(514) 482-6574

Hemophilia

WORLD FEDERATION OF HEMOPHILIA
1310 Greene Avenue, Ste. 500
Montreal, Quebec H3Z 2B2
(514) 933-7944

Kidney

KIDNEY FOUNDATION OF CANADA
2300 René LeVesque Blvd.
Montreal, Quebec H3Z 2Z3
(514) 938-4515

Liver

CANADIAN LIVER FOUNDATION
365 Bloor Street E, Ste. 200
Toronto, Ontario M4W 3L4
(416) 964-1953

Mental Health

CANADIAN MENTAL HEALTH ASSOCIATION
1560 Yonge Street
Toronto, Ontario M4S 2Z3
(416) 484-7750

Neurological Disorders

ALS SOCIETY OF CANADA
220 - 6 Adelaide Street E
Toronto, Ontario M5C 1H6
(416) 362-0269
(800) 267-4ALS

CANADIAN ASSOCIATION OF FRIEDREICH'S ATAXIA
5620, rue C.A. Jobin
Montreal, Quebec H1P 1H8
(514) 321-8684

Organ Donation

M.O.R.E. OF ONTARIO
984 Bay Street, Ste. 503
Toronto, Ontario M5S 2A5
(416) 921-1130
(800) 263-2833

Reproductive Disorders

CANADIAN PELVIC INFLAMMATORY DISEASE SOCIETY
P.O. Box 33804, Sta. D
Vancouver, British Columbia V6J 4L6

INFERTILITY AWARENESS ASSOCIATION OF CANADA
774 Echo Drive, Ste. 523
Ottawa, Ontario K7S 5N8
(613) 730-1322

Respiratory Disorders

INTERNATIONAL CYSTIC FIBROSIS (MUCOVISCIDOSIS) ASSOCIATION
323 Lippens Avenue
Montreal, Quebec H2M 1H7
(514) 381-0922

LUNG ASSOCIATION
Three Raymond Street
Ottawa, Ontario K1R 1A3
(613) 230-4200

Visual Impairment

CANADIAN COUNCIL OF THE BLIND
405-396 Cooper Street
Ottawa, Ontario K2P 2H7
(613) 567-0311

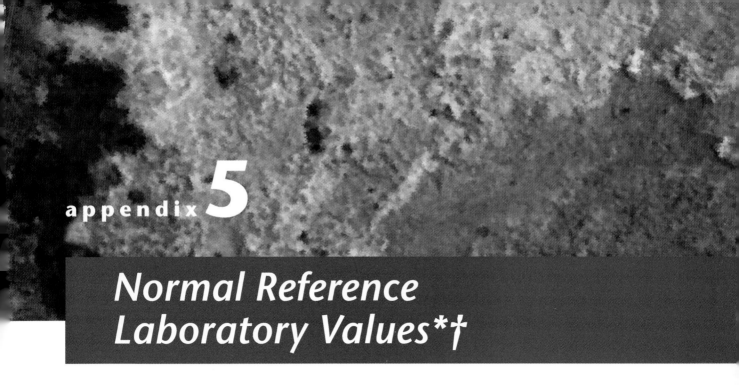

Normal Reference Laboratory Values*†

Blood, Plasma, or Serum Values

Determination	Reference Range Conventional	SI	Minimal ml Required	Note
Acetoacetate plus acetone	Negative		1-B	
Aldolase	1.3–8.2 U/L	22–137 nmol · sec⁻¹/L	2-S	Use unhemolyzed serum
Ammonia	12–55 μmol/L	12–55 μmol/L	2-B	Collect in heparinized tube; deliver *immediately* packed in ice
Amylase	4–25 units/ml	4–25 arb. unit	1-S	
Ascorbic acid	0.4–1.5 mg/100 ml	23–85 μmol/L	7-B	Collect in heparinized tube before any food is given
Bilirubin	Direct: up to 0.4 mg/ 100 ml	Up to 7 μmol/L	1-S	
	Total: up to 1.0 mg/ 100 ml	Up to 17 μmol/L		
Blood volume	8.5–9.0% of body weight in kg	80–85 ml/kg		
Calcium	8.5–10.5 mg/100 ml (slightly higher in children)	2.1–2.6 mmol/L	1-S	
Carbamazepine	4.0–12.0 μg/ml	17–51 μmol/L		
Carbon dioxide content	24–30 mEq/L	24–30 mmol/L	1-S	Fill tube to top
Carbon monoxide	Less than 5% of total hemoglobin		3-B	Fill tube to top

Table continued on following page

*From Scully, RE (ed): Case Records of the Massachusetts General Hospital. N Engl J Med 314:39–49, 1986, with permission.

†Abbreviations used: SI = Système International d'Unités; P = plasma; S = serum; B = blood; and U = urine.

Blood, Plasma, or Serum Values (*Continued*)

Determination	Reference Range		Minimal ml Required	Note
	Conventional	SI		
Carotenoids	0.8–4.0 µg/ml	1.5–7.4 µmol/L	3-S	Vitamin A may be done on same specimen
Ceruloplasmin	27–37 mg/100 ml	1.8–2.5 µmol/L	2-S	
Chloramphenicol	10–20 µg/ml	31–62 µmol/L	0.2-S	
Chloride	100–106 mEq/L	100–106 mmol/L	1-S	
CK isoenzymes	5% MB or less		0.2-S	
Copper	Total: 100–200 µg/ 100 ml	16–31 µmol/L	1-S	
Creatine kinase (CK)	Female: 10–79 U/L	167–1317 nmol · sec^{-1}/L	1-S	
	Male: 17–148 U/L	283–2467 nmol · sec^{-1}/L		
Creatinine	0.6–1.5 mg/100 ml	53–133 µmol/L	1-S	
Ethanol	0 mg/100 ml	0 mmol/L	2-B	Collect in oxalate and refrigerate
Glucose	Fasting: 70–110 mg/ 100 ml	3.9–5.6 mmol/L	1-P	Collect with oxalate–fluoride mixture
Iron	50–150 µg/100 ml (higher in males)	9.0–26.9 µmol/L	1-S	
Iron-binding capacity	250–410 µg/100 ml	44.8–73.4 µmol/L	1-S	
Lactic acid	0.6–1.8 mEq/L	0.6–1.8 mmol/L	2-B	Collect with oxalate– fluoride; deliver immediately packed in ice
Lactic dehydro-genase	45–90 U/L	750–1500 nmol · sec^{-1}/L	1-S	Unsuitable if hemolyzed
Lead	50 µg/100 ml or less	Up to 2.4 µmol/L	2-B	Collect with oxalate–fluoride mixture
Lipase	2 units/ml or less	Up to 2 arb. unit	1-S	
Lipids				
Cholesterol	120–220 mg/100 ml	3.10–5.69 mmol/L	1-S	Fasting
Triglycerides	40–150 mg/100 ml	0.4–1.5 g/L	1-S	Fasting
Lipoprotein elec-trophoresis (LEP)			2-S	Fasting, do not freeze serum
Lithium	0.5–1.5 mEq/L	0.5–1.5 mmol/L	1-S	
Magnesium	1.5–2.0 mEq/L	0.8–1.3 mmol/L	1-S	
5′ Nucleotidase	1–11 U/L	17–183 nmol · sec^{-1}/L	1-S	
Osmolality	280–296 mOsm/ kg water	280–296 mmol/kg	1-S	
Oxygen saturation (arterial)	96–100%	0.96–1.00	3-B	Deliver in sealed heparinized syringe packed in ice
PCO$_2$	35–45 mm Hg	4.7–6.0 kPa	2-B	Collect and deliver in sealed heparinized syringe
pH	7.35–7.45	Same	2-B	Collect without stasis in sealed heparinized syringe; deliver packed in ice
PO$_2$	75–100 mm Hg (dependent on age) while breathing room air Above 500 mm Hg while on 100% O$_2$	10.0–13.3 kPa	2-B	
Phenobarbital	15–50 µg/ml	65–215 µmol/L	1-S	

Table continued on following page

Blood, Plasma, or Serum Values (*Continued*)

| Determination | Reference Range | | Minimal ml Required | Note |
	Conventional	SI		
Phenytoin (Dilantin)	5–20 µg/ml	20–80 µmol/L	1-S	
Phosphatase (acid)	Male—Total: 0.13–0.63 sigma U/ml	36–175 nmol · sec⁻¹/L	1-S	Must always be drawn just before analysis or stored as frozen serum; avoid hemolysis
	Female—Total: 0.01–0.56 sigma U/ml	2.8–156 nmol · sec⁻¹/L		
	Prostatic: 0–0.5 Fishman–Lerner U/100 ml			
Phosphatase (alkaline)	13–39 U/L, infants and adolescents up to 104 U/L	217–650 nmol · sec⁻¹/L, up to 1.26 µmol · sec⁻¹/L	1-S	
Phosphorus (inorganic)	3.0–4.5 mg/100 ml (infants in first year up to 6.0 mg/100 ml)	1.0–1.5 mmol/L	1-S	
Potassium	3.5–5.0 mEq/L	3.5–5.0 mmol/L	1-S	Serum must be separated promptly from cells
Primidone (Mysoline)	4–12 µg/ml	18–55 µmol/L	1-S	
Procainamide	4–10 µg/ml	17–42 µmol/L	1-S	
Protein: Total	6.0–8.4 g/100 ml	60–84 g/L	1-S	
Albumin	3.5–5.0 g/100 ml	35–50 g/L	1-S	
Globulin	2.3–3.5 g/100 ml	23–35 g/L		Globulin equals total protein minus albumin
Electrophoresis	(% of total protein)		1-S	Quantitation by densitometry
Albumin	52–68			
Globulin:				
Alpha₁	4.2–7.2			
Alpha₂	6.8–12			
Beta	9.3–15			
Gamma	13–23			
Pyruvic acid	0–0.11 mEq/L	0–0.11 mmol/L	2-B	Collect with oxalate fluoride. Deliver immediately packed in ice
Quinidine	1.2–4.0 µg/ml	3.7–12.3 µmol/L	1-S	
Salicylate:	0		2-P	
Therapeutic	20–25 mg/100 ml;	1.4–1.8 mmol/L		
	25–30 mg/100 ml to age 10 yr 3 hr post dose	1.8–2.2 mmol/L		
Sodium	135–145 mEq/L	135–145 mmol/L	1-S	
Sulfonamide	5–15 mg/100 ml		2-P	
Transaminase, aspartate amino-transferase	7–27 U/L	117–450 nmol · sec⁻¹/L	1-S	
Transaminase, alanine amino-transferase	1–21 U/L	17–350 nmol · sec⁻¹/L	1-S	
Urea nitrogen (BUN)	8–25 mg/100 ml	2.9–8.9 mmol/L	1-S	
Uric acid	3.0–7.0 mg/100 ml	0.18–0.42 mmol/L	1-S	
Vitamin A	0.15–0.6 µg/ml	0.5–2.1 µmol/L	3-S	

Table continued on following page

Urine Values

Determination	Reference Range Conventional	SI	Minimal ml Required	Note
Acetone plus aceto-acetate (quantitative)	0	0 mg/L	2 ml	
Amylase	24–76 units/ml	24–76 arb. unit		
Calcium	300 mg/day or less	7.5 mmol/day or less	24-hr specimen	Collect in special bottle with 10 ml of concentrated HCl
Catecholamines	Epinephrine: under 20 µg/day	<109 nmol/day	24-hr specimen	Should be collected with 10 ml of concentrated HCl (pH should be between 2.0 and 3.0)
	Norepinephrine: under 100 µg/day	<590 nmol/day		
Chorionic gonado-tropin	0	0 arb. unit	1st morning void	
Copper	0–100 µg/day	0–1.6 µmol/day	24-hr specimen	
Coproporphyrin	50–250 µg/day	80–380 nmol/day	24-hr specimen	Collect with 5 g of sodium carbonate
	Children under 80 lb (36 kg): 0–75 µg/day	0–115 nmol/day		
Creatine	Under 100 mg/day or less than 6% of creatinine. In pregnancy: up to 12%. In children under 1 yr: may equal creatinine. In older children: up to 30% of creatinine.	<0.75 mmol/day	24-hr specimen	Also order creatinine
Creatinine	15–25 mg/kg of body weight/day	0.13–0.22 mmol · kg^{-1}/day	24-hr specimen	
Cystine or cysteine	0	0	10 ml	Qualitative
Hemoglobin and myoglobin	0		Freshly voided sample	Chemical examination with benzidine
5-Hydroxyindole-acetic acid	2–9 mg/day (women lower than men)	10–45 µmol/day	24-hr specimen	Collect with 10 ml of concentrated HCl
Lead	0.08 µg/ml or 120 µg/day or less	0.39 µmol/L or less	24-hr specimen	
Phosphorus (inorganic)	Varies with intake; average, 1 g/day	32 mmol/day	24-hr specimen	Collect with 10 ml of concentrated HCl
Porphobilinogen	0	0	10 ml	Use freshly voided urine
Protein: Quantitative	<150 mg/24 hr	<0.15 g/day	24-hr specimen	
Steroids: 17-Ketosteroids (per day)			24-hr specimen	Not valid if patient is receiving meprobamate

Age	Male	Female		
10	1–4 mg	1–4 mg	3–14 µmol	3–14 µmol
20	6–21	4–16	21–73	14–56
30	8–26	4–14	28–90	14–49
50	5–18	3–9	17–62	10–31
70	2–10	1–7	7–35	3–24

Determination	Conventional	SI	Minimal ml Required	Note
17-Hydroxysteroids	3–8 mg/day (women lower than men)	8–22 µmol/day as tetrahydro-cortisol	24-hr specimen	Keep cold; chlorpromazine and related drugs interfere with assay

Table continued on following page

Urine Values (*Continued*)

Determination	Reference Range Conventional	SI	Minimal ml Required	Note
Sugar: Quantitative glucose	0	0 mmol/L	24-hr or other timed specimen	
Urobilinogen	Up to 1.0 Ehrlich U	To 1.0 arb. unit	2-hr sample (1–3 p.m.)	
Uroporphyrin	0–30 μg/day	<36 nmol/day	See *Coproporphyrin*	
Vanillylmandelic acid (VMA)	Up to 9 mg/24 hr	Up to 45 μmol/day	24-hr specimen	Collect as for catecholamines

Special Endocrine Tests

Steroid Hormones

Determination	Reference Range Conventional	SI	Minimal ml Required	Note
Aldosterone	Excretion: 5–19 μg/24 hr	14–53 nmol/day	5/day	Keep specimen cold
	Supine: 48 ± 29 pg/ml	133 ± 80 pmol/L	3-S, P	Fasting, at rest, 210-mEq sodium diet
	Upright (2 hr): 65 ± 23 pg/ml	180 ± 64 pmol/L		Upright, 2 hr, 210-mEq sodium diet
	Supine: 107 ± 45 pg/ml	279 ± 125 pmol/L		Fasting, at rest, 110-mEq sodium diet
	Upright (2 hr): 239 ± 123 pg/ml	663 ± 341 pmol/L		Upright, 2 hr, 110-mEq sodium diet
	Supine: 175 ± 75 pg/ml	485 ± 208 pmol/L		Fasting, at rest, 10-mEq sodium diet
	Upright (2 hr): 532 ± 228 pg/ml	1476 ± 632 pmol/L		Upright, 2 hr, 10-mEq sodium diet
Cortisol	8 a.m.: 5–25 μg/100 ml	0.14–0.69 μmol/L	1-P	Fasting
	8 p.m.: Below 10 μg/100 ml	0–0.28 μmol/L	1-P	At rest
	4-hr ACTH test: 30–45 μg/100 ml	0.83–1.24 μmol/L	1-P	20 U ACTH, IV per 4 hr
	Overnight suppression test: Below 5 μg/100 ml	0.14 nmol/L	1-P	8 a.m. sample after 0.5 mg dexamethasone by mouth at midnight
	Excretion: 20–70 μg/24 hr	55–193 nmol/day	2/day	Keep specimen cold
Dehydroepiandrosterone (DHEA)	Male: 0.5–5.5 ng/ml	1.7–19 nmol/L	2-S, P	
	Female: 1.4–8.0 ng/ml	4.9–28 nmol/L		Adult
	0.3–4.5 ng/ml	1.0–15.6 nmol/L		Postmenopausal

Table continued on following page

Special Endocrine Tests (*Continued*)

Steroid Hormones

Determination	Reference Range		Minimal ml Required	Note
	Conventional	SI		
Dehydroepiandro-sterone sulfate (DHEA-S)	Male:		2-S, P	
	151–446 µg/100 ml	3.9–11.4 µgmol/L		
	Female:			
	84–433 µg/100 ml	2.2–11.1 µmol/L		Adult
	1.7–177 µg/100 ml	0.04–4.5 µmol/L		Postmenopausal
11-Deoxycortisol	Responsive:		1-P	8 a.m. sample, preceded by 4.5 g of metyrapone by mouth per 24 hr or by single dose of 2.5 g by mouth at midnight
	Over 7.5 µg/100 ml	>0.22 µmol/L		
Estradiol	Male: <50 pg/ml	<184 pmol/L	5-S, P	
	Female: 23–361 pg/ml	84–1325 pmol/L		Adult
	<30 pg/ml	<110 pmol/L		Postmenopausal
	<20 pg/ml	<73 pmol/L		Prepubertal
Progesterone	Male: <1.0 ng/ml	<3.2 nmol/L	5-S, P	
	Female:			
	0.2–0.6 ng/ml	0.6–1.9 nmol/L		Follicular phase
	0.3–3.5 ng/ml	0.95–11 nmol/L		Midcycle peak
	6.5–32.2 ng/ml	21–102 nmol/L		Postovulatory
Testosterone	Adult male:		1-P	a.m. sample
	300–1100 ng/100 ml	10.4–38.1 nmol/L		
	Adolescent male:			
	Over 100 ng/100 ml	>3.5 nmol/L		
	Female:			
	25–90 ng/100 ml	0.87–3.12 nmol/L		
Unbound testos-terone	Adult male:		2-P	a.m. sample
	3.06–24.0 ng/100 ml	106–832 pmol/L		
	Adult female:			
	0.09–1.28 ng/100 ml	3.1–44.4 pmol/L		

Polypeptide Hormones

Determination	Reference Range		Minimal ml Required	Note
	Conventional	SI		
Adrenocorticotropin (ACTH)	15–70 pg/ml	3.3–15.4 pmol/L	5-P	Place specimen on ice and send promptly to laboratory. Use EDTA tube only.
Alpha subunit	<0.5–2.5 ng/ml	<0.4–2.0 nmol/L	2-S	Adult male or female
	<0.5–5.0 ng/ml	<0.4–4.0 nmol/L		Postmenopausal female

Table continued on following page

Special Endocrine Tests (*Continued*)

Polypeptide Hormones

Determination	Reference Range		Minimal ml Required	Note
	Conventional	SI		
Calcitonin	Male: 0–14 pg/ml	0–4.1 pmol/L	5-S	Test done only on known or suspected cases of medullary carcinoma of the thyroid
	Female: 0–28 pg/ml	0–8.2 pmol/L		
	>100 pg/ml in medullary carcinoma	>29.3 pmol/L		
Follicle-stimulating hormone (FSH)	Male: 3–18 mU/ml	3–18 arb. unit	5-S, P	Same sample may be used for LH
	Female: 4.6–22.4 mU/ml	4.6–22.4 arb. unit		Pre- or postovulatory
	13–41 mU/ml	13–41 arb. unit		Midcycle peak
	30–170 mU/ml	30–170 arb. unit		Postmenopausal
Growth hormone	Below 5 ng/ml	<233 pmol/L	1-S	Fasting, at rest
	Children: Over 10 ng/ml	>465 pmol/L		After exercise
	Male: Below 5 ng/ml	<233 pmol/L		
	Female: Up to 30 ng/ml	0–1395 pmol/L		
	Male: Below 5 ng/ml	<233 pmol/L		After glucose load
	Female: Below 5 ng/ml	<233 pmol/L		
Insulin	6–26 µU/ml	43–187 pmol/L	1-S	Fasting
	Below 20 µU/ml	<144 pmol/L		During hypoglycemia
	Up to 150 µU/ml	0–1078 pmol/L		After glucose load
Luteinizing hormone (LH)	Male: 3–18 mU/ml	3–18 arb. unit	5-S, P	Same sample may be used for FSH
	Female:			
	2.4–34.5 mU/ml	2.4–34.5 arb. unit		Pre- or postovulatory
	43–187 mU/ml	43–187 arb. unit		Midcycle peak
	30–150 mU/ml	30–150 arb. unit		Postmenopausal
Parathyroid hormone	<25 pg/ml	<2.94 pmol/L	5-P	Keep blood on ice, or plasma must be frozen if it is to be sent any distance; a.m. sample
Prolactin	2–15 ng/ml	0.08–6.0 nmol/L	2-S	
Renin activity	Supine:		4-P	EDTA tubes, on ice, normal diet
	1.1 ± 0.8 ng/ml/hr	0.9 ± 0.6 nmol/L/hr		
	Upright:			
	1.9 ± 1.7 ng/ml/hr	1.5 ± 1.3 nmol/L/hr		
	Supine:			Low-sodium diet
	2.7 ± 1.8 ng/ml/hr	2.1 ± 1.4 nmol/L/hr		
	Upright:			
	6.6 ± 2.5 ng/ml/hr	5.1 ± 1.9 nmol/L/hr		
	Diuretics:			Low-sodium diet
	10.0 ± 3.7 ng/ml/hr	7.7 ± 2.9 nmol/L/hr		
Somatomedin C (Sm-C, IGF-1)	0.08–2.8 U/ml	0.08–2.8 arb. unit	2-P	EDTA plasma Prepubertal
	0.9–5.9 U/ml	0.9–5.9 arb. unit		During puberty
	0.34–1.9 U/ml	0.34–1.9 arb. unit		Adult males
	0.45–2.2 U/ml	0.45–2.2 arb. unit		Adult females

Special Endocrine Tests (*Continued*)

Thyroid Hormones

Determination	Reference Range		Minimal ml Required	Note
	Conventional	SI		
Thyroid-stimulating hormone (TSH)	0.5–5.0 μU/ml	0.5–5.0 arb. unit	2-S	
Thyroxine-binding globulin capacity	15–25 μg T$_4$/100 ml	193–322 nmol/L	2-S	
Total triiodothyronine (T$_3$)	75–195 ng/100 ml	1.16–3.00 nmol/L	2-S	
Reverse triiodothyronine (rT3)	13–53 ng/ml	0.2–0.8 nmol/L	2-S	
Total thyroxine by RIA (T$_4$)	4–12 μg/100 ml	52–154 nmol/L	1-S	
T$_3$ resin uptake	25–35%	0.25–0.35	2-S	
Free thyroxine index (FT$_4$I)	1–4		2-S	

Vitamin D Derivatives

Determination	Reference Range		Minimal ml Required	Note
	Conventional	SI		
1,25-Dihydroxyvitamin D	26–65 pg/ml	62–155 pmol/L	1-S	
25-Hydroxyvitamin D	8–55 ng/ml	19.4–137 nmol/L	1-S	

Hematologic Values

Determination	Reference Range		Minimal ml Required	Note
	Conventional	SI		
Coagulation factors:				
Factor I (fibrinogen)	0.15–0.35 g/100 ml	4.0–10.0 μmol/L	4.5-P	Collect in Vacutainer containing sodium citrate
Factor II (prothrombin)	60–140%	0.60–1.40	4.5-P	Collect in plastic tubes with 3.8% sodium citrate
Factor V (accelerator globulin)	60–140%	0.60–1.40	4.5-P	Collect as in factor II determination
Factor VII-X (proconvertin-Stuart)	70–130%	0.70–1.30	4.5-P	Collect as in factor II determination
Factor X (Stuart factor)	70–130%	0.70–1.30	4.5-P	Collect as in factor II determination
Factor VIII (antihemophilic globulin)	50–200%	0.50–2.0	4.5-P	Collect as in factor II determination
Factor IX (plasma thromboplastic cofactor)	60–140%	0.60–1.40	4.5-P	Collect as in factor II determination

Table continued on following page

Special Endocrine Tests *(Continued)*

Hematologic Values

Determination	Reference Range Conventional	SI	Minimal ml Required	Note
Factor XI (plasma thromboplastic antecedent)	60–140%	0.60–1.40	4.5-P	Collect as in factor II determination
Factor XII (Hageman factor)	60–140%	0.60–1.40	4.5-P	Collect as in factor II determination
Coagulation screening tests:				
Bleeding time (Simplate)	3–9.5 min	180–570 sec		
Prothrombin time	Less than 2-sec deviation from control	Less than 2-sec deviation from control	4.5-P	Collect in Vacutainer containing 3.8% sodium citrate
Partial thromboplastin time (activated)	25–38 sec	25–38 sec	4.5-P	Collect in Vacutainer containing 3.8% sodium citrate
Whole-blood clot lysis	No clot lysis in 24 hr	0/day	2.0-whole blood	Collect in sterile tube and incubate at 37°C
Fibrinolytic studies:				
Euglobin lysis	No lysis in 2 hr	0/2 hr	4.5-P	Collect as in factor II determination
Fibrinogen split products	Negative reaction at >1:4 dilution	0 (at 1:4 dilution)	4.5-S	Collect in special tube containing thrombin and epsilon aminocaproic acid
Thrombin time	Control ± 5 sec	Control ± 5 sec	4.5-P	Collect as in factor II determination
"Complete" blood count:				
Hematocrit	Male: 45–52% Female: 37–48%	Male: 0.45–0.52 Female: 0.37–0.48	1-B	Use EDTA as anticoagulant; the seven listed tests are performed automatically on the Ortho ELT 800, which directly determines cell counts, hemoglobin (as the cyan-methemoglobin derivative), and MCV and computes hematocrit, MCH, and MCHC
Hemoglobin	Male: 13–18 g/100 ml Female: 12–16 g/100 ml	Male: 8.1–11.2 mmol/L Female: 7.4–9.9 mmol/L		
Leukocyte count	4300–10,800/mm^3	4.3–10.8 × 10^9/L		
Erythrocyte count	4.2–5.9 million/mm^3	4.2–5.9 × 10^{12}/L		
Mean corpuscular volume (MCV)	86–98 μm^3/cell	86–98 ft		
Mean corpuscular hemoglobin (MCH)	27–32 pg/RBC	1.7–2.0 pg/cell		
Mean corpuscular hemoglobin concentration (MCHC)	32–36%	0.32–0.36		
Erythrocyte sedimentation rate	Male: 1–13 mm/hr Female: 1–20 mm/hr	Male: 1–13 mm/hr Female: 1–20 mm/hr	5-B	Use EDTA as anticoagulant
Erythrocyte enzyme:				
Glucose-6-phosphate dehydrogenase	5–15 U/g Hb	5–15 U/g	9-B	Use special anticoagulant (ACD solution)

Table continued on following page

Special Endocrine Tests (*Continued*)

Hematologic Values

Determination	Reference Range Conventional	SI	Minimal ml Required	Note
Pyruvate kinase	13–17 U/g Hb	13–17 U/g	8-B	Use special anticoagulant (ACD solution)
Ferritin (serum)				
Iron deficiency	0–12 ng/ml	0–4.8 nmol/L		
	13–20 Borderline	5.2–8 nmol/L Borderline		
Iron excess	>400 ng/L	>160 nmol/L		
Folic acid				
Normal	>3.3 ng/ml	>7.3 nmol/L	1-S	
Borderline	2.5–3.2 ng/ml	5.75–7.39 nmol/L	1-S	
Haptoglobin	40–336 mg/100 ml	0.4–3.36 g/L	1-S	
Hemoglobin studies:				
Electrophoresis for abnormal hemoglobin			5-B	Collect with anticoagulant
Electrophoresis for A_2 hemoglobin	3.0%	0.015–0.035	5-B	Use oxalate as anticoagulant
Borderline	0.3–3.5%	0.03–0.035		
Hemoglobin F (fetal hemoglobin)	Less than 2%	<0.02	5-B	Collect with anticoagulant
Hemoglobin, met- and sulf-	0	0	5-B	Use heparin as anticoagulant
Serum hemoglobin	2–3 mg/100 ml	1.2–1.9 μmol/L	2-S	
Thermolabile hemoglobin	0	0	1-B	Any anticoagulant
Lupus antico-agulant	0	0	4.5-P	Collect as in factor II determination
LE (lupus erythema-tosus) preparation:				
Method I	0	0	5-B	Use heparin as anticoagulant
Method II	0	0	5-B	Use defibrinated blood
Leukocyte alkaline phosphatase:			20-Isolated blood leukocytes	Special handling of blood necessary
Qualitative method	Males: 33–188 U	33–188 U	Smear-B	
	Females (off contra-ceptive pill): 30–160 U	30–160 U		
Muramidase	Serum, 3–7 μg/ml	3–7 mg/L	1-S	
	Urine, 0–2 μg/ml	0.2 μg/L	1-U	
Osmotic fragility of erythrocytes	Increased if hemolysis occurs in over 0.5% NaCl; decreased if hemolysis is incomplete in 0.3% NaCl		5-B	Use heparin as anti-coagulant
Peroxide hemolysis	Less than 10%	0.10	6-B	Use EDTA as anticoagulant
Platelet count	150,000–350,000/ mm³	$150–350 \times 10^9$/L	0.5-B	Use EDTA as anticoagulant; counts are performed on Clay Adams Ultraflow; when counts are low, results are confirmed by hand counting

Table continued on following page

Special Endocrine Tests (*Continued*)

Hematologic Values

| Determination | Reference Range | | Minimal ml Required | Note |
	Conventional	SI		
Platelet function tests:				
Clot retraction	50–100%/2 hr	0.50–1.00/2 hr	4.5-P	Collect as in factor II determination
Platelet aggregation	Full response to ADP, epinephrine, and collagen	1.0	18-P	Collect as in factor II determination
Platelet factor 3	33–57 sec	33–57 sec	4.5-P	Collect as in factor II determination
Reticulocyte count	0.5–2.5% red cells	0.005–0.025	0.1-B	
Vitamin B_{12}	205–876 pg/ml	150–674 pmol/L	12-S	
Borderline	140–204 pg/ml	102.6–149 pmol/L		

Cerebrospinal Fluid Values

| Determination | Reference Range | | Minimal ml Required | Note |
	Conventional	SI		
Bilirubin	0	0	2	
Cell count	0–5 mononuclear cells		0.5	
Chloride	120–130 mEq/L	120–130 mmol/L	0.5	
Colloidal gold	0000000000–0001222111	Same	0.1	
Albumin	Mean: 29.5 mg/100 ml	0.295 g/L	2.5	
	±2 SD: 11–48 mg/100 ml	± 2 SD: 0.11–0.48		
IgG	Mean: 4.3 mg/100 ml	0.043 g/L		
	±2 SD: 0–8.6 mg/100 ml	±2 SD: 0–0.086		
Glucose	50–75 mg/100 ml	2.8–4.2 mmol/L	0.5	
Pressure (initial)	70–180 mm of water	70–180 arb. unit		
Protein:				
Lumbar	15–45 mg/100 ml	0.15–0.45 g/L	1	
Cisternal	15–25 mg/100 ml	0.15–0.25 g/L	1	
Ventricular	5–15 mg/100 ml	0.05–0.15 g/L	1	

Miscellaneous Values

| Determination | Reference Range | | Minimal ml Required | Note |
	Conventional	SI		
Carcinoembryonic antigen (CEA)	0–2.5 ng/ml	0–2.5 µg/L	20-P	Must be sent on ice
Chylous fluid				Use fresh specimen
Digitoxin	17 ± 6 ng/ml	22 ± 7.8 nmol/L	1-S	Medication with digitoxin or digitalis
Digoxin	1.2 ± 0.4 ng/ml	1.54 ± 0.5 nmol/L	1-S	Medication with digoxin 0.25 mg per day
	1.5 ± 0.4 ng/ml	1.92 ± 0.5 nmol/L	1-S	Medication with digoxin 0.5 mg per day

Table continued on following page

Special Endocrine Tests (*Continued*)

Miscellaneous Values

Determination	Reference Range		Minimal ml Required	Note
	Conventional	SI		
Duodenal drainage				pH should be in proper range with minimal amount of gastric juice
pH (urine)	5–7	5–7		
Gastric analysis	Basal:			
	Females: 2.0 ± 1.8 mEq/hr	0.6 ± 0.5 μmol/sec		
	Males: 3.0 ± 2.0 mEq/hr	0.8 ± 0.6 μmol/sec		
	Maximal (after histalog or gastrin):			
	Females: 16 ± 5 mEq/hr	4.4 ± 1.4 μmol/sec		
	Males: 23 ± 5 mEq/hr	6.4 ± 1.4 μmol/sec		
Gastrin-I	0–200 pg/ml	0–95 pmol/L	4-P	Heparinized sample
Immunologic tests:				
Alpha-fetoprotein	Undetectable in normal adults		2-S	
Alpha-I-antitrypsin	85–213 mg/100 ml	0.85–2.13 g/L	10-B	
Rheumatoid factor	<60 IU/ml		10 ml clotted blood	Fasting sample preferred
Antinuclear antibodies	Negative at a 1:8 dilution of serum		2-S	Send to laboratory promptly
Anti-DNA antibodies	Negative at a 1:10 dilution of serum		2-S	
Antibodies to Sm and RNP (ENA)	None detected		10 ml clotted blood	
Antibodies to SS-A (Ro) and SS-B (La)	None detected		10 ml clotted blood	
Autoantibodies to:				
Thyroid colloid and microsomal antigens	Negative at a 1:10 dilution of serum		2-S	Low titers in some elderly normal women
Gastric parietal cells	Negative at a 1:20 dilution of serum		2-S	
Smooth muscle	Negative at a 1:20 dilution of serum		2-S	
Mitochondria	Negative at a 1:20 dilution of serum		2-S	
Interstitial cells of the testes	Negative at a 1:10 dilution of serum		2-S	
Skeletal muscle	Negative at a 1:60 dilution of serum		2-S	
Adrenal gland	Negative at a 1:10 dilution of serum		2-S	
Bence Jones protein	No Bence-Jones protein detected in a 50-fold concentrate of urine		50-U	
Complement, total hemolytic	150–250 U/ml		10-B	Must be sent on ice

Table continued on following page

Special Endocrine Tests (*Continued*)

Miscellaneous Values

| Determination | Reference Range | | Minimal ml Required | Note |
	Conventional	SI		
Cryoprecipitable proteins	None detected	0 arb. unit	10-S	Collect and transport at 37°C
C3	Range, 83–177 mg/100 ml	0.83–1.77 g/L	2-S	
C4	Range, 15–45 mg/100 ml	0.15–0.45 g/L	2-S	
Factor B	12–30 mg/100 ml		5 ml clotted blood	
C1 esterase inhibitor	13.2–24 mg/100 ml		5 ml clotted blood	
Hemoglobin A_{1e}	3.8–6.4%	0.038–0.064	5-P	Send EDTA tube on ice promptly to laboratory
Hypersensitivity pneumonitis screen	No antibodies to those antigens assayed		5 ml clotted blood	
Immunoglobulins:				
IgG	639–1349 mg/100 ml	6.39–13.49 g/L	2-S	
IgA	70–312 mg/100 ml	0.7–312 g/L	2-S	
IgM	86–352 mg/100 ml	0.86–3.52 g/L	2-S	
Viscosity	1.4–1.8 relative viscosity units		10-B	Expressed as the relative viscosity of serum compared with water
Iontophoresis	Children: 0–40 mEq sodium/L	0–40 mmol/L		Value given in terms of sodium
	Adults: 0–60 mEq sodium/L	0–60 mmol/L		
Propranolol (includes bioactive 4-OH metabolite)	100–300 ng/ml	386–1158 nmol/L	1-S	Obtain blood sample 4 hr after last dose of beta-blocking agent
Stool fat	Less than 5 g in 24 hr or less than 4% of measured fat intake in 3-day period	<5 g/day	24-hr or 3-day specimen	
Stool nitrogen	Less than 2 g/day or 10% of urinary nitrogen	<2 g/day	24-hr or 3-day specimen	
Synovial fluid:				
Glucose	Not less than 20 mg/100 ml lower than simultaneously drawn blood sugar	See Blood Glucose	ml of fresh fluid	Collect with oxalate–fluoride mixture
D-Xylose absorption	5–8 g/5 hr in urine; 40 mg per	33–53 mmol/day	5-U	For directions see Benson et al.: N Engl J Med 256:335, 1957
	100 ml in blood 2 hr after ingestion of 25 g of D-xylose	2.7 mmol/L	5-B	

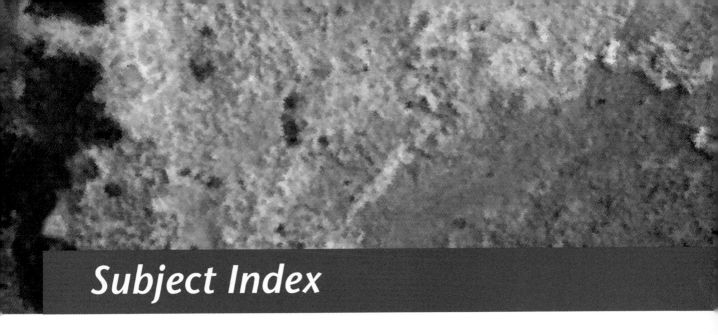

Subject Index

Numbers followed by an "f" indicate figures; numbers followed by a "t" indicate tabular material.

A

Abdominal artery aneurysm, 199–200, 199f
Abdominal hernia, 140–141
Abdominopelvic trauma, 11
ABGs. *See* Arterial blood gas(es)
ABO incompatibility, 60
Abortion, spontaneous, 118
Abrasion, 293
  definition of, 347
Abruptio placentae, 121
Abscess
  brain, 232–233, 233f
  lung, 163–165, 164f
Acetabulum, 65
  definition of, 347
Acetylcholine, 277, 330
  definition of, 347
Acidosis
  definition of, 347
  in osteoporosis, 269
  respiratory, 175
Acne vulgaris, 288, 289f
Acquired immunity, 15
Acquired immunodeficiency
     syndrome (AIDS), 17, 25t, 27t,
     30–32, 162t, 169
Acral-lentiginous melanoma, 303–304
Acromegaly, 247–248, 248f
ACTH. *See* Adrenocorticotropic
     hormone
Acupressure, 225
Acupuncture, 333
Acute disease, definition of, 347

Acute infection, 26
Acute lymphoblastic leukemia (ALL), 208
Acute lymphocytic leukemia. *See*
     Acute lymphoblastic leukemia
Acute monoblastic leukemia, 208
Acute monocytic leukemia. *See* Acute
     monoblastic leukemia
Acute myeloblastic leukemia (AML),
     47, 207–208
Acute myelogenous leukemia. *See*
     Acute myeloblastic leukemia
Acute pain, 330–331
Acute poststreptococcal
     glomerulonephritis. *See*
     Glomerulonephritis
Acute tubular necrosis (ATN), 81
Acyanotic heart defect(s), 61
Adenocarcinoma, 47
  of kidney, 85
Adenoid hyperplasia, 178
Adenoidectomy, 178
Adenoma, 47
  definition of, 347
  of parathyroid gland, 254
  of pituitary gland, 247
Adolescence, communicable diseases
     of, 33–34
Adrenal gland disease(s), 246t,
     255–256
Adrenocorticotropic hormone
     (ACTH), 238, 249, 255
  definition of, 347
African sleeping sickness, 8
Aganglionic megacolon. *See*
     Hirschsprung's disease

Age, as predisposing factor, 3
Agnosia, 228
  definition of, 347
Agraphia, 228
  definition of, 347
AIDS. *See* Acquired immunodeficiency
     syndrome
Airway obstruction, 13, 175
Alanine aminotransferase, 361
Albumin, urine, 77t
Alcohol use, 18, 46–47, 147
Alexia, 228
  definition of, 347
Alkaline phosphatase, 361
Alkalosis
  in bulimia, 150
  definition of, 347
  respiratory, 175
ALL. *See* Acute lymphoblastic
     leukemia
Allergen, 16
  definition of, 347
Allergy, 15–16, 16f
  food, 16, 151
Allogenic transplantation, 212
Alopecia, 289–291, 290f
  definition of, 347
  in syphilis, 103
  in systemic lupus erythematosus,
     278
Alopecia areata, 290f
ALS. *See* Amyotrophic lateral sclerosis
Alternative medicine
  for cancer, 51–52
  for circulatory system disease, 213
  for colds and flu, 29

Alternative medicine — Continued
for digestive system disease, 152
for headache, 225
for musculoskeletal disease, 274, 276
for pain management, 333–334
Alveolus, 66, 162
definition of, 347
Alzheimer's disease, 236–237
Amblyopia, 318
definition of, 347
Amebic dysentery, 8, 27t
Amenorrhea, 111, 249
definition of, 347
primary, 111
secondary, 111
Amino acid, 4
definition of, 347
AML. *See* Acute myeloblastic leukemia
Ammonia, blood, 212
Amniocentesis, 361
Amniotic fluid, 61
definition of, 347
Amsler's chart, 316
Amyotrophic lateral sclerosis (ALS), 238
ANA. *See* Antinuclear antibody
Analgesia, patient-controlled, 331, 331f
Analgesic(s), 331
for cold temperature disorders, 12
definition of, 347
for headache, 222, 224
for pericarditis, 188
for prostatitis, 105
for sinusitis, 160
for spinal cord deformities, 266
Anaphylactic shock, 16
Anaphylaxis, 16
definition of, 347
Anaplasia, 44, 48
definition of, 347
Anastomosis, 64
definition of, 347
Anemia, 202–207
aplastic, 204f, 205–206
Cooley's. *See* Thalassemia
erythroblastic. *See* Thalassemia
folic acid deficiency, 204–205
hemolytic, 17
iron deficiency, 203–204, 204f
pernicious, 17, 204f, 205
sickle cell, 4–6, 204f, 206
sideroblastic, 202
Anesthetic, 331
Aneurysm, 199–200, 199f
definition of, 348
dissecting, 199, 199f
fusiform, 199, 199f
sacculated, 199, 199f

Angina pectoris, 194–196
unstable, 195
Angiography, 59, 361–362
definition of, 348
Ankylosis, 273
definition of, 348
Anorexia
in celiac sprue, 134
from chemotherapy, 50
definition of, 348
in folic acid deficiency anemia, 205
in glomerulonephritis, 79
in measles, 34
Anorexia nervosa, 18, 149
Anoxia, 57
definition of, 348
ANS. *See* Autonomic nervous system
Anthracosis, 172
Antibiotic(s)
for brain abscess, 233
definition of, 348
Antibody(ies), 15, 32
definition of, 348
to Epstein-Barr virus, 361
Anticholinergic(s)
definition of, 348
for gastritis, 130
for motion sickness, 322
for Parkinson's disease, 237
Antidiarrheal(s)
definition of, 348
for gastroenteritis, 131
Antidiuretic hormone. *See* Vasopressin
Anti-DNA antibody, 361
Antiemetic(s)
for chronic renal failure, 80
definition of, 348
for gastritis, 129–130
in radiation injury, 12
Antigen(s), 15
definition of, 348
Anti-inflammatory agent(s), 331
Antineoplaston therapy, 51
Antinuclear antibody (ANA), 361
Antipruritic(s)
definition of, 348
for rubella, 37
for shingles, 302
Antipyretic(s)
definition of, 348
for measles, 34
for pharyngitis, 161
for prostatitis, 105
for pyelonephritis, 78
Antistreptolysin O test, 187
Anuria, 77t
in toxemias of pregnancy, 120
Aortic insufficiency, 192–193
Aortic stenosis, 192–193, 192f
Aortography, 361

Aphasia, 228
definition of, 348
Aphthous stomatitis, 129
Aplastic anemia, 204f, 205–206
Apnea, 177
definition of, 348
Appendectomy, 136
Appendicitis, acute, 135–136, 136f
Apraxia, 228
definition of, 348
Aqueous humor, 315
Arachnoid membrane, 226
Aromatherapy, 333
Arousal, 95
Arousal dysfunction, in women, 97
Arrhythmia(s)
in cerebrovascular accident, 234
in cystic fibrosis, 66
definition of, 348
in myocardial infarction, 196
in pericarditis, 188
Arterial blood gas(es) (ABGs), 361
Arteriogram. *See* Angiography
Arteriosclerosis, 200–201
Arthralgia
in chronic fatigue syndrome, 30
definition of, 348
Arthrogram, 361
Artificial heart valve, 191, 192f
Asbestosis, 171
Ascites
in colorectal cancer, 141
definition of, 348
in nephrotic syndrome, 80
in pericarditis, 188
ASD. *See* Atrial septal defect
Aspartate aminotransferase, 361
Aspergillus, 7f
Asphyxiation, 13
Aspiration pneumonia, 163
Assay, 361
Associations, concerned with diseases of human body, 381–387
Asthma, 168–169
extrinsic, 169
intrinsic, 169
Astigmatism, 312f, 313
Ataxic cerebral palsy, 57
Atelectasis, 175–176
in cystic fibrosis, 66
definition of, 348
in pneumothorax, 165
Atherosclerosis, 194, 200–201, 200f
Athetoid cerebral palsy, 57
Athlete's foot. *See* Tinea pedis
Atmospheric pressure, extremes of, 12
ATN. *See* Acute tubular necrosis
Atopic dermatitis, 299–301, 300f, 304
Atrial septal defect (ASD), 61–62
Atrophic gastritis, 17

Atropine
definition of, 348
for uveitis, 317
Audiogram, 362
Auscultation, 62, 165–166, 362
definition of, 348
Autohypnosis, 332
Autoimmune disease, 16–17
Autoinoculation, definition of, 348
Autologous transplantation, 212
Autonomic nervous system (ANS),
221, 221f
Autosomal trait
dominant, 5f, 6, 73, 348
recessive, 4–6, 5f, 66, 73, 348
Axon, 221, 223f
Ayurvedic medicine, 274
definition of, 348
Azoospermia, 98
definition of, 348

B

Bacillary dysentery. *See* Shigellosis
Bacillus, 8, 9f
Bacteremia, 27t, 233, 292
definition of, 348
Bacterial disease, 8–9, 9f
Bacterial endocarditis. *See*
Endocarditis
Bacterial meningitis, acute, 230–231,
231f
Bacterial pneumonia, 162t, 163
Barium enema, 362
Barium swallow, 362
Barrel chest, 168
Basal cell carcinoma, 303
Basophil(s), 203f
B-cell lymphocyte(s), 15
BCG vaccine, 35t, 170, 362
Bell's palsy, 234, 234f
Bell's phenomenon, 234, 234f
Benign prostatic hyperplasia (BPH),
107
Benign tumor, 13, 44, 45t
Beriberi, 18
Berylliosis, 171–172
Beta-carotene, 51
Bile, 134
definition of, 348
Biliary colic, 146
Bilirubin
blood, 146, 362, 367
definition of, 348
in erythroblastosis fetalis, 61
Bilirubinuria
definition of, 348
in viral hepatitis, 148
Biofeedback, 332
Biopsy, 17, 49

definition of, 348
Biotherapy. *See* Immunotherapy
Biotin, 177
definition of, 348
Black lung disease. *See* Anthracosis
Bladder
cancer of, 45f, 46t, 85–86
congenital defects of, 64–65
congenital diverticulum of, 65
exstrophy of, 65
neurogenic, 84–85
tumors of, 85–86
Bladder evacuation technique(s)
Credé's method, 85
intermittent self-catheterization, 85
Blast(s), 207
definition of, 349
Blastomycosis, 172–173
North American, 172–173
Bleb, definition of, 349
Blepharitis, 317–318
Blood disease(s), 185, 186f
Blood serum for hormones, 362
Blood test(s), references values for,
389–391
Blood vessel disease(s), 185, 186f,
199–202
Bloodstream infection, 27t
BMT. *See* Bone marrow
transplantation
Bodywork therapy, 225
Bone disease(s), 262–272, 263f
Bone marrow, 203f
Bone marrow biopsy, 362
Bone marrow transplantation (BMT),
51, 212
Bone matrix, 267
BPH. *See* Benign prostatic hyperplasia
Bradycardia
in cardiac arrest, 198
in cerebral concussion, 227
definition of, 349
Brain, 222f
Brain abscess, 232–233, 233f
Brain tumor, 239
primary, 239
secondary, 239
Breast
benign fibroadenoma of, 116
cancer of, 45f, 46t, 48, 51, 116–117,
117f
diseases of, 115–117, 115f
Breast reconstruction, 117
Bronchial stenosis, 165
Bronchiectasis, 176
Bronchiole, 66
definition of, 349
Bronchitis, chronic, 167–168
Bronchodilator(s)
for asthma, 169

for chronic obstructive pulmonary
disease, 167
definition of, 349
Bronchography, 362
Bronchoscopy, 362
Brucellosis, 27t, 162t
Brudzinski's sign, 230, 362
definition of, 349
Bruit(s)
definition of, 349
in essential hypertension, 193
Bulimia, 18, 149–150
Bulla, 286f, 286t
definition of, 349
in impetigo, 291
Burkitt's lymphoma, 48
Burn(s), 13
classification of, 13, 14f
rule of nines, 13, 14f
Bursitis, 275
Butterfly rash, 278, 278f

C

Cachexia
in cancer, 51
in colorectal cancer, 141
definition of, 349
CAD. *See* Coronary artery disease
Calcium
serum, 367
urine, 368
Calculi, renal. *See* Renal calculi
Callus, 296
Calyx
definition of, 349
renal, 81
Cancer, 14, 43–52. *See also* specific
sites and types
cases by site and sex, 45, 45f
classification of, 47–48
deaths by site and sex, 45, 45f
diagnosis of, 49
distant stage of, 46, 46t
etiology of, 48–49
five-year relative survival rates for,
46t
grading and staging of, 46, 48
localized, 46, 46t
preventive measures, 46–47
regional stage of, 46, 46t
risk factors for, 46–47
treatment of, 49–52
chemotherapy, 50
hormonal therapy, 51
immunotherapy, 51
radiation therapy, 50
surgery, 49–50
warning signs of, 49
Canker sore, 129

Carbuncle, 291–292, 292f
Carcinoembryonic antigen (CEA), 362
Carcinogen, 46, 49
    definition of, 349
Carcinogenesis, 49
Carcinoma, 45t, 47
Cardiac advance(s), 198–199
Cardiac arrest, 198
Cardiac catheterization, 362
Cardiac enzyme(s), 362
Cardiogenic shock, 196
    definition of, 349
Cardiomegaly, 62
    definition of, 349
Cardiovascular disease(s), congenital,
    60–64
Carditis, 187–189
    in rheumatic fever, 187
Carpal tunnel syndrome, 3, 275–276
    definition of, 349
Cast(s), urinary, 78
    definition of, 349
Cataract, 314–315
    congenital, 314
    secondary, 314
    senile, 314
    traumatic, 314
Catheterization
    cardiac, 362
    of ejaculatory ducts, 362
    urine, 362
CBC. *See* Complete blood count
CEA. *See* Carcinoembryonic antigen
Celiac sprue, 134–135
Cell-mediated immunity, 15
Cellulitis
    definition of, 349
    of eyelid, 314
    with lymphedema, 211
Central nervous system (CNS),
    220–221, 221–222f
    infections of, 230–233
Cerebral angiography, 362
Cerebral concussion, 10, 227
Cerebral contusion, 10, 227–228
Cerebral disease, 234–236
Cerebral palsy, 57
    ataxic, 57
    athetoid, 57
    postnatal causes of, 57
    prenatal causes of, 57
    spastic, 57
Cerebrospinal fluid (CSF), 224
    definition of, 349
Cerebrospinal fluid (CSF) analysis,
    230, 232, 232f, 362
    references values for, 399
Cerebrovascular accident (CVA),
    234–235
Cerumen, impacted, 319

Cervix
    cancer of, 46t, 49
    conization of, 113
    dysplasia of, 113
    stenosis of, 111
Cervicitis, 98
    definition of, 349
Cesarean birth, 122
CFS. *See* Chronic fatigue syndrome
Chancre, 102–103, 102f
    definition of, 349
CHEM 20 Health Profile, 375, 376t
Chemical agent(s), in disease process,
    11–14
Chemistry screen, 362
Chemotherapy, for cancer, 50
Chest percussion, 176
Chest radiography, 163f, 170f
Chest trauma, 11
Cheyne-Stokes respiration, 235
    definition of, 349
CHF. *See* Congestive heart failure
Chickenpox. *See* Varicella
Chickenpox vaccine, 36t
Chilblain, 12
Children
    circulatory system diseases of,
        212–213
    communicable diseases of, 33–34
    digestive system diseases of,
        150–152
    ear diseases of, 323
    eye diseases of, 318–319
    musculoskeletal diseases of,
        279–280
    respiratory system diseases of,
        177–179
    skin diseases of, 304–306
Chlamydial infection(s), 104
Chlamydial pneumonia, 162t
Cholecystectomy, 146–147
Cholecystitis, acute, 146–147
Cholecystogram, 362
Cholelithiasis, 144–146, 145f
    definition of, 349
    in sickle cell anemia, 206
Cholera, 8, 25t, 27t
Cholera vaccine, 35t
Cholestasis, 147
    definition of, 349
Chondroma, 279
Chondrosarcoma, 279
Chorea
    definition of, 349
    in rheumatic fever, 187
Choriocarcinoma, 50
    definition of, 349
Chromosomal disorder, 6
Chromosome, 4
    definition of, 349

Chronic disease, 4
    definition of, 349
    laboratory tests for, 379–380
Chronic fatigue syndrome (CFS),
    29–30
Chronic illness, 31
Chronic lymphocytic leukemia (CLL),
    47, 209
Chronic myelocytic leukemia (CML),
    47, 208–209
Chronic obstructive pulmonary
    disease (COPD), 167
Chronic pain, 330–331
Chyme, 59
    definition of, 349
Cigarette smoking. *See* Smoking
Cilium
    bronchial, 167
    definition of, 349
Circulatory system disease(s),
    183–213, 186f
    alternative medicine, 213
    blood vessel diseases, 199–202
    carditis, 187–189
    of children, 212–213
    common symptoms of, 213
    coronary diseases, 194–198, 194f
    hypertensive heart disease, 193
    laboratory tests for, 375–376
    leukemias, 207–209, 207f
    lymphatic diseases, 209–211, 210f
    organ function tests for, 369
    red blood cell disorders, 202–207
    rheumatic fever and rheumatic
        heart disease, 185–187
    valvular heart diseases, 190–193,
        190–191f
Cirrhosis, 17, 147
Claudication
    in atherosclerosis, 200
    in congenital heart disease, 62
    definition of, 349
CLL. *See* Chronic lymphocytic
    leukemia
Closed fracture, 270, 271f
Closed reduction, 272
Clotting factor(s), 6
Clubbing, 174
    definition of, 349
Clubfoot, 65
CML. *See* Chronic myelocytic
    leukemia
CNS. *See* Central nervous system
Coarctation of the aorta, 61–62,
    63f
Coccidioidin skin test, 173, 363
Coccidioidomycosis, 8, 172–173
Coccus, 9, 9f
Coitus, 98
    definition of, 349

Cold
  common. *See* Common cold
  extreme temperature, 11–12
Cold sore, 129, 301–302, 301f
Colectomy, 137
  definition of, 349
Colic
  biliary, 146
  infantile, 150
Colitis
  granulomatous. *See* Crohn's disease
  ulcerative. *See* Ulcerative colitis
Colon cancer. *See* Colorectal cancer
Colonoscopy, 363
Color blindness, 4
Colorectal cancer, 45f, 46t, 47–48,
  141–142, 141f
Colostomy, definition of, 349
Coma
  in bacterial meningitis, 230
  definition of, 349
  diabetic, 257
  myxedema, 253
Comedo, 288
  definition of, 350
Comminuted fracture, 270, 271f
Common cold, 8, 26–29, 27t
  alternative medicine, 29
Communicable disease(s), 23–40
  of adolescence, 33–34
  of childhood, 33–34
  incubation period of, 27–28t
  isolation periods for, 27–28t
  reporting to county and state health
    departments, 26
  transmission of, 25–26t
Communicating hydrocephalus,
  58–59
Complement system, 15
Complete blood count (CBC), 363
Complete neurological examination,
  363
Computerized tomography (CT), 363
Conceptus, definition of, 350
Concussion, cerebral, 10, 227
Congenital aganglionic megacolon.
    See Hirschsprung's disease
Congenital disease(s), 55–67
  cardiovascular diseases, 60–64
  definition of, 57
  digestive system diseases, 59–60
  genitourinary diseases, 64–65
  metabolic diseases, 66–67
  musculoskeletal diseases, 65–66
  nervous system diseases, 57–59
Congenital heart defect(s), 6, 61–64,
  62–63f
Congestive heart failure (CHF),
  197–198, 197f
Conization

cervical, 113
  definition of, 350
Conjunctiva, 313
  definition of, 350
Conjunctivitis, 317
Connective tissue disease, 264–265f,
  275–279
Contact dermatitis, 299, 300f
Contagious disease(s). *See*
    Communicable disease(s)
Contracture
  in Bell's palsy, 234
  definition of, 350
  in Duchenne's muscular dystrophy,
    279
  in scleroderma, 298
Contusion, cerebral, 10, 227–228
Convergence testing, 363
Cooley's anemia. *See* Thalassemia
Coombs' test, direct, 363
COPD. *See* Chronic obstructive
    pulmonary disease
Cor pulmonale, 173–174
Cordotomy, 332
  definition of, 350
Corneal abrasion, 314
Corns, 296
Coronary artery disease (CAD),
  194–195, 194f
Coronary bypass procedure, 195
Coronary disease, 194–198, 194f
Corpus luteum, 111
  definition of, 350
Cortisol, 255–256
Coryza
  definition of, 350
  in viral hepatitis, 148
CPK. *See* Creatine phosphokinase
Cradle cap, 298
Craniotomy, 226
  definition of, 350
Creatine phosphokinase (CPK), 363
Creatinine, 80
  definition of, 350
  serum, 367
Credé's method of bladder evacuation,
  85
Crepitation, 272
  definition of, 350
Cretinism, 4, 253
Crohn's disease, 137
Croup, 178
Cryosurgery, 101, 303
  definition of, 350
Cryotherapy, 316
  definition of, 350
Cryptococcus, 7f
Cryptorchidism. *See* Undescended
    testes
CSF. *See* Cerebrospinal fluid

CT. *See* Computerized tomography
Culture and sensitivity test, 363
Curet, 319
  definition of, 350
Cushing's syndrome, 255–256
CVA. *See* Cerebrovascular accident
Cyanosis, 62
  in congestive heart failure, 198
  definition of, 350
  in hypoparathyroidism, 255
  in pneumonia, 163
Cyanotic heart defect(s), 61
Cyst, 286t
  ovarian, 111–112
Cystectomy, 86
  definition of, 350
Cystic fibrosis, 4, 66–67
Cystic mastitis, chronic. *See* Mammary
    dysplasia
Cystitis, 83–84
Cystometry, 363
Cystoscopy, 363
Cystourethrography, 363
Cytology, 363

D & C. *See* Dilation and curettage
Dandruff, 298
Deafness, 323
Débridement, 101, 296
  definition of, 350
Decompression sickness, 12
Decubitus ulcer, 237, 293, 294f
  definition of, 350
Deer tick, 32, 32f
Degenerative disease, of nervous
    system, 236–238
Delivery, cesarean birth, 122
Delivery disorder(s), 116–122
  common symptoms of, 122
Delta hepatitis, 25t
Dementia
  definition of, 350
  neurogenic bladder in, 84
  presenile. *See* Alzheimer's disease
Dendrite, 221, 223f
Dermatitis, 298–301
  atopic, 299–301, 300f, 304
  contact, 299, 300f
  seborrheic, 298–299, 299f
Dermatomyositis, 17, 277–278
Dermatophytosis, 293–296, 294–296f,
  305–306
Dermis, 285, 285f
Dermopathy, 252
Dexamethasone suppression test, low-
    dose, 365
Diabetes insipidus, 6, 249–250

Diabetes mellitus, 6, 17–18, 256–258
acute complications of, 257
gestational, 256
immune-mediated type 1, 256–257
late complications of, 257–258
type 2, 256–257
Diabetic coma, 257
Dialysis, 86, 87f
Dialyzer, 86, 87f
Diaper rash, 304–305, 306f
Diaphoresis
in atelectasis, 176
in congestive heart failure, 198
definition of, 350
in motion sickness, 322
Diaphragmatic hernia, 133f
Diarrhea, 142, 151
acute, 151
chronic, 151
Diastolic pressure, 193
definition of, 350
DIC. *See* Disseminated intravascular coagulation
Diet faddism, 18
Dietary Guide for the United States, 340
Differentiated cell(s), 48
definition of, 350
Digestive system disease(s), 127–152, 130f
alternative medicine for, 152
in children, 150–152
common symptoms of, 152
congenital, 59–60
diseases of accessory organs, 142–149, 143f, 145f
eating disorders, 149–150
laboratory tests for, 378
lower gastrointestinal tract diseases, 134–142
organ function tests for, 371–372
upper gastrointestinal tract diseases, 129–133
Dilatation, of heart, 190
Dilation, definition of, 350
Dilation and curettage (D & C), 363
Diphtheria, 8, 25t, 27t, 28–29
Diphtheria toxoid, 39
Diplopia
definition of, 350
in strabismus, 318
in stroke, 235
Discoid lupus erythematosus (DLE), 297
Disease, definition of, 3
Disease process
hereditary diseases, 3–6
iatrogenic diseases, 19
idiopathic diseases, 19
immune-related factors in, 15–17
infections, 6–9

inflammation in, 6–9
mental and emotional factors in, 17–18, 338
nutritional factors in, 18–19, 340
physical and chemical agents in, 11–14
predisposing factors, 3
trauma and, 9–11
Dissecting aneurysm, 199, 199f
Disseminated intravascular coagulation (DIC), 121
definition of, 350
Distant cancer, 46, 46t
Distress, 340–341
Diuretic(s), 18
definition of, 350
for lymphedema, 211
for myocarditis, 188
for pulmonary edema, 173
Diverticulitis, 138, 139f
Diverticulum
of bladder, 65
of intestine, 138, 139f
DLE. *See* Discoid lupus erythematosus
Dominant trait, autosomal, 5f, 6, 73, 348
Dopamine, 237
Doppler ultrasonography, 201, 363
Down syndrome. *See* Trisomy 21

DPT vaccine, 35t, 39
Drusen, 316
Duchenne's muscular dystrophy, 6, 279–280
Ductus arteriosus, 61
definition of, 350
Duodenal ulcer, 135
Duodenum, 135
Duplicated ureter, 64
Dura mater, 225
Dysentery
amebic, 8, 27t
bacillary. *See* Shigellosis
Dysmenorrhea, 111
primary, 111
secondary, 111
Dyspareunia, 96
Dysphagia
definition of, 351
in goiter, 250
in hiatal hernia, 133
in scleroderma, 298
Dysphasia
definition of, 351
in stroke, 235
Dysplasia, 49
cervical, 113
definition of, 351
hip, 65–66
mammary, 115–116

Dyspnea
in anaphylactic shock, 16
in coarctation of the aorta, 62
definition of, 351
in pericarditis, 188
in pneumonia, 163
Dystonia, definition of, 351
Dysuria
definition of, 351
in pyelonephritis, 78

E

Ear disease(s), 319–323, 320f
of children, 323
common symptoms of, 323
Eardrum, perforated, 10–11
Eating disorder, 149–150
ECG. *See* Electrocardiography
Echocardiogram, 189, 363
definition of, 351
Echoencephalography, 363
Eclampsia. *See* Toxemia(s) of pregnancy
ECM. *See* Erythema chronicum migrans
Ectopic orifice of the ureter, 64–65
Ectopic pregnancy, 118, 119f
Ectopic site, 112
definition of, 351
Eczema. *See* Atopic dermatitis
Edema
in anaphylactic shock, 16
in chronic bronchitis, 167
definition of, 351
in glomerulonephritis, 79
in gonorrhea, 99
peripheral, 197, 197f
pitting, 198, 356
pulmonary. *See* Pulmonary edema
EEG. *See* Electroencephalography
Effacement, 121
definition of, 351
Effusion, definition of, 351
Ejaculatory analysis, 363
Elderly, 3
Electric shock, 12
Electrocardiography (ECG), 364
Electrocautery
for cancer, 50
definition of, 351
for genital warts, 101
Electrodesiccation, 303
definition of, 351
Electroencephalography (EEG), 364
Electrolyte(s)
definition of, 351
serum, 367
Electrolyte analysis, 364
Electrolyte balance, 73, 142

Electromyography (EMG), 364
Electrophoresis, of serum proteins, 367
Embolism
  as cause of stroke, 234
  definition of, 351
  fracture-related, 272
  pulmonary. *See* Pulmonary embolism
  septic, 165
Embolus, 189
  definition of, 351
EMG. *See* Electromyography
Emotion(s)
  in disease process, 17–18
  negative, 338, 341, 341t
Emotional stress, 17, 340–341
Emphysema, chronic pulmonary, 168, 168f
En bloc surgery, 50
  definition of, 351
Encapsulated tumor, 44
Encapsulation, definition of, 351
Encephalitis, 8, 27t, 231–232
Endemic disease, 33, 250
  definition of, 351
Endocarditis, 189, 189f
Endocrine system disease(s), 243–258, 245f, 246t
  adrenal gland disease, 246t, 255–256
  common symptoms of, 258
  endocrine pancreatic disease, 246t, 256–258
  laboratory tests for, 377, 393–401
  organ function tests for, 370–371
  parathyroid gland disease, 246t, 254–255
  pituitary gland disease, 246t, 247–251
  thyroid gland diseases, 246t, 250–253
Endocrine test(s), references values for, 393–401
Endometriosis, 112–113, 112f
Endometrium, 112
  definition of, 351
Endorphin, 330
  definition of, 351
Endoscopic retrograde cholangio-pancreatography (ERCP), 364
Endoscopy, 364
Endotracheal intubation, 179
Entamoeba histolytica, 8f
Enteritis, regional. *See* Crohn's disease
Enterobiasis, 151–152
Enteropathy
  definition of, 351
  gluten-induced. *See* Celiac sprue
Environmental hazard(s), 3

Environmental influence(s), on health, 339–340
Eosinophil(s), 203f
Epidermis, 284–285, 285f
Epididymitis, 105–106
Epididymo-orchitis, 37
  definition of, 351
Epidural hematoma, 225–227, 226f
Epigastric pain, 129
Epigastric region, definition of, 351
Epigastrium, 59
  definition of, 351
Epiglottitis, acute, 178–179
Epilepsy, 235–236
Epispadias, 65
Epistaxis, 160
  in coarctation of the aorta, 62
  definition of, 351
Epithelial layer, 47
  definition of, 351
ERCP. *See* Endoscopic retrograde cholangiopancreatography
Erectile dysfunction, 96–97
  intermittent, 96
  partial, 96
  selective, 96
Erythema
  in allergic reaction, 16
  definition of, 351
  from radiation therapy, 50
  in rheumatic fever, 187
  in urticaria, 287
Erythema chronicum migrans (ECM), 32
Erythematous vesicle, in genital herpes, 100
Erythroblastic anemia. *See* Thalassemia
Erythroblastosis fetalis, 60–61, 60f
Erythrocyte sedimentation rate (ESR), 364
Escherichia coli O157:H7, 32–33
Esophageal cancer, 46t, 47
Esophageal varices, 147
Esotropia, 318, 319f
ESR. *See* Erythrocyte sedimentation rate
Essential hypertension, 193
Ewing's sarcoma, 279
Exchange transfusion, 61
  definition of, 351
Excoriation, 65
  definition of, 351
Excretion, 49
  definition of, 351
Exfoliative cytology, 49, 364
  definition of, 351
Exocrine gland, 4
  definition of, 351
Exophthalmos, 252, 252f

definition of, 351
Exstrophy of the bladder, 65
External hemorrhoid, 139, 140f
External otitis, 319–321
External respiration, 159
Extracorporeal hemodialysis, 86–88, 87f
Extraopia, 318, 319f
Extremity trauma, 11
Extrinsic asthma, 169
Exudate, 166
  definition of, 351
Eye disease(s), 311–318, 312f
  of children, 318–319
  common symptoms of, 319

Faith, 342–343
Farsightedness. *See* Hyperopia
Fecalith, 135, 136f
  definition of, 352
Female infertility, 98
Female reproductive system disease(s), 109–114, 109–110f
  common symptoms of, 114
Femoral head, 65
  definition of, 352
Femoral hernia, 140–141
Ferritin, serum, 367
Fever blister, 301–302, 301f
Fibrillation, ventricular, 193
  definition of, 352
Fibrin, 38
  definition of, 352
Fibroadenoma, benign, of breast, 116
Fibrocystic disease, of breast. *See* Mammary dysplasia
Fibroid, uterine. *See* Leiomyoma, uterine
Fibrosarcoma, 279
First degree burn, 14f
Fissure, 286f, 286t
Fistula
  in Crohn's disease, 137
  definition of, 352
Flu. *See* Influenza
Fluid retention, 18
Fluke, 9, 10f
Fluorescein stain, 364
Fluorescent treponemal antibody-absorption (FTA-ABS) test, 103
Fluoroscopy, 364
Folic acid, serum, 367
Folic acid deficiency anemia, 204–205
Follicle-stimulating hormone (FSH), 114
  definition of, 352
Fontanelle(s), 59
  definition of, 352

Food allergy, 16, 151
Food poisoning. *See* Gastroenteritis
Fracture, 270–272
    closed, 270, 271f
    comminuted, 270, 271f
    greenstick, 270, 271f
    impacted, 270, 271f
    incomplete, 271, 271f
    open, 270, 271f
Friendship, health and, 342–343
Frostbite, 12
FSH. *See* Follicle-stimulating hormone
FTA-ABS test. *See* Fluorescent
        treponemal antibody-
        absorption test
Full thickness burn, 14f
Fungal infection. *See* Mycosis
Fungal pneumonia, 162t
Fungemia, 27t
Furuncle, 291–292
Fusiform aneurysm, 199, 199f

Gallbladder disease(s), 18, 142–149,
        143f, 145f
Gallstone(s). *See* Cholelithiasis
Gamma globulin, 34, 148
    definition of, 352
Ganglion, definition of, 352
Gangrene, 199, 201
    definition of, 352
Gastric analysis, 364
Gastric ulcer, 131–132, 131f
Gastritis, 129–130
    atrophic, 17
Gastroenteritis, 130–131
Gastroscopy, 364
Gate control theory, of pain, 329–330,
        329f
Gene, 4
    definition of, 352
Generalized seizure, 236
Genetic disease(s). *See* Hereditary
        disease(s)
Genital herpes, 99–100, 100f
Genital wart(s), 101, 101f
Genitourinary disease(s), congenital,
        64–65
Genotype, 4
    definition of, 352
German measles. *See* Rubella
Gestational diabetes, 256
Giardia lamblia, 8f
Giardiasis, 27t
Gigantism, 247–248, 247f
Glaucoma, 315
    open-angle, 315
Globulin, in urine, 77t
Glomerulonephritis, acute, 79

Gluten-induced enteropathy. *See*
        Celiac sprue
Glycosuria, 256
    definition of, 352
Goiter, 252
    simple, 250–251, 251f
Goitrogen, 250
    definition of, 352
Gonadotropin, 248–249
Gonococcal disease, 25t
Gonorrhea, 27t, 99
Gout, 6, 274
    metabolic, 274
    renal, 274
Grading, of neoplasms, 48
Gram's stain, 364
Granulocyte(s), 208
Granuloma, 169
    definition of, 352
Granulomatous colitis. *See* Crohn's
        disease
Graves' disease. *See* Hyperthyroidism
Greenstick fracture, 270, 271f
Growth hormone, 247–249, 247–248f
Gutherie screening test. *See*
        Phenylketonuria test

Haemophilus influenzae b vaccine, 35t,
        179
Hair, 285, 285f
Halitosis, definition of, 352
Hashimoto's thyroiditis, 17, 251
HCG. *See* Human chorionic
        gonadotropin
Head trauma, 10–11, 225–228
Headache, 221–225
    acute, 221–224, 224t
    alternative medicine, 225
    chronic, 221–224, 224t
    etiologies of, 224t
    migraine, 224–225
Health, 337–343
    environmental influences on,
        339–340
    holistic, 337–343
    laughter and play and, 341–342
    lifestyle and, 339
    love, friendship, and faith and,
        342–343
    managing negative emotions, 341,
        341t
    mind's connection with, 338
    nutrition and, 340
    personal responsibility for, 339
    stress and distress and, 340–341
Heart attack. *See* Myocardial infarction
Heart defect(s)
    acyanotic, 61

    congenital, 61–64, 62–63f
    cyanotic, 61
Heart disease(s), 185, 186f
    congenital, 6, 61–64, 62–63f
    hypertensive, 193
    obesity and, 18
    rheumatic, 185–187
    valvular, 190–193, 190–191f
Heart murmur. *See* Murmur
Heart valve, artificial, 191, 192f
Heat, extreme, 11–12
Heat cramp(s), 11–12
Heat exhaustion, 11–12
Heatstroke, 11–12
Helminth(s), 9, 151–152
Hematemesis, 129
    definition of, 352
Hematocrit, 204, 206, 364
Hematologic disease(s), 185, 186f
    laboratory tests for, 376–377
    organ function tests for, 370
Hematologic value(s), references
        values for, 396–399
Hematoma, 228
    definition of, 352
    epidural, 225–227, 226f
    subdural, 225–227, 226f
Hematopoietic tissue, 207
    definition of, 352
Hematuria
    definition of, 352
    in polycystic kidney disease, 73
    in sexually transmitted diseases, 104
Hemiparesis, 226
    definition of, 352
Hemiplegia, 228
Hemochromatosis, 147
Hemodialysis, 86–88, 87f
Hemoglobin, 202, 364
    definition of, 352
Hemoglobin S, 206
Hemolysis
    in cirrhosis, 147
    in erythroblastosis fetalis, 60
    definition of, 352
Hemolytic anemia, 17
Hemolytic disease of the newborn. *See*
        Erythroblastosis fetalis
Hemolytic uremic syndrome, 33
Hemophilia, 6
Hemoptysis
    in congestive heart failure, 198
    definition of, 352
    in tuberculosis, 169
Hemorrhoid(s), 139, 140f
    external, 139, 140f
    internal, 139, 140f
Hemorrhoidectomy, 139
Hepatitis
    acute viral, 147–149

chronic active, 17
viral, 8
Hepatitis A, 25t, 27t, 148
Hepatitis B, 25t, 27t, 148–149
Hepatitis B vaccine, 35t, 149
Hepatitis C, 25t, 27t, 148
Hepatitis D, 27t, 148
Hepatitis E, 27t, 148
Hepatitis G, 148
Hepatomegaly
in colorectal cancer, 141
definition of, 352
in pericarditis, 188
Herbal therapy, 225
Hereditary disease(s), 3–6
chromosomal disorders, 6
classification of, 4–6
monogenic disorders, 4–6, 5f
multifactorial disorders, 6
Hernia
abdominal, 140–141
diaphragmatic, 133f
femoral, 140–141
hiatal, 132–133, 132–133f
inguinal, 133f, 140–141
mixed, 133
paraesophageal, 133
sliding, 132–133
strangulated, 133f, 140
umbilical, 133f, 140–141
Herniated intervertebral disk,
266–267, 267f
Herpes, 8, 9f
genital, 99–100, 100f
Herpes zoster, 302, 302f
Herpes-related skin lesion(s), 201–203
Herpetic stomatitis, acute, 129
Heterozygote, 4
definition of, 352
Hiatal hernia, 132–133, 132–133f
Hip dysplasia, congenital, 65–66
Hirschsprung's disease, 59–60
Histamine, 330
definition of, 352
Histoplasmin skin test, 173, 364
Histoplasmosis, 7, 172–173
HIV. *See* Human immunodeficiency
virus
Hives. *See* Urticaria
Hodgkin's disease, 17, 47–48, 50, 211
Holistic health, 337–343
Holistic medicine, 338–339
Homeostasis, 7
definition of, 352
Homozygote, 4
definition of, 352
Hookworm, 25t
Hordeolum. *See* Stye
Hormonal therapy, for cancer, 51
Hormone, 244

Housemaid's knee, 275
Human chorionic gonadotropin
(HCG), serum, 367
Human immunodeficiency virus
(HIV), 30–32
Humor, therapeutic value of, 332–333
Humoral immunity, 15
Humpback. *See* Kyphosis
Hydrazine sulfate, 51
Hydrocele, 98
definition of, 352
Hydrocephalus, 58–59
communicating, 58–59
noncommunicating, 58–59
Hydronephrosis, 82f, 83
definition of, 352
in neurogenic bladder, 85
silent, 83
in stricture of ureter, 65
Hydrotherapy, 225
Hydroureter, 64
definition of, 353
Hydroxyproline, 364
Hypercalcemia. *See*
Hyperparathyroidism
Hypercapnia. *See* Respiratory acidosis
Hyperglycemia
definition of, 353
in diabetes mellitus, 256–258
in pancreatic cancer, 144
Hyperkalemia, 81
Hyperlipemia, 80
definition of, 353
Hypernephroma. *See*
Adenocarcinoma, of kidney
Hyperopia, 311, 312f
Hyperparathyroidism, 81, 254
definition of, 353
Hyperpituitarism, 247–248, 247–248f
Hyperplasia
adenoid, 178
of breast, 115
in chronic bronchitis, 167
definition of, 353
etiology of neoplasms, 49
Hypersecretion, 244
Hypersensitivity reaction, 16
Hypertension, 18
definition of, 353
essential, 193
in polycystic kidney disease, 73
portal, 147
Hyperthyroidism, 251–252, 252f
Hypertrophy, 62, 167, 272
definition of, 353
right ventricular, 190
Hypoalbuminemia, 80
definition of, 353
Hypocalcemia. *See*
Hypoparathyroidism

Hypocapnia. *See* Respiratory alkalosis
Hypoglycemia
definition of, 353
in Reye's syndrome, 212
Hypokalemia
in bulimia, 150
definition of, 353
Hypoparathyroidism, 254–255
Hypophosphatemia, 254
Hypophysectomy, 332
definition of, 353
Hypopituitarism, 248–249
Hyposecretion, 244
Hypospadias, 65
Hypotension
in cerebral concussion, 227
definition of, 353
Hypothermia, 12
Hypothyroidism, 98, 253
definition of, 353
Hypoventilation, 13
definition of, 353
Hypovolemic shock, 11, 118
definition of, 353
Hypoxemia, 13
definition of, 353
Hypoxia
definition of, 353
in respiratory alkalosis, 175
in sickle cell anemia, 206
Hysterosalpingography, 98, 364
definition of, 353

I

Iatrogenic disease, 19, 113, 249, 253,
255
definition of, 353
IBS. *See* Irritable bowel syndrome
Idiopathic disease, 19, 188, 236, 249,
266
definition of, 353
Idiopathic thrombocytopenia, 17
IF. *See* Intrinsic factor
Ileostomy, 137
definition of, 353
Illness, 3
Imagery, 332
Immune globulin, 148
Immune response, 15
Immune system disease(s)
laboratory tests for, 379
organ function tests for, 372
Immunity
acquired, 15
cell-mediated, 15
humoral, 15
natural, 15
Immunization, 15, 26, 33
Immunodeficiency disease, 17

Immunoglobulin, definition of, 353
Immunotherapy, 51
Impacted cerumen, 319
Impacted fracture, 270, 271f
Impetigo, 291, 291f
Impotence. *See* Erectile dysfunction
Incomplete fracture, 271, 271f
Incontinence
    definition of, 353
    urinary. *See* Urinary incontinence
Incubation period, 27–28t
Induration, 201, 296
    definition of, 353
Infant, 3
Infantile colic, 150
Infection(s), 6–9
Infectious disease(s), 23–40. *See also*
        Communicable disease(s)
    laboratory tests for, 379
Infectious mononucleosis, 27t,
        161–162, 162t
Infective endocarditis. *See*
        Endocarditis
Infective tubulointerstitial nephritis.
        See Pyelonephritis
Infertility
    female, 98
    male, 98
Inflammation, 6–9, 15
    acute, 6
    chronic, 6
Influenza, 8, 9f, 25t, 27t, 29, 212
    alternative medicine, 29
Influenza vaccine, 29, 35t
Inguinal hernia, 133f, 140–141
Insect bite, 13, 16
Insidious onset, 73
    definition of, 353
Insulin, 256–258
Insulin shock, 257
Intercostal nerve block, 166
Interferon, 51
Internal hemorrhoid, 139, 140f
Internal respiration, 159–160
Intervertebral disk, herniated,
        266–267, 267f
Intestinal flu. *See* Gastroenteritis
Intraocular lens (IOL), 314
Intravenous pyelogram, 364
Intrinsic asthma, 169
Intrinsic factor (IF), 205
Intromission, definition of, 353
IOL. *See* Intraocular lens
Ionizing radiation, 12
Iron, serum, 367
Iron deficiency anemia, 203–204,
        204f
Iron supplement, 204
Irritable bowel syndrome (IBS),
        136–137

Ischemia
    definition of, 353
    myocardial, 194
    renal, 81
    spinal, 230
Islets of Langerhans, 256
Isoimmunization, 60
    definition of, 353
Isolation period, 27–28t

J

Jaundice
    in cirrhosis, 147
    definition of, 353
Jock itch. *See* Tinea cruris
Joint disease(s), 272–274

K

Kaposi's sarcoma, 31
Keratin, 284–285
    definition of, 353
Keratitis, 318
Keratolytic agent, 288
    definition of, 353
Keratotomy, radial, 313
Kernig's sign, 230, 365
    definition of, 353
Ketoacidosis, 256
    definition of, 353
Ketone(s), 256
Ketosis, 256
Kidney
    adenocarcinoma of, 85
    cancer of, 45f, 46t
    diseases of, 73–83, 75–76f
    transplantation of, 88
Kidney stone(s). *See* Renal calculi
Kidneys, ureters, and bladder (KUB),
        x-ray of, 365, 368
Klinefelter's syndrome, 6
Koplik's spots, 34
    definition of, 354
KUB. *See* Kidneys, ureters, and
        bladder, x-ray of
Kyphoscoliosis, 173–174
    definition of, 354
Kyphosis, 262–266, 266f

L

Laboratory test(s)
    for chronic disorders, 379–380
    for circulatory system diseases,
        375–376
    for digestive system diseases, 378
    for endocrine system diseases, 377
    for hematologic system diseases,
        376–377

for immune system diseases, 379
    for infectious and febrile
        conditions, 379
    for musculoskeletal diseases,
        377–378
    for nervous system diseases, 376
    normal references values for,
        389–401
    for reproductive system diseases,
        378–379
    for respiratory system diseases, 376
    for tumors, 379
    for urinary system diseases, 377
Lactate dehydrogenase (LDH), 365
Laparoscopy, 365
Laryngeal cancer, 46t, 47
Laryngitis
    acute, 161
    chronic, 161
Laryngoscopy, 365
Lassitude
    definition of, 354
    in viral hepatitis, 148
Laughter
    health and, 341–342
    therapeutic value of, 332–333
LDH. *See* Lactate dehydrogenase
LE test. *See* Lupus erythematosus test
Legionella infection, 27t, 162t, 164
Legionnaires' disease. See *Legionella*
        infection
Leiomyoma
    definition of, 354
    uterine, 111, 113
Lentigo maligna melanoma, 303–304,
        304f
Leprosy, 25t
Lesion, definition of, 354
Leukemia, 45f, 45t, 47–48, 207–209,
        207f
    acute lymphoblastic (lymphocytic),
        208
    acute monoblastic (monocytic),
        208
    acute myeloblastic (myelogenous),
        47, 207–208
    chronic lymphocytic, 47, 209
    chronic myelocytic, 47, 208–209
Leukocyte(s), 47
    definition of, 354
Leukocytosis
    in appendicitis, 136
    definition of, 354
    in furuncles and carbuncles, 292
Leukopenia, 17
    from chemotherapy, 50
    in measles, 34
Leukorrhea, 100
    definition of, 354
LH. *See* Luteinizing hormone

Libido, 330
   definition of, 354
Lice. *See* Pediculosis
Lifestyle, health and, 339
Ligation
   definition of, 354
   for pulmonary embolism, 174
Lipid
   abnormalities in, 4
   definition of, 354
Lipiduria, 80
   definition of, 354
Liver
   cancer of, 46t, 47
   diseases of, 142–149, 143f, 145f
Localized cancer, 46, 46t
Lockjaw. *See* Tetanus
Lordosis, 262–266, 266f
Lou Gehrig's disease. *See* Amyotrophic
      lateral sclerosis
Love, health and, 342–343
Low-dose dexamethasone suppression
      test, 365
Lower gastrointestinal tract disease(s),
      134–142
Lower urinary tract disease(s), 83–85
Lumbar pain, 73
Lumbar puncture, 230, 232, 232f, 365
Lumbar region, definition of, 354
Lumen
   of aorta, 61
   of artery, 194
   definition of, 354
Lumpectomy, 116
Lung
   abscess of, 163–165, 164f
   cancer of, 45f, 46t, 47, 176–177
Lupus erythematosus (LE) test, 365
Luteinizing hormone (LH), 114
   definition of, 354
Lyme disease, 27t, 32, 32f
Lymphadenopathy, 17
   in colorectal cancer, 141
   definition of, 354
   in syphilis, 103
Lymphangiography, 365
Lymphangitis, 211
   definition of, 354
Lymphatic system disease(s), 185,
      186f, 209–211, 210f
Lymphedema, 209–211
Lymphoblast(s), 208
Lymphocyte(s), 203f
Lymphocytopenia, 211
   definition of, 354
Lymphoma
   Burkitt's, 48
   non-Hodgkin's. *See* Non-Hodgkin's
      lymphoma
Lymphosarcoma, 17, 211–212

Lysis
   for deep-vein thrombophlebitis, 201
   definition of, 354

M

McBurney's point
   definition of, 354
   pain in appendicitis, 136, 136f
Macrocephaly, 67
   definition of, 354
Macrophage(s), 15
   definition of, 354
Macula, 316
   definition of, 354
Macular degeneration, 316
Macule, 286f, 286t
   definition of, 354
   in impetigo, 291
   in syphilis, 103
   in varicella, 37
Maculopapular lesion
   definition of, 354
   in measles, 34
Magnetic resonance imaging (MRI),
      365
Malabsorption, 18
Malabsorption syndrome, 134
Malaise
   in common cold, 28
   definition of, 354
   in gastroenteritis, 131
   in glomerulonephritis, 79
   in osteomyelitis, 269
   in sinusitis, 160
Malaria, 8, 27t
Male infertility, 98
Male pattern baldness, 289–291
Male reproductive system disease(s),
      104–108, 105–106f
   common symptoms of, 108
Malignant giant-cell tumor, 279
Malignant melanoma. *See* Melanoma
Malignant tumor, 13, 44, 45t. *See also*
      Cancer
Malnourishment, 18
Mammary dysplasia, 115–116
Mammogram, 47, 365
   definition of, 354
Mantoux test, 169
Massage, 225, 332
Mastectomy, total radical, 116
Matrix
   bone, 267
   definition of, 354
Measles, 8, 25t, 27t, 33–34
Measles vaccine, 34
Medicine, holistic, 338–339
Mediterranean disease. *See*
      Thalassemia

Megakaryocyte(s), 203f, 205
   definition of, 354
Megaloblast(s), 204
Megaloblastic anemia. *See* Pernicious
      anemia
Melanin, 285
   definition of, 354
Melanoma, 45f, 46t, 303–304, 304f
   acral-lentiginous, 303–304
   lentigo maligna, 303–304, 304f
   nodular, 303–304
   superficial spreading, 303–304
   warning signs of, 305f
Menarche, 111
   definition of, 354
Mendelian disorder. *See* Monogenic
      disorder
Ménière's disease, 322–323
Meninges, 222, 230, 231f
   definition of, 354
Meningitis
   acute bacterial, 230–231, 231f
   meningococcal, 25t, 27t
Meningocele, 57–58, 58f
Meningococcal meningitis, 25t, 27t
Menopause, 114
Menorrhagia, 113, 203, 253
   definition of, 354
Mental factor(s), in disease process,
      17–18
Metabolic factor(s), 66–67
Metabolic gout, 274
Metastasis, 13, 44, 46, 85, 108
   definition of, 354
Metered-dose inhaler, 169
Metrorrhagia, 113
   definition of, 354
Microorganism(s), pathogenic, 7–9
   definition of, 356
Microscopic urine, 365
Micturition, 84
   definition of, 354
Migraine headache, 224–225
   premonitory symptoms of, 225
Mind-body connection(s), 337–343
Miner's asthma. *See* Anthracosis
Miner's elbow, 275
Mineral deficiency, 19
Mineral excess, 19
Mite, 9
Mitochondria, 202
   definition of, 354
Mitral insufficiency, 190
Mitral regurgitation, 196
   definition of, 354
Mitral stenosis, 190
Mitral valve prolapse, 190
Mixed connective-tissue disease, 17
Mixed hernia, 133
MMR vaccine, 35t

Monoblast(s), 208
Monocyte(s), 203f
Monogenic disorder, 4–6, 5f
Mononucleosis, infectious. *See*
    Infectious mononucleosis
Morphea, 298
Motion sickness, 322
Motor neuron, 223f
MRI. *See* Magnetic resonance imaging
MS. *See* Multiple sclerosis
Multifactorial disorder, 6
Multiple sclerosis (MS), 237–238
Mumps, 8, 25t, 27t, 37
Mumps vaccine, 37
Murmur, 62, 190
Muscular dystrophy, Duchenne's, 6,
    279–280
Musculoskeletal disease(s), 261–280,
    263–265f
    alternative medicine for, 274, 276
    bone disorders, 262–272, 263f
    of children, 279–280
    common symptoms of, 280
    congenital, 65–66
    connective tissue diseases,
        264–265f, 275–279
    joint diseases, 272–274
    laboratory tests for, 377–378
    muscle diseases, 264–265f, 275–279
    organ function tests for, 371
    tumors, 279
Music, therapeutic value of, 333
Mutation, 4, 13, 48
    definition of, 354
Myalgia
    definition of, 355
    in diarrhea, 142
    in influenza, 29
    in prostatitis, 104
Myalgic encephalomyelitis. *See*
    Chronic fatigue syndrome
Myasthenia gravis, 17, 276–277
Mycoplasmal pneumonia, 162t
Mycosis, 7–8, 7f
    respiratory, 172–173
Myelin sheath, 237
Myeloblast(s), 207
Myelography, 365
Myelomeningocele, 57–58, 58f
Myelosuppression, 207
    definition of, 355
Myocardial infarction, 195–196, 196f
Myocarditis, 188–189
Myocardium, 11, 194
    definition of, 355
Myopia, 312f, 313
Myotonia, 95
    definition of, 355
Myringotomy, 321
    definition of, 355

Myxedema, 253
Myxedema coma, 253

 N

Nail(s), 285, 285f
Narcotic(s), definition of, 355
Nasal discharge, purulent, 160
Natural immunity, 15
Near-drowning, 12–13
Nearsightedness. *See* Myopia
Neck trauma, 11
Negative emotion(s), 338, 341, 341t
Neoplasm(s), 14, 43–52
    classification of, 47–48
    definition of, 44, 355
    diagnosis of, 49
    etiology of, 48–49
    grading and staging of, 48
    treatment of, 49–52
        alternative medicine, 51–52
        chemotherapy, 50
        hormonal therapy, 51
        immunotherapy, 51
        radiation therapy, 50
        surgery, 49–50
Nephrectomy, 65, 85
    definition of, 355
Nephritis, 292
    definition of, 355
Nephron, 73, 76f
Nephrosclerosis, 200
    definition of, 355
Nephrotic syndrome, 79–80
Nerve block, intercostal, 166
Nervous system disease(s), 219–239,
    221–223f
    cancer, 239
    cerebral diseases/disorders, 234–236
    common symptoms of, 239
    congenital, 57–59
    degenerative diseases, 236–238
    head trauma, 225–228
    headache, 221–225
    infections of central nervous
        system, 230–233
    laboratory tests for, 376
    organ function tests for, 370
    paralysis, 228–230
    peripheral nerve diseases, 233–234
Neural tube defect(s), 57–58, 58f
Neuritis
    definition of, 355
    peripheral, 233
    in pernicious anemia, 205
Neuroblastoma, definition of, 355
Neurogenic bladder, 84–85
Neuromodulator, 330
    definition of, 355
Neuron, 221, 223f

Neurotomy, 332
    definition of, 355
Neurotransmitter, 330
    definition of, 355
Neutropenia
    in acute myeloblastic leukemia, 208
    definition of, 355
Nevus, 58
    definition of, 355
Nit(s), 292, 293f
Nocturia
    definition of, 355
    in pyelonephritis, 78
Nodular melanoma, 303–304
Nodule, 286f, 286t
Noncommunicating hydrocephalus,
    58–59
Non-Hodgkin's lymphoma, 17, 47–48,
    211–212
Nonvirulent strain, 33
    definition of, 355
Normoblast(s), definition of, 355
North American blastomycosis,
    172–173
Nosebleed. *See* Epistaxis
Nuchal rigidity, 230
    definition of, 355
Nucleus pulposus, 266
Nutrition, 340
Nutritional imbalance, 18–19
Nystagmus, 313
    in cerebral palsy, 57
    definition of, 355
    in toxemias of pregnancy, 120

 O

Obesity, 18
Occult blood, 135, 367
    definition of, 355
Ohio Valley disease. *See*
    Histoplasmosis
Oil aspiration, 162t
Oil gland, 285, 285f
Oligomenorrhea, 114
    definition of, 355
Oligospermia, 98
    definition of, 355
Oliguria, 77t
    definition of, 355
    in glomerulonephritis, 79
    in toxemias of pregnancy, 120
Open fracture, 270, 271f
Open reduction, 272
Open-angle glaucoma, 315
Ophthalmia neonatorum, gonorrheal,
    25t, 99
    definition of, 352
Ophthalmopathy, 252
Ophthalmoscopy, 365

Opportunistic infection, 31
  definition of, 355
Opticokinetic drum test, 365
Oral cavity cancer, 45f, 46t, 47
Orchidectomy, 108
  definition of, 355
Orchitis, 106–107
Organ function test(s)
  for circulatory system diseases, 369
  for digestive system diseases,
    371–372
  for endocrine system diseases,
    370–371
  for hematologic system diseases,
    370
  for immune system diseases, 372
  for musculoskeletal diseases, 371
  for nervous system diseases, 370
  for reproductive system diseases,
    372
  for respiratory system diseases,
    369–370
  for tumors, 372–373
  for urinary system diseases, 371
Orgasmic dysfunction, in women, 97
Orthopnea
  definition of, 355
  in pericarditis, 188
  in pulmonary edema, 173
Ortolani's sign, 66, 365
  definition of, 355
Osteitis deformans. *See* Paget's disease
Osteoarthritis, 272
Osteogenic sarcoma, 279
Osteolytic lesion, 48
  definition of, 355
Osteoma, 47
Osteomalacia, 268–269
Osteomyelitis, 269–270
Osteoporosis, 267–268, 268f
  risk factors for, 269t
Osteosarcoma, 47
Otitis media, 11, 321, 323
  serous, 321
  suppurative, 321
Otologic examination, 365
Otosclerosis, 322
Otoscopy, 365
Ovary
  cancer of, 46t
  cyst of, 111–112
  disease of, endocrine, 246t
  tumors of, 111–112

P

PAC. *See* Pulmonary artery
    catheterization
Paget's disease, 270

Pain
  acute, 330–331
  assessment of, 330
  chronic, 330–331
  definition of, 328–329
  at McBurney's point, 136, 136f
  pathophysiology of, 329–330, 329f
  purpose of, 329
  terminal, 330–331
  treatment of
    alternative medicine, 333–334
    autohypnosis, 332
    biofeedback, 332
    humor, laughter, and play, 332–333
    imagery, 332
    massage, 332
    medications, 331
    music, 333
    relaxation therapy, 332
    surgery, 331–332
    transcutaneous electrical nerve
      stimulation, 332
Painful intercourse. *See* Dyspareunia
Palliative treatment, 50
  definition of, 355
Pallor
  in colorectal cancer, 141
  definition of, 355
  in erythroblastosis fetalis, 61
  in nephrotic syndrome, 80
  in pneumothorax, 166
Pancreatic cancer, 45f, 46t, 144
Pancreatic disease(s), 142–149, 143f
  endocrine, 246t, 256–258
Pancreatitis
  acute, 142–143
  chronic, 143–144
Panhypopituitarism, 249
Panhysterosalpingo-oophorectomy,
    113
  definition of, 355
Pap test. *See* Papanicolaou test
Papanicolaou (Pap) test, 47, 49, 366
  definition of, 355
Papilloma, 101
  definition of, 355
Papillomatosis, 115
  definition of, 355
Papillomavirus, 101
  definition of, 355
Papule, 286f, 286t
  in acne vulgaris, 288
  definition of, 356
  in rubella, 34
  in syphilis, 103
Paraesophageal hernia, 133
Paralysis, 228–230
Paraplegia, 228–230
Parasite(s), 9, 10f
Parasympathetic ganglion, 59

  definition of, 356
Parasympathetic nerve, 221, 221f
Parathyroid gland disease(s), 246t,
    254–255
Parathyroid hormone (PTH), 254–255
Paratyphoid fever, 28t
Parenteral administration, definition
    of, 356
Parenteral hyperalimentation, 143
Parenteral iron supplements, 204
Paresthesia
  definition of, 356
  in herniated intervertebral disk, 266
  in hyperpituitarism, 248
Parity, 113
  definition of, 356
Parkinson's disease, 237
Partial seizure, 236
Partial thickness burn, 14f
Particle beam therapy, 50
Parturition, 113
  definition of, 356
Patch test, 366
Patent blood vessel, definition of,
    356
Patent ductus arteriosus (PDA), 61–62
Pathogenic microorganism(s), 7–9
  definition of, 356
Patient-controlled analgesia (PCA),
    331, 331f
  definition of, 356
PCA. *See* Patient-controlled analgesia
PDA. *See* Patent ductus arteriosus
Pediculosis, 292–293, 293f, 305
Pediculosis capitis, 292
Pediculosis corporis, 292
Pediculosis pubis, 292
Pedigree, 5f
Pelvic examination, 366
Pelvic inflammatory disease (PID),
    113–114
Pelvic trauma, 11
Penile prosthesis, 97
Penlight examination, 366
Peptic ulcer
  of duodenum. *See* Duodenal ulcer
  of stomach. *See* Gastric ulcer
Percussion, 166, 362
  definition of, 356
Percutaneous transluminal coronary
    angioplasty (PTCA), 195
  definition of, 356
Perforated eardrum, 10–11
Pericardial effusion, 188
Pericardiocentesis, 188, 366
  definition of, 356
Pericarditis, 187–188, 188f
Peripheral artery aneurysm, 199–200,
    199f
Peripheral edema, 197, 197f

Peripheral nervous system (PNS), 221, 221f
Peripheral nerve system disease(s), 233–234
Peripheral neuritis, 233
Peristalsis, 59
    definition of, 356
Peritoneal dialysis, 86, 87f
Pernicious anemia, 17, 204f, 205
Personal responsibility, 339
Pertussis, 8, 25t, 28t, 39
    catarrhal stage of, 39
    paroxysmal stage of, 39
Pertussis vaccine, 39
Petechia
    in acute myeloblastic leukemia, 207
    definition of, 356
    in endocarditis, 189
    in erythroblastosis fetalis, 61
pH, 7
    of blood, 175
    definition of, 356
    of urine, 78t
pH studies, 366
Phacoemulsification, 315
    definition of, 356
Phagocytosis, 15, 169
    definition of, 356
Pharyngitis
    acute, 160–161
    chronic, 160–161
    streptococcal, 26t
Phenotype, 4
    definition of, 356
Phenylketonuria (PKU), 4, 67
Phenylketonuria (PKU) test, 366
Philadelphia chromosome, 209
Phlebography, 201, 366
Phlebotomy, 207
Phosphate(s), urine, 368
Phosphorus, serum, 367
Photophobia
    in chronic fatigue syndrome, 30
    definition of, 356
    in uveitis, 317
Phototherapy, 61
    definition of, 356
Physical agent(s), in disease process, 11–14
Physical trauma, 9
PID. *See* Pelvic inflammatory disease
Pinkeye. *See* Conjunctivitis
Pinworm(s), 9, 10f, 151–152
Pitting edema, 198
    definition of, 356
Pituitary gland disease(s), 246t, 247–251
PKU. *See* Phenylketonuria
Placenta previa, 120–121, 120f

Plague vaccine, 36t
Plaque
    atherosclerotic, 195
    definition of, 356
    in discoid lupus erythematosus, 297
Plasma, definition of, 356
Plasma test(s), reference values for, 389–391
Plasmodium, 8f
Platelet(s), 203f
Play
    health and, 341–342
    therapeutic value of, 332–333
Pleura, 11, 166
    definition of, 356
Pleural effusion, 166–167
Pleurectomy, 166
    definition of, 356
Pleurisy, 166
Pleuritis. *See* Pleurisy
Plication
    definition of, 356
    for pulmonary embolism, 174
PMS. *See* Premenstrual syndrome
Pneumococcal pneumonia, 28t
Pneumococcal vaccine, 36t
Pneumoconiosis, 171–173
Pneumocystis carinii, 8f
Pneumoencephalography, definition of, 356
Pneumonia, 8, 26t, 162–163, 163f
    aspiration, 163
    diseases accompanied by, 162t
    microbial causes of, 162t
    not caused by infection, 162t
    pneumococcal, 28t
Pneumothorax, 165–166, 165f
PNS. *See* Peripheral nervous system
Poisoning, 12
Poliomyelitis, 8, 26t, 28t, 33
Poliomyelitis vaccine, 36t
Polyarthritis, 187
Polycystic kidney disease, 73–78
Polycythemia vera, 174, 206–207
    definition of, 356
Polydipsia
    definition of, 356
    in diabetes, 256
Polymorphonuclear leukocyte(s), 6
    definition of, 356
Polymyositis, 277–278
Polypeptide hormone(s), references values for, 394–395
Polyphagia, 256
    definition of, 356
Polyposis, 141
    definition of, 356
Polyposis coli, 48

Polyuria, 77t
    in chronic renal failure, 80
    definition of, 356
    in diabetes insipidus, 249
Portal hypertension, 147
Postmenopausal bleeding, 114
Postnatal period, definition of, 356
Postural drainage, 163, 176
    definition of, 356
PPD tuberculin test, 366
Predisposing factor(s), in disease process, 3
Preeclampsia. *See* Toxemia(s) of pregnancy
Pregnancy
    ectopic, 118, 119f
    rubella during, 37, 62
Pregnancy disorder(s), 116–122
    common symptoms of, 122
Pregnancy test, 367
Premature ejaculation, 97
Premature labor, 121
Premature rupture of membranes (PROM), 121
Premenopausal bleeding, abnormal, 114
Premenstrual syndrome (PMS), 109–111
Premonitory symptom(s), of migraine, 225
Prenatal period, definition of, 357
Presbyopia, 311–313
Presenile dementia. *See* Alzheimer's disease
Preventive surgery, 50
Primigravida, 120
    definition of, 357
Proctoscopy, 366
Projectile vomiting, 59
    definition of, 357
Prolapse
    definition of, 357
    mitral valve, 190
PROM. *See* Premature rupture of membranes
Prostaglandin, 111
    definition of, 357
Prostate cancer, 45f, 46t, 47, 51, 107–108
Prostate-specific antigen (PSA), 366
Prostatitis, 104–105
Prosthesis
    definition of, 357
    penile, 97
Protein electrophoresis, serum, 367
Proteinuria, 77t
    definition of, 357
    in nephrotic syndrome, 79–80
    in viral hepatitis, 148

Protozoa, pathogenic, 8, 8f
Pruritus
in allergic reaction, 16
in chronic renal failure, 80
definition of, 357
in diabetes, 257
in external otitis, 320
in hemorrhoids, 139
in Hodgkin's disease, 211
in psoriasis, 287
PSA. *See* Prostate-specific antigen
Pseudofracture, 269
Psittacosis, 162t
Psoriasis, 287, 287f
Psychosomatic illness, 341
PTCA. *See* Percutaneous transluminal coronary angioplasty
PTH. *See* Parathyroid hormone
Ptosis, 277
definition of, 357
Puerperal fever, 28t
Pulmonary artery catheterization (PAC), 366
Pulmonary edema, 173, 197, 197f
Pulmonary embolism, 174–175, 174f
Pulmonary emphysema, chronic, 168, 168f
Pulmonary function study(ies), 366
Pulmonary infarction, 174–175
definition of, 357
Pulmonary stenosis, 61–62
Pulmonary tuberculosis. *See* Tuberculosis
Pulmonic insufficiency, 192
Pulmonic stenosis, 192
Pulse, thready, 173, 358
Purpura
in aplastic anemia, 205
definition of, 357
Purulent discharge
definition of, 357
nasal, 160
urethral, 99
Pustule, 286f, 286t
in acne vulgaris, 288
definition of, 357
in genital herpes, 100, 100f
Pyelogram
intravenous, 364
retrograde, 366
Pyelonephritis, acute, 78–79
Pyloric sphincter, 59
definition of, 357
Pyloric stenosis, 59
Pyloromyotomy, 59
Pyoderma, 293
definition of, 357
Pyuria
in appendicitis, 136

definition of, 357
in pyelonephritis, 78

Q

Q fever, 162t
Quadriplegia, 228–230

R

RA. *See* Rheumatoid arthritis
Rabies, 8, 9f, 28t
Rabies vaccine, 36t
Radial keratotomy, 313
definition of, 357
Radiation therapy, 50
Radioimmunoassay, 366
Radioisotope, 50, 196
definition of, 357
Radioisotope study(ies), 366
Radioresistant cancer, 50
Rales
definition of, 357
in mitral insufficiency/stenosis, 190
in pneumonia, 163
Rauwolfia, 135
definition of, 357
Raynaud's phenomenon, 278
definition of, 357
Recessive trait, autosomal, 4–6, 5f, 66, 73, 348
Rectal examination, 366
Rectal manometry, 366
Red blood cell disorder(s), 202–207, 203f
Reduction
closed, 272
open, 272
Reed-Sternberg cell, 48, 211
definition of, 357
Reference value(s), for laboratory tests, 389–401
Reflux
definition of, 357
esophageal, 133
urinary, 65
Refraction test, 366
Refractive error(s), 311–313, 312f
Regional cancer, 46, 46t
Regional enteritis. *See* Crohn's disease
Relaxation therapy, 225, 332
Religion, 342–343
Renal calculi, 64, 73, 81–83, 82f
definition of, 357
Renal failure
chronic, 80–81
treatment of, 86–88
dialysis, 86, 87f
hemodialysis, 86–88, 87f

kidney transplantation, 88
peritoneal dialysis, 86, 87f
Renal function test, 366
Renal gout, 274
Reproductive system disease(s), 93–122
breast diseases, 115–117, 115f
female reproductive diseases, 109–114, 109–110f
laboratory tests for, 378–379
male reproductive diseases, 104–108, 105–106f
organ function tests for, 372
pregnancy and delivery disorders, 118–122
sexual dysfunction, 96–98
sexually transmitted diseases, 99–104
Resection
definition of, 357
of ureter, 64
Respiration
external, 159
internal, 159–160
Respiratory acidosis, 175
Respiratory alkalosis, 175
Respiratory mycosis, 172–173
Respiratory system disease(s), 157–179, 159f
of children, 177–179
common symptoms of, 179
laboratory tests for, 376
organ function tests for, 369–370
pneumoconiosis, 171–173
Reticulocyte(s), definition of, 357
Reticulocyte count, 205, 366
Reticulum cell sarcoma, 211
Retinal detachment, 315–316, 315f
Retinoblastoma, 6, 48
Retinopathy
definition of, 357
diabetes-induced, 258
Retrocaval ureter, 64
Retrograde pyelogram, 366
Retrovirus, 30
definition of, 357
Reye's syndrome, 29, 37, 212–213
Rh factor, 60
Rh immune globulin (RhIg), 61
Rheumatic fever, 17, 162t, 185–187
Rheumatic heart disease, 185–187
Rheumatoid arthritis (RA), 6, 272–273, 273f
Rheumatoid factor, 366
RhIg. *See* Rh immune globulin
Rhinitis
definition of, 357
epistaxis and, 160
in measles, 34

Rhizopus, 7f
Rhonchus, 172
    definition of, 357
    in toxemias of pregnancy, 120
Rickets, 18, 268
Rickettsiae, 8, 162t
Right ventricular hypertrophy, 190
Ringed sideroblast(s), 202
Ringworm. *See* Tinea corporis
Rinne test, 322, 366
Risking, 343
Rocky Mountain spotted fever, 8, 162t
Round back. *See* Kyphosis
Roundworm(s), 9, 151–152
Rubella, 26t, 28t, 34–37
    definition of, 357
    maternal, 62
Rubella vaccine, 37
Rubeola. *See* Measles
Rule of nines, 13, 14f

S

Sacculated aneurysm, 199, 199f
Salicylate(s), 131–132
    definition of, 357
    for herniated intervertebral disk,
        267
Salmonellosis, 28t
Sarcoma, 45t, 47
    Ewing's, 279
    Kaposi's, 31
    osteogenic, 279
    reticulum cell, 211
Scabies, 28t
Scale, 286f, 286t
Scarlet fever, 28t
Schilling test, 205, 366
Schilling's leukemia. *See* Acute
        monoblastic leukemia
Scintiscan, 367
Scleroderma, 17, 298
    morphea, 298
    systemic, 298
Sclerotherapy, 202
Scoliosis, 262–266, 266f
Scurvy, 18
Seborrhea, 318
    definition of, 357
Seborrheic dermatitis, 298–299, 299f
Second degree burn, 14f
Seizure, 235–236
    generalized, 236
    partial, 236
Semen analysis, 363
Senile cataract, 314
Sensory neuron, 223f
Septic embolism, 165
Septic organism, definition of, 357

Septicemia
    definition of, 358
    in pelvic inflammatory disease, 114
Septum
    definition of, 358
    ventricular, 61
Sequential multiple analyzer (SMA),
        375
Seroconversion, 31
    definition of, 358
Serological study, 367
Serous otitis media, 321
Serum test(s), 367
    references values for, 389–391
714X treatment, 51
Sex, as predisposing factor, 3
Sex therapy, 97
Sex-linked trait, 6
Sexual dysfunction, 96–98
Sexual health, 95
Sexual response cycle, 95
Sexually transmitted disease(s) (STD),
        99–104
    common symptoms of, 104
SGOT. *See* Aspartate aminotransferase
SGPT. *See* Alanine aminotransferase
Shigellosis, 27t
Shingles. *See* Herpes zoster
Shock
    anaphylactic, 16
    cardiogenic, 196, 349
    hypovolemic, 11, 118, 353
    insulin, 257
Shock wave lithotripsy, 146
    extracorporeal, 82
Shunt
    definition of, 358
    for hydrocephalus, 59
Sickle cell anemia, 4–6, 204f, 206
Sickle cell trait, 206
Sideroblast(s), ringed, 202
Sideroblastic anemia, 202
SIDS. *See* Sudden infant death
        syndrome
Sigmoidoscopy, 367
Silicosis, 171
Silo-filler's disease, 162t
Sinusitis, 160
    acute, 160
    chronic, 160
Skin cancer, 303
    basal cell carcinoma, 303
    squamous cell carcinoma, 303
Skin disease(s), 283–306, 285f
    acne vulgaris, 288, 289f
    alopecia, 289–291, 290f
    carbuncles, 291–292, 292f
    of children, 304–306
    common symptoms of, 306
    corns and calluses, 296

    decubitus ulcers, 293, 294f
    dermatitis, 298–301
    dermatophytosis, 293–296,
        294–296f
    discoid lupus erythematosus, 297
    furuncles, 291–292
    herpes-related lesions, 301–302
    impetigo, 291, 291f
    pediculosis, 292–293, 293f
    psoriasis, 287, 287f
    scleroderma, 298
    ulcer of, 49
    urticaria, 287–288, 288f
    warts, 296–297, 297f
Skin lesion(s), 285–287, 286f, 286t
    in genital herpes, 100, 100f
Skin test, 367
Skull fracture, 10
SLE. *See* Systemic lupus erythematosus
Sliding hernia, 132–133
Slipped disk, 266
Slit-lamp examination, 367
SMA. *See* Sequential multiple analyzer
Smoking, 46–47, 176–177
Snake bite, 13
Snellen's chart, 367
Spastic cerebral palsy, 57
Spastic colon. *See* Irritable bowel
        syndrome
Specific gravity, of urine, 78t
Specific surgery, 50
Spider bite, 13
Spina bifida, 57–58, 58f
Spina bifida occulta, 57–58
Spinal cord injury, 11, 228–230,
        229f
Spinal trauma, 11
Spine, deformities of, 262–266, 266f
Spirillum, 8, 9f
Spirituality, 342–343
Spirochete, 32
    definition of, 358
Spirometry, 176
Splenomegaly
    in cirrhosis, 147
    definition of, 358
Spontaneous abortion, 118
Sporadic condition, 250
Sprain, 275
Sprue, celiac, 134–135
Sputum, 163
    definition of, 358
Sputum culture, 367
Sputum study, 169–170
Squamous cell carcinoma, 303
Staghorn calculi, 82f
Staging, of cancer, 46, 48
Stapedectomy, 322
    definition of, 358
Starvation, 18

Stasis pigmentation, 202
  definition of, 358
STD. *See* Sexually transmitted
       disease(s)
Stenosis
  bronchial, 165
  definition of, 358
  valvular, 190, 191f
Steroid hormone(s), references values
       for, 393–394
Stomach cancer, 46t
Stomatitis, 129
  acute herpetic, 129
  aphthous, 129
Stool culture, 367
Stool occult blood. *See* Occult blood
Strabismus, 318–319, 319f
Strain, 275
Stratum corneum, 296
  definition of, 358
Streptococcal pharyngitis, 26t
Stress, 340–341
Stridor
  in acute epiglottitis, 178
  in allergic reaction, 16
  in aneurysms, 199
  definition of, 358
Stroke. *See* Cerebrovascular accident
Stupor, 230
  definition of, 358
Stye, 313–314
Subcutaneous layer, 285, 285f
Subcutaneous nodule(s), in rheumatic
       fever, 187
Subdural hematoma, 225–227, 226f
Substantia gelatinosa, definition of,
       358
Sudden infant death syndrome (SIDS),
       177
Superficial spreading melanoma,
       303–304
Suppurative lesion, definition of, 358
Suppurative otitis media, 321
Surgery
  en bloc, 50, 351
  palliative, 50
  preventive, 50
  specific, 50
  treatment of neoplasms, 49–50
Sweat gland, 285, 285f
Swimmer's ear. *See* External otitis
Sympathectomy, 201
  definition of, 358
Sympathetic nerve, 221, 221f
Synapse, 330
  definition of, 358
Syncope
  definition of, 358
  in goiter, 250
  in heart disease, 11

in tricuspid stenosis, 191
Synovial fluid analysis, 368
Syphilis, 8, 26t, 28t, 101–103, 102f,
       162t
  latent, 103
  primary, 102
  secondary, 103
  tertiary, 103
Systemic disease, 6
  definition of, 358
Systemic lupus erythematosus (SLE),
       17, 278–279, 278f
Systemic scleroderma, 298
Systemic sclerosis. *See* Scleroderma
Systolic pressure, 193
  definition of, 358

T

T_3. *See* Triiodothyronine
T_4. *See* Tetraiodothyronine
Tachycardia
  in chest trauma, 11
  definition of, 358
  in menopause, 114
  in pericarditis, 188
  in pulmonary edema, 173
Tachypnea
  in chronic bronchitis, 167
  in coarctation of the aorta, 62
  definition of, 358
Talipes calcaneus, 65
Talipes equinus, 65
Talipes valgus, 65
Talipes varus, 65
Tapeworm, 9, 10f
Taxol, 50
Tay-Sachs disease, 4
TB. *See* Tuberculosis
T-cell lymphocyte(s), 15, 30
Tendonitis, 276
Tennis elbow, 275
TENS. *See* Transcutaneous electrical
       nerve stimulation
Teratogen, 58
  definition of, 358
Teratoma, 112
  definition of, 358
Terminal pain, 330–331
Testes
  cancer of, 46t, 108
  disease of, endocrine, 246t
  undescended, 64, 108, 350
Tetanus, 8, 28t, 39–40
Tetanus immune globulin (TIG), 40
Tetanus toxoid, 40
Tetany
  in celiac sprue, 134
  definition of, 358
  in hypoparathyroidism, 255

Tetraiodothyronine (T_4), 250–253
Tetralogy of Fallot, 61–62
Thalassemia, 202
Therapeutic touch, 333
Thermography, 368
Third degree burn, 14f
Thoracentesis, 166–167, 368
  definition of, 358
Thoracic artery aneurysm, 199–200,
       199f
Thoracotomy, 166
  definition of, 358
Thready pulse, 173
  definition of, 358
Thrill, 62
  definition of, 358
Thrombocytopenia
  in acute myeloblastic leukemia, 208
  definition of, 358
  idiopathic, 17
Thrombocytosis, 174
  definition of, 358
Thromboendarterectomy, 201
  definition of, 358
Thrombophlebitis, 201–202
Thrombosis, 234
  definition of, 358
Thrombus, 199
  definition of, 358
Thrush, 8
Thymoma, 277
Thyroid cancer, 45f, 46t
Thyroid function test(s), 368
Thyroid gland disease(s), 246t,
       250–253
Thyroid hormone(s), references values
       for, 396
Thyroid storm, 252
Thyroiditis, Hashimoto's, 17, 251
Thyroid-stimulating hormone (TSH),
       249, 253
Thyrotoxicosis, 17, 251–252
TIA. *See* Transient ischemic attack
TIG. *See* Tetanus immune globulin
Tight chest, 169
Tinea capitis, 293–296, 294f, 305–306
Tinea corporis, 7f, 8, 293–296, 295f,
       305–306
Tinea cruris, 293–296, 296f
Tinea pedis, 8, 293–296, 295f
Tinea unguium, 293–296, 295f
Tinel's sign, 276
Tinnitus
  definition of, 358
  in essential hypertension, 193
  in impacted cerumen, 319
  in migraine, 225
TNM system, 48
Tonometer, 315
  definition of, 359

Tonometry, 368
Tonsillectomy, 178
Tonsillitis, acute, 177–178
Tophus, 274, 368
  definition of, 359
Total radical mastectomy, 116
Total serum protein, 367
Toxemia, 138
  definition of, 359
Toxemia(s) of pregnancy, 57, 118–120
Toxic shock syndrome, 28t
Toxocariasis, 151–152
Toxoplasma gondii, 8f
Trabecular meshwork, 315
Tracheostomy, 179
Trachoma, 26t, 28t
Transcutaneous electrical nerve
    stimulation (TENS), 332
Transfusion, exchange, 61, 351
Transfusion reaction, 16
Transient ischemic attack (TIA), 235
Transient visual scotomata, 30
  definition of, 359
Transillumination
  definition of, 359
  of sinuses, 160
Transposition of the great vessels, 62
Transudate, 166
  definition of, 359
Transurethral prostate resection
    (TURP), 107
Transurethral resection, 86
  definition of, 359
Transurethral thermo-ablation
    therapy, 107
Trauma, 9–11. *See also* specific organs
  head, 225–228
Traumatic cataract, 314
Traveler's diarrhea. *See* Gastroenteritis
Trench fever, 8
Trendelenburg's test, 368
Trichiniasis, 162t
Trichomonas, 8
Trichomoniasis, 8, 103–104
Tricuspid insufficiency, 191
Tricuspid stenosis, 191
Trigger point, 332
  definition of, 359
Triiodothyronine (T$_3$), 250–253
Trisomy 21, 6
  definition of, 350
Trypanosoma, 8f
TSH. *See* Thyroid-stimulating
    hormone
Tuberculin test, 170
Tuberculosis (TB), 8, 26t, 28t,
    169–170, 170f
Tularemia, 28t, 162t

Tumor(s), 44, 286t. *See also*
    Neoplasm(s)
  benign, 13, 44, 45t
  brain, 239
  encapsulated, 44
  laboratory tests for, 379
  malignant, 13, 44, 45t. *See also*
    Cancer
  of musculoskeletal system, 279
  organ function tests for, 372–373
  of urinary system, 85–86
Turner's syndrome, 6
TURP. *See* Transurethral prostate
    resection
Tympanoplasty, 321
  definition of, 359
Typhoid fever, 8, 26t, 28t, 162t
Typhoid vaccine, 36t
Typhus, 8, 28t, 162t

U

Ulcer
  decubitus, 237, 293, 294f
  duodenal, 135
  gastric, 131–132, 131f
  skin, 49, 286t
Ulcerative colitis, 17, 137–138
Ultrasonic cutaneous lithotripsy, 82
Ultrasonography, 368
Umbilical hernia, 133f, 140–141
Undescended testes, 64, 108
  definition of, 350
Universal precautions, 31–32
  definition of, 359
Unstable angina, 195
Upper gastrointestinal endoscopy, 368
Upper gastrointestinal tract disease(s),
    129–133
Urate crystals in joint fluid, 368
Urea, 80
  definition of, 359
Uremia, 78. *See also* Renal failure,
    chronic
  definition of, 359
Ureter
  congenital defects of, 64–65
  duplicated, 64
  ectopic orifice of, 64–65
  retrocaval, 64
  stricture or stenosis of, 65
Ureterocele, 65
Urethra, congenital defects of, 64–65
Urethral discharge, purulent, 99
Urethritis, 83–84
Urinalysis, 73, 77–78t, 368
  references values for, 392–393
  significance of changes in urine,
    77–78t

Urinary bladder. *See* Bladder
Urinary incontinence, 16, 84
Urinary system disease(s), 71–88,
    74–76f
  common symptoms of, 88
  congenital, 64–65
  kidney diseases, 73–83
  laboratory tests for, 377
  lower urinary tract diseases, 83–85
  organ function tests for, 371
  tumors, 85–86
Urine
  catheterization, 362
  microscopic, 365
Urine catch, 24-hour, 368
Urine concentration and dilution test,
    368
Urine culture, 368
Urolith. *See also* Renal calculi
  definition of, 359
Urticaria, 15, 287–288, 288f
  definition of, 359
Uterus
  cancer of, 49
  leiomyoma of, 111, 113
Uveitis, 317

V

Vaccine, 33–34, 35–36t
Vaginal smear, 368
Vagotomy, 135
Valley fever. *See* Coccidioidomycosis
Valvotomy, 190
  definition of, 359
Valvular heart disease, 190–193,
    190–191f
Valvular stenosis, 190, 191f. *See also*
    specific valves
Varicella, 8, 27t, 37–38, 38f, 212
Varicella-zoster immune globulin
    (VZIG), 38
Varices
  definition of, 359
  esophageal, 147
Varicocele, 98
  definition of, 359
Varicose vein(s), 201f, 202
Vascular endothelial growth factor
    (VEGF), 198
Vasoconstriction, 95
  definition of, 359
Vasodilator, 201
  definition of, 359
Vasopressin, 249–250
  definition of, 359
VDRL test. *See* Venereal Disease
    Research Laboratory test

Vegetation(s), on heart valves, 189, 189f
VEGF. *See* Vascular endothelial growth factor
Vein(s), varicose, 201f, 202
Venereal Disease Research Laboratory (VDRL) test, 368
Venereal herpes. *See* Genital herpes
Ventricle
    of brain, 58
    definition of, 359
Ventricular fibrillation, 193
    definition of, 352
Ventricular septal defect (VSD), 61–62, 62f
Ventricular septal rupture, 196
    definition of, 359
Ventriculography, definition of, 359
Verrucae. *See* Wart(s)
Vertebral column, 228–230, 229f
Vertigo, 322
    definition of, 359
Vesicle, 286f, 286t
    definition of, 359
    in impetigo, 291
    in varicella, 37
Villi, intestinal, 134
    definition of, 359

Viral disease(s), 8, 9f
Viral hepatitis, acute, 147–149
Viral pneumonia, 162t, 163, 163f
Virulence of pathogen, 269
    definition of, 359
Visual acuity test, 368
Vitamin B$_1$, 18
Vitamin B$_{12}$, 205
    serum, 367
Vitamin C, 18
Vitamin D, 18, 268–269
Vitamin D derivative(s), references values for, 396
Vitamin deficiency, 18–19
Vitamin excess, 18–19
Vitreous humor, 316
Vomiting, 151
    projectile, 59, 357
VSD. *See* Ventricular septal defect
VZIG. *See* Varicella-zoster immune globulin

Wart(s), 296–297, 297f
    genital, 101, 101f
WBC. *See* White blood count

Weaver's bottom, 275
Wheal(s), 15, 16f, 286f, 286t
    definition of, 359
    in urticaria, 287, 288f
White blood count (WBC), 368
Whooping cough. *See* Pertussis
Wood's light, 294–296, 368
Worm(s). *See* Helminth(s)
Worship, 342–343

X-linked trait, 6

Yeast, 7f
Yellow fever, 8
Yellow fever vaccine, 36t
Yoga therapy, 333–334, 343

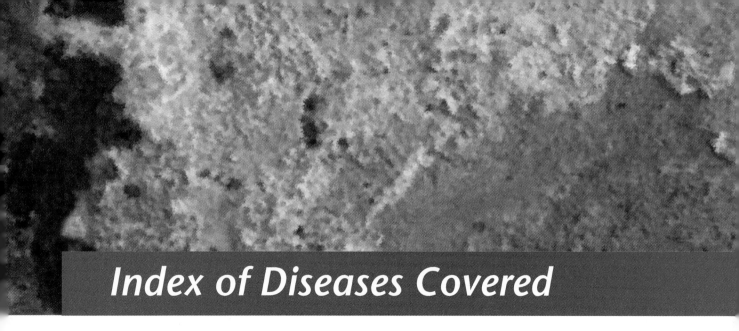

Index of Diseases Covered

A

Abdominal aneurysm, 199–200
Abdominal hernia, 140–141
Abortion, spontaneous, 118
Abruptio placentae, 121
Abscess
  brain, 232–233
  lung, 164–165
Acidosis, respiratory, 175
Acne vulgaris, 288
Acquired immunodeficiency
    syndrome (AIDS), 30–32
Acromegaly. *See* Hyperpituitarism
Acute lymphoblastic (lymphocytic)
    leukemia (ALL), 208
Acute monoblastic (monocytic)
    leukemia, 208
Acute myeloblastic (myelogenous)
    leukemia (AML), 207–208
Acute tubular necrosis (ATN), 81
Adenocarcinoma of the kidney
    (hypernephroma), 85
Adenoid hyperplasia, 178
Alkalosis, respiratory, 175
Allergy, food, 151
Alopecia, 289–291
Alzheimer's disease, 236–237
Amenorrhea, 111
Amyotrophic lateral sclerosis (ALS),
    238
Anemia
  aplastic, 205–206
  folic acid deficiency, 204–205
  iron deficiency, 203–204
  pernicious, 205
  sickle cell, 206
Aneurysms, abdominal, 199–200

Angina pectoris, 195
Anorexia nervosa, 149
Anthracosis, 172
Aortic insufficiency/stenosis, 192–193
Aplastic anemia, 205–206
Appendicitis, acute, 135–136
Arousal dysfunction, in women, 97
Arteriosclerosis, 200–201
Asbestosis, 171
Asthma, 168–169
Atelectasis, 175–176
Atherosclerosis, 200–201
Atopic dermatitis (eczema), 299–301,
    304

B

Bacterial meningitis, acute, 230–231
Bell's palsy, 234
Benign prostatic hyperplasia (BPH),
    107
Berylliosis, 171–172
Bladder
  congenital defects of, 64–65
  tumors of, 85–86
Blepharitis, 317–318
Brain
  abscess of, 232–233
  tumor of, 239
Breast
  benign fibroadenoma of, 116
  cancer of, 116–117
  fibrocystic disease of, 115–116
Bronchiectasis, 176
Bronchitis, chronic, 167–168
Bulimia, 149–150
Bursitis, 275

C

Calluses, 296
Cancer
  breast, 116–117
  colorectal, 141–142
  lung, 176–177
  pancreatic, 144
  prostatic, 107–108
  skin, 303
  testicular, 108
Carbuncles, 291–292
Cardiac arrest, 198
Carpal tunnel syndrome, 275–276
Cataract, 314–315
Celiac sprue (gluten-induced
    enteropathy), 134–135
Cerebral concussion, 227
Cerebral contusion, 227–228
Cerebral palsy, 57
Cerebrovascular accident (stroke),
    234–235
Cerumen, impacted, 319
Chickenpox. *See* Varicella
Chlamydial infections, 104
Cholecystitis, acute, 146–147
Cholelithiasis, 144–146
Chronic fatigue syndrome, 29–30
Chronic lymphocytic leukemia (CLL),
    209
Chronic myelocytic leukemia (CML),
    208–209
Chronic obstructive pulmonary
    disease (COPD), 167
Chronic renal failure (uremia), 80–
    81
Cirrhosis, 147
Clubfoot (talipes), 65

Cold, common, 26–29
Cold sores, 301–303
Colic, infantile, 150
Colitis
  granulomatous. *See* Crohn's disease
  ulcerative, 137–138
Colorectal cancer, 141–142
Common cold, 26–29
Concussion, cerebral, 227
Congenital aganglionic megacolon.
    See Hirschsprung's disease
Congenital defects of ureter, bladder,
    and urethra, 64–65
Congenital heart defects, 61–64
Congenital hip dysplasia, 65–66
Congestive heart failure (CHF),
    197–198
Conjunctivitis, 317
Contact dermatitis, 299
Contusion, cerebral, 227–228
Cor pulmonale, 173–174
Corneal abrasion, 314
Corns, 296
Coronary artery disease, 194–195
Cretinism. *See* Hypothyroidism
Crohn's disease (granulomatous
    colitis, regional enteritis), 137
Croup, 178
Cryptorchidism. *See* Undescended
    testes
Cushing's syndrome, 255–256
Cyst, ovarian, 111–112
Cystic fibrosis, 66–67
Cystitis, 83–84

D

Deafness, 323
Decubitus ulcer, 293
Dermatitis
  atopic, 299–301, 304
  contact, 299
  seborrheic, 298–299
Dermatophytoses, 293–296, 305–306
Diabetes insipidus, 249–250
Diabetes mellitus, 256–258
Diaper rash, 304–305
Diarrhea, 142, 151
Diphtheria, 38–39
Discoid lupus erythematosus, 297
Diverticulitis, 138
Duchenne's muscular dystrophy,
    279–280
Duodenal ulcer (peptic ulcer of the
    duodenum), 135
Dysmenorrhea, 111
Dyspareunia (painful intercourse),
    96

E

Eclampsia. *See* Toxemias of pregnancy
Ectopic pregnancy, 118
Eczema. *See* Atopic dermatitis
Emphysema, chronic pulmonary,
    168
Encephalitis, 231–232
Endocarditis, 189
Endometriosis, 112–113
Epididymitis, 105–106
Epidural hematoma, 225–227
Epiglottitis, acute, 178–179
Epilepsy, 235–236
Epistaxis (nosebleed), 160
Erectile dysfunction (impotence),
    96–97
Erythroblastosis fetalis (hemolytic
    disease of the newborn), 60–61
Escherichia coli O157:H7, 32–33
Essential hypertension, 193
External otitis (swimmer's ear),
    319–321

F

Female infertility, 98
Fever blisters, 301–303
Fibroadenoma, benign, of breast, 116
Fibrocystic disease of breast, 115–116
Folic acid deficiency anemia, 204–205
Food allergy, 151
Fractures, 270–272
Furuncles, 291–292

G

Gastric ulcer (peptic ulcer of the
    stomach), 131–132
Gastritis, 129–130
Gastroenteritis, 130–131
Genital herpes, 99–101
Genital warts, 101
German measles. *See* Rubella
Gigantism. *See* Hyperpituitarism
Glaucoma, 315
Glomerulonephritis, acute, 79
Gluten-induced enteropathy. *See*
    Celiac sprue
Goiter, simple, 250–251
Gonorrhea, 99
Gout, 274
Granulomatous colitis. *See* Crohn's
    disease
Graves' disease. *See* Hyperthyroidism

H

Hashimoto's thyroiditis, 251

Headache
  acute, 211–224
  chronic, 221–224
  migraine, 224–225
Heart attack. *See* Myocardial infarction
Heart defects, congenital, 61–64
Heart disease, rheumatic, 185–187
Helminths (worms), 151–152
Hematoma
  epidural, 225–227
  subdural, 225–227
Hemiplegia, 228
Hemolytic disease of the newborn. *See*
    Erythroblastosis fetalis
Hemorrhoids, 139
Hepatitis, viral, 147–149
Hernia
  abdominal, 140–141
  hiatal, 132–133
Herniated intervertebral disk, 266–267
Herpes, genital, 99–101
Herpes zoster (shingles), 302
Hiatal hernia, 132–133
Hip, congenital dysplasia of, 65–66
Hirschsprung's disease (congenital
    aganglionic megacolon), 59–60
Hives. *See* Urticaria
Hodgkin's disease, 211
Hordeolum. *See* Stye
Hydrocephalus, 58–59
Hydronephrosis, 83
Hypercalcemia. *See*
    Hyperparathyroidism
Hypercapnia. *See* Respiratory acidosis
Hypernephroma. *See* Adenocarcinoma
    of the kidney
Hyperparathyroidism
    (hypercalcemia), 254
Hyperpituitarism (acromegaly,
    gigantism), 247–248
Hypertension, essential, 193
Hyperthyroidism (Graves' disease),
    251–252
Hypocalcemia. *See*
    Hypoparathyroidism
Hypocapnia. *See* Respiratory alkalosis
Hypoparathyroidism (hypocalcemia),
    254–255
Hypopituitarism, 248–249
Hypothyroidism (cretinism,
    myxedema), 253

I

Impacted cerumen, 319
Impetigo, 291
Impotence. *See* Erectile dysfunction
Infantile colic, 150

Infectious mononucleosis, 161–162
Infertility, male and female, 98
Influenza, 29
Intervertebral disk, herniated, 266–267
Iron deficiency anemia, 203–204
Irritable bowel syndrome (IBS), 136–137

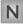

K

Keratitis, 318
Kidney, adenocarcinoma of, 85
Kidney stones. *See* Renal calculi
Kyphosis, 262–266

L

Laryngitis
    acute, 161
    chronic, 161
Legionella infections (Legionnaires' disease), 164
Legionnaires' disease. See *Legionella* infections
Leiomyoma, uterine, 113
Leukemia
    acute lymphoblastic, 208
    acute monoblastic, 208
    acute myeloblastic, 207–208
    chronic lymphocytic, 209
    chronic myelocytic, 208–209
Lockjaw. *See* Tetanus
Lordosis, 262–266
Lung
    abscess of, 164–165
    cancer of, 176–177
Lyme disease, 32
Lymphedema, 209–211
Lymphosarcoma, 211–212

M

Macular degeneration, 316
Malabsorption syndrome, 134
Male infertility, 98
Malignant melanoma, 303–304
Mammary dysplasia, 115–116
Measles (rubeola), 34
Ménière's disease, 322–323
Meningitis, bacterial, 230–231
Meningocele, 57–58
Menopause, 114
Migraine headache, 224–225
Mitral insufficiency/stenosis, 190
Motion sickness, 322
Multiple sclerosis, 237–238
Mumps, 37

Muscular dystrophy, Duchenne's, 279–280
Myasthenia gravis, 276–277
Mycoses, respiratory, 172–173
Myelomeningocele, 57–58
Myocardial infarction (heart attack), 195–196
Myocarditis, 188–189
Myxedema. *See* Hypothyroidism

N

Nephrotic syndrome, 79–80
Neural tube defects, 57–58
Neuritis, peripheral, 233
Neurogenic bladder, 84–85
Nosebleed. *See* Epistaxis
Nystagmus, 313

O

Orchitis, 106–107
Orgasmic dysfunction, in women, 97
Osteitis deformans. *See* Paget's disease
Osteoarthritis, 272
Osteomalacia, 268–269
Osteomyelitis, 269–270
Osteoporosis, 267–268
Otitis media, 321, 323
Otosclerosis, 322
Ovarian cysts and tumors, 111–112

P

Paget's disease (osteitis deformans), 270
Painful intercourse. *See* Dyspareunia
Pancreatic cancer, 144
Pancreatitis
    acute, 142–143
    chronic, 143–144
Paraplegia, 228–230
Parkinson's disease, 237
Pediculosis, 292–293, 305
Pelvic inflammatory disease (PID), 113–114
Peptic ulcer of the duodenum. *See* Duodenal ulcer
Peptic ulcer of the stomach. *See* Gastric ulcer
Pericarditis, 187–188
Peripheral artery aneurysm, 199–200
Peripheral neuritis, 233
Pernicious anemia, 205
Pertussis (whooping cough), 39
Pharyngitis
    acute, 160–161
    chronic, 160–161
Phenylketonuria (PKU), 67

Placenta previa, 120–121
Pleural effusion, 166–167
Pleurisy (pleuritis), 166
Pleuritis. *See* Pleurisy
Pneumonia, 162–163
Pneumothorax, 165–166
Polycystic kidney disease, 73–78
Polycythemia vera, 206–207
Polymyositis, 277–278
Preeclampsia. *See* Toxemias of pregnancy
Pregnancy, ectopic, 118
Premature ejaculation, 97
Premature labor/premature rupture of membranes (PROM), 121
Premenstrual syndrome (PMS), 109–111
Prostatic cancer, 107–108
Prostatitis, 104–105
Psoriasis, 287
Pulmonary edema, 173
Pulmonary embolism, 174–175
Pulmonary emphysema, chronic, 168
Pulmonary tuberculosis (TB), 169–170
Pulmonic insufficiency/stenosis, 192
Pyelonephritis, acute, 78–79
Pyloric stenosis, 59

Q

Quadriplegia, 228–230

R

Refractive errors, 311–313
Regional enteritis. *See* Crohn's disease
Renal calculi (kidney stones, uroliths), 81–83
Renal failure, chronic, 80–81
Respiratory acidosis (hypercapnia), 175
Respiratory alkalosis (hypocapnia), 175
Respiratory mycoses, 172–173
Retinal detachment, 315–316
Reye's syndrome, 212–213
Rheumatic fever, 185–187
Rheumatic heart disease, 185–187
Rheumatoid arthritis (RA), 272–273
Rubella (German measles), 34–37
Rubeola. *See* Measles

S

Scleroderma, 298
Scoliosis, 262–266
Seborrheic dermatitis, 298–299
Shingles. *See* Herpes zoster
Sickle cell anemia, 206

Silicosis, 171
Sinusitis, 160
Skin carcinoma, 303
Spina bifida, 57–58
Spinal cord injury, 228–230
Spine, deformities of, 262–266
Spontaneous abortion, 118
Sprains, 275
Stomatitis, 129
Strabismus, 318–319
Strains, 275
Stroke. *See* Cerebrovascular accident
Stye (hordeolum), 313–314
Subdural hematoma, 225–227
Sudden infant death syndrome (SIDS),
    177
Swimmer's ear. *See* External otitis
Syphilis, 101–103
Systemic lupus erythematosus (SLE),
    278–279

Talipes. *See* Clubfoot
Tendonitis, 276

Testicular cancer, 108
Tetanus (lockjaw), 39–40
Thoracic aneurysm, 199–200
Thrombophlebitis, 201–202
Thyroiditis, Hashimoto's, 251
Tonsillitis, acute, 177–178
Toxemias of pregnancy (preeclampsia
    and eclampsia), 118–120
Transient ischemic attack (TIA), 235
Trichomoniasis, 103–104
Tricuspid insufficiency/stenosis, 191
Tuberculosis, pulmonary, 169–170
Tumors
    bladder, 85–86
    brain, 239
    musculoskeletal system, 279
    ovarian, 111–112

Ulcer
    decubitus, 293
    duodenal, 135
    gastric, 131–132
Ulcerative colitis, 137–138

Undescended testes (cryptorchidism),
    64
Uremia. *See* Chronic renal failure
Ureter, congenital defects of, 64–65
Urethra, congenital defects of, 64–65
Urethritis, 83–84
Uroliths. *See* Renal calculi
Urticaria (hives), 287–288
Uterine leiomyoma, 113
Uveitis, 317

Varicella (chickenpox), 37–38
Varicose veins, 202
Viral hepatitis, acute, 147–149
Vomiting, 151

Warts, 296–297
    genital, 101
Whooping cough. *See* Pertussis
Worms. *See* Helminths